WORLD HEALTH ORGANIZATION

INTERNATIONAL AGENCY FOR RESEARCH ON CANCER

ONCOGENESIS AND HERPESVIRUSES III

Part 1: DNA of Herpesviruses, Viral Antigens, Cell-Virus Interaction

*Proceedings of the Third International Symposium
on Oncogenesis and Herpesviruses
held in Cambridge, Mass., USA
25–29 July 1977*

(3rd : 1977 :
Cambridge, Mass.)

EDITORS

G. DE THE   W. HENLE

F. RAPP

RC267
A1
I5
no.24:1
1978

TECHNICAL EDITOR FOR IARC

W. DAVIS

IARC Scientific Publications No. 24

INTERNATIONAL AGENCY FOR RESEARCH ON CANCER

LYON

1978

The International Agency for Research on Cancer (IARC) was established in 1965 by the World Health Assembly as an independently financed organization within the framework of the World Health Organization.   The headquarters of the Agency are at Lyon, France, and it has Research Centres in Iran, Kenya and Singapore.

The Agency conducts a programme of research concentrating particularly on the epidemiology of cancer and the study of potential carcinogens in the human environment.   Its field studies are supplemented by biological and chemical research carried out in the Agency's laboratories in Lyon and, through collaborative research agreements, in national research institutions in many countries.   The agency also conducts a programme for the education and training of personnel for cancer research.

The publications of the Agency are intended to contribute to the dissemination of authoritative information on different aspects of cancer research.

ISBN 92 832 1124 3

PRINTED IN SWITZERLAND

CONTENTS

DNA OF HERPESVIRUSES - STRUCTURE AND ASSOCIATION WITH CELL DNA

CELL-VIRUS INTERACTION:
MOLECULAR EVENTS IN PERMISSIVE AND SEMI-PERMISSIVE CYCLES

CELL-VIRUS INTERACTIONS:
INTEGRATION AND EXPRESSION OF THE VIRAL GENOME

CONTENTS OF PART 2

CELL VIRUS INTERACTIONS:
TRANSFORMATION AND PROPERTIES OF TRANSFORMED CELLS

HOST RESPONSE TO HERPESVIRUS INFECTION
(PRIMARY-LATENCY-REACTIVATION, ROLE OF GENETIC FACTORS)

COMPARATIVE HOST RESPONSE TO HERPESVIRUS ASSOCIATED TUMOURS

SUMMARY OF DISCUSSION ON RESEARCH PRIORITIES

Foreword

The studies of viral oncogenesis in the Agency have been focussed on the etiology of Burkitt's lymphoma and nasopharyngeal carcinoma, but the field of research related to the herpesviruses has extended beyond this specific goal. A great many of the papers presented at the Third International Symposium on Oncogenesis and Herpesviruses are contributing to a fundamental understanding of the mechanisms of viral action and of cell transformation, which will perhaps have repercussions on the whole question of viral involvement in human cancer.

Meanwhile the Agency's prospective study in Uganda has reached the stage where it is clear that the Epstein-Barr virus plays a causal role in the etiology of Burkitt's lymphoma, but investigation especially of malarial infection as a co-factor is continuing with an intervention trial in Tanzania.

Thanks are due to the National Cancer Institute, National Institutes of Health, USA, and the College of Medicine, Hershey, PA, USA, for generous financial support and to all those who collaborated in the organization of the Symposium and the preparation of the proceedings. I want to thank especially the editors, Dr G. de-Thé, Dr Henle and Dr Rapp and the local organizing committee, Professor J.L. Strominger, Professor T.H. Weller, Professor A.S. Evans and Dr G.E. Foley for all their work that has had such a successful outcome.

John HIGGINSON, M.D.

Director

International Agency
for Research on Cancer,
Lyon, France

INTRODUCTION

At the time that Oncogenesis and Herpesviruses II was published in 1975, the editors stressed that the central question was whether any herpesvirus was oncogenic in man, and a considerable effort has been devoted to attempts to find the answer.

The present volume includes reviews and selected papers of all the experimental areas related to these viruses. The first part deals with herpesvirus DNA, and its interaction with cellular DNA. Strain differences and their antigenicity are discussed in the next group of papers, followed by an extensive section on cell-virus interaction - covering molecular events, integration of the viral genome, control of transcription and translation, cellular transformation and properties of the transformed cells. In the section dealing with the host response to herpesvirus infection and associated tumours, particular attention has naturally been focussed on those diseases known to be closely associated with Epstein-Barr virus: infectious mononucleosis, Burkitt's lymphoma and nasopharyngeal carcinoma.

Although the nature of the association of this virus with nasopharyngeal carcinoma still remains to be determined, recently published results of a prospective study on Burkitt's lymphoma have shown that the Epstein-Barr virus is a causative agent for at least this human malignancy.

This raises, with increasing urgency, the question of whether effective intervention against the Epstein-Barr virus could be developed in order to prevent the associated diseases, and the reported attempts at vaccination against herpesvirus infection, and of its tentative control by chemotherapy may point the way for the future.

G. de-Thé
W. Henle
F. Rapp

PARTICIPANTS

D.V. ABLASHI

National Cancer Institute, National Institutes
of Health, Room B904, Landow Building,
Bethesda, Maryland 20014, USA

B.G. ACHONG

Department of Pathology, Medical School,
University of Bristol, University Walk,
Bristol, BS8 1TD, UK

A. ADAMS

Department of Tumor Biology, Karolinska
Institutet, S-104 01 Stockholm 60, Sweden

H.K. ADLDINGER

College of Veterinary Medicine, University
of Missouri, Columbia, Missouri 65201, USA

R. ADLER

Department of Human Genetics, University of
Michigan, Ann Arbor, Michigan 48103, USA

S. ALEXANDER

Sidney Farber Cancer Institute, Harvard
Medical School, 44 Binney Street, Boston,
Massachusetts 02115, USA

C.A. ALFORD

Department of Pediatrics, Room 609, CDLD
Building, UAB Medical Center, University
Station, Birmingham, Alabama 35294, USA

G.P. ALLEN

Department of Microbiology, University of
Mississippi Medical Center, 2500 North State
Street, Jackson, Mississippi 39216, USA

W.S. AL-NAKIB

Department of Microbiology, Faculty of Medicine,
University of Kuwait, Kuwait

M. ANDERSSON-ANVRET

Department of Tumor Biology, Karolinska
Institutet, S-104 01 Stockholm 60, Sweden

A.P. ANDRESE

Litton Bionetics Inc., 5516 Nicholson Lane,
Kensington, Maryland 20795, USA

A.M. ARVIN

Division of Infectious Diseases, Stanford
University School of Medicine, Stanford,
California 94305, USA

L. AURELIAN   Division of Comparative Medicine, Department of Biochemistry and Biophysics, The Johns Hopkins University Schools of Medicine and Hygiene and Public Health, Baltimore, Maryland 21205, USA

L.A. BABIUK   Department of Veterinary Microbiology, W.C.V.M. University of Saskatchewan, Saskatoon, Saskatchewan S7N 0W0, Canada

S. BACCHETTI   Department of Pathology, McMaster University, 1200 Main Street West, Hamilton, Ontario L8S 4J9, Canada

S.L. BACHENHEIMER   Department of Bacteriology and Immunology, University of North Carolina, 123 McNider 202H, Chapel Hill, North Carolina 27514, USA

R.F. BAKER   Department of Biological Sciences, University of Southern California, Los Angeles, California 90007, USA

R. BARZILAI   Hebrew University, Hadassah Medical School, Jerusalem, Israel

Y. BECKER   Laboratory for Molecular Virology, Hebrew University, Hadassah Medical School, Jerusalem, Israel

S.H. BENEDICT   Department of Microbiology, School of Medicine, Vanderbilt University, Nashville, Tennessee 37240, USA

Z.H. BENGALI   National Cancer Institute, National Institutes of Health, Building 41, Room S-100, Bethesda, Maryland 20014, USA

T. BEN-PORAT   Department of Microbiology, Vanderbilt University School of Medicine, Nashville, Tennessee 37232, USA

M.I. BERNHARD   Sloan-Kettering Institute for Cancer Research, 1275 York Avenue, New York, New York 10021, USA

E. BETH   Sloan-Kettering Institute for Cancer Research, 1275 York Avenue, New York, New York 10021, USA

R.J. BIGGAR   BTP/NIH Accra, Department of State, Washington, DC 20520, USA

C.A. BIRON   Cancer Research Center, Box 3, 217H Swing
                     Building, University of North Carolina, Chapel
                     Hill, North Carolina 27514, USA

K.A. BIRON   Cancer Research Center, University of North
                     Carolina, Box 3, 217H Swing Building, Chapel
                     Hill, North Carolina 27514, USA

H. BLOUGH   Scheie Eye Institute, Myrin Circle, 51 North
                     39th Street, Philadelphia, Pennsylvania 19104,
                     USA

M. BODEMER   Department of Radiology, Yale University School
                     of Medicine, New Haven, Connecticut 06510, USA

W.W. BODEMER   Department of Radiology, Yale University School
                     of Medicine, New Haven, Connecticut 06510, USA

J.F. BOECKER   The Joseph Stokes Jr. Research Institute of The
                     Children's Hospital of Philadelphia, 34th Street
                     & Civic Center Boulevard, Philadelphia,
                     Pennsylvania 19174, USA

J.A. BOEZI   Department of Biochemistry, Michigan State
                     University, East Lansing, Michigan 48824, USA

J.B. BOOKOUT   Section of Immunology and Cell Biology,
                     Baltimore Cancer Research Center, 3100 Wyman
                     Park Drive, Baltimore, Maryland 21211, USA

W. BOTO   University of Massachusetts Medical School,
                     Boston, Massachusetts 02115, USA

A. BOURKAS   Pediatric Research Centre, Ste-Justine Hospital,
                     3175 chemin Ste-Catherine, Montreal H3T 1C5,
                     Quebec, Canada

M.K. BRADLEY   Upstate Medical Center, SUNY - Syracuse,
                     1000 Ackerman Avenue, Syracuse, New York
                     13210, USA

P.E. BRANTON   Department of Pathology, McMaster University,
                     1200 Main Street West, Hamilton, Ontario
                     L8S 4J9, Canada

M.K. BREINIG   Department of Microbiology, Medical College of
                     Virginia, MCV Station 847, Richmond, Virginia
                     23298, USA

L. BREWER   Herpes Research Laboratory, USPHS Hospital, 1131 14th Avenue South, Seattle, Washington 98114, USA

S.M. BROWN   Medical Research Council Virology Unit, Institute of Virology, University of Glasgow, Church Street, Glasgow G11 5JR, UK

G. BURTONBOY   7, Place de la Neuville, 1348 Louvain-la-Neuve, Belgium

R. BUTTYAN   Committee on Virology, University of Chicago, Marjorie B. Kovler Viral Oncology Laboratories, 910 East 58th Street, Chicago, Illinois 60637, USA

A. CAMACHO   Microbiology Department, University of Chicago, 939 East 57th Street, Chicago, Illinois 60637, USA

W.F. CAMPBELL   Department of Microbiology, Mayo Clinic/ Foundation, 200 SW 1st Street, Rochester, Minnesota 55901, USA

J.P. CAMPIONE   McMaster University, 1200 Main Street West, Hamilton, Ontario L8S 4J9, Canada

E.M. CANTIN   National Institutes of Health, NIDR, Bethesda, Maryland 20014, USA

C. CARTER   Sidney Farber Cancer Institute, 44 Binney Street, Boston, Massachusetts 02115, USA

L. CAUCHY   National Institute of Agronomy Research, Station of Avian Pathology, Tours-Nouzilly, 37380 Monnaie, France

Y.M. CENTIFANTO   Department of Ophthalmology, University of Florida, Box J-284, JHMHC, Gainesville, Florida 32610, USA

K.C. CHADHA   Department of Medical Viral Oncology, Roswell Park Memorial Institute, 666 Elm Street, Buffalo, New York 14263, USA

V.L. CHAN   Department of Microbiology and Parasitology, University of Toronto, Toronto M5S 1A1, Canada

Y. CHARDONNET — Virology Unit, National Institute of Health and Medical Research (INSERM), 1 place Pr. Joseph Renaut, 69008 Lyon, France

W.A. CHECK — Medical News, JAMA, 1765 E. 55th Street, Chicago, Illinois 60615, USA

A.B. CHEN — Department of Microbiology, Vanderbilt University School of Medicine, Nashville, Tennessee 37232, USA

Y.-C. CHENG — Department of Experimental Therapeutics, Roswell Park Memorial Institute, 666 Elm Street, Buffalo, New York 14263, USA

T.D.Y. CHIN — University of Kansas Medical Center, Department of Community Health, 39th and Rainbow, Kansas City, Kansas 66103, USA

S. CHOUSTERMAN — Viral Physiology Laboratory, Institute for Scientific Research on Cancer (IRSC) B.P. 8, 94800 Villejuif, France

B.L. CHRISTENSON — Department of Virology, National Bacteriological Laboratory, S-105 21 Stockholm, Sweden

M.A. CICCONI — Department of Tropical Public Health, Harvard University School of Public Health, 665 Huntington Avenue, Boston, Maryland 02115, USA

D.P. CLARK — Upstate Medical Center, SUNY - Syracuse, 766 Irving Avenue, Syracuse, New York 13210, USA

J.B. CLEMENTS — Institute of Virology, University of Glasgow, Church Street, Glasgow G11 5JR, UK

W. CLOUGH — Sidney Farber Cancer Institute, 44 Binney Street, Boston, Massachusetts 02115, USA

G.H. COHEN — University of Pennsylvania, Philadelphia, Pennsylvania 19104, USA

F. COLBERE-GARAPIN — Virology Department, Institut Pasteur, 25 rue du Dr Roux, 75015 Paris, France

A.M. COLBERG — Department of Microbiology, The Milton S. Hershey Medical Center, The Pennsylvania State University College of Medicine, Hershey, Pennsylvania 17033, USA

B.A. COLBY	Cancer Research Center, Box 3, 217H Swing Building, University of North Carolina, Chapel Hill, North Carolina 27514, USA
A.W. CONFER	College of Veterinary Medicine, University of Missouri, Columbia, Missouri 65201, USA
J. COPPEY	Biology Division, Fondation Curie-Institut du Radium, 26 rue d'Ulm, 75231 Paris, France
C.D. COPPLE	Cold Spring Harbor Laboratory, P.O. Box 100, Cold Spring Harbor, New York 11724, USA
L. COREY	Herpes Research Laboratory, USPHS Hospital, 1131 14th Avenue South, Seattle, Washington 98114, USA
E.P. CORTHOUT	Dambruggestraat 39, B-2000 Antwerp, Belgium
O. COSTA	International Agency for Research on Cancer, 150 cours Albert-Thomas, 69372 Lyon Cédex 2, France
F. COUDERT	National Institute of Agronomy Research, Station of Avian Pathology, Tours-Nouzilly, 37380 Monnaie, France
R.J. COURTNEY	Department of Virology and Epidemiology, Baylor College of Medicine, 1200 Moursund Avenue, Houston, Texas 77030, USA
R. COUTINHO	Laboratory of Health Sciences, University of Amsterdam, Mauritskade 57, Amsterdam, The Netherlands
D. CRAWFORD	Department of Pathology, Medical School, University of Bristol, Bristol BS8 1TD, UK
K.J. CREMER	Radiobiology Laboratories, Yale University Medical School, 333 Cedar Street, New Haven, Connecticut 06510, USA
C.S. CRUMPACKER	Division of Infectious Diseases, Beth Israel Hospital, 330 Brookline Avenue, Boston, Massachusetts 02115, USA
J.R. CRUZ	Department of Tropical Public Health, Harvard School of Public Health, 665 Huntington Avenue, Boston, Massachusetts 02115, USA

J.C. DAHLBERG	National Cancer Institute, National Institutes of Health, Room 37, Building 1C21, Bethesda, Maryland 20014, USA
T.R. DAMBAUGH	Section of Infectious Disease, Department of Medicine, University of Chicago, 950 East 59th Street, Chicago, Illinois 60637, USA
G.J. DAMMIN	Department of Pathology, Harvard Medical School, Boston, Massachusetts 02115, USA
M.D. DANIEL	New England Regional Primate Research Center, Harvard Medical School, One Pine Hill Drive, Southborough, Massachusetts 01772, USA
G. DARAI	Institute of Medical Virology, Heidelberg University, Im Neuenheimer Feld 324, 6900 Heidelberg, Federal Republic of Germany
G. DARBY	Division of Virology, Department of Pathology, University of Cambridge, Addenbrooke's Hospital, Hills Road, Cambridge CB2 1QP, UK
G.F. DEBOER	Central Veterinary Institute, Virology Department, 39 Houtribweg, Lelystad, The Netherlands
N.C. DE DE LA PENA	Research Department, Institute of Oncology Angel H. Roffo, University of Buenos Aires, Avenida San Martin 5481, 1417 Buenos Aires, Argentina
F. DEINHARDT	Max v. Pettenkofer-Institute of Hygiene and Medical Microbiology of the University of Munich, D-8000 Munich 2, Federal Republic of Germany
J.M. DEMARCHI	Department of Microbiology, Vanderbilt University School of Medicine, Nashville, Tennessee 37232, USA
J.G. DERGE	Frederick Cancer Research Center, P.O. Box B, Frederick, Maryland 21701, USA
C. DESGRANGES-BLANC	International Agency for Research on Cancer, 150 cours Albert-Thomas, 69372 Lyon, Cédex 2, France
G.B. DE-THÉ	International Agency for Research on Cancer, 150 cours Albert-Thomas, 69372 Lyon, Cédex 2, France

V. DIEHL — Medical University, Karl-Wiechert-Allee 9, 3 Hannover-Kleefeld, Federal Republic of Germany

F.W. DOANE — Department of Microbiology and Parasitology, Fitzgerald Building, University of Toronto, Toronto M5S 1A1, Canada

R. DOLIN — National Institutes of Health, Building 10, Room 11N214, NIAID, Bethesda, Maryland 20014, USA

J.P. DONAHOE — Ohio State University, Columbus, Ohio 43210, USA

V. DOSTAL — Institute for Cancer Research, Department of Virology, Borschkegasse 8a, A 1095 Wien, Austria

R.G. DUFF — Department of Virology, Abbott Laboratories, North Chicago, Illinois 60064, USA

K. DUNN — Department of Bacteriology and Immunology, 123 MacNider 202H, University of North Carolina, Chapel Hill, North Carolina 27514, USA

P.S. ECKLUND — Children's Hospital of Michigan, 3901 Beaubien Boulevard, Detroit, Michigan 48201, USA

C.M. EDSON — Sidney Farber Cancer Institute, 44 Binney Street, Boston, Massachusetts 02115, USA

J.M.B. EDWARDS — Virus Reference Laboratory, Central Public Health Laboratory, Colindale Avenue, London NW9 5HT, UK

F.A. ENNIS — Bureau of Biologics, Food and Drug Administration, Bethesda, Maryland 20014, USA

M.A. EPSTEIN — Department of Pathology, University of Bristol Medical School, Bristol BS8 1TD, UK

A.S. EVANS — Department of Epidemiology, Yale University, 333 Cedar Street, New Haven, Connecticut 06510, USA

L.A. FALK — Departments of Chemistry and Tumor Biology, Karolinska Institutet, S 104 01 Stockholm, Sweden

L.T. FELDMAN
Department of Microbiology, Vanderbilt University School of Medicine, Nashville, Tennessee 37232, USA

P.M. FEORINO
Viral Oncology Branch, Center for Disease Control, 1600 Clifton Road, N.E., Atlanta, Georgia 30333, USA

M. FIALA
Department of Medicine, Martin Luther King, Jr. General Hospital, 12021 S. Wilmington Avenue, Los Angeles, California 90050, USA

M.E. FIGUEROA
Department of Microbiology, The Milton S. Hershey Medical Center, The Pennsylvania State University College of Medicine, Hershey, Pennsylvania 17033, USA

B. FLECKENSTEIN
New England Regional Primate Research Center, Harvard Medical School, One Pine Hill Drive, Southborough, Massachusetts 01772, USA

R.M. FLÜGEL
Institute for Virus Research, German Cancer Research Center, Im Neuenheimer Feld 280, 6900 Heidelberg, Federal Republic of Germany

C.K.Y. FONG-CHENG
Virology Laboratory/151B, Veterans Administration Hospital, West Haven, Connecticut 06516, USA

M. FONT, Jr
Wayne State University School of Medicine, Detroit, Michigan 48201, USA

B.R. FRANCKE
The Salk Institute, Tumor Virology Laboratory, P.O. Box 1809, San Diego, California 92112, USA

T.N. FREDRICKSON
Department of Pathobiology, University of Connecticut, Storrs, Connecticut 06268, USA

L.D. FRENKEL
Department of Pediatrics, Medical College of Ohio, CS No. 10008, Toledo, Ohio 43699, USA

N. FRENKEL
Department of Biology, University of Chicago, 1103 East 57th Street, Chicago, Illinois 60637, USA

K.O. FRESEN
Institute of Virology, Albert-Ludwig University, Hermann Herderstrasse 11, Postfach 820, D-7800 Freiburg in Brisgau, Federal Republic of Germany

A. FRIEDMANN Department of Genetics, Hebrew University, Hadassah Medical School, Jerusalem, Israel

E.H. FROST Montreal Cancer Institute, Notre Dame Hospital, 1560 Est Sherbrooke, Montreal H2L 4M1, Quebec, Canada

D.A. FUCCILLO Litton Bionetics Inc., 5516 Nicholson Lane, Kensington, Maryland 20795, USA

J. FUNDERBURGH Department of Ophthalmology, University of Washington School of Medicine, Health Sciences Building, RJ-10, Seattle, Washington 98195, USA

M. FUNDERBURGH Department of Pathobiology, School of Public Health and Community Medicine, SC-38, University of Washington, Seattle, Washington 98195, USA

P.A. FURMAN Burroughs Wellcome Co., 3030 Cornwallis Road, Research Triangle Park, North Carolina 27709, USA

T. FURUKAWA The Wistar Institute, 36th Street at Spruce, Philadelphia, Pennsylvania 19104, USA

J.A. FYFE Wellcome Research Laboratories, Research Triangle Park, North Carolina 27709, USA

H.E. GADLER National Bacteriological Laboratory, S-105 21 Stockholm, Sweden

W.M. GALLATIN Department of Immunology, University of Alberta, Edmonton, Alberta T6G 2M7, Canada

L. GEDER Department of Microbiology, The Milton S. Hershey Medical Center, The Pennsylvania State University College of Medicine, Hershey, Pennsylvania 17033, USA

J.L.M.C. GEELEN Laboratory of Health Sciences, University of Amsterdam, Mauritskade 57, Amsterdam, The Netherlands

L.D. GELB Division of Infectious Diseases, Box 8051, Department of Medicine, Washington University School of Medicine, St. Louis, Missouri 63110, USA

G.A. GENTRY   Department of Microbiology, University of Mississippi Medical Center, 2500 North State Street, Jackson, Mississippi 39216, USA

P. GERBER   Building 29A, National Institutes of Health, Bethesda, Maryland 20014, USA

F. GERVAIS   Pediatric Research Centre, Ste-Justine Hospital, 3175 chemin Ste-Catherine, Montreal H3T 1C5, Quebec, Canada

D.W. GIBSON   Johns Hopkins University School of Medicine, 725 North Wolfe Street, Baltimore, Maryland 21205, USA

D.G. GILMOUR   Department of Microbiology, New York University Medical Center, 550 First Avenue, New York, New York 10016, USA

G. GIRALDO   Immunovirology Section, Sloan-Kettering Memorial Institute, 1275 York Avenue, New York, New York 10021, USA

D.B. GIVEN   Section of Infectious Disease, Department of Medicine, University of Chicago, 950 East 59th Street, Chicago, Illinois 60637, USA

R. GLASER   Department of Medical Microbiology, College of Medicine, 333 West Tenth Avenue, Columbus, Ohio 43210, USA

J.C. GLORIOSO   Unit for Laboratory Animal Medicine, University of Michigan, 010 Animal Research Facility, Ann Arbor, Michigan 48109, USA

R.J. GOLDBERG   National Cancer Institute, National Institutes of Health, Building 37, room 1C27, Bethesda, Maryland 20014, USA

N. GOLDBLUM   The Chanock Centre for Virology, Hebrew University, Hadassah Medical School, Jerusalem, Israel

K. GOLDSTEIN   George Washington University, Washington, DC 20007, USA

E. GÖNCZÖL   Imperial Cancer Research Fund, Lincoln's Inn Fields, P.O. Box No. 123, London WC2A 3PX, UK

S.R. GOODMAN   Sidney Farber Cancer Institute, 44 Binney Street, Boston, Massachusetts 02115, USA

A. GRANOFF   St. Jude Children's Research Hospital,
Box 318, Memphis, Tennessee 38101, USA

P. GUNVÉN   Department of Tumor Biology, Karolinska
Institutet, S-104 01 Stockholm 60, Sweden

P. GUPTA   Department of Microbiology, The Milton S.
Hershey Medical Center, The Pennsylvania State
University, Hershey, Pennsylvania 17033, USA

M.L. GUSS   Landow Building, Room C306, National Cancer
Institute, National Institutes of Health,
Bethesda, Maryland 20014, USA

D.P. GUSTAFSON   School of Veterinary Medicine, Purdue University, West Lafayette, Indiana 47907, USA

N. GUTENSOHN   Department of Epidemiology, Harvard School of
Public Health, 677 Huntington Avenue, Boston,
Massachusetts 02115, USA

D.C. HALSTEAD-MCFARLAND Allentown General Hospital, Allentown,
Pennsylvania 18102, USA

C. HAMELIN   Virology Research Centre, Institut Armand-
Frappier, P.O. Box 100, Laval, Quebec H7N 4Z3,
Canada

B. HAMPAR   Frederick Cancer Research Center, Fort Detrick,
Building 560, Frederick, Maryland 21701, USA

J.-P. HARDY   Montreal Cancer Institute, Notre Dame Hospital,
1560 Est Sherbrooke, Montreal H2L 4M1, Quebec,
Canada

V. HARDY   Montreal Cancer Institute, Notre Dame Hospital,
1560 Est Sherbrooke, Montreal H2L 4M1, Quebec,
Canada

G.S. HAYWARD   Department of Pharmacology, Johns Hopkins
University Medical School, 725 North Wolfe
Street, Baltimore, Maryland 21205, USA

S.D. HAYWARD   Department of Pharmacology, Johns Hopkins
University Medical School, 725 North Wolfe
Street, Baltimore, Maryland 21205, USA

R.L. HEBERLING   Division of Microbiology and Infectious Disease,
Southwest Foundation for Research and Education,
P.O. Box 28147, San Antonio, Texas 78284, USA

U.I. HEINE   National Cancer Institute, National Institutes
                    of Health, Building 37, Room IC-15, Bethesda,
                    Maryland 20014, USA

M.R. HELLER   Committee on Virology, University of Chicago,
                    Marjorie B. Kovler Viral Oncology Laboratories,
                    910 East 58th Street, Chicago, Illinois 60637,
                    USA

A. HELLMAN   Building 41, National Cancer Institute, National
                    Institutes of Health, Bethesda, Maryland 20014,
                    USA

K.B. HELLMAN   Department of Health, Education and Welfare
                    24211 Peach Tree Road, Clarksburg, Maryland
                    20734, USA

G. HENLE   The Joseph Stokes, Jr Research Institute of The
                    Children's Hospital of Philadelphia, 34th Street
                    & Civic Center Boulevard, Philadelphia, Penn-
                    sylvania 19174, USA

W. HENLE   The Joseph Stokes, Jr. Research Institute of The
                    Children's Hospital of Philadelphia, 34th Street
                    & Civic Center Boulevard, Philadelphia, Penn-
                    sylvania 19174, USA

J.F. HEWETSON   Department of Microbiology, Medical College of
                    Pennsylvania, 3300 Henry Avenue, Philadelphia,
                    Pennsylvania 19129, USA

J. HILFENHAUS   Behringwerke AG, Auf'm Gebrande 24, D-3550
                    Marburg, Federal Republic of Germany

M.D. HILTY   Children's Hospital, 561 S. 17th Street,
                    Columbus, Ohio 43205, USA

Y. HINUMA   Department of Microbiology, Kumamoto University
                    Medical School, Kumamoto 860, Japan

K. HIRAI   Department of Molecular Biology, Tokai Univer-
                    sity School of Medicine, Bohseidai, Isehara
                    259-11, Japan

R.G. HIRST   Department of Virology, Wellcome Research
                    Laboratories, Beckenham, Kent BR3 3BS, UK

H.E. HOFFMAN   Stine Laboratory, E.I. DuPont de Nemours & Co.,
                    Inc., Newark, Delaware 19711, USA

P.J. HOFFMAN

Department of Experimental Therapeutics, Hoswell Park Memorial Institute, 666 Elm Street, Buffalo, New York 14263, USA

T.C. HOLLAND

Biophysics Laboratories, Department of Biochemistry and Biophysics, The Pennsylvania State University, University Park, Pennsylvania 16802, USA

K.K. HOLMES

Herpes Research Laboratory, USPHS Hospital, 1131 14th Street, Seattle, Washington 98114, USA

M.K. HOWETT

Department of Microbiology, The Milton S. Hershey Medical Center, The Pennsylvania State University College of Medicine, Hershey, Pennsylvania 17033, USA

G.D. HSIUNG

Department of Laboratory Medicine, Yale University School of Medicine, New Haven, Connecticut 06510, USA

E.-S. HUANG

Department of Medicine and Cancer Research Center, Box 3 217H Swing Building, University of North Carolina, Chapel Hill, North Carolina 27514, USA

Y.-S. HUANG

Cancer Research Center, University of North Carolina, Box 3 217H Swing Building, Chapel Hill, North Carolina 27514, USA

R.D. HUNT

New England Regional Primate Research Center, One Pine Hill Drive, Southborough, Massachusetts 01772, USA

L.M. HUTT

Cancer Research Center, University of North Carolina, Box 3, 217H Swing Building, Chapel Hill, North Carolina 27514, USA

R.W. HYMAN

Department of Microbiology, The Milton S. Hershey Medical Center, The Pennsylvania State University College of Medicine, Hershey, Pennsylvania 17033, USA

J. ICART

CHU Rangueil, 62 rue de Metz, 31000 Toulouse, France

J.P. ILTIS

Department of Microbiology, The Milton S. Hershey Medical Center, The Pennsylvania State University College of Medicine, Hershey, Pennsylvania 17033, USA

J. IRWIN   National Institutes of Health, 6206 41st Avenue, Hyattsville, Maryland 20782, USA

H.C. ISOM   Department of Microbiology, The Milton S. Hershey Medical Center, The Pennsylvania State University College of Medicine, Hershey, Pennsylvania 17033, USA

R.J. JACOB   Committee on Virology, University of Chicago, Marjorie B. Kovler Viral Oncology Laboratories, 910 East 58th Street, Chicago, Illinois 60637, USA

B. JACQUEMONT   Virology Unit, National Institute of Health and Medical Research (INSERM), 1, place Pr. Joseph Renaut, 69008 Lyon, France

R.J. JARIWALLA   Division of Biophysics, The Johns Hopkins University, 725 North Wolfe Street, Baltimore, Maryland 21205, USA

M.A. JERKOFSKY   Department of Microbiology, University of Maine, 254 Hitchner Hall, Orono, Maine 04473, USA

L.D. JOHNSON   New England Regional Primate Research Center, Harvard Medical School, One Pine Hill Drive, Southborough, Massachusetts 01772, USA

J.H. JONCAS   Pediatric Research Centre, Ste-Justine Hospital, 3175 chemin Ste-Catherine, Montreal H3T 1C5, Quebec, Canada

C.V. JONGENEEL   Department of Bacteriology and Immunology, University of North Carolina, 123 McNider 202H, Chapel Hill, North Carolina 27514, USA

M.C. JORDAN   Department of Medicine, University of California School of Medicine, Los Angeles, California 90024, USA

O.R. KAADEN   Federal Research Institute for Animal Virus Disease, Pl Ehrlichstrasse 28, P.O. Box 1149, D-74 Tübingen, Federal Republic of Germany

H.C. KAERNER   Institute for Virus Research, German Cancer Research Centre, Im Neuenheimer Feld 280, 6900 Heidelberg, Federal Republic of Germany

E.F. KALETA — Institute of Poultry Diseases, The Hannover School of Veterinary Medicine, D-3000 Hannover, Federal Republic of Germany

S.S. KALTER — Division of Microbiology and Infectious Diseases, Southwest Foundation for Research and Education, P.O. Box 28147, San Antonio, Texas 78284, USA

A.S. KAPLAN — Department of Microbiology, Vanderbilt University School of Medicine, Nashville, Tennessee 37232, USA

R.A. KARMALI — Clinical Research Institute, 110 Pine Avenue West, Montreal, Quebec H2W 1R7, Canada

S. KATO — Department of Pathological Research, Institute of Microbial Diseases, University of Osaka, Osaka 565, Japan

B. KAYIBANDA — Institute of Cancer and Immunogenetics, 94800 Villejuif, France

R.A. KEENLYSIDE — Viral Diseases Division, Center for Disease Control, Bureau of Epidemiology, Building 1, Room 6125, Atlanta, Georgia 30333, USA

A.D. KELMAN — Boston University School of Medicine, Harrison Avenue, Boston, Massachusetts 02118, USA

A.J. KENYON — Sloan-Kettering Memorial Institute, 1275 York Avenue, New York, New York 10021, USA

E.R. KERN — Department of Pediatrics, University of Utah College of Medicine, Salt Lake City, Utah 84132, USA

A. KESSOUS — Montreal Cancer Institute, Notre Dame Hospital, 1560 Est Sherbrooke, Montreal H2L 4M1, Quebec, Canada

E. KIEFF — Section of Infectious Disease of the Department of Medicine University of Chicago, 950 East 59th Street, Chicago, Illinois 60637, USA

R.A. KILLINGTON — Department of Microbiology, School of Medicine, University of Leeds, Leeds LS2 9NL, UK

B.A. KILPATRICK — Department of Medicine and Cancer Research Center, University of North Carolina, Box 3 217H Swing Building, Chapel Hill, North Carolina 27514, USA

K.S. KIM

Department of Microbiology, New York State Institute for Research in Mental Retardation, 1050 Forest Hill Road, Staten Island, New York 10314, USA

R. KIMES

Monsanto Company, 800 N. Lindbergh Boulevard, St. Louis, Missouri 63166, USA

W. KING

Committee on Virology, University of Chicago, Marjorie B. Kovler Viral Oncology Laboratories, 910 East 58th Street, Chicago, Illinois 60637, USA

H. KIRCHNER

Institute for Virus Research, German Cancer Research Center, Im Neuenheimer Feld 280, 6900 Heidelberg, Federal Republic of Germany

S. KIRWIN

Scheie Eye Institute, 51 North 39th Street, Philadelphia, Pennsylvania 19104, USA

G. KLEIN

Departments of Chemistry and Tumor Biology, Karolinska Institutet, S-104 01 Stockholm, Sweden

M. KLEIN

Department of Microbiology, Temple University Medical School, Philadelphia, Pennsylvania 19104, USA

G.E. KNOX

Department of Pediatrics, Room 609, CDLD Building, UAB Medical Center, University Station, Birmingham, Alabama 35294, USA

E.N. KRAISELBURD

Comprehensive Cancer Center, University of Puerto Rico Medical Sciences Campus, G.P.O. Box 5067, San Juan, Puerto Rico 00936, USA

E.S. KUCERA

Department of Microbiology and Immunology, Bowman Gray School of Medicine, Winston-Salem, North Carolina 27103, USA

M.-P. KUNG

Department of Experimental Therapeutics, Roswell Park Memorial Institute, 666 Elm Street, Buffalo, New York 14263, USA

E. KURSTAK

Comparative Virology Research Group, Faculty of Medicine, Université de Montréal, Montreal, Quebec, Canada

B.F. LADIN

Vanderbilt University, Nashville, Tennessee 37232, USA

P.K. LAI	Department of Microbiology, Rush-Presbyterian-St. Luke's Medical Center, 1753 West Congress Parkway, Chicago, Illinois 60612, USA
F.D. LAKEMAN	Department of Medical Microbiology, University of Wisconsin Medical School, 470 North Charter Street, Madison, Wisconsin 53706, USA
J.-P. LAMELIN	International Agency for Research on Cancer, 150 cours Albert Thomas, 69372 Lyon, Cédex 2, France
Y. LANGELIER	Cellular Genetics Unit, Molecular Biological Research Institute, 2 place Jussieu, 75221 Paris, Cédex 05, France
V.M. LARSON	Merck Institute for Therapeutic Research, West Point, Pennsylvania 19486, USA
J. LAU	Life Sciences Research Laboratories, 2900 72nd Street North, St. Petersburg, Florida 33710, USA
R.N. LAUSCH	Department of Microbiology, The Milton S. Hershey Medical Center, The Pennsylvania State University College of Medicine, Hershey, Pennsylvania 17033, USA
J.F. LAVENDER	Lilly Research Laboratories, Indianapolis, Indiana 46206, USA
W.C. LAWRENCE	School of Veterinary Medicine, University of Pennsylvania, 3800 Spruce Street, Philadelphia, Pennsylvania 19104, USA
L.F. LEE	Science and Education Administration-Federal Research, United States Department of Agriculture, Regional Poultry Research Laboratory, 3606 East Mount Hope Road, East Lansing, Michigan 48823, USA
Y.-S. LEE	Life Sciences Research Laboratories, 2900 72nd Street North, St. Petersburg, Florida 33710, USA
J.M. LEIDEN	Committee on Virology, University of Chicago, Marjorie B. Kovler Viral Oncology Laboratories, 910 East 58th Street, Chicago, Illinois 60637, USA
S.S. LEINBACH	Department of Biochemistry, Michigan State University, East Lansing, Michigan 48824, USA

S.L. LEMASTER   Scheie Eye Institute, 51 39th Street North, Room 608, Philadelphia, Pennsylvania 19104, USA

S.M. LEMON   Department of Infectious Diseases, University of North Carolina, Box 3, 217H Swing Building, Chapel Hill, North Carolina 27514, USA

E.T. LENNETTE   The Joseph Stokes Jr Research Institute of The Children's Hospital of Philadelphia, 34th Street & Civil Center Boulevard, Philadelphia, Pennsylvania 19174, USA

G. LENOIR   International Agency for Research on Cancer, 150 cours Albert-Thomas, 69372 Lyon, Cédex 2, France

M. LEVINE   Department of Human Genetics, University of Michigan, Ann Arbor, Michigan 48105, USA

P. LEVINE   National Cancer Institute, National Institutes of Health, Bethesda, Maryland 20014, USA

M. LEYRITZ-WILLS   Pediatric Research Center, Ste-Justine Hospital, 3175 chemin Ste-Catherine, Montreal H3T 1C5, Quebec, Canada

J.-L. H. LI   University of North Carolina, Chapel Hill, North Carolina 27514, USA

T. LINDAHL   Departments of Chemistry and Biology, Karolinska Institutet, S-104 01 Stockholm 60, Sweden

S. LITTLE   Harvard Medical School, 665 Huntington Avenue, Boston, Massachusetts 02115, USA

H. LOCKER   Department of Biology, University of Chicago, 1103 East 57th Street, Chicago, Illinois 60637, USA

B.M. LONGENECKER   Department of Immunology, University of Alberta, Edmonton, Alberta T6G 2M7, Canada

C. LOPEZ   Sloan-Kettering Cancer Center, 1275 York Avenue, New York, New York 10021, USA

H. LUDWIG   Institute of Virology, Justus-Liebig-University, Frankfurter Strasse 107, D-6300 Giessen, Federal Republic of Germany

D. LUU — Pediatric Research Centre, Ste-Justine Hospital, 3175 chemin Ste-Catherine, Montreal H3T 1C5, Quebec, Canada

N. MACHTIGER — Sidney Farber Cancer Institute, 44 Binney Street, Boston, Massachusetts 02115, USA

J. MACNAB — Department of Virology, University of Glasgow, Church Street, Glasgow G11 5JR, UK

I.T. MAGRATH — National Cancer Institute, National Institutes of Health, Building 10, Room 2B50, Bethesda, Maryland 20014, USA

N.J. MAITLAND — Cold Spring Harbor Laboratory, P.O. Box 100, Cold Spring Harbor, New York 11724, USA

S. MAK — Department of Biology, McMaster University, Hamilton, Ontario L8X 4K1, Canada

G. MAKARI — Sidney Farber Cancer Institute, 44 Binney Street, Boston, Massachusetts 02115, USA

M.M. MANAK — The Johns Hopkins University School of Hygiene and Public Health, Division of Biophysics, 615 North Wolfe Street, Baltimore, Maryland 21205, USA

R. MANAKER — National Cancer Institute, National Institutes of Health, Building 37, Room 1B14, Bethesda, Maryland 20014, USA

R.A. MÄNTYJÄRVI — Department of Clinical Microbiology, University of Kuopio, P.O. Box, 70101 Kuopio, Finland

E.-C. MAR — Cancer Research Center, University of North Carolina, Box 3, 217H Swing Building, Chapel Hill, North Carolina 27514, USA

B.M. MARCZYNSKA — Rush Presbyterian-St. Luke's Medical Center, 1753 West Congress Parkway, Chicago, Illinois 60612, USA

W. MARK — McArdle Laboratory, University of Wisconsin, 450 N. Randall Avenue, Madison, Wisconsin 53706, USA

N.G. MAXTON — Deputy Controller's Office, The Pennsylvania State University College of Medicine, Hershey, Pennsylvania 17033, USA

S.A. MAYYASI   Pfizer Inc., 199 Maywood Avenue, Maywood, New
                    Jersey 07607, USA

B.A. MCCARTHY   Department of Microbiology, The Milton S. Hershey
                    Medical Center, The Pennsylvania State University
                    College of Medicine, Hershey, Pennsylvania 17033,
                    USA

J.K. MCDOUGALL   Cold Spring Harbor Laboratory, P.O. Box 100,
                    Cold Spring Harbor, New York 11724, USA

M.S. MCGUIRE   Department of Microbiology, The Milton S. Hershey
                    Medical Center, The Pennsylvania State University
                    College of Medicine, Hershey, Pennsylvania 17033,
                    USA

M.A. MCKINLAY   Rensselaer Polytechnic Institute, 2150 Rosa Road,
                    Apt. B-18-A, Schenectady, New York 12309, USA

J.C. MCKITRICK   Hospital of the University of Pennsylvania,
                    3400 Spruce Street, Philadelphia, Pennsylvania
                    19104, USA

J.L. MELNICK   Department of Virology and Epidemiology, Baylor
                    College of Medicine, 1200 Moursund Avenue, Houston,
                    Texas 77030, USA

L.N. MENDIS   Department of Virology, St. Thomas' Hospital,
                    London SE1 7HT, UK

J. MENEZES   Pediatric Research Centre, Ste-Justine Hospital,
                    3175 chemin Ste-Catherine, Montreal H3T 1C5,
                    Quebec, Canada

T.C. MERIGAN   Division of Infectious Diseases, Stanford
                    University School of Medicine, Stanford, Califor-
                    nia 94305, USA

A. MEYMANDI   Cancer Research Center, University of North
                    Carolina, Box 3, 217H Swing Building, Chapel
                    Hill, North Carolina 27514, USA

J.H. MICHAELSON   University of Connecticut, Department of
                    Pathobiology, Schenectady, New York 12309, USA

F.J. MICHALSKI   St. Michael's Hospital, Dun Laoghaire,
                    Dublin, Ireland

S. MICHELSON-FISKE   Medical Virology and Viral Vaccines Unit, Institut Pasteur, 25 rue du Dr Roux, 75015 Paris, France

R.H. MILLER   Department of Microbiology, The Milton S. Hershey Medical Center, The Pennsylvania State University College of Medicine, Hershey, Pennsylvania 17033, USA

R.L. MILLER   Department of Microbiology, The Milton S. Hershey Medical Center, The Pennsylvania State University College of Medicine, Hershey, Pennsylvania 17033, USA

R.L. MILLETTE   Department of Immunology and Microbiology, Wayne State University School of Medicine, 540 East Canfield, Detroit, Michigan 48201, USA

A.C. MINSON   Department of Pathology, University of Cambridge, Addenbrooke's Hospital, Hills Road, Cambridge CB2 1QP, UK

J. MITCHELL   International Agency for Research on Cancer, 150 cours Albert-Thomas, 69372 Lyon, Cédex 2, France

M. MIZELL   Laboratory of Tumor Cell Biology, Tulane University, New Orleans, Louisiana 70118, USA

H.-H. MOON   Department of Microbiology, New York State Institute for Research in Mental Retardation, 1050 Forest Hill Road, Staten Island, New York 10314, USA

P.S. MORAHAN   Department of Microbiology, Medical College of Virginia, MCV Station 847, Richmond, Virginia 23298, USA

L.J. MORDAN   Department of Biology, Notre Dame University, Notre Dame, Indiana 46556, USA

D.G. MORGAN   Department of Pediatrics, Laboratory of Clinical Investigation (LCI 407), Yale University Medical School, 333 Cedar Avenue, New Haven, Connecticut 06510, USA

L.S. MORSE   Committee on Virology, University of Chicago, Marjorie B. Kovler Viral Oncology Laboratories, 910 East 58th Street, Chicago, Illinois 60637, USA

C. MULDER   Department of Pharmacology, University of
                     Massachusetts Medical School, 55 Lake Avenue
                     North, Worcester, Massachusetts 01605, USA

K. MUNK   Institute for Virus Research, German Cancer
                     Research Centre, Im Neuenheimer Feld 280,
                     D-6900 Heidelberg, Federal Republic of Germany

B.K. MURRAY   Department of Microbiology, Medical College of
                     Virginia, MCV Station 847, Richmond, Virginia
                     23298, USA

A. NAHMIAS   Division of Infectious Diseases and Immunology,
                     Department of Pediatrics, Emory University
                     School of Medicine, Atlanta, Georgia 30303, USA

K. NAZERIAN   Science and Education Administration-Federal
                     Research United States Department of Agriculture,
                     Regional Poultry Research Laboratory, 3606 East
                     Mount Hope Road, East Lansing, Michigan 48823,
                     USA

J.G. NEDRUD   Cancer Research Center, University of North
                     Carolina, Box 3, 217H Swing Building, Chapel
                     Hill, North Carolina 27514, USA

B.J. NEFF   Merck, Sharpe and Dohme, West Point, Pennsylvania
                     19486, USA

R.H. NEUBAUER   Frederick Cancer Research Center, P.O. Box B,
                     Building 560, Frederick, Maryland 21701, USA

P. NEWMAN   National Cancer Institute, National Institutes
                     of Health, Bethesda, Maryland 20014, USA

A.A. NEWTON   Department of Biochemistry, University of
                     Cambridge, Tennis Court Road, Cambridge CB2 1QP,
                     UK

J.C. NIEDERMAN   Yale University School of Medicine, 333 Cedar
                     Street, New Haven, Connecticut 06510, USA

J. NIKOSKELAINEN   Santa Clara Valley Medical Center, Stanford,
                     California 94305, USA

K. NILSSON   Department of Tumor Biology, The Wallenberg
                     Laboratory, University of Uppsala, P.O. Box 562,
                     S-751 22 Uppsala, Sweden

D.B. NIMMO   68 Channon Street, Gympie, Queensland 4570, Australia

M. NONOYAMA   Life Sciences Research Laboratories, 2900 72nd Street North, St. Petersburg, Florida 33710, USA

B. NORRILD   Department of Pediatrics, Emory University School of Medicine, 69 Butler Street, Atlanta, Georgia 30303, USA

O. NYORMOI   Sidney Farber Cancer Institute, 44 Binney Street, Boston, Massachusetts 02115, USA

B.F. ÖBERG   Astra Läkemedel, Fack, S-151 85 Södertälje, Sweden

D. O'CALLAGHAN   Department of Microbiology, University of Mississippi Medical Center, 2500 North State Street, Jackson, Mississippi, 39216, USA

W. OKADA   Pediatric Research Centre, Ste-Justine Hospital, 3175 chemin Ste-Catherine, Montreal H3T 1C5, Quebec, Canada

G.F. OKASINSKI   Cancer Research Center, University of North Carolina, Box 3, 217H Swing Building, Chapel Hill, North Carolina 27514, USA

T. OOKA   Departement de Biologie Générale et Appliquée, Université Claude Bernard (Lyon-I), 69 Villeurbanne, France

H. OPENSHAW   National Institute of Dental Research, Laboratory of Oral Medicine, National Institutes of Health, Bethesda, Maryland 20013, USA

T.D. ORELLANA   Section of Infectious Disease, Department of Medicine, University of Chicago, 950 East 59th Street, Chicago, Illinois 60637, USA

T. OSATO   Department of Virology, Cancer Institute, Hokkaido University School of Medicine, Sapporo N15 W7, Japan

J.E. OSBORN   Department of Medical Microbiology, University of Wisconsin, 330 Bascom Hall, Madison, Wisconsin 53706, USA

J.S. PAGANO   Cancer Research Center, University of North Carolina, Box 3, 217H Swing Building, Chapel Hill, North Carolina 27514, USA

B. PANCAKE   Sidney Farber Cancer Institute, 44 Binney Street, Boston, Massachusetts 02115, USA

D.S. PARRIS   Sidney Farber Cancer Institute, 44 Binney Street, Boston, Massachusetts 02115, USA

P.-P. PASTORET   Laboratory of Virology, 45 rue des Vétérinaires, 1000 Brussels, Belgium

P. PATEL   Pediatric Research Centre, Ste-Justine Hospital, 3175 chemin Ste-Catherine, Montreal H3T 1C5, Quebec, Canada

G.R. PEARSON   Department of Microbiology, Mayo Clinic/Foundation, S-6 Plummer Building, Rochester, Minnesota 55901, USA

A. PECHACZEK   Hans Kolb Weg 1, 7830 Ehingen (Donau), Federal Republic of Germany

M.M. PEDERSEN   Department of Immunology and Microbiology, Wayne State University School of Medicine, 540 East Canfield, Detroit, Michigan 48201, USA

P. PERIMAN   Texas Technical University School of Medicine, Amarillo, Texas 79100, USA

S. PERSON   Pennsylvania State University, 618 Life Science Building, University Park, Pennsylvania 16802, USA

G.M. PIKLER   Mayo Clinic/Foundation, S-6 Plummer Building, Rochester, Minnesota 55901, USA

L.I. PIZER   Department of Microbiology, University of Pennsylvania School of Medicine, Philadelphia, Pennsylvania 19104, USA

P.A. PIZZO   National Cancer Institute, National Institutes of Health, Building 10, Room 2B50, Bethesda, Maryland 20014, USA

W. PLOWRIGHT   The Royal Veterinary College, University of London, Royal College Street, London NW1 0TU, UK

J.H. POPE   Oncology Unit, Queensland Institute of Medical Research, Bramston Terrace, Herston, Brisbane 4600, Queensland, Australia

A.L.T. POWELL — Section of Infectious Disease, Department of Medicine, University of Chicago, 950 East 59th Street, Chicago, Illinois 60637, USA

K.L. POWELL — Department of Virology and Epidemiology, Baylor College of Medicine, 1200 Moursund Avenue, Houston, Texas 77030, USA

I. PRASAD — Public Health Research Institute of New York City, 455 First Avenue, New York, New York 10016, USA

K. PRESSLER — Astawerke AG, D-4800 Bielefeld, Federal Republic of Germany

C.M. PRESTON — Medical Research Council Institute of Virology, University of Glasgow, Church Street, Glasgow G11 5JR, UK

C. PREZYNA — Sidney Farber Cancer Institute, 44 Binney Street, Boston, Massachusetts 02115, USA

R.W. PRICE — Sloan-Kettering Memorial Institute, 1275 York Avenue, New York, New York 10021, USA

D.K. PRIGNOLI — Department of Virology, Boston University School of Medicine, Boston, Massachusetts 02115, USA

W.H. PRUSOFF — Department of Pharmacology, Yale University School of Medicine, New Haven, Connecticut 06510, USA

D.J.M. PURIFOY — Department of Virology and Epidemiology, Baylor College of Medicine, 1200 Moursund Avenue, Houston, Texas 77030, USA

D.T. PURTILO — University of Massachusetts Medical School, 39 Spring Street, Shrewsbury, Massachusetts 01545, USA

L.F. QUALTIERE — Department of Microbiology, Mayo Clinic, S-6 Plummer Building, Rochester, Minnesota 55901, USA

G. QUINNAN — Bureau of Biologics, National Institutes of Health, Bethesda, Mayrland 20014, USA

H. RABIN — Frederick Cancer Research Center, P.O. Box B, Frederick, Maryland 21701, USA

C. RANDALL   Department of Microbiology, University of
Mississippi Medical Center, 2500 North State
Street, Jackson, Mississippi 39216, USA

F. RAPP   Department of Microbiology, The Milton S. Hershey
Medical Center, The Pennsylvania State University
College of Medicine, Hershey, Pennsylvania 17033,
USA

L.E. RASMUSSEN   Division of Infectious Diseases, Stanford
University School of Medicine, Stanford, Califor-
nia 94305, USA

S. READ   Pennsylvania State University, 618 Life Science
Building, University Park, Pennsylvania 16802,
USA

M.C. REESE   Department of Microbiology, The Milton S. Hershey
Medical Center, The Pennsylvania State University
College of Medicine, Hershey, Pennsylvania 17033,
USA

W.C. REEVES   Department of Epidemiology, School of Public
Health SC-36, University of Washington, Seattle,
Washington 98195, USA

C.M. REINKE   Dental Research Institute, School of Dentistry,
University of Michigan, Ann Arbor, Michigan
48109, USA

H.E. RENIS   Experimental Biology, The Upjohn Co., Kalamazoo,
Michigan 49001, USA

A.B. RICKINSON   Department of Pathology, University of Bristol
Medical School, Bristol BS8 1TD, UK

F.J. RIXON   Vanderbilt University, 2112 Fairfax Avenue,
Nashville, Tennessee 37212, USA

P.R. ROANE   Department of Microbiology, College of Medicine,
Howard University, 520 W. Street NW, Washington,
DC 20059, USA

B. ROIZMAN   Committee on Virology, University of Chicago,
Marjorie B. Kovler Viral Oncology Laboratories,
910 East 58th Street, Chicago, Illinois 60637,
USA

H.M. ROSEMOND-HORNBEAK   Department of Microbiology, College of Medicine, University of South Alabama, Mobile, Alabama 36608, USA

K. ROSENTHAL   Sidney Farber Cancer Institute, 44 Binney Street, Boston, Massachusetts 02115, USA

H. ROUHANDEH   Southern Illinois University, Carbondale, Illinois 62901, USA

B. ROUSE   Department of Microbiology, Walters Life Sciences Building, University of Tennessee, Knoxville, Tennessee 37916, USA

A.S. RUBENSTEIN   Abbott Laboratories, Department 900, North Chicago, Illinois 60064, USA

L. RYMO   Department of Clinical Chemistry, Sahlgren's Hospital, 413 45 Gothenburg, Sweden

S. SAIDI   School of Public Health, Teheran University, P.O. Box 1310, Teheran, Iran

R.M. SANDRI   Sidney Farber Cancer Institute, 44 Binney Street, Boston, Massachusetts 02115, USA

B.K. SCHAEFFER   Department of Virology, Boston University School of Medicine, Boston, Massachusetts 02115, USA

P.A. SCHAFFER   Sidney Farber Cancer Institute, 44 Binney Street, Boston, Massachusetts 02115, USA

A.J. SCHEFFER   Laboratory of Medical Microbiology, State University of Groningen, 20 Moddermanlaan, Groningen GN 9721, The Netherlands

L.E. SCHNIPPER   Beth Israel Hospital, 330 Brookline Avenue, Boston, Massachusetts 02115, USA

C.H. SCHRÖDER   Institute for Virus Research, German Cancer Research Centre, Im Neuenheimer Feld 280, D-6900 Heidelberg, Federal Republic of Germany

M. SCRIBA   Sandoz Research Institute, Brunner Strasse 59, A-1325 Wien, Austria

P.J. SEIGEL	Sidney Farber Cancer Institute, 44 Binney Street, Boston, Massachusetts 02115, USA
J.-M. SEIGNEURIN	Laboratoire de Virologie, Hôpital des Sablons, B.P. 217X, 38043 Grenoble, Cedex, France
M. SEVOIAN	Department of Veterinary and Animal Science, University of Massachusetts, Amherst, Massachusetts 01003, USA
O.S. SETTNES	Institute of Medical Microbiology, Juliane Mariesvej 22, DK-2100 Copenhagen, Denmark
J.E. SHAW	Cancer Research Center, University of North Carolina, Box 3, 217H Swing Building, Chapel Hill, North Carolina 27514, USA
P. SHELDRICK	Institute for Scientific Research on Cancer (IRSC), B.P. 8, 94800 Villejuif, France
G.P. SHIBLEY	Pfizer, Inc., 199 Maywood Avenue, Maywood, New Jersey 07607, USA
E.J. SHILLITOE	Department of Oral Immunology and Microbiology, Guy's Hospital Medical and Dental Schools, London, UK
C. SHIPMAN, Jr	Dental Research Institute, University of Michigan, Ann Arbor, Michigan 48109, USA
T.C. SHOPE	Department of Pediatrics, Wayne State University, 3901 Beaubien Boulevard, Detroit, Michigan 48201, USA
S.S. SILVER	Life Sciences Research Laboratories, 2900 North 72nd Street, St. Petersburg, Florida 33710, USA
S. SILVERSTEIN	Department of Microbiology, Columbia University, Health Sciences Center, 680 West 168th Street, New York, New York 10032, USA
J. SKARE	Sidney Farber Cancer Institute, 44 Binney Street, Boston, Massachusetts 02115, USA
C.C. SMITH	Division of Comparative Medicine, The Johns Hopkins University Schools of Medicine and Hygiene and Public Health, Baltimore, Maryland 21205, USA

J.W. SMITH   Department of Microbiology, Louisiana State University Medical Center, New Orleans, Louisiana 70112, USA

M.C. SMITH   Cancer Research Center, University of North Carolina, Box 3, 217H Swing Building, Chapel Hill, North Carolina 27514, USA

R.A. SONSTEGARD   Department of Microbiology, College of Biological Science, University of Guelph, Guelph, Ontario N1G 2W1, Canada

P.G. SPEAR   Committee on Virology, University of Chicago, Marjorie B. Kovler Viral Oncology Laboratories, 910 East 58th Street, Chicago, Illinois 60637, USA

S. SPRECHER   Institut Pasteur du Brabant, 28 rue du Remorqueur, 1040 Brussels, Belgium

C.F. SPRINGGATE   Tulane Medical School, 1430 Tulane Avenue, New Orleans, Louisiana 70112, USA

J. STACZEK   Wistar Institute, 36th Street at Spruce, Philadelphia, Pennsylvania 19104, USA

S. STAGNO   Department of Pediatrics, Room 609, CDLD Building, UAB Medical Center, University Station, Birmingham, Alabama 35294, USA

P.G. STANSLY   National Cancer Institute, National Institutes of Health, Building WB Room 855, Bethesda, Maryland 20014, USA

T.G. STEMATSKY   Central Virus Laboratory, P.O. Box 8255, Tel-Aviv-Yafo, Israel

H. STERN   Virus Laboratory, St. George's Medical School, Hyde Park Corner, London SW1, UK

J.G. STEVENS   Reed Neurological Research Center, University of California School of Medicine, Los Angeles, California 90024, USA

M.F. STINSKI   Department of Microbiology, College of Medicine, University of Iowa, Iowa City, Iowa 52240, USA

S.C. ST. JEOR   Department of Microbiology, The Milton S. Hershey Medical Center, The Pennsylvania State University College of Medicine, Hershey, Pennsylvania 17033, USA

J.R. STRINGER   Department of Molecular Biology and Biochemistry, University of California, Irvine, California 92717, USA

B.C. STRNAD   Division of Comparative Medicine, Department of Biochemistry and Biophysics, The John Hopkins University Schools of Medicine and Hygiene and Public Health, Baltimore, Maryland 21205, USA

J. STROMINGER   Sidney Farber Cancer Institute, 44 Binney Street, Boston, Massachusetts 02115, USA

J. SUBAK-SHARPE   Department of Virology, Institute of Virology, University of Glasgow, Church Street, Glasgow G11 5JR, UK

M.H.-J. SUH   Montreal Cancer Institute, Notre Dame Hospital, 1560 Est Sherbrooke, Montreal H2L 4M7, Canada

W.C. SUMMERS   Radiobiology Laboratories, Yale University Medical School, 333 Cedar Street, New Haven, Connecticut 06510, USA

W.P. SUMMERS   Radiobiology Laboratories, Yale University Medical School, 333 Cedar Street, New Haven, Connecticut 06510, USA

M.S. SWARTZ   Harvard University - MIT Program, 2 Ridgewood Road, Malden, Massachusetts 02148, USA

P. TALBOT   Wellcome Research Laboratories, Langley Court, Beckenham, Kent BR3 3BS, UK

S. TALLEY-BROWN   Department of Immunology and Microbiology, Wayne State University School of Medicine, Detroit, Michigan 48201, USA

M. TAKAHASHI   Research Institute for Microbial Diseases, Osaka University, Yamuda-Kami, Suita, Osaka, Japan

A. TANAKA   Life Sciences Research Laboratories,
                            2900 North 72nd Street, St. Petersburg,
                            Florida 33710, USA

M.J. TEMPLE   Department of Biology, Georgetown University,
                            406 Reiss, Washington, DC 20057, USA

R.B. TENSER   Department of Neurology, The Milton S. Hershey
                            Medical Center, The Pennsylvania State
                            University College of Medicine, Hershey,
                            Pennsylvania 17033, USA

S.S. TEVETHIA   Tufts University School of Medicine,
                            Department of Pathology, Boston, Massachusetts
                            02115, USA

G.A. THEIS   Department of Microbiology, New York Medical
                            College, Valhalla, New York 10595, USA

L. THIRY   Institut Pasteur du Brabant, 104 Avenue
                            Herronière, 1040 Brussels, Belgium

D.A. THORLEY-LAWSON   Sidney Farber Cancer Institute, 44 Binney
                            Street, Boston, Massachusetts 02115, USA

M. TOCCI   Department of Microbiology, The Milton S.
                            Hershey Medical Center, The Pennsylvania State
                            University College of Medicine, Hershey,
                            Pennsylvania 17033, USA

I. TOPLIN   455 E. Saddle River Road, Ridgewood, New
                            Jersey 07450, USA

M.G. TOVEY   Laboratory of Viral Oncology, Institute for
                            Scientific Research on Cancer (IRSC), B.P. 8,
                            94800 Villejuif, France

N.R. TRAUB   Committee on Virology, University of Chicago,
                            Marjorie B. Kovler Viral Oncology Laboratories,
                            910 East 58th Street, Chicago, Illinois
                            60637, USA

P.A. TRUMPER   Department of Pathology, Medical School,
                            University of Bristol, Bristol BS8 1TD, UK

M.-R. TSAI   Frederick Cancer Research Center, P.O. Box B,
                            Frederick, Maryland 21701, USA

K.S. TWEEDELL   Department of Biology, University of Notre
                            Dame, Notre Dame, Indiana 46556, USA

L.F. VELICER
Department of Microbiology and Public Health, Michigan State University, East Lansing, Michigan 48824, USA

R.W. VELTRI
West Virginia University Medical Center, Division of Otolaryngology, Morgantown, West Virginia 26506, USA

J.B. VER PLANCK
Department of Virology, Boston University School of Medicine, Boston, Massachusetts 02115, USA

D.W. VERWOERD
Molecular Biology Section, Veterinary Research Institute, P.O. Box 12501, Onderstepoort 0110, South Africa

B.F. VESTERGAARD
Department of Clinical Virology, Institute of Medical Microbiology, Juliane Mariesvej 22, DK-2100 Copenhagen, Denmark

V. VONKA
Institute of Sera and Vaccines, 101 03 Prague 10, W. Pieck 108, Czechoslovakia

E.K. WAGNER
Department of Molecular Biology and Biochemistry, University of California, Irvine, California 92717, USA

M.J. WAGNER
Radiobiology Laboratories, Yale University School of Medicine, 333 Cedar Street, New Haven, Connecticut 06510, USA

W.C. WALLEN
National Cancer Institute, National Institutes of Health, Bethesda, Maryland 20014, USA

J.L. WANER
Department of Tropical Public Health, Harvard School of Public Health, 665 Huntington Avenue, Boston, Massachusetts 02115, USA

K.G. WARREN
The Multiple Sclerosis Research Center of the Wistar Institute, University of Pennsylvania, Philadelphia, Pennsylvania 19104, USA

A.L. WATKINS
Department of Pathobiology, University of Washington, Seattle, Washington 98195, USA

R.J. WATSON
Institute of Virology, University of Glasgow, Church Street, Glasgow G11 5JR, UK

R. WEINMANN
The Wistar Institute, 36th Street at Spruce, Philadelphia, Pennsylvania 19104, USA

T.H. WELLER   The Department of Tropical Public Health,
Harvard School of Public Health, 665 Huntington
Avenue, Boston, Massachusetts 02115, USA

S. WELLING   Medical Microbiology Department, Oostersingel 59,
Groningen, The Netherlands

R.J. WHITLEY   Department of Pediatrics, Room 609 CDLD Building,
UAB Medical Center, University Station, Birmingham,
Alabama 35294, USA

P. WILDY   Department of Pathology, University of Cambridge,
Addenbrooke's Hospital, Hills Road, Cambridge
CB2 1QP, UK

J.A. WILHELM   Medical Microbiology Institute, Immunology
Department, Frohbergstrasse 3, 9000 St. Gallen,
Switzerland

N.M. WILKIE   Medical Research Council Virology Unit, Institute
of Virology, University of Glasgow, Church Street,
Glasgow G11 5JR, UK

A. WILLS   Pediatric Research Centre, Ste-Justine Hospital,
3175 chemin Ste-Catherine, Montreal H3T 1C5,
Quebec, Canada

T.G. WISE   Bureau of Biologics, Food and Drug Administration,
Bethesda, Maryland 20014, USA

R.L. WITTER   Science and Education Administration-Federal
Research United States Department of Agriculture,
Regional Poultry Research Laboratory, 3606 East
Mount Hope Road, East Lansing, Michigan 48823, USA

C. WOHLENBERG   National Institutes of Health, Bethesda, Maryland
20014, USA

H. WOLF   Max v. Pettenkofer-Institute of Hygiene and
Medical Microbiology of the University of Munich,
D-8000 Munich 2, Federal Republic of Germany

A. YABROV   Department of Medical Microbiology, Banting
Institute, Room 220, 100 College Street, Toronto,
Ontario, Canada

Y. YAJIMA   Department of Microbiology, Rush-Presbyterian-
St Luke's Medical Center, 1753 West Congress
Parkway, Chicago, Illinois 60612, USA

K. YAMANISHI   Department of Microbiology, The Milton S. Hershey
                    Medical Center, The Pennsylvania State University
                    College of Medicine, Hershey, Pennsylvania 17033,
                    USA

K. YANAGI   Department of Biochemistry, New York University
                    Medical Center, 550 First Avenue, New York, New
                    York 10016, USA

E. YEFENOF   Department of Tumor Biology, Karolinska Institutet,
                    S-104 01 Stockholm 60, Sweden

T.O. YOSHIDA   Hamamatsu University School of Medicine, Hamamatsu,
                    Japan

K.K.-Y. YU   Biology Department, University of New Brunswick,
                    Fredericton, New Brunswick E3B 5A3, Canada

H. ZUR HAUSEN   Institute of Virology, Albert-Ludwig University,
                    Hermann Herderstrasse 11, Postfach 820, D-7800
                    Freiburg im Brisgau, Federal Republic of Germany

M. ZWEIG   Department of Viral Oncology, Frederick Cancer
                    Research Center, Frederick, Maryland 21701, USA

DNA OF HERPESVIRUSES – STRUCTURE AND ASSOCIATION WITH CELL DNA

EPSTEIN-BARR VIRUS GENOMES AND THEIR BIOLOGICAL FUNCTIONS: A REVIEW

H. ZUR HAUSEN, K.-O. FRESEN & G.W. BORNKAMM

Institut für Virologie,
Zentrum für Hygiene, Universität Freiburg,
Freiburg im Breisgau, Federal Republic of Germany

The structural organization of herpesvirus DNA and, in particular, the structure of herpes simplex virus DNA, has been analysed in detail by Sheldrick. Since, in addition, space does not permit the inclusion of all the information gathered during the past two or more years with regard to the structure and mode of persistence of herpesvirus DNA, this review will be restricted to the discussion of recent work on the organization of Epstein-Barr virus (EBV) DNA. Comparisons will be made with other oncogenic herpesviruses whenever possible.

Nucleic acid hybridizations showed that multiple copies of EBV DNA were commonly present in non-producer cell lines transformed by this virus, as well as in tumour cells of biopsy material from Burkitt's lymphomas and nasopharyngeal carcinomas (Nonoyama & Pagano, 1971, 1973; zur Hausen & Schulte-Holthausen, 1970; zur Hausen et al., 1970). The number of genome equivalents per cell ranged between 1-2, up to approximately 200 (zur Hausen, 1975), but was most frequently between 20 and 50. From this, it may be calculated that viral DNA in transformed cells may amount to up to 0.25% of the total cellular DNA. Similar concentrations of viral DNA copies per transformed cell have been observed in three other systems of herpesvirus-transformed cells: Fleckenstein et al., (1977) were able to demonstrate multiple genome equivalents of herpesvirus saimiri and of herpesvirus ateles DNA in transformed cells and tumour biopsy material transformed or induced by the respective viruses, while Nazerian and his co-workers (1973) found multiple copies of Marek's disease herpesvirus in lymphatic tumour material of diseased chickens by nucleic acid hybridization.

The presence of a large number of viral DNA copies within each individual tumour cell raised the question of the mode of persistence of this DNA. The first studies were undertaken by Nonoyama & Pagano (1973) and resulted in the remarkable demonstration of non-integrated EBV DNA sequences in cells of the Raji line of Burkitt tumour origin. These observations were confirmed and extended by Adams and Lindahl and their co-workers (Kaschka-Dierich et al., 1976; Lindahl et al., 1976[1]). The Swedish group demonstrated the persistence of EBV DNA as circular plasmids by biophysical methods and revealed these molecules by electron microscopy. Banding of EBV DNA from cells of EBV-carrying lymphoblastoid lines in isopycnic caesium chloride gradients revealed trailing patterns suggestive of a covalent linkage of viral DNA with the host-cell genome (Adams et al., 1973). These studies were extended to additional lines with similar results, although EBV-transformed cells of human umbilical cord-blood origin seemed to lack "integrated" sequences (Adams et al., 1977).

In view of the recent demonstration of the intracellular hetero-geneity of EBV DNA in individual lines (see below), the integration of EBV DNA and the quantitation of the integrated, as compared to the plasmid state, requires further investigation. Circular viral DNA was also demonstrated in herpesvirus saimiri and herpesvirus ateles-transformed cells[2].

The discovery of 10-15% smaller circular molecules in lympho-blastoid cord-blood cells obtained after transformation with 883-L-EBV, as compared to circular and linear EBV DNA from other sources, deserves attention (Adams et al., 1977). Since the B95-8 line of marmoset cells, which produces EBV DNA of unit length, was established after infection with EBV from 883-L cells (Miller & Lipman, 1973), this may indicate the existence of intracellular heterogeneity of EBV DNA in this line, although other interpretations are possible.

The existence of strain variations in various EBV isolates was initially investigated by studying the kinetics of reassociation between EBV DNA isolated from the P3HR-1 strain, and viral DNA origi-nating from the marmoset line B95-8 (Pritchett et al., 1975; Sugden et al., 1976). According to the data of Pritchett et al. (1975) the transforming EBV strain derived from B95-8 cells lacked about 15% of the DNA sequences of the non-transforming P3HR-1 EBV strain. These authors interpreted their data to mean that EBV from B95-8 cells is derived from a parental EBV through loss of genetic complexity.

One general problem in performing these renaturation kinetics experiments is the use of *in vitro* labelled DNA. Only 34% of the labelled species formed duplexes with large excesses of homologous

---

[1] See also p. 113

[2] See p. 125

DNA (Sugden et al., 1976). This seems to be due to the *in vitro* labelling conditions.

More detailed information on the existence of strain variations in EBV of different origins is derived from analyses of the restriction-enzyme cleavage patterns of such preparations (Delius & Bornkamm, 1978; Hayward & Kieff, 1977; Lee et al., 1977; Sugden et al., 1976). EBV DNA from P3HR-1, B95-8 and Jijoye cells and, in addition, EBV DNA recovered from Raji cells after superinfection with P3HR-1 EBV, were analysed. All the restriction-enzyme patterns reveal the existence of differences in the molecular weight of certain fragments, as between the P3HR-1 and B95-8 viruses. These are particularly striking after *Eco*RI, *Hsu*I and *Sal*I cleavage, but less pronounced after cleavage of this DNA by the *Bam*HI endonuclease. It is interesting to note that the virus isolated from the Jijoye line, from which the P3HR-1 clone originated, showed certain differences in the cleavage pattern when compared to the P3HR-1 EBV (Hayward & Kieff, 1977). Strain-specific differences in the cleavage patterns have been noted in herpes simplex virus isolates and various strains of human cyto-megalovirus (Kilpatrick & Huang, 1977; Skare et al., 1975), but do not provide an explanation for observed differences in biological behaviour.

The structural organization of the EBV genome derived from different cell lines is still far from being elucidated. The number of bands observed in multimolar and submolar quantities renders an interpretation extremely difficult. In most instances, the sum of the molecular weights of the fragments is in excess of 10^8; this led to the suggestion by Hayward & Kieff (1977) that EBV from P3HR-1 and B95-8 cells contains two populations of molecules which differ in sequence arrangement.

The analysis is further complicated by the observation that virus recovered from Raji cells after superinfection with P3HR-1 EBV possesses a more heterogenous DNA population than the P3HR-1 input virus (Lee et al., 1977). In contrast to the superinfecting virus, this agent also possesses transforming properties.

Attempts to gain further insight into the structural details of different EBV strains by partial denaturation mapping (Delius & Bornkamm, 1978) have not yet yielded unequivocal results. They indicate that the terminal sequences of EBV do show some variability, and suggest that there exist no extended regions of inverted sequences in the DNA of B95-8 EBV.

It should also be pointed out here that molecular biological studies of EBV DNA do reveal heterogeneities in DNA preparations from different EBV strains. They are as yet, however, far from providing a comparable understanding of the structural organization of this DNA as that obtained, for instance, from studies of herpes simplex virus or herpesvirus saimiri DNA.

Some clarification of the complicated picture emerging from the biochemical analysis of EBV DNA appears to result from more biologically oriented experiments, and the remaining part of this review will be devoted to their discussion.

Fresen & zur Hausen (1976) noted that infection of cells of the human B-lymphoma lines BJA-B and Ramos with P3HR-1 virus resulted in the appearance of two characteristic patterns of EBV nuclear antigen (EBNA) expression: whereas some nuclei gave a faint granular pattern, others showed brilliant staining. Even prolonged cultivation of such cells did not alter this heterogenous EBNA expression. If, in contrast, BJA-B or Ramos cells were infected with the B95-8 virus, these cells uniformly gave a brilliant EBNA pattern.

Cloning of BJA-B cells, converted to EBNA expression by the P3HR-1 virus, resulted in three types of clones (Fresen et al., 1977). The first gave the same pattern as the parental line, and was excluded from further studies since it may have represented a pick-up of more than one cell. The second type showed exclusively the faint granular pattern, thus revealing a remarkable homogeneity in EBNA expression.

The third type gave the brilliant EBNA pattern, but, in addition, always contained EBNA-negative cells at varying frequencies. Subcloning of such cells resulted in clones with similar properties, containing, apart from brilliant EBNA-positive cells, a number of EBNA-negative segregants. One entirely EBNA-negative subclone was also obtained which did not contain detectable traces of EBV DNA when studied by reassociation kinetics hybridization. Even one year of continuous propagation of one of the brilliantly EBNA-expressing subclones did not result in either the disappearance of EBNA-positive or EBNA-negative cells, the latter representing by then about 70% of the total cell population. We interpreted these data to mean that the P3HR-1 virus preparations contain two populations of molecules: one inducing the faint granular EBNA type and leading to a stable conversion of infected cells, the other being responsible for the brilliant EBNA conversion. This second type of molecule appears to be defective in P3HR-1 cells in that it is unable to guarantee its uniform distribution and persistence during cell mitosis. In the parental P3HR-1 cell, it may require the helper function of the faint granular EBNA-expressing genomes for its maintenance, and it is possible that this defect may be related to the inability of P3HR-1 virus to transform cells *in vitro*. The heterogeneity of P3HR-1 virus preparations was further underlined by studies on early antigen (EA) induction in non-converted BJA-B and Ramos cells and their converted clones and subclones (zur Hausen & Fresen, 1977). Infection of EBV genome-carrying cells converted by P3HR-1 EBV resulted on average in a 15-fold higher EA induction, as compared to the EBV-negative parental BJA-B or Ramos lines.

Infection of P3HR-1 virus-converted BJA-B cells and their clones and subclones with the transforming (but usually not EA-inducing) B95-8 virus yielded some EA-positive cells in the P3HR-1 virus-converted line; this was more pronounced in the faint granular EBNA-expressing subclones. No increase in EA induction was found in brilliantly EBNA-expressing clones after infection with B95-3 virus. These data suggested complementation of the different types of EBV genomes. This view received further support from studies of the kinetics of EA induction in genome-carrying and genome-negative susceptible cells after infection with different dilutions of the P3HR-1 virus. In genome-carrying cells, EA induction followed first-order kinetics, whereas in genome-negative cells, EA was induced according to second-order kinetics. These data strongly support the view that P3HR-1 cells, at least, contain two subtypes of EBV genome which, upon co-infection, complement each other in EA induction.

We were recently able to show that the transforming EBV strains from B95-3 and Nuevo cells induce a nuclear antigen in Ramos, but not in BJA-B cells, which can be easily demonstrated by indirect immunofluorescence (Fresen et al., 1973). In other cells, only EBNA is induced. P3HR-1 virus is unable to induce this nuclear antigen, although it leads to EBNA expression in Ramos cells. This result may point to a heterogeneity also in the biological functions of the B95-3 and Nuevo-EBV preparations.

Lee et al. (1977) and Fresen et al. (1973[1]) recently observed the recovery of transforming virus from non-producer Raji and NC37 cells after superinfection with the P3HR-1 virus. In view of the previously reported data on complementation in EA induction (zur Hausen & Fresen, 1977), it seems unlikely that the non-transforming heterogenous P3HR-1 virus was converted in the Raji and NC37 cells into a transforming agent. It is much more probable that a transforming virus has been rescued by the superinfecting P3HR-1 virus mixture. Based on these results, it is tempting to speculate that at least a number of transforming EBV strains are helper-dependent in some early and late functions, and require complementation by an as yet poorly defined component in the P3HR-1 cells, which may be represented by the faint granular EBNA-expressing genomes in P3HR-1 virus-converted BJA-B and Ramos cells. On this basis, the system would show certain analogies to the dependence of sarcoma virus replication on helper effects mediated by leukaemia and mammalian oncornavirus infections. The lack of transforming virus in the P3HR-1 virus preparations could then be attributed to a defect regulating the persistence within the transformed cells of those molecules inducing brilliant EBNA expression. This may be visualized by the segregation of EBNA-negative cells from brilliantly EBNA-expressing subclones of P3HR-1 virus-converted BJA-B cells. Abortive transformation by P3HR-1 virus has been observed (Aya & Osato, 1978).

---

[1] Unpublished data

The foregoing detailed discussion of biological data in a review of
the biochemical aspects of herpesvirus genomes is intended to demonstrate that the interpretation of the structural organization, at least
of Epstein-Barr virus DNA, is still at a level at which the clues provided by biological experiments are essential.

REFERENCES

Adams, A., Lindahl, T. & Klein, G. (1973)   Linear association between
    cellular DNA and Epstein-Barr virus DNA in a human lymphoblastoid
    cell line.   *Proc. nat. Acad. Sci. (Wash.), 70*, 2888-2892

Adams, A., Bjursell, C., Kaschka-Dierich, C. & Lindahl, T. (1977)
    Circular Epstein-Barr virus genomes of reduced size in a human
    lymphoid cell line of infectious mononucleosis origin.   *J. Virol.,
    22*, 373-380

Aya, T. & Osato, T. (1978)   Abortive growth of human lymphocytes
    carrying a dormant Epstein-Barr viral genome.   *Med. Microbiol.
    Immunol., 164*, 255-266

Delius, H. & Bornkamm, G.W. (1978)   Heterogeneity of Epstein-Barr
    virus.   III. Comparison of a transforming and a non-transforming
    virus by partial denaturation napping of their DNA.
    J. Virol. (in press)

Fleckenstein, B., Müller, I. & Werner, J. (1977)   The presence of
    Herpesvirus saimiri genomes in virus-transformed cells.   *Int.
    J. Cancer, 19*, 546-554

Fresen, K.O. & zur Hausen, H. (1976)   Establishment of EBNA-expressing
    cell lines by infection of Epstein-Barr virus (EBV) genome-negative
    human lymphoma cells with different EBV strains.   *Int. J. Cancer,
    17*, 161-166

Fresen, K.O., Merkt, B., Bornkamm, G.W. & zur Hausen, H. (1977)
    Heterogeneity of Epstein-Barr virus originating from P3HR-1 cells.
    I. Studies on EBNA induction.   *Int. J. Cancer, 19*, 317-323

Fresen, K.O., Cho, M.-S. & zur Hausen, H. (1978)   Heterogeneity of
    Epstein-Barr virus.   IV. Induction of a specific antigen by EBV
    from two transformed marmoset cell lines in Ramos cells.   *Int. J.
    Cancer* (in press)

Hayward, S.D. & Kieff, E. (1977)   DNA of Epstein-Barr virus.   II.
    Comparison of the molecular weights of restriction endonuclease
    fragments of the DNA of Epstein-Barr virus strains and identifica-
    tion of end fragments of the B95-8 strain.   *J. Virol., 23*, 421-429

Kaschka-Dierich, C., Adams, A., Lindahl, T., Bornkamm, G.W., Bjursell,
    G., Klein, G., Giovanella, B.C. & Singh, S. (1976)   Intracellular
    forms of Epstein-Barr virus DNA in human tumour cells *in vivo*.
    Nature (Lond.), 260, 302-306

Kilpatrick, B.A. & Huang, E.-S. (1977)   Human cytomegalovirus genome:
    partial denaturation map and organization of genome sequences.
    J. Virol., 24, 261-276

Lee, Y.S., Yajima, Y. & Nonoyama, M. (1977)   Mechanism of infection
    by Epstein-Barr virus. II. Comparison of viral DNA from HR-1 and
    superinfected Raji cells by restriction enzymes.   *Virology, 81*
    17-24

Lindahl, T., Adams, A., Bjursell, B., Bornkamm, G.W., Kaschka-Dierich,
    C. & Jehn, U. (1976)   Covalently closed circular duplex DNA of
    Epstein-Barr virus in a human lymphoid cell line.   *J. molec. Biol.,
    102*, 511-530

Miller, G. & Lipman, M. (1973)   Release of infectious Epstein-Barr
    virus by transformed marmoset leukocytes.   *Proc. nat. Acad. Sci.
    (Wash.), 70*, 190-194

Nazerian, K., Lindahl, T., Klein, G. & Lee, L.F. (1973)   Deoxyribo-
    nucleic acid of Marek's disease virus in virus induced tumors.
    J. Virol., 12, 841-846

Nonoyama, M. & Pagano, J.S. (1971)   Detection of Epstein-Barr virus
    genome in non-productive cells.   *Nature new Biol., 233*, 103-106

Nonoyama, M. & Pagano, J.S. (1973)   Homology between Epstein-Barr
    virus DNA and viral DNA from Burkitt's lymphoma and nasopharyngeal
    carcinoma determined by DNA-DNA reassociation kinetics.   *Nature
    (Lond.), 242*, 44-47

Pritchett, R.F., Hayward, S.D. & Kieff, E.D. (1975)   DNA of Epstein-
    Barr virus. I. Comparative studies of the DNA of Epstein-Barr
    virus from HR-1 and B95-8 cells: size, structure, and relatedness.
    J. Virol., 15, 556-569

Skare, J., Summers, W.P. & Summers, W.C. (1975)   Structure and
    function of herpesvirus genomes. I. Comparison of five HSV-1 and
    two HSV-2 strains by cleavage of their DNA with Eco Rl restriction
    endonuclease.   *J. Virol., 15*, 726-732

Sugden, B., Summers, W.C. & Klein, G. (1976)   Nucleic acid renatura-
    tion and restriction endonuclease cleavage analyses show that the
    DNAs of a transforming and a nontransforming strain of Epstein-
    Barr virus share approximately 90% of their nucleotide sequences.
    J. Virol., 18, 765-775

zur Hausen, H. (1975)   Oncogenic herpes viruses.   *Biochim. Biophys.
    Acta, 417*, 25-53

zur Hausen, H. & Fresen, K.O. (1977)   Heterogeneity of Epstein-Barr
    virus. II. Induction of early antigens (EA) by complementation.
    Virology, 81, 138-143

zur Hausen, H. & Schulte-Holthausen, H. (1970)   Presence of EB virus
    nucleic acid homology in a "virus-free" line of Burkitt tumour
    cells.   *Nature (Lond.), 227*, 245-248

zur Hausen, H., Schulte-Holthausen, H., Klein, G., Henle, W., Henle,
    G., Clifford, P. & Santesson, L. (1970)   EBV DNA in biopsies of
    Burkitt tumours and anaplastic carcinomas of the nasopharynx.
    Nature (Lond.), 228, 1056-1058

PHYSICAL MAPPING OF HERPES SIMPLEX VIRUS-CODED FUNCTIONS AND POLYPEPTIDES BY MARKER RESCUE AND ANALYSIS OF HSV-1/HSV-2 INTERTYPIC RECOMBINANTS

N.M. WILKIE, N.D. STOW, H.S. MARSDEN, V. PRESTON,
R. CORTINI, M.C. TIMBURY & J.H. SUBAK-SHARPE

*Department of Virology
and Medical Research Council Virology Unit,
Institute of Virology,
University of Glasgow,
Glasgow, UK*

Knowledge of the genome locations of virus-specified functions is essential for the understanding of viral gene expression and its regulation. The polynucleotide sequence arrangement of the DNA of a number of herpesviruses has been studied in recent years and physical maps of the DNA of herpes simplex virus types 1 and 2 (HSV-1 and HSV-2) have been constructed for several restriction endonucleases (Clements et al., 1977; Cortini & Wilkie, 1978; Hayward et al.[1]; Skare & Summers, 1977; Wilkie, 1976). Although a number of conditional lethal temperature-sensitive (*ts*) mutants of HSV-1 and HSV-2 have been isolated and ordered into genetic maps (Benyesh-Melnick et al., 1974; Brown et al., 1973; Schaffer et al., 1974; Timbury & Calder, 1976), the only reported function so far located on the physical map is the viral thymidine kinase (Maitland & MacDougal, 1977; Wigler et al., 1977). Genetic markers can be located on physical maps by means of marker rescue experiments (Hutchison & Edgell, 1971; Lai & Nathans, 1974, 1975; Miller & Fried, 1976; Weissbeek et al., 1976) and a general approach for HSV has previously been suggested (Wilkie et al., 1974).

---

[1] Personal communication

In the present communication this approach is refined and
extended and used to identify the physical map locations of a number
of *ts* mutants of HSV-1.   The physical mapping of most of these *ts*
mutations is confirmed by the identification of the crossover regions
in the genomes of intertypic recombinants between HSV-1 and HSV-2.
Quite independently analysis of the polypeptides synthesized in cells
infected by these intertypic recombinants also allows the tentative
assignment of physical map locations to a number of HSV-specified
polypeptides.   The results are summarized and compared to the immediate early transcription map (Clements et al., 1977;   Watson &
Clements[1]) and to the genetic map (Brown et al., 1973;   Brown &
Jamieson[2]).

MARKER RESCUE

The rationale for mapping of *ts* mutants of HSV-1 by marker rescue
arises from these considerations: Following infection of permissive
cells at the restrictive temperature with intact genomes of *ts* mutants
no infectious progeny is produced.   Similarly, cells infected with
fragments of wild-type DNA produce no infectious progeny.   In a
mixed infection using intact *ts* DNA and fragments of wild-type DNA,
replication to produce infectious progeny is possible by marker
rescue through interaction between the intact *ts* genome and wild-type
DNA fragments containing the normal counterpart of the *ts* mutation.
This interaction, which could be at the level of complementation or
of genetic recombination, occurs entirely within the mixedly infected
cell.   In either case the production of infectious progeny (all *ts*
in the case of complementation, but wild-type in the case of recombination) upon co-infection with a *ts* genome and an isolated restriction
endonuclease fragment of wild-type DNA allows the allocation of the *ts*
mutation to a map position within that fragment.

In our earlier report (Wilkie et al., 1974) *ts* genomes were introduced into the cell as virus particles.   However, the use of infectious virus, which was not very efficient in marker rescue, led to
problems due to cytotoxicity and the presence of revertants in mutant
stocks.   These problems have been largely overcome by using *ts* DNA
instead of *ts* virus to infect cells.   Therefore, in the present
series of experiments BHK (C13) cells were infected at the restrictive
temperature with intact *ts* DNA and wild-type restriction endonuclease
fragments using the modified calcium orthophosphate precipitation
technique described by Stow & Wilkie (1976)

---

[1] Unpublished data

[2] See p. 33

Figure 1 summarizes two experiments which define map co-ordinates for the HSV-1 mutant ts K.   Cells co-infected with ts K DNA and isolated BglII or $Hind$III/Xba double-digest fragments were harvested after three days at 38.5°C.   Progeny virus was detected by plating at 38.5°C and 31°C and the infectious titres at both temperatures are shown.

FIG. 1.   RESCUE OF ts (HSV-1) WITH ts^+ DNA FRAGMENTS

Confluent monolayers of BHK (C13) cells were infected at 38.5°C with 0.2 - 0.4 µg of intact ts K DNA and similar genome equivalents of BglII or $Hind$III/Xba fragments of ts^+ DNA (strain 17), by the method described by Stow & Wilkie (1976).   After three days the cells were harvested by scraping into the culture medium, sonicated and progeny virus titrated at 38.5°C and 31°C.   The DNA fragment maps are also depicted.

	HindIII/Xba 38 5°C	HindIII/Xba 31°C		BglII 38 5°C	BglII 31°C
1	3.6×10^2	5.2×10^2	a	8.4×10^2	1.4×10^3
2	8.0×10^2	3.2×10^3	b	3.2×10^2	6.4×10^2
3	<40	<40	c	2.1×10^3	1.5×10^4
4*	3.2×10^2	1.9×10^3	d	<40	<40
5	1.2×10^2	2.8×10^2	e	9.6×10^2	5.6×10^3
6	2.2×10^3	2.2×10^4	f	<40	<40
7	<40	<40	gh	1.2×10^2	1.4×10^3
8*	"	"	i	<40	<40
9	"	"	j	"	"
10	"	"	k	"	"
11*	4.8×10^2	1.1×10^4	l	5.2×10^2	3.4×10^3
12	<40	<40	m	<40	<40
13	"	"	n	"	"
14	"	"	o	"	"
15	"	"	p	"	"

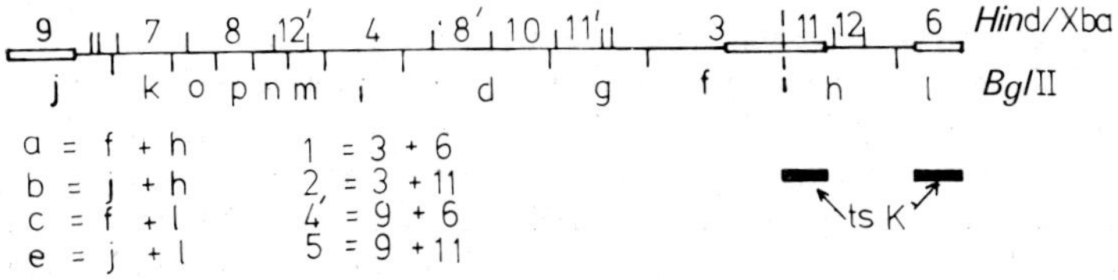

a = f + h   1 = 3 + 6
b = j + h   2 = 3 + 11
c = f + l   4 = 9 + 6
e = j + l   5 = 9 + 11

The results were quite clear-cut: Progeny were detected only after co-infection with *Hind*III/*Xba* bands *1, 2, (4 + 4'), 5, 6* and *(11 + 11')* and in *Bgl*II bands *a, b, c, e, (g + h)* and *l*.   The only nucleotide sequences these bands have in common are those of the repetition bounding the S region, and it can be concluded that the mutation in *ts* K lies in this region of HSV-1 DNA.   It can be seen from the data presented in Figure 1 that recombination accounts for a substantial proportion of the rescue progeny.   Analysis of the progeny from individual plaques following marker rescue indicates the presence of both recombinant wild-type and complemented (*ts*) virus.   The number and precise sequence of distinct events which ultimately result in marker rescue remain unknown and will clearly need to be elucidated.   Using the same approach as outlined above, map locations have also been obtained for HSV-1 mutants *ts* A, *ts* D, *ts* F, *ts* J and *ts* S.   These results will be documented and analysed in detail elsewhere.   Figure 8, given later, summarizes our current map co-ordinates for these mutants.

The marker rescue approach is not restricted to *ts* mutations and can be used to map any mutant for which there is a suitable selection system, for example mutations which lead to loss of viral deoxypyrimidine kinase activity.   Schildkraut et al. (1975) have reported that bromodeoxycytidine (BCDR) inhibits the replication of wild-type HSV. However, the replication of HSV mutants deficient in the synthesis of active virus-specified deoxypyrimidine kinase (dPyK: often only referred to as TK) is resistant to the presence of the drug (Brown & Jamieson[1]).   We have carried out marker rescue experiments with one particular mutant of HSV-1, dPyK^{-7} (isolated by A.T. Jamieson), which appears to be defective in viral thymidine kinase activity (TK) because of mutation in the structural gene for the viral deoxypyrimidine kinase (Jamieson & Subak-Sharpe, 1978).   Initial experiments showed that the yield of progeny virus from BHK cells infected with DNA from wild-type virus in the presence of 100 µg/ml of BCDR in the culture medium was reduced by a factor of about 10^6, whereas the virus yield from cells infected with DNA from dPyK^{-7} was virtually unaffected. It was therefore tested whether cells co-infected with intact wild-type DNA and DNA fragments which contained the dPyK^{-7} mutation might produce recombinant genomes containing a defective TK gene, which could replicate in the presence of BCDR to produce infectious progeny.

BHK cells were infected with intact DNA from wild-type virus and isolated *Xba* fragments of DNA from dPyK^{-7} in the presence of 100 µg/ml BCDR.   The yield of progeny virus after co-infection with each *Xba* fragment is shown in Figure 2.   Only *Xba f* gave a marked increase in the levels of progeny virus.   In other experiments it was shown that a marked increase in progeny virus yield using *Hind*III fragments was obtained only with *Hind*III *a + b*.   Only *Hind*III *a* overlaps with *Xba f*

---

[1] See p. 33

FIG. 2.   RESCUE OF dPyK^{-7} GENE FROM DNA FRAGMENTS OF
dPyK^{-7} DNA IN THE PRESENCE OF 5-BROMODEOXYCYTIDINE

Confluent monolayers of BHK (C13) cells were co-infected at 37°C with
Xba fragments of dPyK^{-7} DNA and intact wild-type HSV-1 DNA as for
Figure 1.   The culture medium contained 100 µg/ml of 5-bromodeoxy-
cytidine and was replaced every 24 hours.   Progeny virus was titrated
in the absence of the drug.

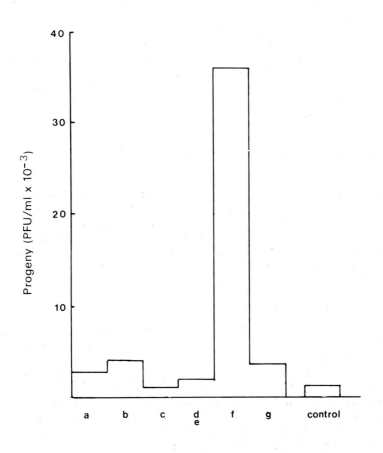

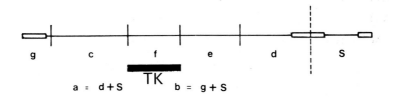

(Wilkie, 1976).   Clonally purified stocks of virus resulting from
rescue with *Xba f* and *Hin*dIII *a + b* were tested by plating in the
presence and absence of BCDR.   The results indicated that 24 out of
25 plaques picked from the progeny of five separate plate harvests had
a TK⁻ phenotype.

The results can be interpreted to mean that the structural gene
for HSV-1 TK lies in *Xba f*, providing the mutation in dPyK⁻⁷ is in
the structural gene for virus-specified deoxypyrimidine kinase.   Wigler
et al. (1977) and Silverstein et al.[1] have shown that a small *Bam*H1
fragment from the L region of HSV-1 contains the information sufficient
and necessary to effect the transformation of TK⁻ L cells to a TK⁺
phenotype and that the viral TK activity is expressed in the transformants.   Our current mapping data place this fragment at the left-hand
end of *Xba f* (Davidson & Wilkie[2]).   The physical map positions of
virus-specific thymidine kinase deduced from the work reported in this
communication, and from the data of Wigler et al. (1977) and Silverstein
et al.[1] are shown later in Figure 8.

ANALYSIS OF CROSSOVERS IN INTERTYPIC RECOMBINANTS

HSV-1 and HSV-2 appear to share 40-50% base sequence homology in
their DNAs (Sheldrick[2]).   Moreover this shared homology
extends also to gene sequences and their functional equivalence, as
demonstrated by efficient complementation and recombination between
HSV-1 and HSV-2 (Esparza et al., 1976; Timbury & Subak-Sharpe, 1973).
Similarly, after mixed infection with *ts* mutants of HSV-1 and HSV-2,
clones of *ts*⁺ virus have been obtained, some of which code for both
HSV-1 and HSV-2 proteins as detected by specific neutralizing antisera
(Halliburton et al., 1977).

Preliminary comparative hybridization studies using restriction
endonuclease fragments (Wilkie & Cortini[2]) indicate that the homologous
regions in the DNA of HSV-1 and HSV-2 appear to be distributed widely
throughout the long (L) and short (S) unique regions of the genome.
It was therefore possible to align the physical maps of the long and
short regions of HSV-1 and HSV-2, as shown later in Figure 4 for six
restriction endonucleases.   Since the restriction site maps for HSV-1
and HSV-2 are different the fragment profiles can be used to analyse
the crossover points in recombinant genomes.

---

[1] See p. 501

[2] Unpublished data

Figure 3 shows six restriction endonuclease analyses of clone R13, derived from a cross between *ts* B (HSV-1) and *ts* 1 (HSV-2).   The profiles of R13 show DNA fragments derived from each of the parental genomes, indicating that R13 is indeed a recombinant.   Figure 4 shows how the crossover points in R13 were identified from the data of Figure 3.   Characteristic fragments of HSV-2 DNA are shown as clear

FIG. 3. AUTORADIOGRAMS OF ^{32}P-ORTHOPHOSPHATE-LABELLED DNA OF RECOMBINANT R13 AND PARENTAL VIRUSES *ts* 1 (HSV-2) AND *ts* B (HSV-1)

The DNA samples were digested with restriction endonucleases *Xba*, *Hind*III, *Eco*Rl, *Bgl*II, *Hpa*I and *Kpn* and the fragments separated by electrophoresis on slab gels of agarose (0.3%, 0.7% or 1.0%).   The letters refer to specific DNA fragments for which the physical maps are given in Figure 4. ■   HSV-1 DNA fragments;   ○   HSV-2 DNA fragments; *   Novel DNA fragments produced upon digestion of the recombinant DNA.

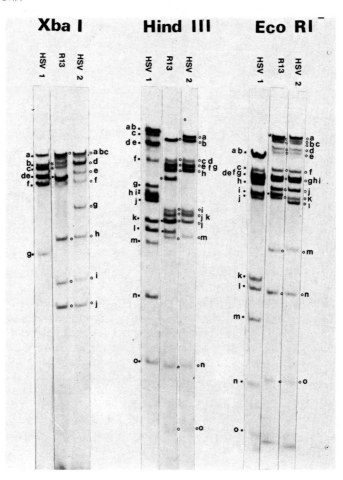

Fig. 3. (continued)

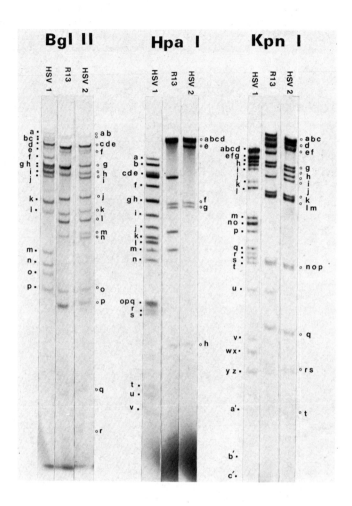

regions and those of HSV-1 DNA as black regions.   Regions in which
the parental nature of the DNA sequences is uncertain are indicated
by hatched lines.   Each region of uncertainty varies with the enzyme
used in the analysis but by aligning the results from all the enzymes
it can be concluded that R13 contains an insertion of HSV-1 genetic
material with maximum map co-ordinates of 54 and 70 and minimum co-
ordinates of 56 and 69.   Since R13 is ts^+ it follows that the mutation in ts 1 (HSV-2) must lie in this region of the map.   Because of
the uncertainty in the location of the crossover points the maximum
map co-ordinates are used to delimit the possible map location of ts
mutants by this method.   (As a corollary it also follows that the

FIG. 4. ANALYSIS OF THE CROSSOVER POINTS IN RECOMBINANT R13

The restriction endonuclease data depicted in Figure 3 are shown in terms of the *Hind*III, *Xba*, *Eco*R1, *Bgl*II, *Hpa*1 and *Kpn* fragments of HSV-1 and HSV-2 DNA.   The HSV-1 maps are shown above and the HSV-2 maps below, the DNA models.   The HSV-1, *Hind*III, *Xba*, *Eco*R1, *Bgl*II and *Hpa*1 maps are taken from published data (Clements et al., 1977; Skare & Summers, 1977; Wilkie, 1976) and the HSV-1 *Kpn* map is from Stow et al. (unpublished data).   The HSV-2 *Hind*III, *Xba*, *Eco*R1, *Bgl*II and *Hpa*1 maps are from the data of Cortini & Wilkie (1978) and the HSV-2 *Kpn* map from the data of Hayward et al. (personal communication).   The black regions depict known HSV-1 DNA fragments and the clear regions HSV-2 DNA fragments.   The hatched regions indicate DNA sequences in which a crossover has occurred.

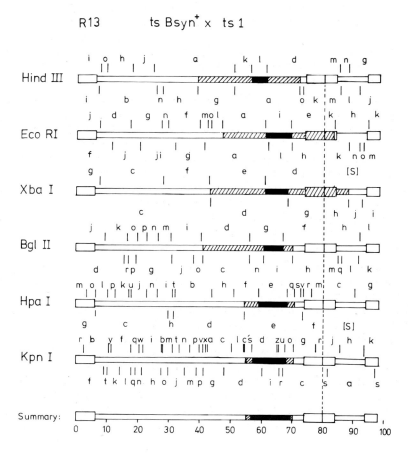

ts B mutation of HSV-1 must lie outside the minimum map co-ordinate region).   A large number of recombinants derived from different genetic crosses between HSV-1 and HSV-2 have been analysed by the six restriction endonucleases and the crossover points in some of those are shown later in Figure 7, for one orientation of the S and L regions.

It should be noted that all such restriction fragment analyses suffer from inherent drawbacks: (1) Double crossover events which span a short region of the map might go undetected at the level of sensitivity currently available.   For example, clone 15a (Timbury & Subak-Sharpe, 1973), derived from a cross between HSV-1 *ts* D and HSV-2 *ts* 1, has identical restriction endonuclease maps to the DNA of HSV-1, and could therefore be either a revertant of *ts* D or a recombinant with undetected crossovers.   (2) Crossovers might also occur which are independent of the selected events which remove the *ts* lesion.   In such cases more than one region is replaced but comparison of data from several independently obtained recombinants usually allows the relevant and irrelevant regions to be pinpointed.   (3) Recombinants can be isolated with crossovers unrelated to the sites of *ts* lesions: recombinant 3134 (*ts* B × *ts* 1), is still *ts* and therefore the insertion of HSV-2 DNA sequences around map position 42 need not be related to the lesion in *ts* B (HSV-1).

Notwithstanding the recognized drawbacks to recombinant analysis, the results show a consistent pattern.   Recombinants derived from crosses involving HSV-2 *ts* 1 (2Sa, 34NSd, 34Sd, 2444, 2853 and R13) all contain insertions of HSV-1 DNA sequences which overlap.   The overlap region lies between map positions 62 and 69 which we conclude must include the precise map location of the lesion in *ts* 1.   In the same way, maximum map co-ordinates for HSV-1 *ts* mutants A, D, F, H, K and S have been determined.   The map co-ordinates for these mutants lie within those determined by the marker rescue studies and therefore confirm and refine them.   Figure 8, given later, summarizes the combined data for the physical location of the mutants.

From the summary shown later in Figure 7, it can be seen that crossovers have been detected in every region of the genome, including the repetitive sequences bounding both the L and S regions.   Some recombinants exhibit heterozygosity for the TR_S and/or TR_L repetitive sequences (2Sa, 2853, 3135, B x 6 and RD2).   With the single exception of 2853, restriction fragment profiles show that all of the recombinant DNA samples have approximately equal amounts of the four major genome arrangements.   Thus such heterozygosity *per se* is no bar to genome rearrangement.   2853 appears to contain a high proportion of the orientation of L depicted in Figure 4, and therefore does not invert the L sequence at the same frequency as HSV-1, HSV-2 or the other recombinants.   These results will be analysed in detail elsewhere.

The HSV DNA structures shown in Figures 1, 2 and 4, and later
in Figures 7 and 8, all depict the same orientation of the L and S
regions of the genome.   As illustrated in Figure 5, the number of
apparent crossovers in some recombinants where one or both repeat
regions show heterozygosity could be affected by drawing the genomes
with inverted L and S regions.   This would be the case for 2Sa, 2853,
3145 and B x 6.   All of these recombinants show a minimum number of
apparent crossovers when drawn in the orientations of S and L shown
in Figure 4.   This orientation of L is also the one found to be the
most frequent in recombinant 2853.   While we do not wish to draw any
conclusions about the configuration of the DNA which actually participated in the original recombination events, we have decided to standard-
ize on this orientation of the genome throughout.

FIG. 5.   DIAGRAMATIC REPRESENTATION OF HOW INVERSIONS OF THE
L AND S SEGMENTS OF HSV DNA COULD AFFECT THE APPARENT NUMBER
OF CROSSOVERS IN RECOMBINANT GENOMES

It should be noted that there is yet another arrangement of the lower
model recombinant which would also show three apparent crossovers.

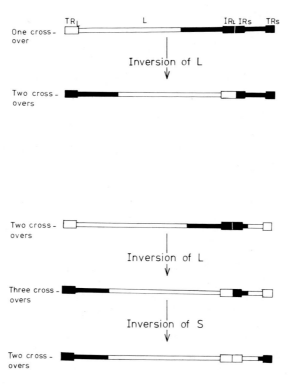

ANALYSIS OF POLYPEPTIDES SYNTHESIZED BY RECOMBINANTS

Comparative analyses of polypeptides induced in cells infected
with HSV-1 and HSV-2 show that, although the overall composition of
the polypeptide profiles in HSV-1 and HSV-2 infected cells is similar,
slight differences in the mobilities of individual proteins are
apparent, enabling them to be characterized as being from type 1 or
type 2 (Cassai et al., 1975; Halliburton et al., 1977).   Halliburton
et al. (1977) have exploited this observation to demonstrate type-
specific polypeptides as well as type-specific antigens encoded in
recombinants between type 1 and type 2.

By combining information about the type-specific composition of
polypeptides encoded by recombinants with information about the map
locations of type-specific DNA sequences in their genomes, it is
possible to infer the physical map location of the structural genes
coding for these polypeptides and/or genes which control the production or mobility of these peptides by some processing event.

Cells infected with recombinants or parental virus were labelled
with ^{35}S-methionine, ^{14}C-glucosamine or ^{32}P-orthophosphate and the
labelled proteins analysed on acrylamide gels under denaturing
conditions.   A virus-induced polypeptide with an apparent molecular
weight of X × 10^3 daltons is defined as V_{mw} X.   In some experiments
the immediate early (IE) polypeptides were analysed.   Immediate early
proteins are defined as those derived from mRNA which accumulates when
infection takes place in the presence of inhibitors of polypeptide
synthesis such as cycloheximide (Honess & Roizman, 1974; Rakusanova
et al., 1971).   When cycloheximide is removed, and translation
permitted in the presence of actinomycin D to block further RNA
synthesis, in the case of HSV-1 the production of four IE polypeptides
with estimated molecular wieghts of 175 000, 136 000, 110 000 and
63 000 (IE V_{mw} 175, 136, 100 and 63) is usually observed.   Additional
minor components are often seen.   IE V_{mw} 175, 110 and 63 probably
correspond to the polypeptides ICPα 4, 0 and 27 respectively, as described by Honess & Roizman (1974).

Figure 6 shows polypeptides of less than about 100 000 daltons,
synthesized in cells infected with 2Sa, 15Sa, 34NSd and 34Sd, the
parental viruses ts D (HSV-1) and ts 1 (HSV-2) and mock-infected cells.
Inspection of the polypeptides induced by 2Sa and 34Sd shows all to
be type 1 except for V_{mw} 22 and 21 which have been replaced by V_{mw}
20.5 and 20 from type 2.   Clone 15Sa is indistinguishable from HSV-1,
in agreement with the finding that its DNA structure is indistinguishable
from that of HSV-1 DNA.   Clone 34NSd also shows that recombinants can
induce polypeptides with mobilities which do not correspond to either
of the parental types.   (These altered bands are indicated with an
asterisk).

FIG. 6.   AUTORADIOGRAPH OF ^{35}S-METHIONINE-LABELLED POLYPEPTIDES

The polypeptides were separated by electrophoresis through a 5-12½% gradient of acrylamide under denaturing conditions, as described by Marsden et al. (1976).   The autoradiograph was cut to show only poly-peptides of less than approximately 100 000 daltons.   ■ HSV-1 poly-peptides; ○ HSV-2 polypeptides.

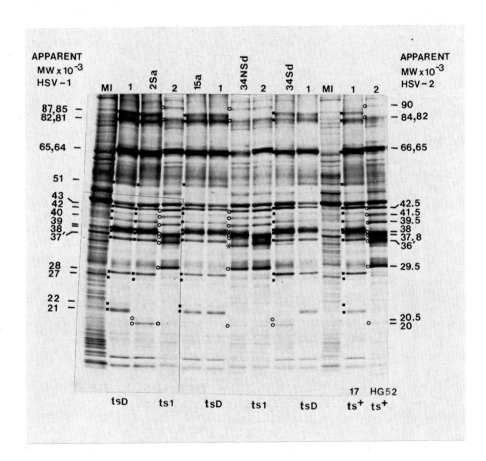

Figure 7, in addition to showing the crossover points of the recombinants, illustrates the method used to map polypeptides.   The example shown is for V_{mw} 21 (HSV-1) and the type 2 equivalent V_{mw} 20. Since clone RD2 contains an insertion of HSV-2 DNA with maximum map co-ordinates 92-96.5, it follows that the genetic information for some part of the V_{mw} 20 maps in this region.   The data from all the other recombinants are consistent with this interpretation.   It should be noted that the DNA sequences present between map co-ordinates 92-96.5 include part of TR$_S$ as well as the unique S sequence.

FIG. 7. SUMMARY OF THE GENOME STRUCTURES OF FIFTEEN
RECOMBINANTS AND AN ILLUSTRATION OF THE METHOD USED TO PHYSICALLY
MAP THE GENES CODING FOR POLYPEPTIDES

The genome structure is illustrated at the top of the figure.
Vertical dotted lines correspond to the ends of the long and short
repeat sequences.   The sequences in a recombinant derived from the
type 1 and type 2 parent are shown by a thick continuous horizontal
line superimposed on the upper and lower respectively of the two
horizontal dotted lines.   A crossover region is shown by two vertical
lines between the thick continuous horizontal lines.   The distance
apart of the two lines indicates the region of uncertainty of the
crossover event.   Where the uncertainty is small the crossover appears
as a single vertical line.   The units on the bottom are daltons $\times$ 10^{-3}.
The numbers (1 or 2) at the right-hand end of each recombinant genome
structure indicate that the recombinant induces V_{mw} 21 (HSV-1) or
V_{mw} 20 (HSV-2) respectively.   Thus the arrow indicates the maximum
map co-ordinates for the location of the gene coding for that polypeptide.   The bar indicates the map position for the polypeptide
(see text).

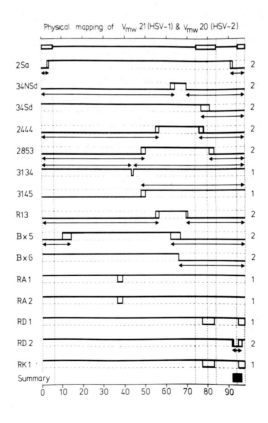

Although HSV-1 and HSV-2 polypeptides can be mapped independently, we assume as a working hypothesis that those which appear to be related on the basis of mobility on polyacrylamide gels will in fact be functionally equivalent.   Supportive evidence for equivalence of polypeptides comes from one or more of the following properties: (*a*) amount;   (*b*) kinetics of synthesis;   (*c*) behaviour in pulse-chase experiments;   (*d*) glycosylation: and (*e*) phosphorylation.   The assumption is probably valid in most cases since, except in certain situations which will be discussed in detail elsewhere, a recombinant virus induces either the type 1 or the type 2 protein but not both.

Figure 8 summarizes our present state of knowledge of the map co-ordinates of the immediate-early, glycosylated, phosphorylated and ^{35}S-methionine-labelled polypeptides.   In interpreting these data it should be borne in mind that the mobility of an individual polypeptide is a function of the molecular weight of the primary protein product and any subsequent modification by post-translation events such as cleavage, glycosylation, acetylation, sulfation or phosphorylation, etc.   The current mapping technique would not discriminate between these possibilities.   Even where the data map the structural gene, it cannot be taken for granted that the whole of the polypeptide is encoded within that region of recombinant DNA which leads to changes in mobility.

INTERPRETATION OF MAPPING DATA

Figure 8 gives the map co-ordinates derived for immediate-early glycosylated, phosphorylated and ^{35}S-methionine-labelled polypeptides, seven HSV-1 *ts* lesions, one HSV-2 *ts* lesion (*ts* 1) and the HSV-1 TK gene (derived from the data presented here and from that reported by Wigler et al., 1977).   Figure 8 also shows the map loci for immediate-early HSV-1 transcripts (Watson & Clements[1]) and the genetic map for the HSV-1 *ts* mutants as determined by three-factor crosses (Brown et al., 1973; Brown & Jamieson[2]).

The inherent drawbacks in the polypeptide mapping technique should be borne in mind when interpreting the protein mapping data.   Map locations for the immediate-early polypeptides were obtained as follows: (1) The data show that when the entire short region is transferred between HSV-1 and HSV-2 then IE V_{mw} 175 (HSV-1) and IE V_{mw} 182 (HSV-2) exchange also   Moreover crossovers within the short repeat (e.g., 2853, RD1, RD2, RK1) affect the mobility of IE V_{mw} 175 and 182 such that the resulting polypeptide can have mobility higher than, intermediate between or less than the parental types.   We

---

[1] Unpublished data

[2] See p. 33

FIG. 8. SUMMARY DIAGRAM OF THE PHYSICAL MAPPING DATA
PRESENTED IN THIS REPORT

The genetic map is derived from the published data of Brown et al.
(1973), Brown & Jamieson (see p.33) and the unpublished observations
of Dargan & Subak-Sharpe (personal communication).

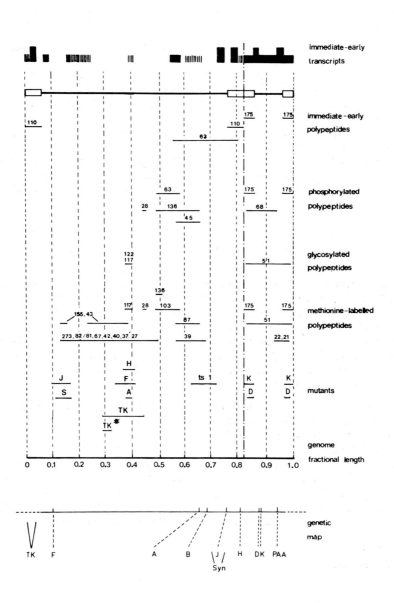

conclude that part of IE V_{mw} 175 probably maps within the short
repetition.   (2) The tentative map location for IE V_{mw} 110 was
obtained from the observation that recombinants completely heterozygous for the long repetition (e.g., 2853) induce both IE V_{mw} 110
(HSV-1) and the HSV-2 equivalent IE V_{mw} 118.   (3) The map location
for IE V_{mw} 63 was obtained in a manner analogous to that described
for V_{mw} 21.   These data show that immediate-early polypeptides are
coded for by both the long and short regions of the genome.

Both long and short regions of the genome also code for major
late polypeptides, e.g., V_{mw} 155 (L) and V_{mw} 21 (S), phosphoproteins,
e.g., P 136 (L) and P 175 (S), and glycoproteins, e.g., V_{mw} 117 (L)
and V_{mw} 51 (S).   We conclude that the functional organization of
the HSV genome does not restrict any of the four groups of polypeptides
examined here to either the long or the short region.

Figure 8 shows the map locations of eight HSV-1 mutants.   The
combined data from marker rescue experiments and from analysis of
intertypic recombinants unambiguously place ts D and ts K in the
inverted repetitive sequences bounding the S region of the genome.
These mutants appear to be in elements which affect the transcription of
the viral genome and the polypeptides induced in infected cells
(Marsden et al., 1976; Watson & Clements[1]).   The question then arises
as to whether there are one or two copies per genome of the sequences
affected by the D and K lesions.   The observations that both TR_S
and IR_S can rescue D and K (e.g., Fig. 1), and that the DNA from ts D
cannot rescue itself (Stow et al.[2]) tend to support two copies per
genome.   If this is so, the genesis of such mutants could be explained
either by independent mutations being produced in both copies (most
probably at different sites), or by subsequent intermolecular TR_S-IR_S
recombination to produce two (identical) mutant sequences following the
initial single mutagenic event in one sequence only.

Inspection of the physical map position of the HSV-1 mutants and
comparison with the genetic map reveals several interesting anomalies.
These can be briefly summarized as follows:

(1) The recombination frequencies do not reflect physical map
distances accurately: for example ts F, A and H map very close to one
another physically, but are separated by large distances on the genetic
map.   It is too soon to speculate whether or not this suggests the
presence of definable "hot spots" for recombination on the HSV genome.

(2) The order of markers in the L unique region may not be the
same in the genetic and physical maps: the close physical map locations of ts A, F and H make this analysis difficult since they behave
as one locus at the present level of resolution.   Physically the

---

[1] See p. 313

[2] Unpublished data

order is therefore (J), (TK), (AFH).   Genetically the order is
(dPyK^{-7}), (F), (A), (J), (H).   The positions of the TK gene and
of *ts* J are therefore critical.   The marker rescue data for dPyK^{-7}
did not resolve this locus from that of A, F and H.   However, Wigler
et al. (1977), on the basis of biochemical transformation experiments,
placed the wild-type structural gene for TK in a restriction endonuclease fragment which we know to map between the loci for *ts* J and
ts A, F and H.   The situation is somewhat unsatisfactory since we
have to assume equivalence between the TK locus as determined by biochemical transformation and that of the dPyK^{-7} lesion.   More detailed
resolution of the physical maps and mapping of further mutants will be
necessary to definitively interrelate the genetic and physical maps.

(3) *Ts* D and *ts* K can be arranged into a linear genetic map with
the other mutants: Mutants like D or K, which map in the repetitive
regions bounding the S unique sequences, would be expected to have
the same recombination frequency with all markers in the L unique
region, provided all four genome arrangements were infectious and
entered freely into intermolecular recombination events (Clements et
al., 1976; Skare & Summers, 1977; Subak-Sharpe & Timbury, 1977).
The ability to order *ts* D and *ts* K into a linear genetic map with
mutants which lie in the L unique region could therefore be interpreted as suggesting that all four major rearrangements of the
genome are not equally infectious.   Although we find that the
recombinant 2853 is at least partially "frozen" into the same
orientation of L which exhibits a minimum number of crossovers in
three other recombinants, we do not feel this is sufficient evidence
by itself to resolve the question.   The analysis of further recombinants between HSV-1 and HSV-2 will furnish the needed further data,
and it is clearly also essential to determine the physical arrangement of HSV DNA in the intracellular pools in which intermolecular
recombination occurs.

SUMMARY

A number of temperature-sensitive (*ts*) mutants and one pyrimidine
deoxyribonucleoside kinase-deficient mutant of herpes simplex virus
(HSV), have been located on the physical map of the genome by means
of marker rescue experiments and by the analysis of the crossover
points in intertypic recombinants between HSV types 1 and 2.   The
physical map is compared to the genetic map and certain anomalies
identified.   Analysis of infected-cell polypeptides specified by
intertypic recombinants has allowed tentative map co-ordinates to
be assigned to the structural genes (or genes which cause post-
translational modification) for many of the polypeptides.

Immediate-early, phosphorylated, glycosylated and structural as well
as non-structural polypeptides have been analysed in this way and it
can be concluded that there is no restriction of any of these groups
of polypeptides to either the long or the short regions of the
genome.   One of the recombinants, 2853, is at least partially
"frozen" in one orientation of the long region.   This orientation
is also the one which exhibits a minimum number of crossovers in three
other recombinants.

ACKNOWLEDGEMENTS

During the course of this work N.D. Stow was the recipient of
a Medical Research Council Grant for training in research
techniques, V. Preston a Commonwealth Scholarship, and
R. Cortini a long-term EMBO research fellowship.
N.M. Wilkie and H.S. Marsden are members of the
Medical Research Council Virology Unit.
The authors wish to thank G. Hope,
A. Davidson and M. Murphy for
their excellent technical
assistance.

REFERENCES

Benyesh-Melnick, M., Schaffer, P.A., Courtney, R.J., Esparza, J.
& Kimura, S. (1974)   Viral gene functions expressed and detected
by temperature-sensitive mutants of herpes simplex virus.
Cold Spring Harb. Symp. quant. Biol., *39*, 731-746

Brown, S.M., Ritchie, D.A. & Subak-Sharpe, J.H. (1973)   Genetic
studies with herpes simplex type 1: The isolation of temperature-
sensitive mutants, their arrangement into complementation groups
and recombination analysis leading to a linkage map.   *J. gen.
Virol.*, *18*, 329-346

Cassai, E.N., Sarmiento, M. & Spear, P.G. (1975)   Comparison of the
Virion Proteins specified by herpes simplex virus types 1 and 2.
J. Virol., *16*, 1327-1331

Clements, J.B., Cortini, R. & Wilkie, N.M. (1976)   Analysis of herpes-
    virus DNA substructure by means of restriction endonucleases.
    J. gen. Virol., *31*, 243-256

Clements, J.B., Watson, R.J. & Wilkie, N.M. (1977)   Temporal regula-
    tion of HSV type 1 transcription: Location of transcripts on the
    viral genome. *Cell*, *12*, 275-286

Cortini, R. & Wilkie, N.M. (1978)   Physical maps for HSV type 2 DNA
    with five restriction endonucleases. *J. gen. Virol.* (in press)

Esparza, J., Benyesh-Melnick, M. & Schaffer, P.A. (1976)   Intertypic
    complementation and recombination between temperature-sensitive
    mutants of herpes simplex virus types 1 and 2. *Virology*, *70*,
    372-384

Halliburton, I.W., Randall, R.E., Killington, R.A. & Watson, D.H.
    (1977)   Some properties of recombinants between type 1 and type
    2 herpes simplex viruses. *J. gen. Virol.*, *36*, 471-484

Honess, R.W. & Roizman, B. (1974)   Regulation of herpesvirus macro-
    molecular synthesis I Cascade regulation of the synthesis of
    three groups of viral proteins. *J. Virol.*, *14*, 8-19

Hutchison, C.A. III & Edgell, M.H. (1971)   Genetic assay for small
    fragments of bacteriophage ØX 174 deoxyribonucleic acid.   *J.
    Virol.*, *8*, 181-189

Jamieson, A.T. & Subak-Sharpe, J.H. (1978)   Interallelic complementa-
    tion of mutants of herpes simplex virus deficient in deoxypyrimi-
    dine kinase activity. *Virology* (in press)

Lai, C.-J. & Nathans, D. (1974)   Mapping temperature-sensitive
    mutants of simian virus 40: Rescue of mutants by fragments of
    viral DNA. *Virology*, *60*, 466-475

Lai, C.-J. & Nathans, D. (1975)   A map of temperature-sensitive
    mutants of simian virus 40. *Virology*, *66*, 70-81

Maitland, N.J. & McDougall, J.K. (1977)   Biochemical transformation
    of mouse cells by fragments of herpes simplex virus DNA. *Cell*,
    11, 233-241

Marsden, H.S., Crombie, I.K. & Subak-Sharpe, J.H. (1976)   Control
    of protein synthesis in herpesvirus-infected cells: Analysis of
    the polypeptides induced by wild type and sixteen temperature-
    sensitive mutants of HSV strain 17. *J. gen. Virol.*, *31*, 347-372

Miller, L.K. & Fried, M. (1976)   Construction of the genetic map of
    the polyoma genome. *J. Virol.*, *18*, 824-832

Rakusanova, T., Ben-Porat, T., Himeno, M. & Kaplan, A.S. (1971)
    Early functions of the genome of herpesvirus I.   Characterization
    of the RNA synthesized in cycloheximide-treated infected cells.
    Virology, *46*, 877-889

Schaffer, P.A., Tevethia, M.J. & Benyesh-Melnick, M. (1974) Recombination between temperature-sensitive mutants of herpes simplex virus type 1. *Virology, 58,* 219-228

Schildkraut, I., Cooper, G.M. & Greer, S. (1975)   Selective inhibition of the replication of herpes simplex virus by 5-halogenated analogues of deoxycytidine. *Molec. Pharmacol., 11,* 153-158

Skare, J. & Summers, W.C. (1977)   Structure and function of herpesvirus genomes.   II Eco RI, XbaI and Hind III endonuclease cleavage sites on herpes simplex virus type 1 DNA. *Virology, 76,* 581-595

Stow, N.D. & Wilkie, N.M. (1976)   An improved technique for obtaining enhanced infectivity with herpes simplex virus type 1 DNA. *J. gen. Virol., 33,* 447-458

Subak-Sharpe, J.H. & Timbury, M.C. (1977)   *Genetics of herpesviruses.* In: Fraenkel-Conrat, H. & Wagner, R.R., eds, *Comprehensive Virology,* vol. 9, New York, Plenum Press, pp. 89-131

Timbury, M.C. & Calder, L. (1976)   Temperature-sensitive mutants of herpes simplex virus type 2: A provisional linkage map based on recombination analysis. *J. gen. Virol., 30,* 179-186

Timbury, M.C. & Subak-Sharpe, J.H. (1973)   Genetic interactions between temperature-sensitive mutants of types 1 and 2 herpes simplex virus. *J. gen. Virol., 18,* 347-357

Weissbeek, P.J. Vereyken, J.M., Baas, P.D., Jansz, H.S. & Van Arkel, G. A. (1976)   The genetic map of bacteriophage ØX 174 constructed with restriction enzyme fragments. *Virology, 72,* 61-71

Wigler, M., Silverstein, S., Lee, L.-S., Pellicer, A., Cheng, Y.-C. & Axel, R. (1977)   Transfer of purified herpes virus thymidine kinase gene to cultured mouse cells. *Cell, 11,* 223-232

Wilkie, N.M. (1976)   Physical maps for herpes simplex virus type 1 DNA for restriction endonucleases Hind III, Hpa-I and Xba. *J. Virol., 20,* 222-233

Wilkie, N.M., Clements, J.B., Macnab, J.C.M. & Subak-Sharpe, J.H. (1974)   The structure and biological properties of herpes simplex virus DNA. *Cold Spring Harb. Symp. quant. Biol., 39,* 657-666

LOCATION OF NON-TEMPERATURE-SENSITIVE GENES ON THE GENETIC MAP OF HERPES SIMPLEX VIRUS TYPE 1

S.M. BROWN & A.T. JAMIESON

Medical Research Council Virology Unit,
Institute of Virology,
Glasgow, UK

INTRODUCTION

Conditional lethal mutants of the temperature-sensitive variety (*ts*) have proved to be useful tools in the construction of genetic maps of animal viruses. Recombination between two different mutants produces wild-type recombinants which can be easily selected from the total progeny virus from mixedly infected cells. This approach has been used to provide the genetic map of herpes simplex virus type 1 (HSV-1). The use of the plaque-morphology marker (*syn*) has permitted the construction of three-factor crosses, thus allowing more accuracy in the determination of recombination frequency and in the ordering of markers (Brown et al., 1973). By constructing crosses involving the genes coding for the enzyme deoxypyrimidine kinase and for resistance to the drug phosphonoacetic acid (PAA), it has been possible both to extend the genetic analysis of HSV-1 such that the eight possible progeny genotypes which arise from a three-factor cross can be identified and also to precisely locate the plaque-morphology marker.

METHODS

The wild-type (ts^+) and *ts* mutants of HSV-1 used were as described by Brown et al. (1973). Deoxypyrimidine-kinaseless mutants ($dPyK^-$) of HSV-1 have been selected for resistance to 1 mg/ml bromodeoxyuridine (BUDR) in thymidine-kinaseless cells (Jamieson et al., 1974). Phosphonoacetic acid-resistant virus (PAA^r) (Hay & Subak-Sharpe, 1976) was resistant to 200 µg/ml PAA. Cells, growth of virus, virus assay and recombination tests were as described by Brown et al. (1973).

Recombination analysis was by three-factor crosses of the type *ts* Y *syn*⁺ *PAA*ˢ × *ts*⁺ *syn Paa*ʳ or the reciprocal and *ts* Y *syn dPyK*⁺ × *ts*⁺ *syn*⁺ *dPyK*⁻. Figure 1A details the eight possible progeny classes which can arise from such a cross. The individual progeny can be identified by their growth properties at the permissive (31°C) and non-permissive temperatures (38°C) in the presence or absence of PAA (100 µg/ml) or in the presence or absence of 5'-bromo-2'-deoxycytidine (BrdC) (100 µg/ml). Progeny which arise from three-factor crosses of the type *PAA*ʳ *syn dPyK*⁺ × *PAA*ˢ *syn*⁺ *dPyK*⁻ can be distinguished by titrating the progeny in the presence and absence of both PAA and BrdC.

FIG. 1. RECOMBINATION ANALYSIS BY THREE-FACTOR CROSSES

Cross *ts* Y *syn*⁺ *PAA*ˢ × *ts*⁺ *syn PAA*ʳ

(A) *Progeny classes*

Progeny	Growth of progeny			
	31°C		38°C	
	- PAA	+ PAA (100 µg/ml)	- PAA	+ PAA
P1 *ts* Y *syn*⁺ *PAA*ˢ	+	-	-	-
P2 *ts*⁺ *syn PAA*ʳ	+	+	+	+
r1 *ts* Y *syn PAA*ʳ	+	+	-	-
r2 *ts*⁺ *syn*⁺ *PAA*ˢ	+	-	+	-
r3 *ts* Y *syn*⁺ *PAA*ʳ	+	+	-	-
r4 *ts*⁺ *syn PAA*ˢ	+	-	+	-
r5 *ts* Y *syn PAA*ˢ	+	-	-	-
r6 *ts*⁺ *syn*⁺ *PAA*ʳ	+	+	+	+

(B) *Progeny titres*

Plate	Plaque morphology	Progeny titre
38°C + PAA	*syn* *syn*⁺	P2 r6
38°C - PAA	*syn*⁺ *syn*	P2 + r4 r6 + r2
31°C + PAA	*syn*⁺ *syn*	P2 + r1 r6 + r3
31°C - PAA	*syn* *syn*⁺	P2 + r1 + r4 + r5 P1 + r6 + r2 + r3

(C) *Calculation of recombination frequencies*

$$RF \% \; ts - syn = \frac{r1 + r2 + r5 + r6}{r1 + r2 + r5 + r6 + r3 + r4 + P1 + P2} \times 100$$

$$RF \% \; syn - PAA^r = \frac{r3 + r4 + r5 + r6}{r1 + r2 + r3 + r4 + r5 + r6 + P1 + P2} \times 100$$

$$RF \% \; ts - PAA^r = \frac{r1 + r2 + r3 + r4}{r1 + r2 + r3 + r4 + r5 + r6 + P1 + P2} \times 100$$

By using the plaque-morphology marker, the amount of each single progeny genotype arising from a three-factor cross can be obtained (Fig. 1B). The recombination frequencies between the different markers are calculated as shown (Fig. 1C).

RESULTS

If a genetic cross of the type ts^+ syn PAA^r $\times$ ts Y syn^+ PAA^s is constructed, there are, as already mentioned, eight possible progeny genotypes. By using the procedure detailed in Figure 1, the titre of each resulting progeny class can be calculated. Using a number of different ts mutants, values of the recombination frequencies (RF) between these markers and the PAA^r gene have been obtained (Table 1).

Table 1. Values for recombination frequencies (RF) between different ts genes and the PAA^r gene

Parent 1	Parent 2	RF (%)		
		PAA^r/ts	ts/syn	PAA^r/syn
PAA^r syn ts^+	PAA^s syn^+ ts A	2.26 0.63	0.66 0.29	1.63 0.03
	PAA^s syn^+ ts B	0.85	0.68	0.79
	PAA^s syn^+ ts D	1.75 2.31	0.29 2.07	2.17 2.03
	PAA^s syn^+ ts F	16.0	10.2	5.3
	PAA^s syn^+ ts I	21.4 9.91	18.9 5.95	3.9 5.0
	PAA^s syn^+ ts J	11 7.42	2 2.4	9.0 6.7
PAA^r syn^+ ts^+	PAA^s syn ts D	0.36 0.46	0.14 0.085	0.22 0.37
	PAA^s syn ts E	12 1.34	0.33 0.04	10.0 1.3
	PAA^s syn ts I	7.2 14.8	3.9 11.6	3.7 3.3
	PAA^s syn ts J	1.72 3.3	1.28 0.34	2.74 2.9
	PAA^s syn ts H	5.0 1.38	0.3 0.22	5.1 1.45

A number of sets of data are given for each *ts* mutant.   The recombination frequency between any *ts* gene and the *PAA*[r] gene can vary. As the RF between the *ts* and the *syn* gene and the *syn* gene and the *PAA*[r] gene calculated from the same set of data also varies, it seems that this is due to a difference in the efficiency of overall recombination.   However, for any one *ts* mutant, the order of the three genes is consistent.   Similarly, using a number of *ts* mutants in a cross of the type *ts*[+] *syn*[+] *dPyK*- × *ts* Y *syn* *dPyK*[+], values for the recombination frequencies between different *ts* genes and the *dPyK* gene have been obtained (Table 2).   In this analysis, two different

Table 2. Values for recombination frequencies (RF) between different *ts* genes and the *dPyK* gene

Parent 1	Parent 2	RF (%)		
		dPyK/ts	*ts/syn*	*dPyK/syn*
dPyK-7 *syn*[+] *ts*[+]	*dPyK*[+] *syn* *ts* A	14.6	3.6	17
dPyK-MDK *syn*[+] *ts*[+]	*dPyK*[+] *syn* *ts* A	16.5	9.5	22
dPyK-7 *syn*[+] *ts*[+]	*dPyK*[+] *syn* *ts* E	12.6	3.0	15
dPyK-MDK *syn*[+] *ts*[+]	*dPyK*[+] *syn* *ts* E	8.4	7.2	12.6
dPyK-7 *syn*[+] *ts*[+]	*dPyK*[ts] *syn* *ts* D	11.3	1.0	10
dPyK-MDK *syn*[+] *ts*[+]	*dPyK*[ts] *syn* *ts* D	22.1	2.7	18.4
dPyK-7 *syn*[+] *ts*[+]	*dPyK*[+] *syn* *ts* I	14.0	3.6	14.6
dPyK-MDK *syn*[+] *ts*[+]	*dPyK*[+] *syn* *ts* I	11.7	3.4	16.0
dPyK-7 *syn*[+] *ts*[+]	*dPyK*[+] *syn* *ts* J	25.3	0.75	25.5
dPyK-MDK *syn*[+] *ts*[+]	*dPyK*[+] *syn* *ts* J	8.0	3.7	12.5
dPyK-7 *syn*[+] *ts*[+]	*dPyK*[+] *syn* *ts* H	22.4	0.44	22.2
dPyK-MDK *syn*[+] *ts*[+]	*dPyK*[+] *syn* *ts* H	34.0	0.22	34.0
dPyK-MDK *syn*[+] *ts*[+]	*dPyK*[+] *syn*[+] *ts* F	6.3	-	-
dPyK-MDK *syn*[+] *ts*[+]	*dPyK*[+] *syn* *ts* F	5.8	2.5	6.6

dPyK- mutants have been used, *dPyK*[-7] and *dPyK*[-MDK].   Although these were separately isolated, there is no difference in the way these mutants behave in genetic crosses.   Variability in recombination frequencies from experiment to experiment is again apparent, but the orders of magnitude are consistent.   With crosses involving both the *PAA*[r] marker and the *dPyK* marker it is possible to calculate the recombination frequencies between the *PAA* and *syn* genes, the *PAA* and *dPyK* genes, and the *syn* and *dPyK* genes.   Recombination values obtained from such a cross were: RF, *PAA-syn* = 9.2%; RF, *dPyK-syn* = 22%;   and RF, *PAA-dPyK* = 35%.

From these data, a linkage map has been constructed which includes the *ts* genes, the *dPyK* gene, the *PAA*[r] gene and the *syn* gene.   Because of the closeness of the *PAA*[r] gene to the *ts* D gene, it is not possible to determine unambiguously on which side of *tsD* the *PAA* gene lies. However, taking the data as a whole, we feel justified in placing *PAA*[r] to the right of *tsD*.   Similarly, it seems reasonable to place the *dPyK* gene slightly to the left of *ts* F.   The average distance between *PAA* and *syn* is 3.4% and between *dPyK* and *syn* is 15.7% (Fig. 2).   Throughout, *ts* X *syn* × *ts* Y *syn*[+] crosses and reciprocals have been used as internal controls.

FIG. 2. LINKAGE MAP OF HSV-1

The map shows the positions of various *ts* genes, the plaque morphology gene *syn*, the gene for thymidine kinase (*dPyK*) and the gene for resistance to phosphonoacetic acid (*PAA*).

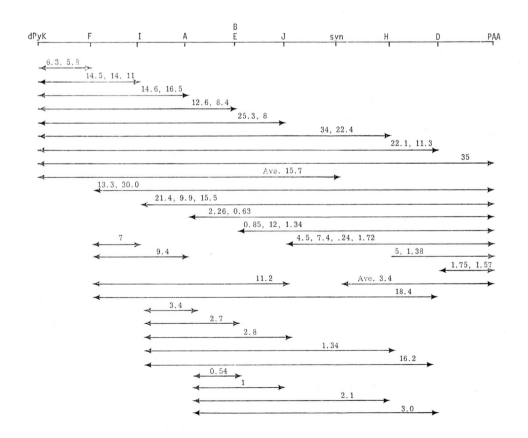

DISCUSSION

This study provides the first detailed analysis of all the
different progeny types arising from three-factor genetic crosses
involving herpes simplex virus.   Thus, not only is it possible to
calculate three recombination frequencies from one genetic cross, but
also for the first time, the plaque-morphology marker can be precisely
located on the genetic map.   Location of the enzyme markers PAA^r and
$dPyK$, which are taken to be the genes coding for the HSV-1 specified
DNA-dependent DNA polymerase and deoxypyrimidine kinase, on the genetic
map of HSV-1 expands the original ts linkage map to cover a total of
35 recombination units, such that any markers lying outside those
present on the genetic map may well appear to be essentially unlinked.

SUMMARY

By constructing crosses involving the genes coding for the enzyme
deoxypyrimidine kinase and for resistance to the drug phosphonoacetic
acid, it has been possible both to extend the genetic analysis of
HSV-1 such that the eight possible progeny genotypes which arise from
a three-factor cross can be identified and also to precisely locate
the gene for the plaque-morphology marker syn, the gene for deoxypyrimidine kinase $dPyK$ and the gene for resistance to phosphonoacetic
acid PAA^r.

REFERENCES

Brown, S.M., Ritchie, D.A. & Subak-Sharpe, J.H. (1973)   Genetic
    studies with herpes simplex virus type 1. The isolation of
    temperature-sensitive mutants, their arrangement into complementa-
    tion groups and recombination analysis leading to a linkage map.
    J. gen. Virol., *18*, 329-346

Hay, J. & Subak-Sharpe, J.H. (1976)   Mutants of herpes simplex virus
    types 1 and 2 that are resistant to phosphonoacetic acid induce
    altered DNA polymerase activities in infected cells.   *J. gen.*
    Virol., *31*, 145-148

Jamieson, A.T., Gentry, G.A. & Subak-Sharpe, J.H. (1974)   Induction
    of both thymidine and deoxycytidine kinase activity by herpes
    virus.   *J. gen. Virol.*, *24*, 465-480

THE USE OF INTERTYPIC RECOMBINANTS FOR ANALYSIS OF GENE ORGANIZATION IN HERPES SIMPLEX VIRUS

L.S. MORSE, L. PEREIRA & B. ROIZMAN

Marjorie B. Kovler Viral Oncology Laboratories,
University of Chicago,
Chicago, Ill., USA

P.A. SCHAFFER

Sidney Farber Cancer Institute,
Harvard Medical School,
Boston, Mass., USA

OBJECTIVE

The purpose of these studies was two-fold. The first was to take advantage of the lack of correspondence of herpes simplex virus type 1 and type 2 (HSV-1, HSV-2) restriction endonuclease cleavage sites and of the differences in the electrophoretic mobility of HSV-1 and HSV-2 specific polypeptides to map the location of templates specifying the polypeptides on the HSV genome by analysing HSV-1 × HSV-2 recombinants. This technique has been used in an elegant manner to map adenovirus temperature-sensitive (*ts*) mutations and the templates specifying polypeptides on the physical map of the DNA (Grodzicker et al., 1974; Mautner et al., 1975). The second objective was to determine whether all four arrangements of HSV DNA participate in the generation of recombinants. The formation of recombinants was predicted by the observation that HSV-1 and HSV-2 DNA share at least 47% DNA homology with good matching of base pairs (Kieff et al., 1972). In addition, HSV-1 and HSV-2 *ts* mutants have been shown genetically to complement efficiently and form recombinants (Benyesh-Melnick et al., 1974; Esparaza et al., 1976; Schaffer, 1975).

Previous reports from this laboratory have shown that HSV-1 and HSV-2 DNAs are linear double-stranded molecules of approximately $97-99 \times 10^6$ in molecular weight (Kieff et al., 1971). HSV-1 DNA consists of two covalently linked components, L and S, containing 82 and 18% of DNA, respectively. The terminal reiterated sequence bracketing the L component, designated ab and its inverted terminal repeat $b'a'$, each contain 6.0% of the DNA whereas the set of sequences bracketing the S component, designated $a'c'$ and ac each contain 4.3% of the viral DNA (Roizman et al., 1975; Wadsworth et al., 1975). DNA extracted from virions or from infected cells consists of four equimolar populations differing in the orientation of L and S components (Hayward et al., 1975; Roizman et al., 1975). Studies of HSV-2 DNA with restriction endonucleases indicate that it has a similar structure (Hayward et al.[1]).

Pertinent to the analysis of HSV polypeptides is the observation that HSV-1 specifies in infected cells at least 48 polypeptides ranging from 20 000 to greater than 200 000 in molecular weight (Honess & Roizman, 1973). Several additional polypeptides less than 20 000 in molecular weight were reported by Marsden et al. (1976). A similar list of HSV-2 polypeptides was reported by Powell & Courtney (1975). Studies by Courtney & Powell (1975), Pereira et al. (1977), Gibson & Roizman (1972) and by Cassai et al. (1975) showed that many HSV-1 and HSV-2 virion polypeptides and infected-cell polypeptides (ICP) differ in electrophoretic mobility but only a few of these polypeptides were identified as functionally identical.

The identification of polypeptides specified by the recombinants was facilitated by the fact that the synthesis of HSV polypeptides is regulated. Specifically, on the basis of the temporal pattern and requirements for their synthesis, HSV-1 ICPs were shown to form at least three groups designated as α, β, and γ whose synthesis is coordinately regulated and sequentially ordered in a cascade fashion (Honess & Roizman, 1974, 1975; Roizman et al., 1974, 1975).

FUNCTIONAL SIGNIFICANCE OF RECOMBINANT DNA ARRANGEMENT

The DNA sequence arrangement of the 26 recombinant DNAs analysed with five restriction endonucleases is summarized in Figure 1 (Morse et al., 1977). The functional significance of the structure of the recombinant DNAs stems from the following considerations:

(i) Recombinants with heterologous L and S components or with heterologous portions of the inverted repeats (e.g., D1E1, A1E2, A2D, A4D, and D5E2) are viable.

---

[1] Unpublished data

FIG. 1. PROVENANCE OF THE DNA SEQUENCES
IN THE INTERTYPIC RECOMBINANTS

The upper and lower line of each doublet represent HSV-1 and HSV-2
DNA respectively.   The heavy line identifies the DNA sequences present
in the recombinant virus.   The diagonal line spans the boundaries of
the crossover sites as defined by the five restriction endonucleases.
Hatch marks at or near the diagonal lines identify critical endonuclease cleavage sites which define the boundaries of the crossover
event.   The hatch marks with a knob identify the restriction sites
retained in recombinant DNA, whereas those without knobs represent
parental cleavage sites that are absent in the recombinant DNA.   The
boxes on the map unit line represent the reiterated sequences of L and
S components of HSV DNA.

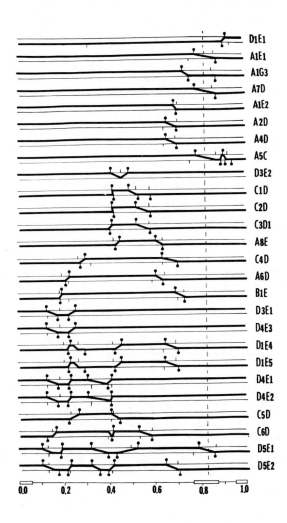

(ii) The linear order of the genes of HSV-1 and HSV-2 essential for the replication of the virus must be at least grossly identical and functionally equivalent. By this we mean that the genes contained in the transposed region of the DNA must specify the same functions as those in the replaced region. This became apparent with the observation that wide and extensive interchange of genomic regions in and between the L and S components can occur. However, without additional analysis of the large transposed regions, we cannot be certain that the order of the genes is actually identical in all functionally homologous HSV-1 and HSV-2 regions.

(iii) The structure of recombinant DNAs suggests that one or at most two arrangements of HSV DNA are replicated. Pertinent to the discussion on this point which will follow is the observation that all recombinants could be drawn in a single arrangement of the DNA which displays the minimum number of crossover events. If those recombinants containing an odd number of crossover events were displayed in the arrangement whereby the L component was inverted from that shown in Figure 1, the consequence would be to increase the number of crossovers by 1. Assuming that the least number of crossovers is most likely in the generation of intertypic recombinants, the central question we wish to pose, is whether all arrangements of HSV-1 DNAs could have participated in the generation of recombinants observed in this study. Our arguments are illustrated in Figure 2.

Let us assume that the parental types have one marker in the L and S components respectively, and that selection against the markers yields a recombinant generated by single crossover events in the L component. As Figure 2 illustrates, if the recombinant event occurs in all arrangements of HSV-1 and HSV-2 DNAs and if all these recombinants are then replicated, the display of the resulting recombinants in the P arrangement should show a single crossover event in the P and I_S arrangement and a double crossover event if recombination occurred in the L_L and I_{SL} arrangement. This diagram further illustrates that recombinants formed from an even number of multiple crossover events are indistinguishable if drawn in the P arrangement.

This argument can be extended to any number of crossover events provided that they are odd in number. In principle, the argument predicts that, if recombination occurs in all four arrangements, then there should be no single arrangement of recombinant DNA showing an odd number of crossover events. As mentioned earlier, all recombinants could be shown in one arrangement of the DNA which displays the minimal number of crossover events. Analysis of the recombinants obtained so far indicates that they fall into two classes. The majority have an even number of recombinational events and neither support nor contradict our argument. The others show an odd number and all fall into one arrangement. The arrangement common to all is the P arrangement in which we have chosen to display our data.

FIG. 2. PREDICTED RECOMBINANT DNA STRUCTURE GENERATED BY SELECTION AGAINST MARKERS IN THE L AND S COMPONENTS

The diagram illustrates the predicted recombinant DNA structure for single or double crossover events generated if all arrangements of HSV-1 and HSV-2 DNAs could have participated in the recombinational event.   The X present in either the L or S components of parental DNAs indicates the position of the hypothetical markers.   The solid lines represent a portion of DNA unique to one parent, whereas the broken lines designate the DNA sequences of the second parent.

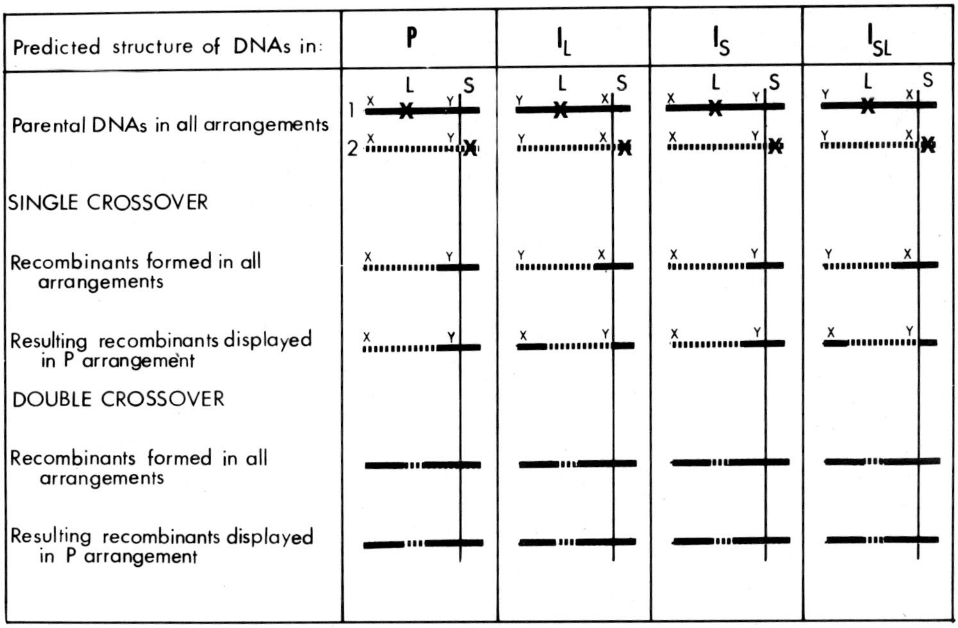

Predicted structure of DNAs in:	P	I_L	I_S	I_{SL}
Parental DNAs in all arrangements				
SINGLE CROSSOVER				
Recombinants formed in all arrangements				
Resulting recombinants displayed in P arrangement				
DOUBLE CROSSOVER				
Recombinants formed in all arrangements				
Resulting recombinants displayed in P arrangement				

These data suggest, then, that there exists a unique orientation of L with respect to S and support the hypothesis that one or at most two arrangements of HSV DNA are replicated.   These arrangements correspond to the P and I_S arrangement.   The data also suggest that the rearrangements of HSV DNA occur during an obligatory post-synthesis repair event of unit length DNA for the simplistic reason that a non-obligatory event could not account for the equimolar concentrations of the four arrangements of DNA (Jacob & Roizman, 1977; Jacob et al.[1]).

MAPPING OF HSV POLYPEPTIDES

The identification of the corresponding HSV-1 and HSV-2 poly-peptides was based on analysis of ICPs specified by the recombinants and rested on two criteria. First, with one exception to be discussed below, the presence in the cell lysate of a polypeptide specified by one serotype excluded the presence of the other. Second, each ICP specified by HSV-1 or HSV-2 could be mapped inde-pendently as either present or absent, and in each instance the corresponding ICPs mapped in the same location.

The HSV-1 and HSV-2 genes that were amenable to mapping by the procedures employed in this study are those that differ in apparent molecular weight of their product. The genes whose products do not differ in apparent molecular weight or in immunological specificity, will have to be mapped by other procedures.

In principle, by correlating the segregation patterns of the polypeptides specified by the recombinant viruses with the DNA sequence arrangement of the recombinants, it has been possible to map the physical location of the templates specifying viral poly-peptides on the HSV genome. The experimental procedure utilized was designed to take advantage of the temporal expression of HSV-1 and HSV-2 polypeptides. Accordingly, cells infected with parental strains, or with recombinants, were pulse-labelled at three time intervals after infection as described in the legends to Figures 3 to 5. The mapping of the template specifying ICP 5 illustrates the mapping procedure. Thus, examination of the ICP 5 specified by recombinants C4D and A6D (Fig. 5, Table 1) indicates that the template (Fig. 1) is to the left of the left crossover site of C4D (0.30 map units) but to the right of the left crossover site of A6D (0.22 map units). The map position of the ICP 5 template is more precisely defined by the crucial recombinants D1E4 and D1E5, each of which specifies an ICP 5 with an electrophoretic mobility inter-mediate between those of HSV-1 and HSV-2 (Fig. 5). This suggests the possibility of an intragenic recombination event. Comparison with the ICP 5 specified by D4E1, D4E3 and C5D indicates that the left boundary of the template for ICP 5 does not extend to the left beyond 0.23 map units, which indicates that the right crossover site of D1E4 and D1E5 is most likely responsible for the aberrant electro-phoretic properties of ICP 5 produced by these recombinants.

---

[1] Unpublished data

FIG. 3. AUTORADIOGRAPHIC IMAGES OF ELECTROPHORETICALLY SEPARATED
POLYPEPTIDES LABELLED WITH ^{14}C-ISOLEUCINE, LEUCINE, AND VALINE IN
HEp-2 CELLS INFECTED WITH SERIES D INTERTYPIC RECOMBINANTS FOR
1-3 HOURS POST INFECTION AT 39°C

Parental strains for series D intertypic recombinants were HSV-1
(KOS *tsE6*) and HSV-1 (186 *tsB5*).   The conditions for polyacrylamide
gel electrophoresis and sample preparation were as previously described
(Heine et al., 1974; Spear & Roizman, 1972) except that we used
20 cm separation gels in this study.

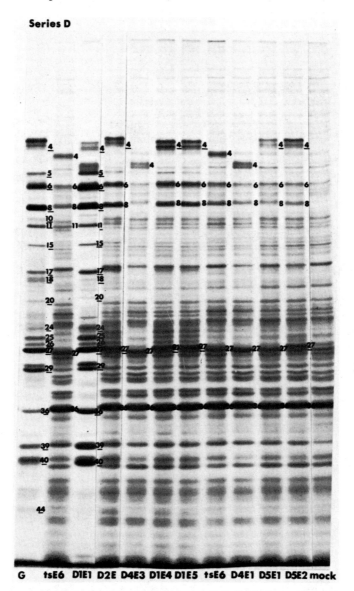

FIG. 4. AUTORADIOGRAPHIC IMAGES OF ELECTROPHORETICALLY SEPARATED
POLYPEPTIDES LABELLED IN HEp-2 CELLS INFECTED WITH SERIES C INTER-
TYPIC RECOMBINANTS FROM 1 TO 3 HOURS POST INFECTION AT 39°C

Parental strains for series C intertypic recombinants were HSV-1
(HFEM *ts* $N10_2$) and HSV-2 (186).

Series C

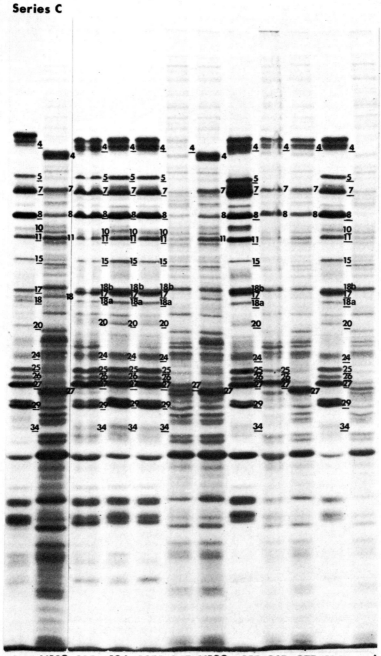

G   N102 C2D   186 C3D1 C4D N102   C5D C6D C7D 186 mock

FIG. 5. AUTORADIOGRAPHIC IMAGES OF ELECTROPHORETICALLY SEPARATED
POLYPEPTIDES LABELLED IN HEp-2 CELLS INFECTED WITH SERIES D INTER-
TYPIC RECOMBINANTS FROM 9 TO 10 HOURS POST INFECTION AT 34°C

Parental strains for series D intertypic recombinants were HSV-1
(KOS *tsE6*) and HSV-1 (186 *tsB5*).

Series D

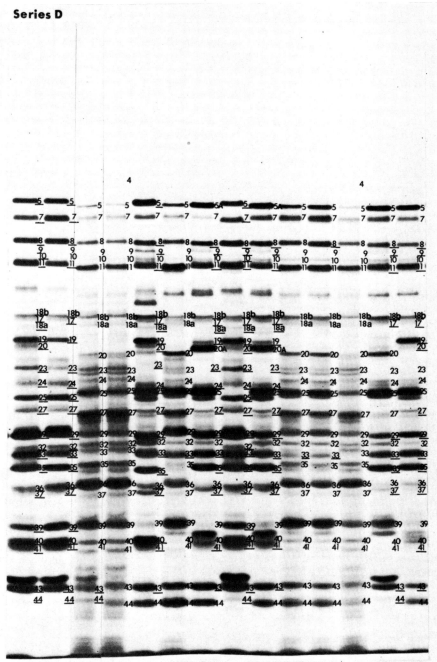

tsB5 D1E1 D3E2 tsE6 A8E D4E3 D1E4 tsB5 D1E5 D4E1 D4E2 tsE6 D5E1 D5E2

Table 1. HSV-1 and HSV-2 infected-cell polypeptides[a]

Recombinant designation	2	4	5	7	8	9	10	11	15	18	19	20	23	24	25	27	29	32	33	35	36	39	40	41	43	44
D1E1	2	1.2	2	2	2	2	2	2	2	2	2	2	2	2	2	2	2	2	2	2	2	2	2	2	2	2
A1E1	1	2	1	1	1	1	1	1	1	1	1	1	1	1	1	1	2	2	1	1	1	1	1	1	1	1
A1G3	1	2	1	1	1	1	1	1	1	1	1	1	1	1	1	2	2	1	1	1	1	1	1	1	1	1
A7D	1	2	1	1	1	1	1	2*	1	1	1	1	1	1	1	1	2	1	1	A	1	1	1	1	1	1
A1E2	1	2	1	1	1	1	1	1	1	1	1	1	1	1	1	2	2	1	1	1	1	1	1	1	1	1
A2D	1	2	1	1	1	2*	1	1	1	1	1	1	1	1	1	2	2	1	1	1	1	2*	1	2*	1	1
A4D	1	2	1	1	1	1	1	1	1	1	2	A	1	1	1	2	2	1	1	1	1	1	1	1	1	1
A5C	1	2	1	1	1	1	1	1	1	1	1	1	1	1	1	2	1	1	1	1	1	1	1	1	1	1
D3E2	1	1	1	1	1	1	1	1	1	1	1	1	1	1	1	1	1	1	1	1	1	1	1	1	2	2
C1D	2	2	2	2	2	2	2	2	2	2	2	2	2	2	2	2	2	2	2	2	2	2	2	2	1	1
C2D	2	2	2	2	2	2	2	2	2	2	2	2	2	2	2	2	1	2	2	2	2	2	2	2	1	1
C3D1	2	2	2	2	2	2	2	2	2	2	2	2	2	2	2	2	1	2	2	2	2	2	2	2	1	1
A8E	1	2	2	1	2	2	2	2	2A	2	2	2	2	2	2	2	2	1	2	2	2	2	2	2	2	1
C4D	1	2	2	1	1	2A	1	1	2	2	2	2	2	1	1	2	2	A	2	1	1	2	2	2	1	1
A6D	1	2	1	1	1	2	1	1	1	2	2	2	2	1	1	2	2	1	2	1	1	1A	1	2	1	1
B1E	1	2	1	1	1	2	1	1	1	2	2	1	1	1	1	2	2	1	2	1	1	1	1	2	1	1
D3E1	1	1	1	1	1	1	1	1	1	1	1	1	1	1	1	1	1	1	2	1	1	1	1	1	1	1
D4E3	1	1	1	1	1	1	1	1	1	1	1	1	1	1	1	1	1	1	2	1	1	1	1	1	1	1
D1E4	1	2	A	1	2	2	1	2	2A	2	2	2	2	1	2	2	1	2	2	2	2	A	1	2	2	1
D1E5	1	2	A	1	2	2	1	2	2A	2	2	2	2	1	2	2	1	2	2	2	2	A	1	2	2	1
D4E1	1	1	1	1	1	1	1	1	1	1	1	1	1	1	1	1	1	1	2A	1	1	1	1	1	1	1
D4E2	1	1	1	1	2	1	1	1	1	1	1	1	1	1	1	1	1	1	2A	1	1	1	1	1	1	1
C5D	1	2	1	2	1	2	1	1	1	1	2	2	1	2	2	2	1	1	1	1	2	2	2	2	2	2
C6D	1	2	1	2	1	2	1	1	1	1	2	2	1	2	2	2	1	1	1	1	1	1	1	1	1	1
D5E1	1	2	1	1	2	2	1	2	1	2	1	1	1	1	1	2	2	1	2	2	1	1	1	1*	2	2
D5E2	1	2	1	1	2	2	1	2	1	2	2	2	1	1	2	2	1	2	2	1	1	1A	2	1	1	1

[a] Identification of infected-cell polypeptides specified by series A, B, C and D intertypic recombinants. Polypeptides identified as HSV-1 are labelled as 1 while those of HSV-2 are labelled as 2. The asterisk identifies the few instances in which the polypeptides produced by the cells infected with the recombinants did not co-segregate with the DNA sequences predicted by other recombinants. The letter A denotes polypeptides with an aberrant electrophoretic mobility.

The map position of the template for ICP 5 was thus determined to be between 0.23 and 0.30 map units. The DNA sequence arrangements and the ICP 5 specified by all other recombinants are consistent with this conclusion.

The segregation patterns of the polypeptides mapped in this study are summarized in Table 1. The table identifies two sets of inconsistencies. The first, identified with an asterisk, comprises a few instances in which the polypeptides produced by the cells infected with the recombinants did not co-segregate with the DNA sequences predicted by other recombinants. Possible explanations for these inconsistencies are: (i) intragenic recombination events resulting in a recombinant gene specifying a polypeptide with an electrophoretic mobility characteristic of one of the parental types; (ii) DNA heteroduplex mismatch repair; and (iii) undetected double crossover events in regions of the DNA lacking restriction enzyme sites. Analysis of Figure 1 shows that small double crossovers have occurred in several recombinants (Morse et al., 1977) and were detected only because they bracketed a restriction enzyme cleavage site. The second type of inconsistency, identified with the letter A, denotes polypeptides with an aberrant electrophoretic mobility. In some instances (e.g., ICP 5 of D1E4 and D1E5), the electrophoretic mobility was intermediate

between those of the parental types.   In other instances, the polypeptide migrated faster than the corresponding parental polypeptides.

Using the approach described above, the linear map positions of
26 HSV polypeptides are summarized in Figure 6.   No polypeptides
were mapped in map positions 0.10 and only one polypeptide was unambiguously shown to arise from a template in the S component.
Figure 6 also shows that the locations of some polypeptides are quite
broad and may have to be refined by other techniques.   The map positions of two polypeptides of special interest are elaborated upon
below.

FIG. 6.   LOCATION OF TEMPLATES SPECIFYING HSV MARKERS
AND POLYPEPTIDES DETERMINED FROM AN ANALYSIS
OF HSV-1 × HSV-2 RECOMBINANTS

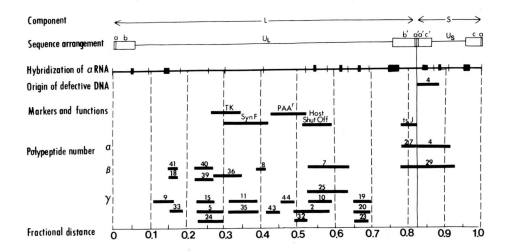

ICP 4

Analysis of the segregation pattern of ICP 4 shows the following:

(i) The template specifying the synthesis of ICP 4 must lie to
the right of 0.787 map units and is located in the S component.   This
became clear from recombinants A1E1, A7D, A5C, and D1E1, all of which
specified the HSV-2 ICP 4.

(ii) The template specifying the synthesis of ICP 4 may be located
partially within the reiterated DNA sequences and therefore a portion

of this template would be duplicated.   This suggestion was supported
by the observation that one recombinant specified both the fully
processed HSV-2 ICP 4 (4c) and the unprocessed HSV-1 ICP (4a).

(iii) Some recombinants (D4E1, D4E2, D4E3, D1E1) aberrantly processed the HSV-1 ICP 4 yet were still viable.   This conclusion became
apparent from the observation that, even under the three different
labelling intervals used for analysing HSV ICP 4, no ICP 4b or 4c was
detected.   While this does not imply that no processing of ICP 4
occurred, it does suggest that only a small amount is required and
that processing must be a viral specified event.

Several observations bear upon the mapping of ICP 4.   A more
precise localization of the template for ICP 4 in the parental DNAs
hinges on the interpretation of the observation that D1E1 (Fig. 3)
specifies both the fully processed form of HSV-2 ICP 4 (4c) and the
unprocessed form of HSV-1 ICP 4 (4a).   In this recombinant, the only
detected HSV-1 sequences were located between map positions 0.93-1.0
indicating that the template for HSV-1 ICP 4 is in the S component and
by extension, that the template for HSV-2 ICP 4 must also be in the S
component.   It would follow, therefore, that in D1E1, HSV-1 ICP 4
maps between 0.93 and 1.000 and HSV-2 ICP 4 maps between 0.83 and 0193.
The map position of HSV-1 ICP 4 determined from analysis of D1E1 is
shown in Figure 6.   There is evidence, however, that the HSV-1 DNA
is diploid for the ICP 4 gene and that D1E1 is an example of a hetero-
ploid recombinant.   This conclusion emerges from the observation that
recombinants formed between intact HSV-1 DNA and the *Xba*I fragment I
of HSV-2 DNA also specify both HSV-1 and HSV-2 ICP 4.   In these
recombinants, the HSV-2 sequences are in map positions 0.945-1.000 and
are therefore reciprocal to those of the D1E1 recombinant (Knipe et
al.[1]).

Several other studies bear upon the mapping of ICP 4.   Specifically,
although viral RNA extracted from polyribosomes primed for synthesis of
α polypeptides hybridizes to restriction endonuclease fragments of the S
component, the amount of reiterated sequences represented in this RNA
was too small (by a factor of two) to contain the entire ICP 4 template.
However, the sum of the sequences in the reiterated and unique sequences
that are represented in the α RNA could contain the ICP 4 template
(Jones et al., 1977).   Additional evidence supporting the second
hypothesis derives from studies on defective virus generated by serial
passage of HSV-1 (Justin).   Cells infected with certain populations
containing defective particles overproduce ICP 4.   The defective DNA
was shown to consist of a reiterated segment arising from the $a'c'$ and
unique sequences of S located between map positions of 0.93 and 1.0 in
the arrangement of HSV DNA shown in Figure 6 (Frenkel et al., 1975,
1976).   Analyses of the sequences of the defective DNA that hybridize

---

[1] Unpublished data

with α RNA (Frenkel & Locker[1]) also show that the amounts of reiterated *ac* sequences of the S component represented in α RNA are not sufficient to specify ICP 4.   Thus, although the evidence clearly indicates that HSV is at least partially diploid for the ICP 4 gene, we cannot at this time determine whether the putative remainder of the ICP 4 gene extends into the unique sequences of S or into the L component.

ICP 27

Analysis of the segregation pattern of ICP 27 permitted the following conclusions:

(i) Our data place ICP 27 within the reiterated sequence *ab* of the L component.

(ii) Recombinants containing heterologous *ab* sequences (e.g., A1G3, A2D, A4D, A1E2, D5E2) do not produce both HSV-1 and HSV-2 ICP 27.

(iii) DNA sequences arising from the region containing the templates for the polypeptide ICP 27 are represented in αRNA, as shown by Jones et al. (1977).

The data supporting the location of the template for ICP 27 are summarized below.

Because A7D, A5C, D5E1, D4E1 and D4E2 all specified ICP 27 of HSV-1 (Table 1), and because the right crossover site in A7D and A5C near the L-S junction had to be to the left of 0.84 map units as determined by *Kpn*I digestion (Morse et al., 1977), the template specifying this polypeptide most likely maps within the L component of the DNA.   By similar reasoning, analyses of recombinants A1E1, A5C, A7D, A1G3 and A2D suggest that ICP 27 maps at the right-hand end of the L component between 0.787 and 0.83 map units.   In support of this location for the template specifying ICP 27 is the observation that the parental strains used to construct the recombinants in series A were a phosphonoacetate-resistant (PAA[r]) mutant of HSV-1 (Honess & Watson, 1974) *ts J* and wild-type HSV-2 (GP6) and that selection was for PAA[r] *ts*[+] progeny.   From those experiments, we previously concluded that *ts J* maps between 0.78 and 0.84 map units (Morse et al., 1977). Marker rescue experiments (Knipe et al.[2]) showed that the temperature-sensitive lesion of *ts J* is located between map positions 0.70 and 0.83 and that therefore the selection is consistent with a requirement for the replacement of HSV-1 sequences with HSV-2 sequences in the L component.

---

[1] Personal communication

[2] Unpublished data

PRESENCE OF GENE TEMPLATES IN REITERATED SEQUENCES OF VIRAL DNA

As indicated above, ICP 27 maps entirely within the $b'a'$ region of
the DNA whereas ICP 4 maps at least in part in the reiterated $a'c'$ and
ac sequence of the S component (Fig. 6).   These observations would
indicate that HSV is diploid for ICP 27 and at least partially diploid
for ICP 4.   However, whereas ICP 4 heteroploidy was readily demonstrable in recombinants with heterotypic ac sequences (e.g., D1E1), it
was not demonstrable for ICP 27 in recombinants with heterotypic ab
sequences (A1G3, A1E2, A2D, A4D, D5E2).

At least two hypothesis could explain the absence of heterotypic
ICP 27.   The first is that the ICP 27 template in the left end of
the L component lacks a promoter site and is not transcribed.   It
should be noted that, if the promoter for transcription of ICP 27 were
in S, then both the right and left templates of ICP 27 would be transcribed off the P and I_L arrangements of HSV DNA, respectively.

The second hypothesis would require that the terminal sequences of
the L and S components be identical but inverted and that the ICP 27
gene lies entirely within such sequences whereas the ICP 4 gene does not.
This hypothesis would be correct if, as we suspect, the inversions of L
and S components relative to each other arise as a consequence of an
obligatory post-synthesis event in which the terminal ab and ac sequences
are regenerated using the reiterated $b'a'a'c'$ junction as a template.
In order to evaluate this hypothesis, we reexamined the data indicating
that the recombinants A1G3, A1E2, A4D and D5E2 have heterotypic ab regions.
The conclusions are based on analyses of the DNAs of recombinant viruses
with the restriction endonuclease HpaI which cleaves HSV-1 DNA within the
ab sequences at map positions 0.037 and 0.787.   The ICP 27 template was
mapped between map positions 0.787 and 0.83.   Since we have no restriction enzyme cleavage sites in the ab sequences between 0.000 and 0.037
and 0.787 and 0.83, we cannot exclude the possibility that these regions
are in fact homotypic and consequently, only one ICP 27 would be expected.

MAPPING SPECIFIC VIRAL FUNCTIONS

The locations of templates specifying viral functions in HSV DNA are
largely unknown.   Analysis of the intertypic recombinants in this study,
however, permitted the physical mapping of some HSV markers and functions.
Their most probable boundaries are shown in Figure 6 and are discussed
below.

HSV-1 (HFEM) Syn⁻ Locus

The biological properties of the intertypic recombinants are
reported in Table 2 (Morse et al., 1977), from which it is observed
that intertypic recombinants (C3D2, C4D, C5D, C6D and C7D expressed
the *syn⁻* plaque morphology phenotype characterized by fusion of cells

Table 2. Biological properties of HSV-1 × HSV-2 intertypic recombinants[a]

Series	Parental strains and phenotypes		Recombinant phenotype selected	Recombinant designation	Plaque morphology in Vero cells	Efficiency of plating 38.5/33.5
	HSV-1	HSV-2				
A	17 tsJ (ts-$PAA^r syn^-$)	GP6 ($ts^+ PAA^s syn^-$)	$ts^+ PAA^r$	A1E1	syn^+	1.0
				A1E2	syn^+	1.0
				A2D	syn^+	1.0
				A4D	syn^+	1.0
				A5C	syn^+	0.01
				A6D	syn^+	0.8
				A1G3	syn^-	0.9
				A7D	syn^+	0.01
				A8E	syn^+	1.0
B	17 tsJ (ts-$PAA^r syn^+$)	186 ($ts^+ PAA^s syn^+$)	$ts^+ PAA^r$	B1E	syn^+	1.2
C	HFEM $tsN10_2$ (ts-$PAA^r syn^-$)	186 ($ts^+ PAA^s syn^+$)	$ts^+ PAA^r$	C1D	syn^+	1.0
				C2D	syn^+	1.0
				C3D1	syn^-	1.0
				C3D2	syn^-	0.85
				C4D	syn^-	0.1
				C5D	syn^-	0.003
				C6D	syn^-	0.06
				C7D	syn^-	0.75
D	KOS $tsE6$ (ts $PAA^s syn^+$)	186 $tsB5$ (ts-$PAA^s syn^+$)	$ts^+ PAA^s$	D1E1	syn^+	0.01
				D1E4	partial syn^-	1.0
				D1E5	partial syn^-	1.0
				D3E1	syn^+	b
				D3E2	syn^+	b
				D4E1	syn^+	b
				D4E2	syn^+	b
				D4E3	syn^+	4.0
				D5E1	syn^+	1.0
				D5E2	partial syn^-	1.0

[a] The virus strains in this study were: (i) HSV-1 (KOS $tsE6$), a DNA[+] ts mutant described elsewhere (Benyesh-Melnick et al., 1974; Courtney et al., 1976; Schaffer, 1975); (ii) HSV-1 (17 tsJ), a DNA[-] ts mutant kindly provided by Professor J. Subak-Sharpe. The properties of this ts mutant have been described (Marsden et al., 1976; Subak-Sharpe et al., 1974); (iii) HSV-1 (HFEM $tsN10_2$), a DNA[-] mutant kindly provided by Dr A. Buchan; (iv) HSV-2 (186 $tsB5$), a DNA[-] ts mutant described elsewhere (Benyesh-Melnick et al., 1974; Schaffer, 1975); (v) HSV-2 (186), the parent strain of HSV-2 (186 $tsB5$); and (vi) HSV-2 (GP6), a syn mutant obtained by Cassai et al. (1976/77) from HSV-2 (G) and kindly furnished to us by Professor M. Terni. Virus stocks were prepared from plaque-purified seed, as previously described (Morse et al., 1977).

[b] Plaques small at 38.5°C and not readily seen at 33.5°C

into polykaryocytes.   Inasmuch as series C recombinants were derived from a cross of HSV-1 (HFEM syn^-) × HSV-2 (186 syn^+), those recombinants expressing the syn^- phenotype most likely contain HFEM DNA sequences specifying this function.   Analysis of recombinant DNAs (Fig. 1) shows that the template responsible for the syn^- phenotype must map to the right of the left crossover site of C4D (0.30) and to the left of the right crossover site of C5D (0.42).

PAA^r

Phosphonoacetate has been shown to selectively inhibit the HSV DNA polymerase (Kieff et al., 1971; Mao et al., 1975).   Resistance to PAA was used for selection of recombinant progeny in series A, B, and C and, therefore, would be consistent with a requirement for HSV-1 DNA sequences in these recombinants.   Based on the DNA sequence arrangements of C1D, C2D and C3D1 (Fig. 1), we conclude that the PAA resistance marker maps between 0.43 and 0.52 map units (Morse et al., 1977).

SHUT-OFF OF HOST PROTEIN SYNTHESIS

HSV-1 and HSV-2 shut off host protein synthesis within a few hours after infection.   Pereira et al. (1977) and Powell & Courtney (1975) noted that HSV-2 shuts off host protein synthesis much more rapidly and efficiently than HSV-1.   We have used this differential property to map the function responsible for the accelerated inhibition of host protein synthesis.

Analysis of HSV-infected HEp-2 cells labelled from one to three hours post infection (Figs 3 & 4) clearly demonstrated that four recombinants (C2D, C3D1, D1E1, C5D) rapidly and efficiently shut off host protein synthesis typical of HSV-2 infected cells.   A correlation of this phenotype with the physical DNA map of the recombinants suggests that the function involved in the accelerated inhibition of host protein synthesis must map between 0.52 and 0.59 map units.   It may be significant that this phenotype correlated with the presence of HSV-2 ICP 7 and 27.   Since we were mapping accelerated inhibition of host protein synthesis, these observations should not be construed to indicate that the number and location of all genes responsible for inhibition of host functions are known.

THYMIDINE KINASE

Three lines of evidence indicate that the gene specifying thymidine kinase (TK) maps between 27 and 35 map units.

(i) The parental HSV-1 mutant (tsE6) used in the construction of the D series recombinants is TK⁻ (Courtney et al., 1976).   Because mutants which are unable to produce thymidine kinase are able to grow in the presence of the drug ara-T (Gentry & Aswell, 1975), we have analysed the ability of recombinants D1E4, D1E5, D5E1 and D5E2 to form plaques in the presence of 100 µg of ara-T per ml of medium.   Only D5E1 and D5E2 were able to plaque in the presence of ara-T and were therefore TK⁻.   This suggests that the TK⁻ gene maps between 0.27 and 0.35 map units (Fig. 1).

(ii) The molecular weight of HSV-1 induced thymidine kinase polypeptide in SDS gels was determined by Honess & Watson (1974) to be 44 000 and by Courtney et al. (1976) to be 43 000.   ICP 35 (molecular weight 42 000) mapped between 0.27 and 0.35 map units whereas the ICP 36, another possible candidate with molecular weight of 47 000, mapped between 0.31 and 0.38 map units.

(iii) These results are consistent with a recent report that the *Hpa*I I DNA fragment contained the genetic information necessary to biochemically transform TK$^-$ cells to the TK$^+$ phenotype (Silverstein[1]; Wigler et al., 1977).

APPARENT GENE ARRANGEMENT IN HSV DNA

Based on Figure 6, derived from this study, two aspects of the arrangement of HSV gene templates are of interest.   First, there appears to be a clear clustering of templates specifying α polypeptides.   Thus, at least two α templates map at the termini of L and S components and are located at least partly within the reiterated regions.   The position of α templates coincides with the map position of some α RNA sequences as reported previously.   The proximity of α templates to the termini of the L and S components suggests the possibility that the promoter for transcription of these functions is at the termini.   Second, although no β or γ polypeptides were unambiguously mapped in the S components, those in the L component do not appear to be clustered.   These observations have several implications and are dealt with in detail in the review by Roizman & Morse[2].

SUMMARY

Analysis of the DNA sequence arrangement and polypeptides specified by 28 HSV-1 × HSV-2 recombinants show the following:

(i) Recombinants with heterogeneous L and S components or with heterogenous inverted repeats are viable.

(ii) HSV-1 and HSV-2 genes appear to be functionally equivalent and with few exceptions co-linearly arranged.   Co-linear DNA maps have been established.

---

[1] Personal communication

[2] See p. 269

(iii) At most two arrangements of HSV DNA are capable of replication. This is consistant with current studies suggesting that sequence arrangements are the consequence of obligatory post-synthesis repair.

(iv) α Polypeptides map at the termini of the L and S components of HSV DNA.   Although α ICP 27 maps entirely within the reiterated region of the L component, the template for α ICP 4 may lie only in part within the reiterated sequences of the S component.   Of note is the finding that cells infected with a recombinant that contains both HSV-1 and HSV-2 DNA sequences in the S component, produced α ICP 4 of both HSV-1 and HSV-2.

(v) Templates specifying β and γ polypeptides map in the L component and appear to be randomly distributed.

(vi) The genes specifying thymidine kinase, resistance to phosphonoacetic acid and syncytial plaque morphology mapped in the L component.   In addition, we have taken advantage of the rapid inhibition of host protein synthesis to map the gene(s) specifying this inhibition in the L component.

ACKNOWLEDGEMENTS

The studies conducted at the University of Chicago were aided by grants from the National Cancer Institute (CA 08494 and CA 19264), the American Cancer Society (VC· 103L), and the National Science Foundation (PCM 76-06254).   The studies at Sidney Farber Cancer Institute, Harvard Medical School, were aided by grants from the National Cancer Institute (CA 10893 and CA 20260).   L.S. Morse is a predoctoral trainee (5-T32 GM07183).

REFERENCES

Benyesh-Melnick, M., Schaffer, P.A., Courtney, R.J., Esparaza, J. & Kimura, S. (1974)   Viral gene functions expressed and detected by temperature-sensitive mutants of herpes simplex virus. *Cold Spring Harb. Symp. quant. Biol.*, *39*, 731-746

Cassai, E., Manservigi, R., Corallini, A. & Terni, M.(1976/77)
    Plaque dissociation of herpes simplex virus: Biochemical and
    biological characters of the viral variants. *Intervirology, 6,*
    212-223

Cassai, E.N., Sarmiento, M. & Spear, P.G. (1975)   Comparison of
    the virion proteins specified by HSV types 1 and 2. *J. Virol.,*
    16, 1327-1331

Courtney, R.J. & Powell, K.L. (1975) *Immunological and biochemical*
    characterization of polypeptides induced by herpes simplex virus
    types 1 and 2.   In: de-Thé, G., Epstein, M.A. & zur Hausen, H.,
    eds, *Oncogenesis and Herpesviruses II, part 1,* Lyon, International
    Agency for Research on Cancer (*IARC Scientific Publications* No. 11),
    pp. 63-73

Courtney, R.J., Schaffer, P.A. & Powell, K. (1976)   Synthesis of
    virus specified polypeptides by temperature-sensitive mutants of
    herpes simplex type 1. *Virology, 70,* 306-318

Esparaza, J., Benyesh-Melnick, M. & Schaffer, P.A. (1976)   Intertypic
    complementation and recombination between temperature-sensitive
    mutants of herpes simplex types 1 and 2. *Virology, 70,* 372-384

Frenkel, N., Jacob, R.J., Honess, R.W., Hayward, G.S., Locker, H. &
    Roizman, B. (1975)   The anatomy of herpes simplex virus DNA.
    III. Characterization of defective DNA molecules and biological
    properties of virus populations containing them. *J. Virol., 16,*
    153-167

Frenkel, N., Locker, H., Batterson, W., Hayward, G. & Roizman, B.
    (1976)   Anatomy of herpes simplex DNA. VI. Defective DNA
    originates from the S component. *J. Virol., 20,* 527-531

Gentry, G.A. & Aswell, J.A. (1975)   Inhibition of herpes simplex
    virus replication by Ara-T. *Virology, 65,* 294-296

Gibson, W. & Roizman, B. (1972)   Proteins specified by herpes simplex
    virus. VIII. Characterization and composition of multiple
    capsid forms of subtypes 1 and 2. *J. Virol., 10,* 1044-1052

Grodzicker, T., Williams, J., Sharp, P. & Sambrook, J (1974)
    Physical mapping of temperature-sensitive mutations of adeno-
    viruses. *Cold Spring Harb. Symp. quant. Biol., 39,* 430-466

Hayward, G.S., Jacob, R.J., Wadsworth, S.C. & Roizman, B. (1975)
    Anatomy of herpes simplex virus DNA: Evidence for four popula-
    tions of molecules that differ in the relative orientations of
    their long and short segments. *Proc. nat. Acad. Sci. (Wash.),*
    72, 4243-4247

Heine, J.W., Honess, R.W., Cassai, E. & Roizman, B. (1974)   Proteins
    specified by herpes simplex virus. XII. The virion polypeptides
    of type I strains. *J. Virol., 14,* 640-651

Honess, R.W. & Roizman, B. (1973)   Proteins specified by herpes simplex virus. XI. Identifications and relative molar rates of synthesis of structural and non-structural herpesvirus polypeptides in infected cells. *J. Virol., 11,* 1346-1365

Honess, R.W. & Roizman, B. (1974)   Regulation of herpesvirus macromolecular synthesis. I. Cascade regulation of the synthesis of three groups of viral proteins. *J. Virol., 14,* 8-19

Honess, R.W. & Roizman, B. (1975)   Regulation of herpesvirus macromolecular synthesis: Sequential translation of polypeptide synthesis requires functional viral polypeptides. *Proc. nat. Acad. Sci. (Wash.), 72,* 1276-1280

Honess, R.W. & Watson, D.H. (1974)   Absence of a requirement for host polypeptides in the herpesvirus thymidine kinase. *J. gen. Virol., 22,* 171-185

Jacob, R.J. & Roizman, B. (1977)   Anatomy of herpes simplex virus DNA. VIII. Properties of replicating DNA. *J. Virol., 23,* 394-411

Jones, P.C., Hayward, G.S. & Roizman, B. (1977)   Anatomy of herpes simplex virus DNA. VI. α RNA is homologous to non-continuous sites in both L and S components of viral DNA. *J. Virol., 21,* 268-276

Kieff, E.D., Bachenheimer, S.L. & Roizman, B. (1971)   Size, composition and structure of the DNA of subtypes 1 and 2 herpes simplex viruses. *J. Virol., 8,* 125-132

Kieff, E.D., Hoyer, B., Bachenheimer, S.L. & Roizman, B. (1972) Genetic relatedness of type 1 and type 2 herpes simplex viruses *J. Virol., 9,* 738-745

Mao, J. C-H., Rabishaw, E.D. & Overby, L.R. (1975)   Inhibition of DNA polymerase from HSV infected W38 cells by phosphonoacetic acid. *J. Virol., 15,* 1281-1283

Marsden, H.S., Crombin, I.K. & Subak-Sharpe, J.H. (1976)   Control of protein synthesis in herpesvirus-infected cells: Analysis of the polypeptides induced by wild-type and sixteen temperature-sensitive mutants of HSV strain 17. *J. gen. Virol., 31,* 347-372

Mautner, V., Williams, J., Sambrook, J., Sharp, P.A. & Grodzicker, T. (1975)   The location of the genes coding for hexon and fiber proteins in adenovirus DNA. *Cell, 5,* 93-99

Morse, L.S., Buchman, T.G., Roizman, B. & Schaffer, P.A. (1977) Anatomy of herpes simplex virus DNA. IX. Apparent exclusion of some parental DNA arrangements in the generation of intertypic (HSV-1 × HSV-2) recombinants. *J. Virol, 24,* 231-248

Overby, L.R., Rabishaw, E.D., Schleicher, J.B., Reuter, A., Shipkowitz, N.L. & Mao, J. C-H. (1974) Inhibition of herpes simplex virus replication by phosphonoacetic acid. *Antimicrob. Agents and Chemother.*, *6*, 360-365

Pereira, L., Wolff, M., Fenwick, M. & Roizman, B. (1977) Regulation of herpesvirus synthesis. V. Properties of α polypeptides specified by HSV-1 and HSV-2. *Virology*, *77*, 733-749

Powell, K. & Courtney, R. (1975) Polypeptides synthesized in herpes simplex virus type 2 infected HEp-2 cells. *Virology*, *66*, 217-228

Roizman, B., Kozak, M., Honess, R.W. & Hayward, G. (1974) Regulation of herpesvirus macromolecular synthesis: Evidence of multilevel regulation of herpes simplex 1 RNA and protein synthesis. *Cold Spring Harb. Symp. quant. Biol.*, *39*, 687-702

Roizman, B., Hayward, G., Jacob, R., Wadsworth, S.W., Frenkel, N., Honess, R.W. & Kozak, M. (1975). *Human herpesviruses I: A model for molecular organization and regulation of herpesviruses - a review.* In: de-Thé, G., Epstein, M.A. & zur Hausen, H., eds, *Oncogenesis and Herpesviruses II, part 1*, Lyon, International Agency for Research on Cancer (*IARC Scientific Publications* No. 11), pp. 3-38

Schaffer, P.A. (1975) Temperature-sensitive mutants of herpesviruses. *Curr. Top. Microbiol. Immunol.*, *70*, 51-100

Spear, P.G. & Roizman, B. (1972) Proteins specified by herpes simplex virus. V. Purification and structural properties of the herpesvirion. *J. Virol.*, *9*, 143-159

Subak-Sharpe, J.H., Brown, J.M., Ritchie, D.A., Timbury, M.C., Macnab, J.C.M., Marsden, J.S. & Hay, J. (1974) Genetic and biochemical studies with herpesvirus. *Cold Spring Harb. Symp. quant. Biol.*, *39*, 717-730

Wadsworth, S.C., Jacob, R.J. & Roizman, B. (1975) Anatomy of herpes simplex virus DNA. II. Size composition and arrangement of inverted terminal repetitions. *J. Virol.*, *15*, 1487-1497

Wigler, M., Silverstein, S., Lee, L., Pellicer, A., Chang, Y. & Axel, R. (1977) Transfer of a purified herpesvirus thymidine kinase gene to cultured mouse cells. *Cell*, *11*, 223-232

CHARACTERIZATION OF THE REPLICATIVE STRUCTURES OF THE DNA OF A HERPESVIRUS (PSEUDORABIES)

T. BEN-PORAT, J.-H. JEAN, M.L. BLANKENSHIP & S. TOKAZEWSKI

Department of Microbiology,
Vanderbilt University School of Medicine,
Nashville, Tennessee, USA

The genome of pseudorabies virus (PRV), one of the herpesviruses, consists of a linear, double-stranded DNA molecule with a molecular weight of approximately 90×10^6. PRV DNA is asymmetric with respect to its G + C content and gives rise to characteristic partial denaturation maps, indicating that it is not circularly permuted (Rubenstein & Kaplan, 1975a). Mature PRV DNA is also nicked and contains an internally inverted repetition of one of the ends (Ben-Porat et al., 1976; Rubenstein & Kaplan, 1975b; Stevely, 1977; Wilkie[1]). In all these respects the DNA of PRV is similar to that of herpes simplex virus (Frenkel & Roizman, 1972; Hirsch et al., 1975; Sheldrick & Berthelot, 1974; Wadsworth et al., 1975; Wilkie, 1973), a closely related virus.

Replication of herpesvirus DNA is semi-conservative (Kaplan & Ben-Porat, 1964) and newly synthesized DNA contains single-stranded regions (Hirsch et al., 1976; Schlomai et al., 1976). Furthermore, part of the newly synthesized viral DNA has been reported to sediment more slowly and part more rapidly than mature viral DNA (Ben-Porat et al., 1976; Hirsch et al., 1976). We have been interested recently in correlating the sedimentation characteristics of viral DNA synthesized at various times after infection with the structures of intracellular viral DNA which can be observed by electron microscopy. This paper describes some of our more recent data on this subject.

---

[1] Personal communication

SEDIMENTATION BEHAVIOUR IN NEUTRAL SUCROSE GRADIENTS OF
PULSE-LABELLED PRV DNA SYNTHESIZED AT VARIOUS TIMES AFTER INFECTION

These experiments were performed in cells pretreated with 5-fluorouracil (FU) which suppresses completely cellular DNA synthesis but affects neither viral DNA synthesis nor virus replication (Kaplan & Ben-Porat, 1961).   The synthesis of viral DNA can thus be followed without the complication of any residual cellular DNA synthesis.

The distribution in a sucrose gradient of viral DNA synthesized during 15-minute labelling periods is illustrated in Figure 1, which shows that PRV DNA synthesis occurs in two phases: early and late. At early times after infection, newly synthesized DNA was associated mainly with molecules that sedimented with S-values up to approximately twice (60-120 S) that of mature viral DNA (54 S).   These structures appeared predominantly between 2 and 3 hours post infection, i.e., during the first round of parental viral DNA replication (Ben-Porat et al., 1977).   At later times after infection, most of the newly synthesized DNA was associated with structures sedimenting with much higher S values, which, in this experiment, were sedimented to the bottom of the tube.

Both at early and late times after infection some of the newly synthesized DNA molecules sedimented more slowly than did mature viral DNA.   However, these probably represent breakage products. We have shown (Ben-Porat & Tokazewski, 1977) that parental viral DNA strands that are transferred to progeny virions retain their integrity. This eliminates the possibility that viral DNA replicates as segments.

STRUCTURES OF VIRAL DNA PRESENT IN INFECTED CELLS
DURING THE FIRST ROUND OF VIRAL DNA REPLICATION

The molecules present in infected cells during the first round of viral DNA replication (when most of the newly synthesized DNA sediments with an S-value of 60-120 S) were analysed by electron microscopy.

The positions of replicative loops on linear, unit-size, molecules and the lengths of the branches on forked molecules observed to date are summarized in Figure 2.   Only molecules with replicative loops larger than 0.5 μm and forked molecules with approximately equal-length branches were included in Figure 2.   Most of the centres of the replicative loops occupy a position approximately 20 μm from one of the ends (Fig. 2A), indicating that initiation of viral DNA replication occurs preferentially at that position.   The lengths of the branches on forked molecules are summarized in Fig. 2B.   Many of the branches are relatively short;   this is inconsistent with internal initiation at approximately 20 μm from one of the ends.

FIG. 1. SEDIMENTATION CHARACTERISTICS OF VIRAL DNA SYNTHESIZED AT VARIOUS TIMES AFTER INFECTION

RK cells, pretreated with FU, were infected with PRV (adsorbed multiplicity, 10 PFU/cell) and incubated further in Eagle's synthetic medium containing 3% dialysed serum (EDS). At various times thereafter the medium was changed to EDS-FUDR containing ³H-thymidine (50 µc/ml). After a 15-minute labelling period, the cells (4 × 10⁵/ml) were scraped into standard saline citrate (SSC) containing 2% Sarkosyl and heated at 60°C for 15 minutes. An equal volume of pronase solution (5 mg/ml) was added and the samples were incubated for 2 hours at 37°C. Aliquots were mixed with purified ¹⁴C-thymidine-labelled viral DNA and were layered on to linear 5-20% sucrose gradients (not more than 2 µg of DNA were layered on each gradient). The gradients were centrifuged in a SW-27 rotor at 10 000 rpm for 16 hours and samples were collected from the top using an ISCO gradient fractionator. The samples were acid precipitated, washed, and the distribution of the acid-precipitable radioactivity was determined. [Identical results were obtained if the samples were deproteinized prior to analysis in sucrose gradients (Ben-Porat et al.,1976a)]. Labelled between: (A) 2 hr 05 min and 2 hr 20 min post infection; (B) 2 hr 15 min and 2 hr 30 min post infection; (C) 4 hr and 4 hr 15 min post infection. The arrow indicates the position of mature viral DNA (54 S).

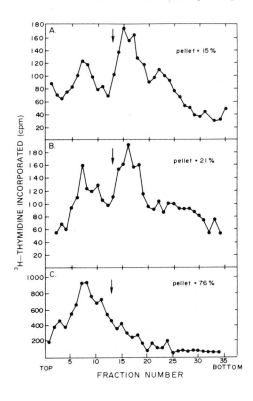

FIG. 2. SUMMARY OF THE POSITIONS OF THE CENTRES
OF REPLICATIVE LOOPS ON UNIT-SIZE MOLECULES AND OF THE LENGTHS
OF BRANCHES ON FORKED MOLECULES

Infected cells were collected at 2 hr 40 min post infection. The DNA
was extracted, viral DNA was separated from cellular DNA by isopycnic
centrifugation in caesium chloride and spread for electron microscopy.
Only unit-size molecules with "eyes" at least 0.5 μm in length and
molecules with equal-size branches were included in this figure.

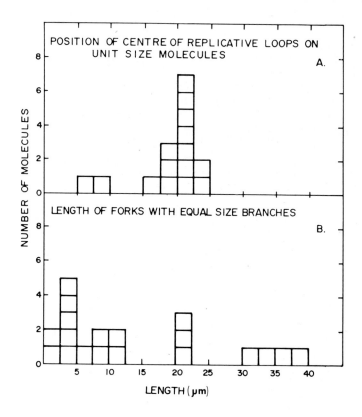

We conclude, therefore, that initiation of DNA replication occurs
also near or at the end of the molecules. Thus PRV DNA synthesis
is initiated at two sites: a site approximately 20 μm from one of
the ends and a site near or at the end of the molecules. An attractive possibility we have considered is that the initiation site is
located near the end of the terminal segment which is also reiterated

internally. We have measured 29 self-annealed molecules and have found that the end of the internally inverted repetition is 12.7 μm from the end of the molecule[1]. These data are similar (but not identical) to the data of others (Powell & Wilkie[2]; Stevely, 1977). Since the internal site of initiation of replication is located at approximately 20 μm from one of the ends, it is unlikely that it is present on the segment of DNA that is internally inverted.

In addition to linear unit-size molecules with replicative eyes or forks, circular molecules with eyes and longer-than-unit-size molecules with replicative forks and eyes were also observed. We have shown (Jean & Ben-Porat, 1976) that upon entering cells parental viral DNA is digested by an exonuclease, the ends of these molecules becoming single-stranded. Circular and concatemeric molecules appear, probably as a result of the exposure of the complementary ends. While replicative eyes and branches are observed on such molecules, the majority of the replicative structures were, however, seen on linear unit-size molecules, indicating that initiation of replication can occur on such molecules. Concatemer formation via exposed complementary ends may occur thereafter, however.

The structures described above did not appear if the infected cells were incubated with an inhibitor of DNA synthesis (fluoro-deoxyuridine). Since, in these experiments, we examined the DNA during the first round of replication, we conclude that these structures are replicative in nature.

STRUCTURES OF VIRAL DNA PRESENT IN INFECTED CELLS
AT LATE TIMES AFTER INFECTION

Figure 1 shows that, during the later phase of viral DNA synthesis (4 hr post infection), newly synthesized molecules are associated with structures which sediment rapidly. These structures sediment with S-values up to 100 times greater than those of mature viral DNA (Ben-Porat[1]); they have been partially characterized (Ben-Porat et al., 1976). Electron microscopic observations of purified intra-cellular viral DNA at 4 hours post infection have revealed the presence of some large "tangles" of DNA with very compact, densely aggregated centres (Ben-Porat et al., 1976) similar to those found in T4 and T7 bacteriophage-infected cells (Hamilton & Luftig, 1976; Huberman, 1968; Paetkau et al., 1977). Longer-than-unit-size, linear viral DNA molecules, as well as some molecules with double-or single-stranded branches were also observed.

---

[1] Unpublished data

[2] Personal communication

The "tangles" of viral DNA are very complex.   However, around
3 hours post infection [a time after infection during which the
second or at the most the third round of DNA replication is occurring
(Ben-Porat et al., 1977)] structures which could represent the
beginning stages in the formation of the "tangles" appear.   An
example of such a structure is illustrated in Figure 3.   This
particular structure, which is characterized by four forks and a
small tangle, was seen in a sample of viral DNA in which fewer than
1% of the molecules were branched.   It is unlikely therefore that it
represents branched viral DNA molecules which have become randomly
tangled.   This type of structure may therefore represent intermediates
in the formation of the concatemeric tangles.   Their nature is unclear.

FIG. 3.   EXAMPLE OF A SMALL "TANGLE"

Infected cells were collected at 2 hr 55 min post infection and treated
as described in the legend to Fig. 2.   The bar represents 1 μm.
The arrows indicate the position of forks.   SS: segment of single-
stranded DNA.

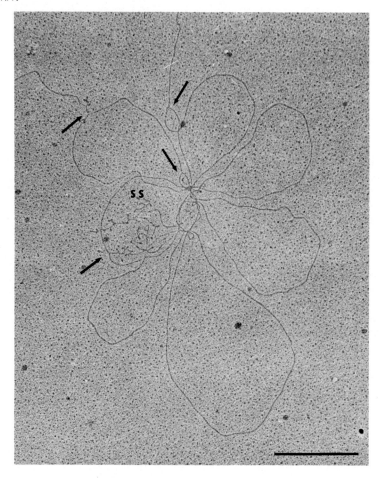

One of the branches of the structures illustrated in Figure 3 is single-stranded. The presence of single-stranded segments of DNA attached to double-stranded molecules has been reported previously by others (Friedman et al., 1977; Rixon, 1977). We have observed them on approximately 2% of the molecules of viral DNA isolated from infected cells.

One of the problems one has to consider when interpreting the structures of replicating herpesvirus DNA molecules is their fragility upon isopycnic centrifugation in caesium chloride or potassium iodide, a procedure essential to their separation from cellular DNA. This is illustrated by the results summarized in Table 1. A considerable reduction in the sedimentation value of "concatemeric" DNA occurs after isopycnic centrifugation in caesium chloride. Similar data are also obtained after isopycnic centrifugation in potassium iodide. Concomitant with the reduction in the sedimentation rate there was also an increase in the amount of DNA sensitive to S_1 nuclease. Whether the two phenomena are related remains to be established.

Table 1. Effects of centrifugation in caesium chloride gradients on sedimentation characteristics and sensitivity to S_1 nuclease of "late" intracellular and mature viral DNA[a]

Type of DNA	Treatment	Size distribution (%)			Sensitivity to S_1 (%)
		<54 S	54 S	>54 S	
Concatemeric	Before caesium chloride	15.6	2.0	82.4	8.5
	After caesium chloride	72.3	7.0	20.7	22.3
Mature	Before caesium chloride	8.0	92.0	-	2.0
	After caesium chloride	6.5	93.5	-	3.0

[a] Concatemeric DNA was obtained as follows: RK cells, pretreated with FU, were infected and incubated at 4 hr post infection in Eagle's medium containing ^{3}H-thymidine (100 μc/ml) for 15 min. Mature viral DNA was obtained from ^{14}C-thymidine-labelled purified virions. The DNA was extracted as described previously (Ben-Porat et al., 1976) and dialysed. Part of each DNA preparation was centrifuged in a caesium chloride gradient and the peak of viral DNA was collected and dialysed. The DNA was sized by centrifugation on sucrose gradients and digested by S_1 nuclease as described previously (Ben-Porat et al., 1976; Jean & Ben-Porat, 1976).

The increase in the amount of DNA that becomes sensitive to the
action of S_1 nuclease after isopycnic centrifugation in caesium
chloride (Table 1) raises the possibility that the segments of single--
stranded DNA observed in preparations of vegetative viral DNA may be
artefacts created during the procedures required to separate cellular
from viral DNA.   We are currently in the process of clarifying this
point.

CHARACTERIZATION OF THE FRAGMENTS GENERATED BY
HindIII RESTRICTION ENDONUCLEASE FROM "CONCATEMERIC" DNA

If PRV DNA is synthesized as true concatemers, i.e., molecules in
which the viral chromosome is tandemly present in linear arrays, one
would not expect the terminal regions of the viral genome to be free.
Upon digestion with restriction enzymes, the two bands consisting of
the two end fragments of the viral DNA should be under-represented
and, instead, a new band consisting of these two fragments joined
together should appear.

HindIII digests PRV DNA into fragments that migrate as three
distinct bands.   A restriction map of PRV has been constructed by
Powell et al.[1], who have shown that the terminal fragments of the
viral DNA molecules are fragment B" (molecular weight 18×10^6) and
fragment C (molecular weight 4.5×10^6) (Table 2).   We have used
this information to determine whether bands C and B" are under-
represented in "concatemeric" DNA.   The results of this experiment,
summarized in Table 2, show that band C is indeed under-represented
in "concatemeric" DNA by almost 75%.   No similar decrease is, however, seen in band B + B", half of which also consists of an end
fragment and which therefore should be reduced by 37.5%;   it is,
however, likely that the joined B" and C fragment was not resolved
from the band containing the B + B" fragments.   The relatively
large decrease in the amount of DNA in the C band obtained from
"concatemeric" viral DNA relative to that obtained from mature viral
DNA indicates that this DNA is present in the infected cells as true
concatemers.

---

[1] Personal communication

Table 2. Distribution of *Hind*III fragments obtained after digestion of mature and concatemeric viral DNA[a]

*Hind*III fragment	Concatemeric DNA (^{3}H)	Mature DNA (^{14}C)	^{3}H/^{14}C
A (internal)	341	449	0.76
B' (internal) + B" (terminal)	288	411	0.70
C (terminal)	10	49	0.20

[a] RK cells, pretreated with FU, were infected and incubated between 4 and 5 hr post infection in Eagle's medium containing ^{3}H-thymidine (50 µc/ml). The DNA was extracted, dialysed, and mixed with ^{14}C-thymidine-labelled DNA extracted from purified virions. The mixture was digested with *Hind*III restriction endonuclease and the DNA was electrophoresed on horizontal agarose (0.7%) slab gels. Strips of the gels were sliced and the number of counts in each of the bands was determined.

SUMMARY

The replication of PRV DNA occurs in two phases, early and late. During the early stages of infection newly synthesized DNA is associated with molecules sedimenting with an S-value up to two-fold greater than that of mature viral DNA. These molecules represent unit-size linear or circular molecules, as well as small concatemers in the process of replication. Initiation of replication occurs at a site situated 20 µm from one of the ends as well as at or near the end of the molecules. At later times, newly synthesized DNA is associated with large, "tangled" concatemers containing single-stranded segments of DNA. Our results indicate that at least some of the single-stranded DNA may be produced during the extraction procedure. Analysis of the large, "tangled" concatemers with restriction enzymes shows that they consist of linear arrays of viral DNA molecules.

ACKNOWLEDGEMENTS

This investigation was supported by a grant from the
National Institutes of Health (AI-10947).

REFERENCES

Ben-Porat, T., Blankenship, M.L., DeMarchi, J. & Kaplan, A.S. (1977)
    Replication of herpesvirus DNA. III. Rate of DNA elongation.
    J. Virol., *22*, 734-741

Ben-Porat, T., Kaplan, A.S., Stehn, B. & Rubenstein, A.S. (1976)
    Concatemeric forms of intracellular herpesvirus DNA. *Virology*,
    69, 547-560

Ben-Porat, T. & Tokazewski, S. (1977)   Replication of herpesvirus
    DNA. II. Sedimentation characteristics of newly-synthesized DNA.
    Virology, *79*, 292-301

Frenkel, N. & Roizman, B. (1972)   Separation of the herpesvirus
    deoxyribonucleic acid duplex into unique fragments and intact
    strands on sedimentation in alkaline gradients.   *J. Virol.*, *10*,
    565-572

Friedman, A., Schlomai, J. & Becker, Y. (1977)   Electron microscopy
    of herpes simplex viral DNA molecules isolated from infected
    cells by centrifugation in CsCl density gradients.   *J. gen.
    Virol.*, *34*, 507-522

Hamilton, D.L. & Luftig, R.B. (1976)   Bacteriophage T4 head morpho-
    genesis. VII. Terminal stages of head maturation.   *J. Virol.*,
    17, 550-567

Hirsch, I., Roubal, J., Vonka, V. & Reischig, J. (1975) *Physical
    structure of herpes simplex virus type 1 DNA*. In: de-Thé, G.,
    Epstein, M.A. & zur Hausen, H., eds, *Oncogenesis and Herpesviruses
    II, Part 1*, Lyon, International Agency for Research on Cancer
    (*IARC Scientific Publications* No. 11), pp. 155-159

Hirsch, I., Roubal, J. & Vonka, V. (1976)   Replicating DNA of herpes
    simplex virus type 1.   *Intervirology*, *7*, 155-175

Huberman, J.A. (1963)   Visualization of replicating mammalian and T4
    bacteriophage DNA.   *Cold Spring Harb. Symp. quant. Biol.*, *33*, 509-
    524

Jean, J.-H. & Ben-Porat, T. (1976)   Appearance *in vivo* of single-stranded complementary ends on herpesvirus DNA.   *Proc. nat. Acad. Sci. (Wash.), 73,* 2674-2678

Kaplan, A.S. & Ben-Porat, T. (1961)   The action of 5-fluorouracil on the nucleic acid metabolism of pseudorabies virus-infected and noninfected rabbit kidney cells.   *Virology, 13,* 78-92

Kaplan, A.S. & Ben-Porat, T. (1964)   Mode of replication of pseudorabies virus DNA.   *Virology, 23,* 90-95

Paetkau, V., Langman, L., Bradley, R., Scraba, D. & Miller, R.C., Jr (1977)   Folded, concatenated genomes as replication intermediates of bacteriophage T7 DNA.   *J. Virol., 22,* 130-140

Rixon, F.J. (1977)   Thesis, Glasgow

Rubenstein, A.S. & Kaplan, A.S. (1975a)   Electron microscopic studies of the DNA of defective and standard pseudorabies virions.   *Virology, 66,* 385-392

Rubenstein, A.S. & Kaplan, A.S. (1975b)   *Electron microscopy of pseudorabies virus DNA.*   In: *Proc. 3rd International Congress for Virology,* Madrid, p. 164

Schlomai, J., Friedland, A. & Becker, Y. (1976)   Replicative intermediates of herpes simplex virus DNA.   *Virology, 69,* 647-659

Sheldrick, P. & Berthelot, N. (1974)   Inverted repetitions in the chromosome of herpes simplex virus.   *Cold Spring Harb. Symp. quant. Biol., 39,* 667-678

Stevely, W.S. (1977)   Inverted repetion in the chromosome of pseudorabies virus.   *J. Virol., 22,* 232-234

Wadsworth, S., Jacob, R.J. & Roizman, B. (1975)   Anatomy of herpes simplex virus DNA. II. Size, composition and arrangement of inverted terminal repetitions.   *J. Virol., 15,* 1487-1497

Wilkie, N.M. (1973)   The synthesis and substructure of herpesvirus DNA: The distribution of alkali labile single-stranded interruptions in HSV-1 DNA.   *J. gen. Virol., 21,* 453-467

THE DNA OF SERIALLY PASSAGED HERPES SIMPLEX VIRUS: ORGANIZATION, ORIGIN, AND HOMOLOGY TO VIRAL RNA

H. LOCKER & N. FRENKEL

Department of Biology,
University of Chicago,
Chicago, Ill., USA

INTRODUCTION

We have previously reported that serial, undiluted passaging of herpes simplex virus type 1 (HSV-1) (Justin) resulted in the evolution of virus populations containing defective DNA molecules and exhibiting altered biological properties (Frenkel et al., 1975, 1976). Analyses of passages 1 (P1) to 14 (P14) revealed a gradual decrease in the yields of infectious virus from P1 to P9, followed by an increase in infectious virus yields between P10 and P14. Changes in other properties of the serially passaged virus were found to correlate with this pattern of viral infectivity. Specifically, P9 and P10, which produced the lowest quantities of infectious virus, also had the lowest PFU to particle ratios and exhibited the highest degree of interference with the replication of indicator virus. These passages also contained the highest proportions of defective DNA molecules, and displayed a highly modified pattern of protein synthesis, characterized predominantly by the overproduction of the α viral polypeptide ICP4 and the reduced synthesis of β and γ viral polypeptides.

Analyses of the DNA extracted from the serially passaged virus populations showed that, in addition to standard HSV DNA, they contained variable proportions of high-density DNA molecules, indistinguishable in size from plaque-purified viral DNA, but composed of multiple repeats of (G + C) rich sequences derived from the S region of standard PO (plaque-purified) HSV-1 DNA. By partial denaturation mapping and by analysis with the restriction enzyme *Eco*RI we were able to recognize two major classes of modified DNA molecules which differed with respect to the size of the repeat units contained in them. In the present communication we would like to report on further studies concerning the structural and functional organization of these defective DNA molecules.

RESULTS

Structural organization of defective DNA

The first set of experiments concerning the structural organization of defective DNA involved restriction enzyme analyses of the high-density DNA molecules contained in P15 virus (P15 HD DNA). Whereas high-density P15 DNA was found to be resistant to the restriction endo-nucleases HindIII, BglII, XbaI, and HpaI, the digestion of this DNA with EcoRI, SalI, or BamHl endonucleases (Fig. 1A) yielded fragments ranging in molecular weight from 1.2 to 5.4 × 10^6 (Frenkel et al., 1975; Hayward[1]). The maps of the fragments generated by digestion of P15 HD DNA with these enzymes were deduced from studies employing either simultaneous digestion with two enzymes, or the sequential digestion of individual restriction endonuclease fragments with a second restriction enzyme. These studies revealed the following: (i) P15 virus appears to contain three major classes of defective DNA molecules (I, II, and III; Fig. 1B), consisting of repeat units of sizes 5.4, 5.3, and 5.1 × 10^6 respectively. (ii) The difference between the three classes of P15 HD DNA molecules appears to be localized in a small region, diagrammed in Fig. 1C at the left-hand end of the repeat unit (positions 5.1 - 5.4 × 10^6). (iii) Our previous data, based upon partial denaturation mapping, showed that a given P14 defective DNA molecule contained tandem repetitions of either the large or the small repeat units, but not both (Frenkel et al., 1975). (iv) From the sizes of fragments produced by the EcoRI, SalI, and BamHl endonucleases it is apparent that the repeat units are organized in head-to-tail tandem arrays. This type of arrangement is consistent with the hypothesis that the defective DNA molecules were generated by a rolling circle type of replication. (v) Digestion of P15 HD DNA with BamHl and EcoRI also produces minor fragments of sizes 2.1 and 3.5 × 10^6 respectively. These minor fragments are not present in the gel patterns of defective DNA digested with *E. coli* exonuclease III prior to restriction with EcoRI and BamHl enzymes (data not shown). Therefore, they must arise from one end of the defective DNA molecules.

A second group of studies concerned the identification of those sequences of plaque-purified (PO) Justin DNA which are present in the various defective DNA repeat units. In these experiments, shown in Figure 2, BglII, EcoRI and HpaI fragments of PO DNA were immobilized on nitrocellulose strips by the transfer technique of Southern (1975), and were then hybridized to either labelled P15 HD DNA, or individual

---

[1] Unpublished data

FIG. 1.   PHYSICAL MAPS OF P15 HD DNA

(A) Autoradiogram of an agarose gel of defective DNA cleaved with
*Bam*Hl, *Sal*I, and *Eco*RI.   P15 HD DNA was purified from cells infected
with P15 virus by equilibrium centrifugation in caesium chloride,
labelled *in vitro* with ^{32}P by nick translation and cleaved with the
restriction enzymes shown.   Nick-translated T5 *ts* (0) DNA, that was
cleaved with the *Hind*III endonuclease, served as a size marker in the
same gel; (B) restriction endonuclease cleavage maps of the three
major classes of defective DNA molecules (I, II, III).   The maps were
deduced from studies employing either simultaneous digestion with two
enzymes, or sequential digestion of individual restriction endonuclease
fragments with a second restriction enzyme.   Fragments are designated
by letters according to their mobility in the gel, as shown in A.
The numbers in parentheses correspond to molecular weight $\times$ 10^{-6};
(C) a single repeat unit of each of the three classes of P15 HD DNA
(I, II, III).   *Bam*Hl sites are designated by *B*, *Sal*I sites by *S*, and
*Eco*RI by *E*.   The sizes of I, II and III repeat units correspond to
5.4, 5.3 and 5.1 $\times$ 10^6 respectively.

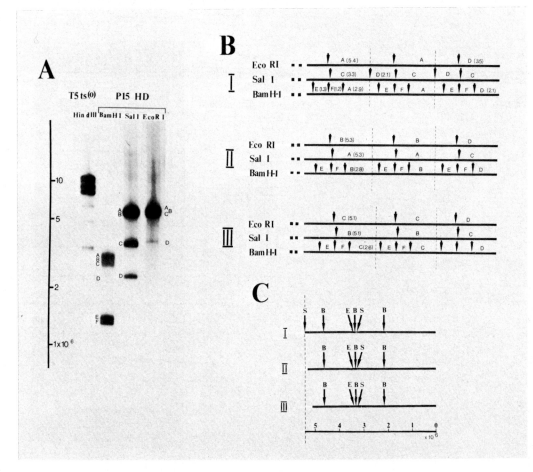

FIG. 2.   ORIGIN OF P15 HD DNA

(A) *Bgl*II, *Eco*RI and *Hpa*I fragments of PO DNA were immobilized on
nitrocellulose strips by the transfer technique of Southern (1975).
Identical strips were then hybridized to ^{32}P-labelled PO DNA, P15 HD
DNA, or to individual fragments which were produced from P15 HD DNA
by double digestion with *Bam*Hl and *Sal*I endonucleases.   The autoradiograms shown were exposed for four days;   (B) diagram showing the
map positions of the *Bam*Hl + *Sal*I double-digest fragments of P15 HD
DNA which were used in the hybridizations shown in A.   Numbers denote
molecular weights × 10^{-6};   (C) schematic representation of the hybridization shown in A.   The cleavage maps of HSV-1 DNA with *Bgl*II,
*Eco*RI or *Hpa*I endonucleases are taken from Hayward, Buckman & Roizman
(unpublished data).   The arrows represent those fragments of HSV-1 DNA
which show hybridization to ^{32}P-labelled P15 HD DNA or the *Bam*Hl + *Sal*I
fragments of P15 HD DNA.   Note that the 0.8 × 10^{6} *Bam*Hl + *Sal*I fragment hybridizes to the right-hand side of S only;   (D) location of the
HSV-1 ac and U$_S$ sequences within the defective DNA repeat units.   The
region of variability between the three types of repeat units lies
within the U$_S$ sequences.

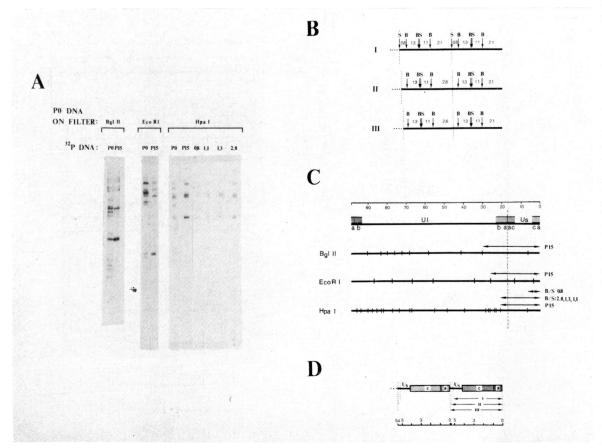

restriction enzyme fragments thereof.   The data indicated the following:
(i) P15 HD DNA contains sequences from the S region of HSV-1 DNA
(Sheldrick & Berthelot, 1974; Wadsworth et al., 1976).   (ii) In the
arrangement defined in Figure 1C, the region 0 to 4.3×10^6 of each of
the three repeat units contains the inverted repetition ac which borders
the S region of HSV-1 DNA.   The region 4.3×10^6 to the end of the
repeat unit contains sequences from the unique region of S (U_s).   The
amount of these unique S sequences varies among the three types of
repeat units.   (iii) The U_s sequences which are contained in the
repetitive HD DNA are those from the right-hand side of S in the prototype arrangement of HSV-1 DNA.

It is noteworthy that the three species of defective DNA molecules
originate from the same region of the parental non-defective HSV-1 DNA
and that each one of these DNA species contains only one type of repeat
unit.   There are two possible models to explain the evolution of these
closely related defective DNA species.   In the first model the non-
defective, parental DNA initially gave rise to defective DNA molecules
containing the largest repeat unit.   In time, this initial defective
DNA gave rise to new DNA molecules containing the smaller repeat units.
In the second model, the various types of defective DNA molecules arose
from the parental HSV DNA independently of one another.   If this was
indeed the case, one could suggest that the region 5.1 to 5.4×10^6
in the prototype HSV-1 DNA (Fig. 2C) contains hot spots for intra-
molecular recombination, possibly facilitating the formation of an
initial circle which could then be extended by a rolling circle-type
replication to give the tandem array of repeats appearing in the
defective DNA molecules.   In this light it is of interest to note that
defective DNA molecules of high density and possibly originating from
the same region of HSV-1 DNA have also been described for several
other strains of HSV-1, which were serially passaged in culture (Bronson
et al., 1973; Murray et al., 1975).

An additional point concerns the amplification of defective DNA
molecules in the population of the serially passaged virus.   It is
reasonable to suggest that each repeat unit contains a site specifying
the initiation of DNA replication, thus enabling defective DNA molecules to replicate faster than the non-defective DNA in the same population.   Whether this same site has the same function in the replication of non-defective HSV-1 DNA is at the moment unknown.   it is noteworthy in this respect that defective variants of SV40 and polyoma
virus have been shown to contain multiple reiterations of the site
specifying the initiation of viral DNA replication (Brockman et al.,
1974; Frenkel et al., 1974; Fried et al., 1974; Martin et al.,
1974).

Sequence homology between defective DNA and cytoplasmic viral RNA

As briefly described above, certain passages of the serially propagated HSV-1 (Justin) exhibit modified patterns of protein synthesis.   Therefore, it was of interest to determine whether the altered DNA molecules present in these virus populations contain sequences capable of specifying viral polypeptides.   In the experiments described below, "early" or "late" cytoplasmic RNAs were extracted from non-defective HSV-1 infected cells and hybridized to purified defective viral DNA.   Early RNA (α RNA) was obtained from the cytoplasm of cells infected for eight hours with HSV-1 (F) in the presence of cycloheximide or canavanine (Honess & Roizman, 1974; Kozak & Roizman, 1974), and late RNA was extracted from the cytoplasm of cells infected for 14 hours with the same virus.   Our data show the following: (i) defective DNA contains sequences complementary to early RNA; (ii) most probably the early RNA corresponding to the defective DNA is that coding for the virus-specified ICP4; and (iii) some portions of the repeat unit correspond to sequences transcribed late in the infection.

Early viral RNA.   Briefly, two sets of hybridization experiments were done.   In the first, trace amounts of labelled PO or P14 defective DNA were hybridized in liquid to excess unlabelled early cytoplasmic RNA.   In the second set of hybridizations, ^{32}P-labelled early RNA was hybridized to unlabelled restriction enzyme fragments of P15 defective DNA which were immobilized on nitrocellulose strips by the transfer technique of Southern (1975).   Both sets of hybridization tests indicate that defective DNA is homologous in part to early RNA.   However, the two studies yielded different estimates of the proportion of the repeat unit which is homologous to this RNA.   On the basis of the liquid hybridizations (Fig. 3A) 30% of the defective DNA, or sequences corresponding to 4900 bases, hybridize to early RNA, while in the filter hybridization test (Fig. 3B) early RNA hybridized only to fragments mapping between 3.3 and 5.4×10^6, i.e., to a maximum of 3200 base pairs.   Thus, the complexity of defective DNA homologous to early RNA, as determined from the filter hybridizations, seems smaller than that found in the liquid hybridization tests.   At present we can suggest two possible explanations for the difference between the two estimates.   The first explanation is trivial and relates to the differences in sensitivity between the two hybridization methods, i.e., it is possible that less abundant RNA species were detected only in the more sensitive liquid hybridization test.   The second and more intriguing, interpretation is based upon the assumption that the data obtained in the filter hybridization tests are complete, i.e., that the early RNA is complementary only to the region 3.3 to 5.4×10^6 of the repeat unit.   This region can in turn be divided into two segments.   The first, mapping from 3.3 to 4.3×10^6, contains the "c" sequences of HSV-1 DNA, and the second, mapping from 4.3 to 5.4×10^6, corresponds to U_s sequences.   These regions are shown schematically in Figure 4.   We would like to suggest that the

FIG. 3.   SEQUENCE HOMOLOGY BETWEEN DEFECTIVE DNA AND CYTOPLASMIC
VIRAL RNA

(A) Hybridization in liquid of nick-translated plaque-purified DNA
and defective DNA, to unlabelled infected cell RNA.   Defective DNA
($HsuR$) was isolated by its resistance to cleavage with HsuI enzyme.
Early unlabelled RNA was extracted from the cytoplasm or the nuclei of
cells infected with HSV-1 (F) for eight hours in the presence of 500 µg/
ml canavanine.   Late RNA was extracted from cells infected for 14 hours
in the absence of canavanine.   The fraction of DNA in hybrid was
estimated by digestion with the single-stranded specific S_1 nuclease.
The data are presented as a plot of the fraction of single-stranded DNA
as a function of the input concentration of RNA (R_0) in moles of nucleotides per litre × the time of hybridization (t) in seconds.   The vertical bars denote the self-annealing of the DNA probe in the presence of
uninfected cell RNA;   (B) autoradiogram of a filter hybridization of
early ^{32}P-labelled RNA to P15 HD DNA.   Identical nitrocellulose strips
containing fragments produced by the double digestion of P15 HD DNA
with BamH1 + SalI restriction endonucleases were hybridized to [32]P-
labelled P15 HD DNA or to ^{32}P-labelled RNA extracted from the cytoplasm of cells infected for eight hours in the presence of 500 µg/ml
canavanine.   The hybridization shows that early RNA hybridizes to the
fragments 1.3, 2.8, 2.6, and 0.8 × 10^6 but not to fragments 2.1 and
1.1 × 10^6.   The diagram shows the location of those fragments within
the largest defective molecule which are complementary to early RNA.

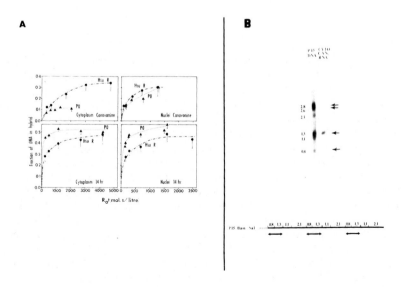

FIG. 4.   TWO MODELS FOR THE GENERATION OF EARLY RNA TRANSCRIPTS
COMPLEMENTARY TO THE DEFECTIVE DNA

RNA complementary to defective DNA could be transcribed from non-
defective HSV-1 DNA either from both ends of S in the same polarity (A),
or from both strands of only one end of S, i.e., symmetrically (B).

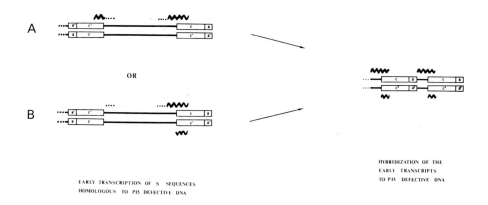

early RNA corresponding to the c portion is entirely symmetrical and
therefore hybridizes to both DNA strands in that region, while RNA
corresponding to U_S is totally asymmetrical and therefore hybridizes
to only one of the DNA strands in the U_S region.   In this model, the
total amount of DNA expected to hybridize to early RNA in liquid would
be 4700 bases, which is in good agreement with the observed value of
4900 bases.   Self-complementary RNA could be transcribed from the c
sequences by one of two mechanisms: (i) symmetrical transcription of
the left- or the right-hand side of the S region of HSV-1 DNA; or
(ii) transcription of both the left- and the right-hand ends of the S
region, in the same polarity.   These two possibilities are diagram-
matically represented in Figure 4.   It is noteworthy that fragments
derived from both the right- and left-hand ends of the S region have
been shown to hybridize to early RNA by other laboratories (Clements
et al., 1977; Jones et al., 1977).   However, further work is needed
to assign strand polarity to the transcripts of this region.

A second question concerns the coding capacity of the early RNA sequences which hybridize to the repeat unit.   As mentioned above, the virus-specified ICP4 is over-produced by some of the passages of the serially propagated HSV-1 (Justin).   In addition, work from other laboratories, involving analysis of recombinants between HSV-1 and HSV-2 (Morse et al.[1]) and mapping of temperature-sensitive mutants of HSV-1 (Wilkie et al.[2]) has shown that the gene for ICP4 maps in the region of HSV-1 DNA contained in the defective DNA.   We would like to suggest, therefore, that the early RNA which hybridizes to the defective DNA corresponds to the mRNA coding for ICP4.   It remains to be determined whether the defective DNA molecules are indeed transcribed during the course of the infection with the serially passaged virus, and whether they contain information sufficient to code for the entire ICP4 or only portions of this protein.

Late viral RNA.   In these experiments trace amounts of labelled PO or P14 defective DNA were hybridized in liquid to unlabelled late RNA. As shown in Figure 3A, the unlabelled cytoplasmic late RNA hybridizes to 50% of the defective DNA, or to a total of 8200 bases.   Because the larger defective DNA repeat unit contains only 8200 base pairs, of which 4900 bases are homologous to early RNA, there would seem to exist an overlap between the sequences hybridizing to the late RNA and those hybridizing to the early RNA.   Alternatively, it is possible that both the early and the late RNAs contain appreciable amounts of symmetrical transcripts, in which case their corresponding templates on the defective DNA need not be overlapping.   Experiments currently under way are designed to unambiguously map the region of defective DNA corresponding to the truly late transcripts, and to determine whether or not the early transcripts are present on cytoplasmic polysomes at late intervals of the infection, when there is no apparent translation of α proteins.

SUMMARY

High-density DNA prepared from serially passaged herpes simplex virus contains three major classes of modified viral DNA molecules. The altered DNA molecules are composed of multiple repetitions of sequences derived from the right-hand side of the S region of the parental plaque-purified viral DNA.   The repeat units contained in

---

[1] See p. 41

[2] See p. 11

the three types of high-density DNA share most of their DNA sequences
but differ with respect to a small region derived from the unique
sequences of the S component of HSV-1 DNA.   Hybridization of the
defective DNA to HSV-infected cell RNA shows that the high-density
DNA contains sequences complementary to both early and late viral
transcripts.

ACKNOWLEDGEMENTS

We thank J. Leiden and Dr B. Roizman for helpful suggestions in
the preparation of this manuscript.   These studies were aided
by grants from the American Cancer Society (VC 204) and from
the National Cancer Institute (University of Chicago Cancer
Research Center, CA-19264, project 404).

REFERENCES

Brockman, W.W., Lee, T.N.H. & Nathans, D. (1974)   Characterization of
cloned evolutionary variants of simian virus 40.   *Cold Spring Harb.
Symp. quant. Biol., 39,* 119-126

Bronson, D.L., Dreesman, G.R., Biswal, N. & Benyesh-Melnick, M. (1973)
Defective virions of herpes simplex virus.   *Intervirology, 1,*
141-153

Clements, J.B., Watson, R.J. & Wilkie, N.W. (1977)   Temporal regulation
of herpes simplex virus type 1 transcription: location of transcripts on the viral genome.   *Cell, 12,* 275-285

Frenkel, N., Rozenblatt, S. & Winocour, E. (1974)   *The repeated
sequences in serially passaged SV40 DNA.*   In: Kolber, A., ed.,
Tumor Virus Host Cell Interaction, Plenum Publishing Co., pp. 39-
58

Frenkel, N., Jacob, R.J., Honess, R.W., Hayward, G.S., Locker, H. &
Roizman, B. (1975)   The anatomy of herpes simplex virus DNA.
III. Characterization of defective DNA molecules and biologic
properties of virus populations containing them.   *J. Virol., 16,*
156-167

Frenkel, N., Locker, H., Batterson, W., Hayward, G.S. & Roizman, B.
(1976)   The anatomy of herpes simplex virus DNA.   VI. Defective
DNA originates from the S component.   *J. Virol., 20,* 527-531

Fried, M., Griffin, B.E., Lund, E. & Robberson, D.L. (1974)
Polyoma virus - A study of wild type, mutant and defective DNAs.
Cold Spring Harb. Symp. quant. Biol., *39*, 45-52

Honess, R.W. & Roizman, B. (1974)   Regulation of herpesvirus macromolecular synthesis. I. Cascade regulation of the synthesis of
three groups of viral proteins.   *J. Virol.*, *14*, 8-19

Jones, P.C., Hayward, G.S. & Roizman, B. (1977)   Anatomy of herpes
simplex virus DNA. VI. αRNA is homologous to non-continuous
sites in both the L and S components of viral DNA.   *J. Virol.*,
21, 268-276

Kozak, M. & Roizman, B. (1974)   Regulation of herpes simplex virus
macromolecular synthesis: nuclear retention of non-translated
viral RNA sequences.   *Proc. nat. Acad. Sci. (Wash.)*, *71*, 4322-
4326

Martin, M.A., Khoury, G. & Fareed, G.C. (1974)   Specific reiteration
of viral DNA sequences in mammalian cells.   *Cold Spring Harb.
Symp. quant. Biol.*, *39*, 129-136

Murray, B.K., Biswal, N., Brookout, J.B., Lanford, R.E., Courtney,
R.J. & Melnick, J.L. (1975)   Cyclic appearance of defective
interfering particles of herpes simplex virus and the concomitant
accumulation of early polypeptide VP 175.   *Intervirology*, *5*,
173-184

Sheldrick, P. & Berthelot, N. (1974)   Inverted repetitions in the
chromosome of herpes simplex virus.   *Cold Spring Harb. Symp.
quant. Biol.*, *39*, 667-678

Southern, E.M. (1975)   Detection of specific sequences among DNA
fragments separated by gel electrophoresis.   *J. molec. Biol.*,
98, 503-517

Wadsworth, S., Hayward, G.S. & Roizman, B. (1976)   Anatomy of
herpes simplex virus. V. Terminally repetitive sequences.
J. Virol., *17*, 503-512

CHARACTERIZATION OF HUMAN VARICELLA-ZOSTER VIRUS DNA

R.W. HYMAN, J.P. ILTIS, J.E. OAKES & F. RAPP

Department of Microbiology and Specialized Cancer Research Center,
The Milton. S. Hershey Medical Center,
The Pennsylvania State University College of Medicine,
Hershey, Penn., USA

Varicella virus, the causative agent of chicken pox, and herpes zoster virus, the causative agent of shingles, have been shown to be immunologically indistinguishable (Taylor-Robinson & Caunt, 1972), and hence the two viruses are referred to as varicella-zoster virus (VZV). The especially close association between VZV and its host cell and the loss of infectivity of the virus following rupture of the infected cell have made it very difficult to obtain cell-free virus particles in sufficient quantity for the study of VZV DNA. One direct result of these difficulties is that, despite the obvious importance of VZV as a human pathogen, particularly in the immunocompromized host (Feldman et al., 1973; Schimpff et al., 1972), very few data have been presented to characterize VZV DNA. We have recently discovered that herpes simplex virus DNA can be isolated from infected cells by release into the Hirt supernatant (Pater et al., 1976), thus removing the need for cell-free virus as a prerequisite for obtaining purified virus DNA. Sufficient quantities of VZV DNA have been obtained by this method (Rapp et al., 1977) to allow us now to begin the characterization of VZV DNA.

Our methods for the radiolabelling and isolation of VZV DNA have been published (Iltis et al., 1977; Oakes et al., 1977). Briefly, VZV-infected cells were mixed with uninfected cells at a ratio of 1:6. At 25% cytopathic effect (CPE) the appropriate radiolabel, ($^{32}PO_4$), ^3H-thymidine, or ^{14}C-thymidine, was added. At maximum CPE the VZV-infected cells were lysed with Hirt lysing buffer (Hirt, 1967), sodium chloride was added, and the precipitate was discarded. The Hirt supernatant was preparatively sedimented on a preformed linear glycerol gradient. Figure 1 illustrates the radioactive profile of a typical gradient which, in this case, is for VZV (Batson) DNA. The DNA band sedimenting halfway down the gradient has been shown to be VZV DNA

FIG. 1. PREPARATIVE GLYCEROL GRADIENT SEDIMENTATION OF
VZV (BATSON) DNA ISOLATED FROM THE HIRT SUPERNATANT

Hirt supernatant (8 ml) obtained from VZV-infected HEL cells labelled
with ^{3}H-thymidine was layered on to a 30 ml preformed linear 10-30%
glycerol gradient (Iltis et al., 1977). Centrifugation was carried
out in a Beckman SW27 rotor for 5 hours at 25 000 rpm at 20°C.
Sedimentation is from right to left. Fractions (1 ml) were collected
from the bottom, and 50-μl aliquots of each fraction were counted in
10 ml of Aquasol (New England Nuclear). The DNA band sedimenting
halfway down the gradient is VZV DNA.

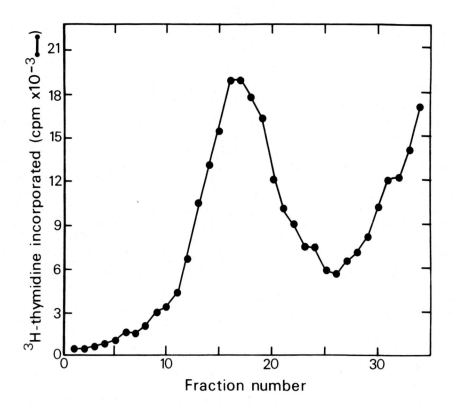

(Rapp et al., 1977). Those fractions corresponding to the peak of
intact VZV DNA were pooled and dialysed. The various VZV isolates
used in this study and the passage number at which their DNAs were

examined are listed in Table 1.   Three sets of measurements were
carried out with the DNAs of these VZV isolates: band velocity
sedimentation, restriction enzyme cleavage, and caesium chloride
buoyant density centrifugation.

Table 1. Passage number of VZV isolates used in this study

Virus isolate	Origin	Source	Passage number at time of examination of:	
			restriction pattern	buoyant density
Batson	Vesicular fluid from an adult case of herpes zoster	N.J. Schmidt	57	71, 76
CaQu	Adult[a] herpes zoster or varicella	N.J. Schmidt	NE[b]	10
Ellen	Childhood varicella	D. Steward	27	NE[b]
Jab	Adult herpes zoster	M.S. Hershey Medical Center	8	4, 8
Kawaguchi	Childhood varicella	M. Takahashi	30	23
Ludwig	Adult herpes zoster	M.S. Hershey Medical Center	NE[b]	8
Oka	Childhood varicella	M. Takahashi	15	13

[a] Diagnosis uncertain as between varicella or herpes zoster
   (N. Schmidt, personal communication)

[b] Not examined

On neutral sucrose gradients, VZV DNA sediments just behind T4 DNA
(Iltis et al., 1977; Rapp et al., 1977).   Different gradients have
yielded slightly different values for the molecular weight of VZV DNA,
but the values have all been about 100×10^6 daltons.   On alkaline
sucrose gradients, VZV DNA sediments heterogeneously.   Both of these
observations are in consonance with what is known about other herpesvirus DNAs (Kieff et al., 1971; Lee et al., 1971; Nonoyama & Pagano,

1972). When the DNAs from two different isolates of VZV are mixed
and sedimented together on a neutral sucrose gradient, their sedimentation behaviour is indistinguishable (Iltis et al., 1977).

The restriction enzyme cleavage patterns of the DNAs from several
VZV isolates have been examined using endonucleases $EcoR_I$ and HindIII
(Oakes et al., 1977). Following an additional purification step of
preparative isopycnic banding in caesium chloride, the VZV DNAs were
dialysed, concentrated by precipitation, and then cleaved with either
$EcoR_I$ or HindIII restriction enzymes. The digestion products were then
separated by electrophoresis through an agarose slab gel. The
dehydrated gel was autoradiographed on medical X-ray film. Figure 2
shows an autoradiograph of the $EcoR_I$-digested DNAs from the Batson,
Ellen, Jab, Kawaguchi and Oka isolates of VZV. Visual examination of
these patterns shows that the number and arrangement of the bands of
the $EcoR_I$-cleaved DNAs from these five isolates are indistinguishable.
Analogous analysis with HindIII-cleaved VZV DNAs shows that those
patterns are also indistinguishable (Oakes et al., 1977).

The final measurements we have accomplished are buoyant density
determinations. ^{14}C-labelled T4 DNA was added to caesium chloride
buoyant density gradients together with ^{3}H-labelled VZV and cell DNAs.
Calculations of the buoyant densities of the DNAs of several VZV
isolates yielded values of 1.709 g/cm^3 for VZV (Batson) DNA, 1.706 g/cm^3
for VZV (Jab) DNA, and 1.703 g/cm^3 for VZV (Kawaguchi) DNA (Iltis et
al., 1977). Each of these three values is within experimental error
of the others and within experimental error of the buoyant density
of 1.705 g/cm^3 for VZV DNA obtained from cell-free virions previously
reported by Ludwig et al. (1972). The buoyant density of VZV (Jab)
DNA, 1.706 g/cm^3, corresponds to a DNA with a content of 47% guanine
plus cytosine (Schildkraut et al., 1962) The DNAs from six isolates
of VZV were mixed in pairs in isopycnic caesium chloride gradients to
determine whether reproducible differences in DNA buoyant density
exist between the DNAs of various VZV isolates. Figure 3A depicts
the radioactivity profile of the gradient containing VZV (Jab) and
VZV (Batson) DNAs, both viruses isolated from herpes zoster, and
demonstrates that the buoyant densities of these two DNAs are indistinguishable. As a control, the radiolabel of the DNAs of the two
VZVs isolated from herpes zoster was reversed so that VZV (Jab) DNA
was ^{3}H-labelled and VZV (Batson) DNA was ^{14}C-labelled. Isopycnic
banding of these DNAs in caesium chloride resulted in a radioactivity
profile identical to Figure 3A (data not shown). Radioactivity
profiles of caesium chloride buoyant density gradients containing
[14]C-labelled VZV (Jab) DNA and ^{3}H-labelled DNAs from three other VZV
isolates are shown in Figure 3B, C and D, and demonstrate that the
DNAs of VZV (Kawaguchi & Oka) both isolated from varicella, and VZV
(CaQu) DNA are slightly less dense than the DNA of VZV (Jab),
isolated from herpes zoster. Figure 4 presents the data for VZV

FIG. 2. COMPARISON OF $EcoR_I$-DIGESTION PRODUCTS OF VZV DNAs
OBTAINED FROM THREE VARICELLA VIRUS ISOLATES AND TWO HERPES
ZOSTER VIRUS ISOLATES

VZV DNA labelled with ^{32}P was isolated from Hirt supernatants of VZV-
infected cells followed by glycerol gradient sedimentation and caesium
chloride buoyant density centrifugation (Oakes et al., 1977).   The
DNA was digested with $EcoR_I$ restriction endonuclease, and the products
separated by electrophoresis on 0.5% agarose gels.   The gels were
dried and placed on medical X-ray film.   (A) Comparison of VZV DNA
from Batson (1), Kawaguchi (2), undigested Batson DNA (3), Jab (4),
and Oka (5) isolates; (B) comparison of VZV DNA from Batson (1) and
Ellen (2) isolates.   A and B represent independent separations of
$EcoR_I$ digestion products.   Reprinted from Oakes, J., Iltis, J.,
Hyman, R. & Rapp, F. (1977) Analysis by restriction enzyme cleavage
of human varicella-zoster virus DNAs. *Virology, 82,* 353-361

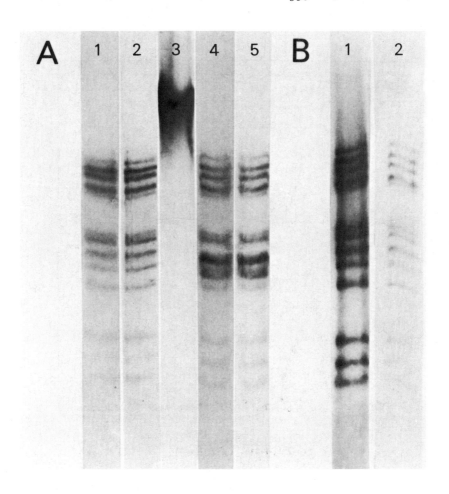

FIG. 3.   ISOPYCNIC BANDING OF PAIRS OF DIFFERENT VZV DNAs
IN CAESIUM CHLORIDE GRADIENTS

Equilibrium sedimentation in caesium chloride of ^{3}H-thymidine-labelled
VZV DNA and a different ^{14}C-thymidine-labelled VZV DNA was carried out
by centrifugation in a Beckman type 40.3 rotor at 36 000 rpm at 20°C
for 65 hours (Iltis et al., 1977).   Sedimentation is from right to
left.   The bottom twenty fractions are not graphed in panels A and B
and the bottom ten fractions are not graphed in panels C and D.
Closed circles, ^{3}H-thymidine-labelled VZV DNA and cell DNA; open
circles, ^{14}C-TdR-labelled VZV DNA.   (A) ^{3}H-labelled VZV (Batson) DNA
and cell DNA and ^{14}C-labelled VZV (Jab) DNA; (B) ^{3}H-labelled VZV
(Kawaguchi) DNA and cell DNA and ^{14}C-labelled VZV (Jab) DNA; (C) ^{3}H-
labelled VZV (Oka) DNA and ^{14}C-labelled VZV (Jab) DNA; (D) ^{3}H-labelled
VZV (CaQu) DNA and cell DNA and ^{14}C-labelled VZV (Jab) DNA.   Reprinted
from Iltis, J., Oakes, J., Hyman, R. & Rapp, F. (1977) Comparison of the
DNAs of varicella-zoster viruses isolated from clinical cases of
varicella and herpes zoster. *Virology, 82,* 343-352

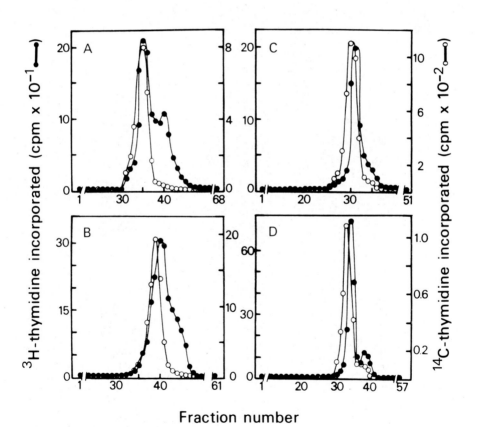

FIG. 4.   ISOPYCNIC BANDING IN CAESIUM CHLORIDE
OF VZV (LUDWIG) DNA

Buoyant density centrifugation in caesium chloride of both a ^{3}H-
thymidine labelled VZV DNA and a ^{14}C-thymidine-labelled VZV DNA was
carried out by centrifugation in a Beckman type 50.3 rotor at 37 000
rpm at 20°C for 65 hours.   Density increases from right to left.
For convenience, the bottom and top fractions of each gradient are not
graphed.   Closed circles, ^{3}H-thymidine-labelled VZV and cell DNAs;
open circles, ^{14}C-thymidine-labelled VZV and cell DNAs.   (A) ^{3}H-
labelled VZV (Ludwig) DNA and cell DNA and ^{14}C-labelled VZV (Ludwig)
DNA and cell DNA;   (B) ^{3}H-labelled VZV (Kawaguchi) DNA and cell DNA
and ^{14}C-labelled VZV (Ludwig) DNA and cell DNA;   (C) ^{3}H-labelled VZV
(Ludwig) DNA and cell DNA and ^{14}C-labelled VZV (Kawaguchi) DNA and
cell DNA.

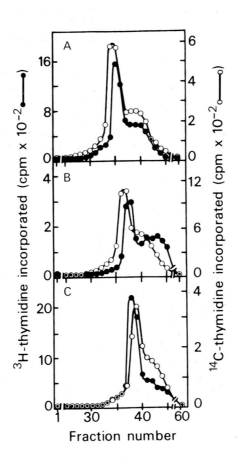

(Ludwig) DNA.   In Figure 4A the buoyant density of ^{14}C-labelled VZV
(Ludwig) DNA is directly compared to that of ^{3}H-labelled VZV (Ludwig)
DNA.   In theory these curves should coincide.   However, this curve,
Figure 4A, shows a one-half fraction displacement of the peaks, which
is presumably caused by the relative heaviness of the ^{14}C-nuclide.
This observation emphasizes again the need to reverse isotopes in
measuring these small differences in DNA buoyant densities.   Figure
4B shows the relative buoyant densities of ^{14}C-labelled VZV (Ludwig)
DNA and ^{3}H-labelled VZV (Kawaguchi) DNA.   Figure 4C shows the same
DNAs but with the radiolabel reversed.   In both cases (Figs 4B & C)
the DNA from the VZV (Ludwig), isolated from herpes zoster, has a higher
buoyant density than the DNA from VZV (Kawaguchi), isolated from varicella.

VZV is not stable cell-free (Taylor-Robinson & Caunt, 1972), so
that it must be passed in a cell-associated state.   Therefore, it is
impossible to control accurately the multiplicity of infection.   When
other herpesviruses are passed at high multiplicity, defective virus
particles containing aberrant DNA are produced (Ben-Porat et al., 1974;
Bronson et al., 1973; Frenkel et al., 1975).   Clearly, the measurements reported here must be repeated when plaque-purified VZV is avail--
able.

The most important observation to arise from these studies is the
small but reproducible difference in the buoyant density of the DNAs
of VZV isolated from varicella as compared to the buoyant density of
those isolated from herpes zoster.   The DNAs from many more isolates
of VZV must be examined before the clinical significance of these
differences in buoyant density can be definitely established.

SUMMARY

The DNA of varicella-zoster virus (VZV) has been characterized by
sucrose gradient sedimentation, restriction enzyme cleavage with either
EcoRI or HindIII site-specific endonucleases, and by isopycnic banding
in caesium chloride.   Comparisons of the DNAs from different clinical
isolates have been made.   DNAs from VZVs isolated from either varicella or herpes zoster are indistinguishable on the basis of size and
restriction enzyme cleavage pattern.   The buoyant density in caesium
chloride of the DNA of VZV isolated from varicella was reproducibly
slightly lower than that of the DNA of VZV isolated from herpes zoster.

ACKNOWLEDGEMENTS

We gratefully acknowledge the generosity of Dr N. Schmidt,
Dr D. Steward, and Dr M. Takahashi, who provided us with VZV
isolates. We also thank Dr Richard Tenser for obtaining the
vesicular fluids from which VZV (Jab) and VZV (Ludwig) were
isolated. This work was conducted under contract
N01-CP-53516 within the Virus Cancer Program of
the National Cancer Institute under Grant
CA 18450 awarded by the National Cancer
Institute and under Grant CA 16498 of
the National Cancer Institute awarded
to R.W. Hyman. J.P. Iltis is the
recipient of a National Institute
of Health Fellowship No. CA 05677.
R.W. Hyman is the recipient of a
Faculty Research Award from the
American Cancer Society
(FRA-158).

REFERENCES

Ben-Porat, T., DeMarchi, J.M. & Kaplan, A.S. (1974)   Characterization
    of defective interfering viral particles present in a population
    of pseudorabies virions. *Virology, 60*, 29-37

Bronson, D.L., Dreesman, G.R., Biswal, N. & Benyesh-Melnick, M. (1973)
    Defective virions of herpes simplex viruses. *Intervirology, 1*,
    141-153

Feldman, S., Hughes, W.T. & Kim, H.Y. (1973)   Herpes zoster in
    children with cancer. *Amer. J. Dis. Child., 126*, 178-184

Frenkel, N.R., Jacob, R.J., Honess, R.W., Hayward, G.S., Locker, H.
    & Roizman, B. (1975)   Anatomy of herpes simplex virus DNA.
    III. Characterization of defective DNA molecules and biological
    properties of virus populations containing them. *J. Virol., 16*,
    153-167

Hirt, B. (1967)   Selective extraction of polyoma DNA from infected
    mouse cell cultures. *J. molec. Biol., 26*, 365-369

Iltis, J.P., Oakes, J.E., Hyman, R.W. & Rapp, F. (1977)   Comparison of the DNAs of varicella-zoster viruses isolated from clinical cases of varicella and herpes zoster.   *Virology, 82*, 345-352

Kieff, E.D., Bachenheimer, S.L. & Roizman, B. (1971)   Size, composition, and structure of the deoxyribonucleic acid of herpes simplex virus subtypes 1 and 2.   *J. Virol., 8*, 125-132

Lee, L.F., Kieff, E.D., Bachenheimer, S.L., Roizman, B., Spear, P.G., Burmester, B.R. & Nazerian, K. (1971)   Size and composition of Marek's disease virus deoxyribonucleic acid.   *J. Virol., 7*, 289-294

Ludwig, H., Haines, H.G., Biswal, N. & Benyesh-Melnick, M. (1972) The characterization of varicella-zoster virus DNA.   *J. gen. Virol., 14*, 111-114

Nonoyama, M. & Pagano, J.S. (1972)   Separation of Epstein-Barr virus DNA from large chromosomal DNA in non-virus-producing cells. *Nature new Biol., 238*, 169-171

Oakes, J.E., Iltis, J.P., Hyman, R.W. & Rapp, F. (1977)   Analysis by restriction enzyme cleavage of human varicella-zoster virus DNAs. *Virology, 82*, 353-361

Pater, M.M., Hyman, R.W. & Rapp, F. (1976)   Isolation of herpes simplex virus DNA from the "Hirt" supernatant.   *Virology, 75* 481-483

Rapp, F., Iltis, J.P., Oakes, J.E. & Hyman, R.W. (1977)   A novel approach to study the DNA of herpes zoster virus.   *Intervirology, 8*, 272-280

Schildkraut, C.L., Marmur, J. & Doty, P. (1962)   Determination of the base composition of deoxyribonucleic acid from its buoyant density in CsCl.   *J. molec. Biol., 4*, 430-443

Schimpff, S., Serpick, A., Stoler, B., Rumack, B., Mellin, H., Joseph, J. & Block, J. (1972)   Varicella-zoster infection in patients with cancer.   *Ann. intern. Med., 76*, 241-254

Taylor-Robinson, D. & Caunt, A.E. (1972)   *Varicella virus*.   In: Gard, S., Hallauer, C. & Meyer, K.F., eds, *Virology Micrographs 12*, New York, Springer-Verlag, pp. 4-71

CHARACTERIZATION OF HUMAN CYTOMEGALOVIRUS DNA: INFECTIVITY AND MOLECULAR WEIGHT

J.L.M.C. GEELEN, C. WALIG, P. WERTHEIM & J. VAN DER NOORDAA

Laboratorium voor de Gezondheidsleer,
University of Amsterdam,
Amsterdam, The Netherlands

Recent evidence suggests that human cytomegalovirus (CMV) may have oncogenic potential (Albrecht & Rapp, 1973; Geder et al., 1976). As we are interested in the state of the genome in productive and non-productive infection, some of the molecular and biological pro- perties of the DNA were studied. In this report data on the infect- ivity and the molecular weight of the viral DNA are presented.

CMV (strain AD 169), plaque purified twice, was propagated in human diploid lung cells (multiplicity of infection: 0.1 PFU/cell). The infectivity was assayed by plaque titration under an agarose overlay (Wentworth & French, 1970). The virus was harvested from the medium when the cells showed an advanced cytopathic effect and purified essentially as described by Huang et al. (1973). Virus concentrates were lysed by incubation with sodium dodecyl sulfate (SDS) and pronase. The released DNA was purified by zone sedimenta- tion in sucrose gradients, as shown in Figure 1. Fractions containing high molecular-weight DNA were pooled and dialysed against 0.01 M tris hydrochloride + 0.005 M EDTA, pH 8.0. When the preparations were analysed for the presence of cellular DNA by centrifugation to equilibrium in caesium chloride gradients, no material could be detected in the area of cellular DNA (1.69–1.70 g/cm^3). As can be seen from Figure 2 only one peak is found with a density of 1.717 g/cm^3. Analysis by electrophoresis on 0.3 and 0.5% horizontal agarose slab gels revealed one sharp band with approximately the mobility of T4 DNA.

The infectivity of the DNA was tested by two methods: the di- ethylaminoethyl dextran (DEAE-dextran) (McCutchan & Pagano, 1968) and the calcium-phosphate technique (Graham & Van der Eb, 1973), combined with dimethyl sulfoxide (DMSO) treatment of the cells (Stow & Wilkie,

FIG. 1.   SEDIMENTATION OF CMV DNA IN A 10-30% (w/v)
LINEAR SUCROSE GRADIENT IN TBS + 0.005 M EDTA

The gradient was centrifuged for 3 hours at 18°C and 35 000 rpm in a
Spinco SW 41 rotor.   TBS: 0.05 M tris hydrochloride + 0.15 M sodium
chloride, pH 7.4.

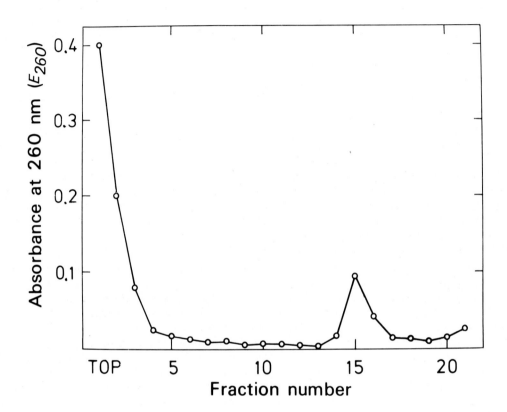

1976).   Plaque titration was performed in human embryonic lung cells
under an agarose overlay.   At 3-6 days after inoculation a cytopathic
effect characteristic for CMV could be seen and CMV-specific antigens
detected by the indirect immunofluorescent staining technique.   Two
to three weeks later the plaques were counted.   As can be seen from
Table 1 the highest number of plaques (± 400 PFU/μg) is found when
the infectivity is assayed by the DMSO-calcium-phosphate technique

FIG. 2. EQUILIBRIUM DISTRIBUTION OF CMV DNA
IN A CAESIUM CHLORIDE GRADIENT

The DNA was centrifuged for 65 hours at 20°C and 40 000 rpm in a
Spinco 65 rotor in 56.5% (w/w) caesium chloride in 0.01 M tris hydrochloride + 0.001 M EDTA, pH 8.0.   The density of the fractions was
measured by the refractive index.   •—•   density (g/cm³)

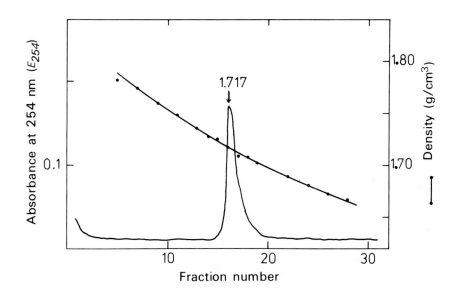

(Stow & Wilkie, 1976).   The infectivity is apparently not due to
residual virus, as incubation with pronase or heating the DNA for
1 hour at 56°C did not have any effect on the infectivity, and a
complete loss of infectivity was found after DNase incubation.

The length of the CMV DNA was measured by electron microscopy.
The preparations were selected on the basis of the following criteria:
a sharp band in agarose gel electrophoresis, a homogeneous peak
upon zone sedimentation in sucrose gradients, and infectivity of
the DNA, indicating the presence of intact CMV DNA.   Mixtures of
CMV DNA and PM_2 DNA (component II) (Espejo et al., 1971) were spread
by the aqueous method of Davis et al. (1971).   The carbon-coated
grids were rotary shadowed with platinum and examined at 60 kV in a
Philips EM-300 electron microscope.   A representative CMV DNA

Table 1. Infectivity of CMV DNA[a]

Technique	Treatment	No. of plaques per dish
DEAE-dextran	None	2, 3, 2
Calcium-phosphate	None	5, 1, 3
Calcium-phosphate + DMSO[b]	None	48, 40, 31
Calcium-phosphate + DMSO[b]	DNase[c]	0, 0, 0
Calcium-phosphate + DMSO[b]	1 hour at 56°C	39, 21, 15

[a] 0.1 µg DNA per dish

[b] Four hours after inoculation the cells were treated for 3 minutes with 25% DMSO in Hepes buffered saline, pH 7.05.

[c] DNase incubation: 2 µg DNA/ml, 10 µg DNase/ml, 0.005 M magnesium chloride, 0.01 M tris hydrochloride, pH 7.4; 1 hour at 37°C

molecule is shown in Figure 3.   The contour lengths of the molecules were measured at a final magnification of approximately 44 000 with a Hewlett Packard calculator equipped with a digitizer.   In one experiment 19 CMV DNA molecules were measured, of which only two were significantly smaller than the other 17 (80% of full size).   Based on the length of PM_2 DNA (35 molecules; 3.30 ± 0.083 µm) the length of CMV DNA was 76.22 ± 3.80 µm.   From the length ratio of CMV DNA to PM_2 DNA and the molecular weight of PM_2 DNA (6.37×10^6; Sol et al., 1975) a molecular weight of $147.13 ± 6.18 \times 10^6$ can be calculated for CMV DNA.   Using a different preparation (nine molecules of CMV DNA and 54 molecules of PM_2 DNA measured) a length of 74.16 µm and a molecular weight of $143.16 ± 9.73 \times 10^6$ was found.   The molecular weight of CMV DNA therefore appears to be significantly higher than the value of 10^8 published previously by Huang et al. (1973) and Sarov & Friedman (1976), but is in the range of murine cytomegalovirus (Mossman & Hudson, 1973).

SUMMARY

Human cytomegalovirus DNA was isolated from purified virions and further purified by sucrose density-gradient centrifugation.   The viral DNA molecules were studied by electron microscopy and found to be linear and to have a length of 76.22 ± 3.80 µm, corresponding to a

FIG. 3.   ELECTRON MICROGRAPH OF CMV DNA
The circular PM$_2$ DNA molecule has a length of 3.30 µm.

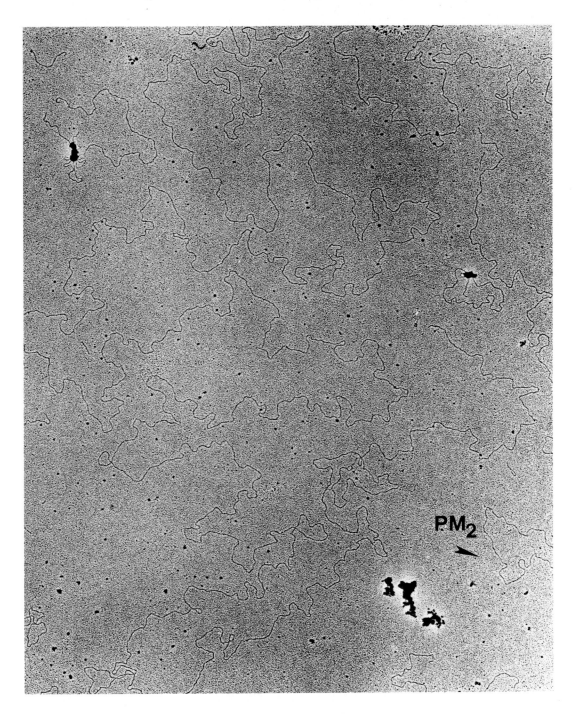

molecular weight of $147.13 \pm 6.18 \times 10^6$.   The DNA was infectious when tested in human embryonic lung cells using the DEAE-dextran and the calcium-phosphate techniques.   The density in caesium chloride was 1.717 g/cm^3.

ACKNOWLEDGEMENTS

We wish to thank Wil Maris for her excellent technical contribution.   T4 DNA was a kind gift of Ms M. Jurkivicova.   These investigations were partly supported by the Koningin Wilhelmina Fonds.

REFERENCES

Albrecht, T. & Rapp, F. (1973)   Malignant transformation of hamster embryo fibroblasts following exposure to cytomegalovirus. *Virology*, *55*, 53-61

Davis, R.W., Simon, M. & Davidson, N. (1971)   Electron microscope heteroduplex methods for mapping regions of base sequence homology in nucleic acids.   *Meth. Enzym.*, *21*, 413-428

Espejo, R.T., Canelo, E.S. & Sinsheimer, R.L. (1971)   Replication of bacteriophage PM$_2$ deoxyribonucleic acid: a closed circular double-stranded molecule.   *J. molec. Biol.*, *56*, 597-621

Geder, L., Lausen, R., O'Neill, F. & Rapp, F. (1976)   Oncogenic transformation of human embryonic lung cells by human cytomegalovirus.   *Science*, *192*, 1134-1137

Graham, F.L. & Van der Eb, A.J. (1973)   A new technique for the assay of infectivity of human adenovirus 5 DNA.   *Virology*, *52*, 465-467

Huang, E.S., Chen, S.T. & Pagano, J.S. (1973)   Human cytomegalovirus. I. Purification and characterization of viral DNA.   *J. Virol.*, *12*, 1473-1481

McCutchan, J.H. & Pagano, J.S. (1968)   Enhancement of the infectivity of simian virus 40 deoxyribonucleic acid with diethylaminoethyl dextran.   *J. nat. Cancer Inst.*, *41*, 351-357

Mossman, T.R. & Hudson, J.B. (1973)   Some properties of the genome
    of murine cytomegalovirus.   *Virology*, *54*, 135-149

Sarov, I. & Friedman, A. (1976)   Electron microscopy of human cyto-
    megalovirus DNA.   *Arch. Virol.*, *50*, 343-347

Sol, C.J.A., Walig, C., Ter Schegget, J. & Van der Noordaa, J. (1975)
    Analysis of defective SV 40 DNA by agarose gel electrophoresis.
    J. gen. Virol., *28*, 285-297

Stow, N.D. & Wilkie, N.M. (1976)   An improved technique for obtaining
    enhanced infectivity with herpes simplex virus type 1 DNA.
    J. gen. Virol., *33*, 447-458

Wentworth, B.B. & French, L. (1970)   Plaque assay of cytomegalovirus
    of human origin.   *Proc. Soc. exp. Biol. (N.Y.)*, *135*, 253-258

STRUCTURAL ORGANIZATION OF HUMAN CYTOMEGALOVIRUS DNA

B.A. KILPATRICK & E.-S.HUANG

*Department of Bacteriology and Immunology,
Department of Medicine and Cancer Research Center,
University of North Carolina School of Medicine,
Chapel Hill, N.C., USA*

The content and order of sequences in human cytomegalovirus (HCMV) DNA has been analysed by DNA reassociation kinetics, restriction endonuclease cleavage, and partial denaturation mapping. The kinetics of DNA reassociation revealed that HCMV isolates share at least 80% genome homology but share no detectable homology with non-human cytomegalovirus isolates nor with other herpes-group viruses such as herpes simplex virus (HSV) types 1 and 2 and Epstein-Barr virus (Huang & Pagano, 1974; Huang et al., 1976). Restriction endonuclease analysis also revealed these relationships and indicated that the order of genome sequences is highly conserved among HCMV isolates (Kilpatrick et al., 1976); restriction digestion by any of several restriction enzymes yields, on a molar basis, both molar fragments (or multiples thereof) and minor fragments, and numerous fragments appear to be common to most or all HCMV isolates. In a previous report we have described the finding of 150-155 × 10^6 daltons for the molecular weight of HCMV DNA (Kilpatrick & Huang, 1977). Here we focus on the general arrangement of HCMV DNA sequences and describe further characterization of HCMV DNA molecules.

HCMV DNA was extracted from purified extracellular virus (Town strain) and was purified by sedimentation gradients (Kilpatrick & Huang, 1977). Molecules from both extreme and intermediate sedimentation positions within the broad sedimentation band were analysed by buoyant density centrifugation and restriction enzyme digestion. These analyses demonstrated that the only significant density species in these preparations was that of HCMV DNA (1.716 g/cm^3), and these molecules yielded *Hin*dIII and *Eco*RI restriction products identical to previously characterized products generated from total HCMV DNA sedimentation band pools.

Contour-length measurements of either intact or partially denatured molecules derived from the faster sedimenting half of such sedimentation

gradients revealed two general size classes of DNA molecules; a low
percentage of molecules had molecular weights of 150–155 × 10⁶ daltons,
and a more abundant population had smaller molecular weights averaging
about 100 × 10⁶ daltons.   Partial denaturation mapping revealed that
molecules of 150–155 × 10⁶ daltons contained essentially the same
sequences (Fig. 1A; molecules above bracket) and that all smaller
molecules (about 100 × 10⁶ daltons) variously contained only these
sequences but in less than the full complement (Fig. 1A, molecules
within bracket).   Thus, all DNA molecules were of viral origin, and
the apparent full complement of sequences was contained in the molecules
of 150–155 × 10⁶ daltons.

FIG. 1.   PARTIAL DENATURATION MAPS
AND ELECTRON MICROGRAPH OF HCMV DNA

(A) Overall alignment of partially denatured HCMV DNA molecules was
determined by maximum overlap of common A+T- and G+C-rich zones.
Each line represents one molecule, and all molecules are arranged in
order of decreasing length from the top downwards.

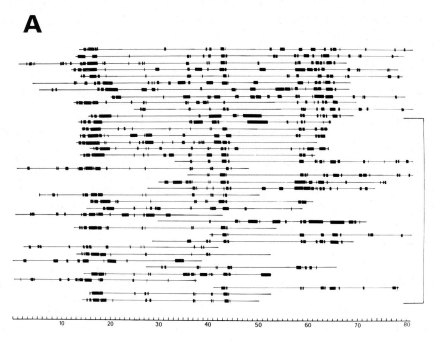

A

Length (μm)

(B) **Partial** denaturation was accomplished in alkaline formaldehyde at pH 11.35 for 5 minutes at 25°C.   This molecule is representative of the 150-155 × 10^6 dalton size class.   The bar shown is 1 μm in length.

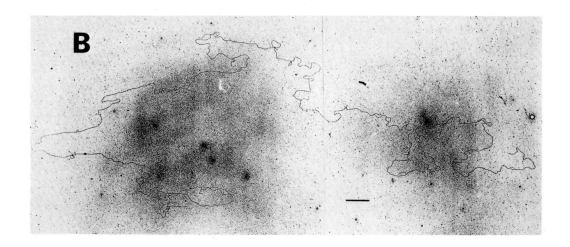

DNA sequences in 78-82% of the genome (molecules of 150-155 × 10^6 daltons) occur in the same linkage arrangement with the same orientation: these sequences are contained between length coordinates 12-15 μm to 65-68 μm in Figure 1.   The remaining 18-22% appears as a terminal region at either end of these sequences but was never found at both ends at once (length coordinates 0 μm to 12-15 μm and 65-68 μm to 80 μm (Fig. 1).   As the right-hand terminus, this region exists in approximately equal numbers of molecules as one of two complete inversions (65-68 μm to 80 μm).   Although as the left-hand terminus this region was found predominantly in one orientation (only one molecule appears to contain a similar inversion), it is likely that further examination of HCMV DNA molecules will reveal a second orientation at this position. A summary of these features is shown in Figure 2A.

The relative arrangement of sequences determined from partial denaturation mapping indicates that HCMV DNA molecules are composed of four overall sequence arrangements as shown in Figure 2B.   These four types of molecules suggest both terminal and internal duplications in HCMV DNA as described for the HSV genome model which may allow specific major inversions of genome sequences (Hayward et al., 1975;   Sheldrick & Berthelot, 1974).

FIG. 2. SUMMARY OF OBSERVED FEATURES AND LENGTHS FROM ALIGNMENTS
OF PARTIALLY DENATURED HCMV DNA MOLECULES

(A) The 65-68 μm (150-155 × 10^6 dalton) length contains all detectable
sequences.   The diagonally dashed lines indicate the general position
of the presumed separation and rejoining which may also be the position
of internal duplications; (B) four possible orientations of HCMV DNA
molecules predicted from partial denaturation map. (orientation 4 may
contain a right end inversion as depicted for orientation 2).

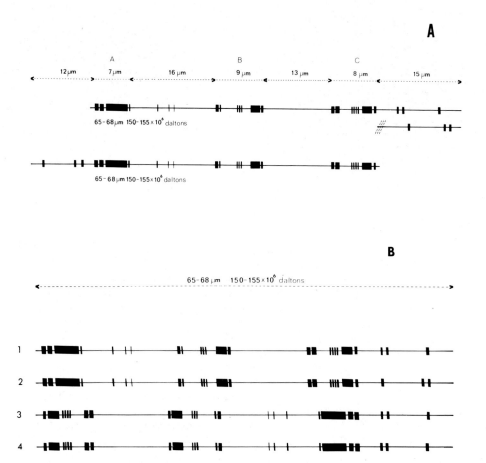

These findings raise several important questions, the answers to which should provide significant insight into the biology of HCMV. The most meaningful biological characterization of HCMV DNA depends upon comparative analysis of carefully defined enriched or purified individual preparations of each of the above two size classes since a total population of molecules contains a mixture of at least both size classes. These analyses may be complicated by a number of factors, however. The total percentage of intact molecules of $150-155 \times 10^6$ daltons in a given virus DNA preparation is low (in numerous previous HCMV DNA preparations most or all molecules had sedimentation values centring around that approximately equivalent to molecules of 100×10^6 daltons, regardless of measures to avoid shearing, and estimations by electron microscope measurements varied between 2-14%; Kilpatrick & Huang, 1977). HCMV DNA molecules contain numerous nicks, gaps, and/or alkali-labile bonds as indicated by susceptibility to S_1 nuclease and ExoIII exonuclease digestion and by partial denaturation, which may indicate increased shear sensitivity of HCMV DNA. Additionally, the total yield of extracellular HCMV particles is characteristically low following a normal virus infection, and of these extracellular particles only about 1/200-1/500 is infectious. It is very likely that the $150-155 \times 10^6$ dalton molecules are most capable of encoding all virus-specified functions in a normal HCMV infection. However, before final conclusions can be reached, both classes of HCMV DNA molecules require separate characterization analyses in order to assign specific biological activities.

To further characterize HCMV DNA size classes, adaptations of purification procedures as shown in Figure 3A were performed which yielded two size components of HCMV DNA. Restriction digestion of these molecules reveals that both size components generate identical cleavage products (Fig. 3B). This further demonstrates the similarity of general sequence content and order in both HCMV DNA size classes and additionally signifies the necessity of distinguishing between size classes during biological characterization of these DNA molecules.

SUMMARY

HCMV DNA preparations in which purity was characterized by sedimentation, buoyant density, and restriction enzyme cleavage contain two molecular weight size classes of HCMV DNA molecules ($150-155 \times 10^6$ and 100×10^6 daltons) in addition to some shear products. Partial denaturation mapping reveals that both size classes contain the same sequences and that molecules of $150-155 \times 10^6$ daltons contain the apparent full complement of sequences which are variously contained in the smaller molecules. The complete genome ($150-155 \times 10^6$ daltons)

FIG. 3.   SEDIMENTATION AND RESTRICTION ENZYME CHARACTERIZATION OF
BOTH SIZE CLASSES OF HCMV DNA MOLECULES

(A) DNA molecules extracted from purified extracellular HCMV, labelled
by adding 30 μCi of carrier-free ^{32}P-orthophosphate per ml of media
during viral DNA replication, and centrifuged to equilibrium at 1.716
g/cm^3, were sedimented in 10-30% sucrose gradients for 1.5 hours at
35 000 rpm in an SW-41 rotor at 20°C;

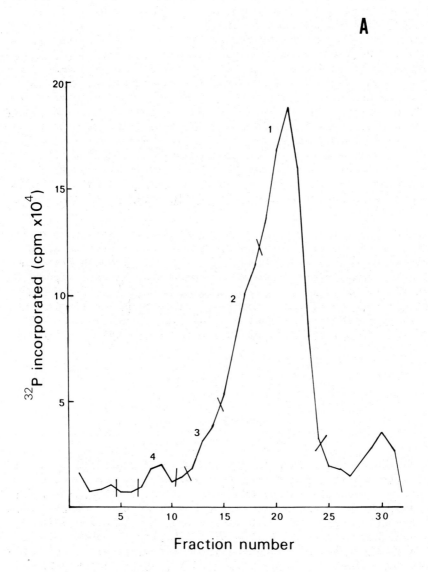

(B) HCMV DNA molecules, pooled and dialysed against TBS, were digested
with *Hind*III in the presence of 10 mM magnesium chloride and 6 mM
β-mercaptoethanol at 37°C for 24 hours and were electrophoresed in
1% agarose slab gels for 8.5 hours at 4 volts/cm. (TBS: 0.15 M sodium
chloride, 0.05 M tris hydrochloride, pH 7.4).

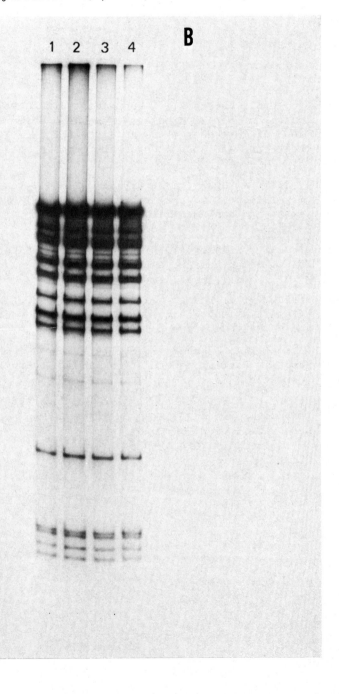

seems to be divisible into two regions of about 78–82% and 18–22%, which undergo complete inversions with respect to one another. Enriched or purified preparations of molecules of 150–155 × 10^6 daltons generate cleavage products identical to those from total HCMV DNA preparations.

REFERENCES

Hayward, G.S., Jacob, R.J., Wadsworth, S.C. & Roizman, B. (1975) Anatomy of herpes simplex virus DNA: Evidence for four populations of molecules that differ in the relative orientations of their long and short components. *Proc. nat. Acad. Sci.(Wash.), 72,* 4243–4247

Huang, E.-S. & Pagano, J.S. (1974) Human cytomegalovirus II. Lack of relatedness to DNA of herpes simplex I and II, Epstein-Barr virus, and nonhuman strains of cytomegalovirus. *J. Virol., 13,* 542–645

Huang, E.-S., Kilpatrick, B.A., Huang, Y.T. & Pagano, J.S. (1976) Detection of human cytomegalovirus and analysis of strain variation. *Yale J. Biol., Med., 49,* 29–43

Kilpatrick, B.A., Huang, E.-S. & Pagano, J.S. (1976) Analysis of cytomegalovirus genomes with restriction endonucleases *Hin*dIII and *Eco*R-I. *J. Virol., 18,* 1095–1105

Kilpatrick, B.A. & Huang, E.-S. (1977) The human cytomegalovirus genome. Partial denaturation map and organization of genome sequences. *J. Virol., 24,* 261–276

Sheldrick, P. & Berthelot, N. (1974) Inverted repetitions in the chromosome of herpes simplex virus. *Cold Spring Harb. Symp. quant. Biol., 39,* 667–678

INTEGRATION OF EPSTEIN-BARR VIRUS DNA

T. LINDAHL, A. ADAMS, M. ANDERSSON-ANVRET & L. FALK

*Departments of Chemistry and Tumor Biology,
Karolinska Institutet,
Stockholm, Sweden*

INTRODUCTION

Cells transformed by tumour viruses consistently retain virus DNA
in their nuclei as shown by nucleic acid hybridization.   It has further
been demonstrated for papovaviruses, adenoviruses, and provirus forms
of RNA tumour viruses that the viral DNA is carried in linearly
integrated form (for reviews, see Doerfler, 1975; Martin & Khoury,
1976).   Very recently, a number of exceptions to this rule have been
found in polyoma virus-transformed rat cells (Prasad et al., 1976),
and in rat hepatoma cells chronically infected with mouse mammary
tumour virus (Ringold et al., 1977), which contain both non-integrated
circular viral DNA molecules and integrated viral DNA.

In the case of oncogenic herpesviruses such as Epstein-Barr virus
(EBV), Marek's disease virus, and herpesvirus saimiri, it has also
been convincingly shown that virus-transformed cells retain virus DNA,
and this has been relatively easy because each cell contains multiple
genome-equivalents of viral DNA in latent form (Fleckenstein et al.,
1977; Nazerian et al., 1973; Nonoyama & Pagano, 1971; zur Hausen &
Schulte-Holthausen, 1970).   On the other hand, studies on the same
viruses with regard to the physical state of the herpesvirus DNA present
in transformed cells have been fraught with difficulties, because most
of the experimental techniques employed in analogous work with smaller
tumour viruses rely on the existence of a marked size difference between
free virus DNA and high molecular-weight cellular DNA isolated by
conventional methods.   Such techniques are not readily applicable to
herpesviruses, which have genomes of molecular weight 100×10^6.
Most of the work on this aspect of herpesvirus biochemistry has been
performed with EBV-transformed cells, and it has been shown that a
large proportion of the latent viral DNA is present in free form

(Nonoyama & Pagano, 1972) and that this viral DNA has a circular conformation (Adams & Lindahl, 1975a).   Similar data have more recently also
been obtained with herpesvirus saimiri-transformed cells (Werner et al.,
1977).   This situation is clearly different from that usually encountered after transformation with smaller tumour viruses, and the existence
of viral episomal DNA makes the search for integrated herpesvirus DNA
sequences particularly complicated, as it has to be performed against a
high "background" of non-integrated viral DNA molecules, which are
recovered as a mixture of covalently closed circles and nicked circles
after DNA purification.   It would still appear that integrated EBV DNA
sequences are regularly present in EBV-transformed cells (Adams &
Lindahl, 1975b; Adams et al., 1973; Andersson-Anvret & Lindahl, 1978;
Kaschka-Dierich et al., 1976, 1977).   In the following, we briefly
discuss various techniques that have been employed to study integration
of tumour virus DNA, and consider their potential application to EBV-
transformed cells.

                    SUCROSE GRADIENT OR GLYCEROL GRADIENT CENTRIFUGATION

     When mammalian cells are lysed on top of alkaline sucrose or
glycerol gradients, the released DNA will sediment rapidly, at about
300 S, on subsequent centrifugation.   This sedimentation rate greatly
exceeds that expected for small monomeric tumour virus genomes, even
if they occur as relatively fast-sedimenting covalently closed circular
DNA molecules.   The technique was employed by Sambrook et al. (1968)
in their classical demonstration of integrated SV40 DNA in virus-transformed 3T3 cells, and is one of the most stringent methods available
for analysis for the presence of short, integrated viral DNA sequences.
The method appears less satisfactory for the demonstration of integrated
DNA of large tumour viruses, however, because in that case non-
integrated, covalently closed circular DNA molecules of viral genome
size sediment at a rate similar to that of the very high molecular-
weight linear cell DNA.   The covalently closed circular EBV DNA
present in EBV-transformed cell lines has a sedimentation coefficient
of 200-250 S in alkaline solution (Lindahl et al., 1976), and it would
be difficult to convincingly demonstrate a sedimentation difference
between such DNA and EBV DNA sequences co-sedimenting with cellular
DNA.   Nonoyama & Pagano (1972) showed by this technique that slow-
sedimenting EBV DNA sequences with the properties of linear single
strands of virus DNA are present in alkaline lysates of Raji cells, and
this viral DNA could be separated from faster sedimenting cellular
DNA.   These data provided early evidence for the existence of non-

integrated EBV DNA in transformed cells, but neither covalently
closed circular EBV DNA nor integrated EBV DNA were detected in the
experiments.   In retrospect, the slow-sedimenting EBV DNA sequences
found by Nonoyama & Pagano were probably derived from nicked circular
DNA (Lindahl et al., 1976).

Sedimentation velocity measurements in neutral solution provide
little advantage over measurements in alkaline solution, as it would
be difficult to separate cellular DNA from both covalently closed and
nicked circular EBV DNA molecules.   Tanaka & Nonoyama (1974) reported
results with this method similar to those previously obtained by
Nonoyama & Pagano (1972) in alkaline solution.   So far, zone-centri-
fugation techniques have not been useful for demonstrating herpesvirus
DNA integration.

CAESIUM CHLORIDE DENSITY-GRADIENT CENTRIFUGATION

For some herpesviruses, e.g., EBV, a large natural density
difference exists between the free viral DNA and host-cell DNA.   In
addition, EBV DNA by itself has little internal density heterogeneity
(Pritchett et al., 1975).   EBV DNA (density 1.718 g/cm^3) and human
cell DNA (density 1.700 g/cm^3) separate well in neutral caesium
chloride gradients, and viral DNA with the expected properties of
integrated DNA can be detected as EBV DNA sequences banding at a
lower density than free viral DNA (Adams et al., 1973; Andersson-
Anvret & Lindahl, 1978).   In a typical experiment, high molecular
weight DNA isolated from lysates of EBV-transformed cells by treatment
with pronase and phenol, plus a trace amount of radioactive bacterial
DNA as an internal density marker, is centrifuged to apparent equilibrium in a neutral caesium chloride gradient, and cellular DNA is then
determined by absorbance (A_{260}) measurements while EBV DNA sequences
are localized by nucleic acid hybridization analysis of individual
gradient fractions.   Several types of control experiments have been
performed to establish that the intracellular viral DNA banding at
an anomalously low density in such experiments represents integrated
DNA.   These EBV DNA sequences remain at the same low density in rebanding experiments at low DNA concentration but shift to a higher
density if the molecular weight of the DNA is reduced by shear treatment;   corresponding viral DNA sequences of low density are not
observed in analogous experiments with mixtures of free EBV DNA from
virus particles and high molecular-weight cellular DNA (Adams et al.,
1973).   We consider neutral caesium chloride density-gradient
centrifugation as the best technique presently available to analyse

EBV DNA integration.   The expected density distribution of integrated viral DNA sequences in such gradients has recently been discussed in detail (Andersson-Anvret & Lindahl, 1978).

Alkaline caesium chloride density-gradient centrifugation is a less satisfactory technique than analysis in neutral gradients, because DNA undergoes a slow, salt-promoted degradation in this solvent (Kiger et al., 1968; Tomizawa & Anraku, 1965).   The reaction mechanism is unknown, but the degradation is due to the caesium chloride itself and not to some contaminating substance.   The resulting reduction in DNA chain length during centrifugation to equilibrium markedly interferes with the analysis of very high-molecular-weight DNA, and in our initial experiments we were unable to demonstrate EBV integration by this method (Adams et al., 1973). In subsequent studies, in which an internal density marker of a density close to that of free EBV DNA was employed, it was found that intracellular EBV DNA that behaved as integrated DNA in neutral caesium chloride gradients also banded at a significantly lower density than free viral DNA in alkaline caesium chloride gradients, although the difference was less marked than in neutral solution because of the background of continuous degradation of the high molecular-weight DNA applied to the gradients in alkaline caesium chloride.   These data showed that the alkali-induced breaks did not occur specifically at the joints between viral and cellular DNA, and it was concluded that EBV DNA quite probably is integrated by regular DNA phosphodiester bonds (Adams & Lindahl, 1975b).   It is noted that alkaline caesium chloride centrifugation is suitable for the analysis of integration of small fragments of viral DNA, such as that apparently occurring during productive infection with herpes simplex virus (Biegeleisen & Rush, 1976).

CENTRIFUGATION IN CAESIUM CHLORIDE GRADIENTS CONTAINING ANTIBIOTICS OR DYES

Several antibiotics, e.g., actinomycin D, bind preferentially to guanine-cytosine base-pairs in DNA and cause an inversion of the usual relation between density and guanine-cytosine content observed for DNA in neutral caesium chloride gradients (Birnstiel et al., 1974; Kersten et al., 1966).   We have employed this technique to show that integrated EBV DNA bands at a higher density than free viral DNA in actinomycin D-caesium chloride gradients (Andersson-Anvret & Lindahl, 1978).   The method seems useful for verifying results obtained by regular caesium chloride density-gradient centrifugation, and demonstrating that the integrated EBV DNA exhibits unusual banding properties because it is associated with DNA of relatively lower guanine-cytosine content and not with non-nucleic-acid material of low density.

Covalently closed circular DNA is conventionally separated from other forms of DNA in caesium chloride gradients containing ethidium bromide or propidium diiodide. The method does not allow a separation of nicked circular EBV DNA and cellular DNA (Lindahl et al., 1976) and does not appear useful for the study of EBV DNA integration.

HIRT FRACTIONATION METHOD

Small tumour-virus DNA molecules in free form remain in the supernatant when high molecular-weight DNA in cell lysates is co-precipitated with a salt-sodium dodecyl sulfate precipitate appearing at low temperatures (Hirt, 1967). The method has recently been used to purify free pseudorabies virus DNA (Ben-Porat et al., 1976) and herpes simplex virus DNA (Pater et al., 1976) from lysates of infected cells, as herpesvirus DNA is enriched in the "Hirt supernatant". In our hands, considerable amounts of large DNA molecules, such as bacteriophage T4 DNA or EBV DNA from virus particles, are also found in the "Hirt precipitate" when they are added to cell lysates in control experiments, so that the presence of herpesvirus DNA sequences in the "Hirt precipitate" of EBV-transformed cells is by itself not sufficient evidence for integration. However, circular EBV DNA molecules present in transformed cells are indeed enriched in the "Hirt supernatant", and we have used this fractionation method to confirm the absence of detectable amounts of circular EBV DNA in the human lymphoma cell line AW-Ramos which contains only one EBV genome-equivalent per cell, present in linearly integrated form (Andersson-Anvret & Lindahl, 1978).

NETWORK TECHNIQUE

This ingenious method depends on the formation of "networks" between reiterated sequences in the host DNA after brief renaturation of denatured DNA. The "networks" of cellular DNA, including inte-grated viral DNA sequences, may be pelleted by centrifugation while free viral DNA stays in solution (Varmus et al., 1973). This technique is unfortunately also complicated by artefacts of trapping in work with high molecular-weight viral DNA, but may conceivably

be used to yield similar information as the Hirt precipitation method.
In its original form, a heat denaturation procedure was used that
causes considerable fragmentation of large DNA molecules (Tomizawa &
Anraku, 1965) and therefore would make an analysis of integration of
herpesvirus DNA meaningless.   When the technique is modified by
using a gentler alkali denaturation procedure (Bellett, 1975), significant trapping of free EBV DNA into "networks" occurs in our
experience[1].

FATE OF PARENTAL VIRUS DNA AFTER INFECTION

Doerfler (1968) showed that fragments of radioactive adenovirus
12 DNA may be recovered covalently linked to cellular DNA after non-
productive infection of baby hamster kidney cells with thymidine-
labelled virus.   In similar experiments with Raji cells superinfected
with ^{3}H-thymidine-labelled EBV, radioactive virus DNA was found in
high molecular-weight form in cell nuclei 40 hours after infection
but integration was not detected (Jehn et al., 1972).   The method has
not been applied to study primary EBV infection of umbilical-cord
leukocytes.

OTHER METHODS

A recent, very convincing way of demonstrating integration of
small tumour-virus DNA molecules also yields information on the sites
of integration.   It consists of treatment of DNA from virus-transformed
cells with a restriction endonuclease that does not cleave the viral DNA,
followed by gel electrophoresis to show that the intracellular viral DNA
retains a higher molecular weight than a free virus genome, presumably
because of the attached cellular DNA sequences (Battula & Temin, 1977;
Botchan et al., 1976).   The method does not seem readily applicable to
large tumour viruses, but DNA fragments containing both cellular DNA and
herpesvirus DNA sequences could perhaps be identified in a similar fashion
after restriction enzyme cleavage.   In another approach, it was shown
that adenovirus type-12 DNA is cleaved much more frequently than host-
cell DNA by the restriction endonuclease *Sal*I, so that fragmented free
virus DNA could be physically separated from integrated viral DNA
sequences (Groneberg et al., 1977).   This method seems less suitable
for the analysis of integrated EBV DNA, because a couple of very large
DNA fragments are obtained after cleavage of free EBV DNA with the
*Sal*I enzyme (Hayward & Kieff, 1977).   In adenovirus-transformed cells,

---

[1] Unpublished data

large mRNA molecules have been found that contain both viral and
cellular sequences providing evidence for linear integration of virus
DNA (Wall et al., 1973).   EBV-transformed cells of the non-producer
type contain EBV RNA transcribed from a surprisingly large part of
the virus genome (Orellana & Kieff, 1977; Sugden, 1975), but viral-
cellular joint transcripts have not been reported and may be difficult
to detect if they occur at all in this system.   In conclusion, it
seems clear that there is a considerable shortage of good methods to
analyse integration of high molecular-weight virus DNA.

OCCURRENCE OF INTEGRATED EBV DNA

   We have searched for integrated EBV DNA in several types of EBV-
transformed cells, primarily by the neutral caesium chloride density-
gradient centrifugation technique, and have regularly detected such
sequences.   Integrated EBV DNA, usually corresponding to several virus
genome-equivalents per cell, was detected in addition to non-integrated
circular EBV genomes in Burkitt's lymphoma-derived cell lines such
as Raji and Rael (Adams et al., 1973; Kaschka-Dierich et al., 1977),
in several lymphoblastoid cell lines, derived from normal individuals,
that do not cause tumours in adult nude mice (Kaschka-Dierich et al.,
1977), in Burkitt's lymphoma tumour biopsies and in human nasopharyngeal carcinomas growing in nude mice (Kaschka-Dierich et al., 1976),
in infectious mononucleosis-derived cell lines (Adams et al., 1977;
Adams et al.[1]), and in at least some human umbilical cord-blood cell
lines immortalized *in vitro* with EBV[1].   The significance of integrated
EBV DNA in relation to the "transformed state" of the cells is unclear,
and it is not presently known if entire virus genomes or large fragments of virus DNA are integrated.   However, there is no simple
correlation between the occurrence of integrated EBV DNA and tumorigenicity (Kaschka-Dierich et al., 1977).   Two types of cells are
of particular interest in the present context: after *in vitro* conversion of the EBV-negative lymphoma line Ramos by EBV infection, stably
EBV-positive sublines have been obtained that contain relatively small
amounts of viral DNA, and all this EBV DNA seems to be present in
integrated form (Andersson-Anvret & Lindahl, 1978).   On the other
hand, certain umbilical cord-blood cell lines derived after immortalization *in vitro* with EBV contained circular EBV DNA, but integrated
virus DNA was not detected and could not account for as much as one
entire virus genome per cell, if present at all (Adams et al., 1977).
In preliminary experiments with cord-blood leukocytes, it has been
observed that pretreatment of the cells with a B-cell mitogen, bacterial
lipopolysaccharide, prior to immortalization with EBV seems to cause

---

[1] Unpublished data

a relatively larger amount of EBV DNA to occur in integrated form in
the resulting transformed cells.   This might explain why integration
is favoured on EBV conversion of the rapidly growing Ramos cell line,
while EBV transformation of essentially non-growing cells *in vivo* or
in vitro preferentially yields virus genomes stabilized in a non-
integrated state.

SUMMARY

    The application to herpesviruses of different standard methods
of measuring tumour-virus integration is discussed.   The evidence
for the presence of integrated virus DNA in EBV-transformed cells
is summarized.

REFERENCES

Adams, A., Bjursell, G., Kaschka-Dierich, C. & Lindahl, T. (1977)
    Circular EB virus genomes of reduced size in a human lymphoid
    cell line of infectious mononucleosis origin.   *J. Virol., 22,*
    373-380

Adams, A. & Lindahl, T. (1975a)   EBV genomes with properties of
    circular DNA molecules in carrier cells.   *Proc. nat. Acad.
    Sci. (Wash.), 72,* 1477-1481

Adams, A. & Lindahl, T. (1975b)   *Intracellular forms of EBV DNA in
    Raji cells.*   In: de-Thé, G., Epstein, M.A. & zur Hausen, H.,
    eds, *Oncogenesis and Herpesviruses II, Part 1,* Lyon, International
    Agency for Research on Cancer (*IARC Scientific Publications* No. 11),
    pp. 125-132

Adams, A., Lindahl, T. & Klein, G. (1973)   Linear association between
    cellular DNA and EBV DNA in a human lymphoblastoid cell line.
    Proc. nat. Acad. Sci. (Wash.), 70, 2888-2892

Andersson-Anvret, M. & Lindahl, T. (1978)   Integrated viral DNA in EBV-
    converted human lymphoma cell lines.   *J. Virol.* (in press)

Battula, N. & Tremin, H.M. (1977)   Infectious DNA of spleen necrosis
    virus is integrated at a single site in the DNA of chronically
    infected chicken fibroblasts.   *Proc. nat. Acad. Sci. (Wash.), 74,*
    281-285

Bellett, A.J.D. (1975)   Covalent integration of viral DNA into cell
    DNA in hamster cells transformed by an avian adenovirus.
    Virology, 65, 427-435

Ben-Porat, T., Kaplan, A.S., Stehn, B. & Rubinstein, A.S. (1976)
    Concatemeric forms of intracellular herpesvirus DNA.   *Virology,
    69*, 547-560

Biegeleisen, K. & Rush, M.G. (1976)   Association of *herpes simplex*
    virus type 1 DNA with host chromosomal DNA during productive
    infection.   *Virology, 69*, 246-257

Birnstiel, M., Telford, J., Weinberg, E. & Stafford, D. (1974)
    Isolation and some properties of the genes coding for histone
    proteins.   *Proc. nat. Acad. Sci. (Wash.), 71*, 2900-2904

Botchan, M., Topp, W. & Sambrook, J. (1976)   The arrangement of
    SV40 sequences in the DNA of transformed cells.   *Cell, 9*, 269-
    287

Doerfler, W. (1968)   The fate of the DNA of adenovirus type 12 in
    baby hamster kidney cells.   *Proc. nat. Acad. Sci. (Wash.), 60*,
    636-643

Doerfler, W. (1975)   Integration of viral DNA into the host genome.
    Curr. Top. Microbiol. Immunol., 71, 1-78

Fleckenstein, B., Müller, I. & Werner, J. (1977)   The presence of
    Herpesvirus saimiri genomes in virus-transformed cells.   *Int. J.
    Cancer, 19*, 546-554

Groneberg, J., Chardonnet, Y. & Doerfler, W. (1977)   Integrated
    viral DNA sequences in adenovirus type 12-transformed hamster
    cells.   *Cell, 10*, 101-111

Hayward, S.D. & Kieff, E. (1977)   Comparison of the molecular
    weights of restriction endonuclease fragments of the DNA of
    strains of EBV and identification of end fragments of the B95-8
    strain.   *J. Virol., 23*, 421-429

Hirt, B. (1967)   Selective extraction of polyoma DNA from infected
    mouse cell cultures.   *J. molec. Biol., 26*, 365-369

Jehn, U., Lindahl, T. & Klein, G. (1972)   Fate of virus DNA in the
    abortive infection of human lymphoid cell lines by EBV.   *J. gen.
    Virol., 16*, 409-412

Kaschka-Dierich, C., Adams, A., Lindahl, T., Bornkamm, G.W.,
    Bjursell, G., Klein, G., Giovanella, B.C. & Singh, S. (1976)
    Intracellular forms of EBV DNA in human tumour cells *in vivo*.
    Nature (Lond.), 260, 302-306

Kaschka-Dierich, C., Falk, L., Bjursell, G., Adams, A. & Lindahl, T.
    (1977)   Human lymphoblastoid cell lines derived from individuals
    without lymphoproliferative disease contain the same latent forms
    of EBV DNA as those found in tumor cells.   *Int. J. Cancer, 20*,
    173-180

Kersten, W., Kersten, H. & Szybalski, W. (1966)   Physico-chemical
    properties of complexes between DNA and antibiotics which affect
    RNA synthesis (Actinomycin, daunomycin, cinerubin, nogalamycin,
    chromomycin, mithramycin, and olivomycin).   *Biochemistry, 5*,
    236-244

Kiger, J.A., Young, E.T. & Sinsheimer, R.L. (1968)   Purification and
    properties of intracellular lambda DNA rings.   *J. molec. Biol.,
    33*, 395-413

Lindahl, T., Adams, A., Bjursell, G., Bornkamm, G.W., Kaschka-
    Dierich, C. & Jehn, U. (1976)   Covalently closed circular
    duplex DNA of EBV in a human lymphoid cell line.   *J. molec.
    Biol., 102*, 511-530

Martin, M.A. & Khoury, G. (1976)   Integration of DNA tumor virus
    genomes.   *Curr. Top. Microbiol. Immunol., 73*, 35-65

Nazerian, K., Lindahl, T., Klein, G. & Lee, L. (1973)   DNA of
    Marek's disease virus in virus-induced tumors.   *J. Virol., 12*,
    841-846

Nonoyama, M. & Pagano, J.S. (1971)   Detection of EB viral genome
    in nonproductive cells.   *Nature new Biol., 233*, 103-106

Nonoyama, M. & Pagano, J.S. (1972)   Separation of EBV DNA from
    large chromosomal DNA in non-virus-producing cells.   *Nature new
    Biol., 238*, 169-171

Orellana, T. & Kieff, E. (1977)   EBV-specific RNA. II. Analysis of
    polyadenylated viral RNA in restringent, abortive and productive
    infections.   *J. Virol., 22*, 321-330

Pater, M.M., Hyman, R.W. & Rapp, F. (1976)   Isolation of *Herpes
    simplex* virus DNA from the "Hirt supernatant".   *Virology, 75*,
    481-483

Prasad, I., Zouzias, D. & Basilico, C. (1976)   State of the viral
    DNA in rat cells transformed by polyoma virus. I. Virus rescue
    and the presence of nonintegrated viral DNA molecules.   *J. Virol.,
    18*, 436-444

Pritchett, R.F., Hayward, S.D. & Kieff, E. (1975)   Comparative
    studies of the DNA of EBV from HR-1 and B95-8 cells.   *J. Virol.,
    15*, 556-569

Ringold, G.M., Yamamoto, K.R., Shank, P.R. & Varmus, H.E. (1977)
    Mouse mammary tumor virus DNA in infected rat cells: character-
    ization of unintegrated forms.   *Cell, 10*, 19-26

Sambrook, J., Westphal, H., Srinivasan, P.R. & Dulbecco, R. (1968)
    The integrated state of viral DNA in SV40-transformed cells.
    Proc. nat. Acad. Sci. (Wash.), 60, 1288-1295

Sugden, B. (1975)   *Viral RNA in cells carrying EBV.*   In: de-Thé, G.,
   Epstein, M.A. & zur Hausen, H., eds, *Oncogenesis and Herpesviruses
   II, Part 1*, Lyon, International Agency for Research on Cancer
   (*IARC Scientific Publications* No. 11), pp. 171-176

Tanaka, A. & Nonoyama, M. (1974)   Latent DNA of EBV: separation from
   high-molecular weight cell DNA in a neutral glycerol gradient.
   Proc. nat. Acad. Sci. (Wash.), 71, 4658-4661

Tomizawa, J.I. & Anraku, N. (1965)   Absence of polynucleotide
   interruption in DNA of T4 and lambda phage particles, with
   special reference to heterozygosis. *J. molec. Biol., 11,*
   509-527

Varmus, H.E., Vogt, P.K. & Bishop, J.M. (1973)   Integration of DNA
   specific for Rous sarcoma virus after infection of permissive
   and non-permissive hosts. *Proc. nat. Acad. Sci. (Wash.), 70,*
   3067-3071

Wall, R., Weber, J., Gage, Z. & Darnell, J.E. (1973)   Production
   of viral mRNA in adenovirus-transformed cells by the post-transcriptional processing of heterogeneous nuclear RNA containing
   viral and cell sequences. *J. Virol., 11,* 953-960

Werner, F.J., Bornkamm, G.W. & Fleckenstein, B. (1977)   Episomal
   viral DNA in a *Herpesvirus saimiri*-transformed lymphoid cell
   line. *J. Virol., 22,* 794-803

zur Hausen, H. & Schulte-Holthausen, H. (1970)   Presence of EBV
   nucleic acid homology in a "virus-free" line of Burkitt tumour
   cells. *Nature (Lond.), 227,* 245-248

EPISOMAL VIRAL DNA IN HERPESVIRUS SAIMIRI-TRANSFORMED LYMPHOID CELL LINES

F.-J. WERNER & G.W. BORNKAMM

Institut für klinische Virologie,
Erlangen, Federal Republic of Germany

B. FLECKENSTEIN

New England Regional Primate Research Center
Harvard Medical School,
Southborough, Mass., USA

C. MULDER

Department of Pharmacology,
University of Massachusetts Medical School,
Worcester, Mass., USA

A number of lymphoid T-cell lines have been established from herpesvirus saimiri (HVS)-induced tumours of primates (Falk et al., 1972). HVS could readily be isolated from most of these lymphoid cell lines. Upon prolonged passage, some of these cell lines lost the ability to produce virus. These non-virus-producing cell lines contained a high number of viral genome copies, though viral antigens have not been detected (Fleckenstein et al., 1977). We want to report here on the structure of viral DNA molecules in two of these non-producer tumour cell lines, No. 1670 and 70N2.

Covalently closed circular viral DNA was isolated from both cell lines. These superhelical DNA molecules were purified from cell extracts by three centrifugation steps: (1) isopycnic banding in caesium chloride; (2) sedimentation in glycerol gradients; and (3) density centrifugation in caesium chloride/ethidium bromide. Alternatively, two subsequent equilibrium centrifugations in caesium chloride/ethidium bromide were employed. The molecular weight of the

viral episomes was determined by measuring the contour length of the
circles in the electron microscope.   The length of the circular DNA
from No. 1670 cells indicated a molecular weight of 131.5 ± 3.6 × 10^6
daltons, and episomes from 70N2 cells had a contour length corresponding to 119.7 ± 2.5 × 10^6 daltons.   Thus, the size of viral episomes from HVS-transformed cells was found to be significantly larger
than that of linear DNA molecules in virus particles (about 100 × 10^6
daltons) (Fig. 1).

FIG. 1.   CONTOUR LENGTHS OF EPISOMAL DNA MOLECULES

The histogram shows the contour lengths of episomal molecules from
tumour cell line 70N2, compared with the average lengths of episomes
from tumour cell line No. 1670 and of linear virion M-DNA (arrows).

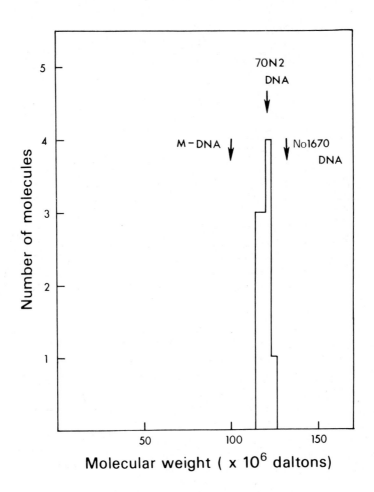

The predominant type of linear DNA molecules of HVS virions (M-DNA, M-genome) consist of about 72% unique DNA (L-DNA, 36% guanine plus cytosine; G + C) and 28% repetitive DNA (H-DNA, 71% G + C) (Fleckenstein & Wolf, 1974; Fleckenstein et al., 1975). The L-DNA (71.6×10^6 daltons) is inserted between two terminal stretches of H-DNA of variable length (Bornkamm et al., 1976).

The structure of the large-sized circular DNA isolated from the tumour cell line was examined by partial denaturation mapping in the electron microscope; this method easily distinguishes between stretches of H-DNA and L-DNA.

Closed circular molecules from No. 1670 cells were partially denatured with 7 M sodium perchlorate and 1.04 M formaldehyde at neutral pH (7.5) and low temperature (30°C).   The denaturation pattern of all 19 episomes in which single-stranded regions were found showed a uniform arrangement of large, partially denatured (L) and duplex (H) stretches. All these circles contained two L-DNA regions (57.8 ± 1.9 and $33.7 \pm 1.4 \times 10^6$ daltons) and two H-DNA regions (22.8 ± 1.9 and $17.2 \pm 0.8 \times 10^6$ daltons respectively).

The correlation between the two L-regions of episomes in No. 1670 cells was determined by comparison of the histograms of the denatured regions of short and long L-pieces.   The histograms were fitted in succession to give optimal correspondence, using a CD3300 computer. This method indicated that the shorter L-region was a subset of the longer L-region, and that both L-regions in each circle were oriented in the same polarity.   This implies that the episomes from tumour cell line No. 1670 were a kind of defective genome containing L-DNA at a complexity of 58×10^6 daltons (81% of the L-region in virions).

As a next step, the L-regions of episomes from No. 1670 cells were correlated with the known physical gene maps of linear DNA from virus particles of HVS strain No. 11.

Cleavage maps of M-genomes have been constructed with the restriction endonucleases *Bam*HI, *Eco*RI, *Kpn*I, *Sac*II, *Sal*I, and *Sma*I (Mulder & Fleckenstein[1]).   *Sal*I cleaved the L-DNA of M-genomes twice (fragment A: 49.5; fragment B: 11.8; and fragment C: 10.3×10^6 daltons). The physical order of these *Sal*I fragments was A-B-C.   Since *Sal*I did not cleave H-DNA, cleavage of M-DNA with this enzyme resulted in a large L-DNA piece (fragment A), contiguous with a duplex H-DNA stretch. A *Sal*I digest of M-DNA was partially denatured, and the denaturation histograms of *Sal*I fragment A were fitted with the aid of a computer into optimal correspondence with the denaturation histograms of L-DNA from the linear molecules.   Figure 2 shows their relative positions.

---

[1] Unpublished data

FIG. 2.   ORIENTATION OF THE TWO L-DNA REGIONS
IN No. 1670 EPISOMES IN CORRELATION WITH THE CLEAVAGE MAPS
OF LINEAR HVS VIRION DNA

The shorter episomal L-region was comprised within *Sal*I fragment A and
represented the left-hand half of the virion L-region.   The longer
episomal L-region probably represented the total fragment A and part
of fragment B.

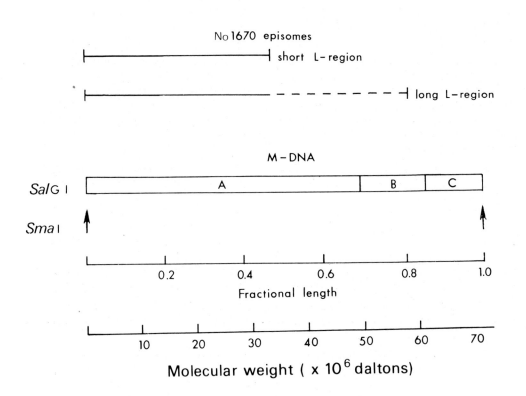

The short L-region of No. 1670 cells fitted best with the left-hand
half of the L-region of M-genomes (0.00 - 0.47 fractional length) and
was completely comprised within *Sal*I fragment A.   The long L-region
of No. 1670 episomes also represented the left-hand side of the
physical map, probably extending from 0.00 to 0.81 fractional length
of virion L-DNA.   This model suggested that the right-hand terminal
19% of the virion L-DNA region (0.81 - 1.00 fractional length) was
missing, an intermediate part (0.47 - 0.81 fractional length) was
present once, and the left-hand 47% (0.00 - 0.47 fractional length) was
duplicated in each episome of No. 1670 cells.

These results implied that the right-hand terminus of the virion
L-DNA region (*Sal*I fragment C) coded for proteins that were not
required to maintain the state of transformation in lymphoid cells,
unless the tumour cell lines contained viral genome copies of different
structure in integrated form in addition to the defective viral episomes
described.

SUMMARY

Structural analysis of episomal viral genomes from two herpesvirus
saimiri (HVS)-transformed tumour cell lines (No. 1670 and 70N2)
showed that both types of episomes have a higher molecular weight than
linear virion DNA.   The arrangement of unique (L) and repetitive (H)
DNA in No. 1670 episomes was studied by partial denaturation mapping.
Part of the L-sequences present in linear virion DNA was found to be
missing, part was found to be duplicated in the episomes.   The episomal
L-DNA regions were correlated with the known physical gene maps of
linear HVS DNA.

ACKNOWLEDGEMENTS

This work was supported by the Deutsche Forschungsgemeinschaft
(Sonderforschungsbereich 118), and (for C. Mulder) by grant
No. VC-121 from the American Cancer Society.
The excellent technical assistance of
Ingrid Müller and Michael Coomey is
greatly appreciated.

REFERENCES

Bornkamm, G.W., Delius, H., Fleckenstein, B., Werner, B.-J. &
    Mulder, C. (1976)   Structure of *Herpesvirus saimiri* genomes:
    arrangement of heavy and light sequences in the M genome.
    J. Virol., *19*, 1954-1961

Falk, L.A., Wolfe, L.G. & Deinhardt, F. (1972)   Demonstration of
    Herpesvirus saimiri-associated antigens in peripheral lymphocytes
    from infected marmosets during *in vitro* cultivation.   *J. nat.
    Cancer Inst.*, *48*, 523-530

Fleckenstein, B. & Wolf, H. (1974)   Purification and properties of
    Herpesvirus saimiri DNA.   *Virology*, *58*, 55-64

Fleckenstein, B., Bornkamm, G.W. & Ludwig, H. (1975)   Repetitive
    sequences in complete and defective genomes of *Herpesvirus saimiri*.
    J. Virol., *15*, 398-406

Fleckenstein, B., Müller, I. & Werner, J. (1977)   The presence of
    Herpesvirus saimiri genomes in virus-transformed cells.   *Int. J.
    Cancer*, *19*, 546-554

HERPESVIRUS PAPIO: STATE OF VIRAL DNA IN BABOON LYMPHOBLASTOID CELL LINES

L. FALK[1], T. LINDAHL & G. KLEIN

Departments of Chemistry and Tumour Biology,
Karolinska Institutet,
Stockholm, Sweden

Herpesvirus papio (HVP) is an indigenous B-lymphotropic virus of baboons sharing cross-reacting viral capsid (VCA) and early antigens (EA) with Epstein-Barr virus (EBV) and about 40% genome homology with EBV DNA. However, EBV nuclear antigen (EBNA) or an analogous nuclear antigen has not been demonstrated in cells of HVP-carrying baboon lymphoblastoid cell lines (LCL) by anticomplement immunofluorescence tests (Falk et al., 1976). HVP transforms marmoset lymphocytes *in vitro* (Falk et al., 1977) and induces a lymphoproliferative disease in some species of marmosets (Deinhardt et al., 1977).

We have examined the state of HVP DNA in baboon LCL established from splenic or circulating lymphocytes of lymphomatous (*P. hamadryas*) or clinically well (*P. anubis*) baboons respectively. High molecular-weight cellular DNA was extracted from the cells by lysis with Sarkosyl and treatment with pronase. DNA was fractionated by caesium chloride density-gradient centrifugation and HVP DNA sequences were localized by nucleic acid hybridization tests as described (Adams & Lindahl, 1975; Lindahl et al., 1976) employing EBV complementary RNA (cRNA) because of EBV-HVP partial genome homology.

Five HVP-producer LCL were analysed and representative data obtained from one cell line, 18C, are presented in Figures 1 and 2. A peak of HVP DNA sequences was localized at a density of 1.715-1.716 g/cm^3 (Fig. 1) probably representing free HVP DNA. Additional evidence for the presence of covalently closed circular viral DNA was

---

[1] Present address: Department of Microbiology, Rush-Presbyterian-St. Luke's Medical Center, 1753 W. Congress Parkway, Chicago, Illinois 60612, USA

FIG. 1. NEUTRAL CAESIUM CHLORIDE DENSITY-GRADIENT
CENTRIFUGATION OF BABOON LCL DNA

High molecular-weight cellular DNA was extracted from 18C baboon cells
with Sarkosyl and treated with pronase.   Solid caesium chloride was
added to a final density of 1.712-1.714 g/cm^3 and *Klebsiella pneumoniae*
^{3}H-DNA (density, 1.717 g/cm^3) was added as an internal density marker.
The DNA was centrifuged in 19-ml aliquots in a Spinco 60 Ti rotor at
33 000 rpm, 21°C, for 65 hours.

●——●——●   cellular DNA (absorbance at 260 nm; A$_{260}$
O---O---O   K. pneumoniae DNA
▲▲▲▲▲▲▲▲   HVP DNA sequences localized by hybridization with EBV
^{32}P-cRNA

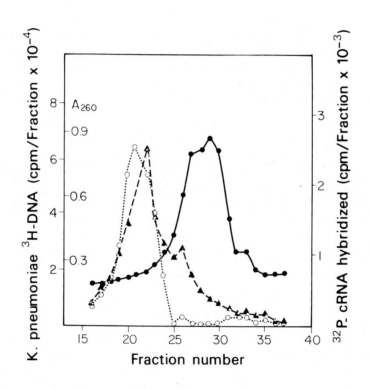

FIG. 2. RECENTRIFUGATION IN CAESIUM CHLORIDE DENSITY GRADIENTS
OF HIGH MOLECULAR-WEIGHT BABOON LCL DNA RECOVERED FROM GRADIENTS
SUCH AS THOSE SHOWN IN FIG. 1

DNA in the density range 1.700-1.710 g/cm^3 recovered from three
caesium chloride gradients (fractions 24-28 in Fig. 1) was diluted
with fresh caesium chloride solution and recentrifuged under the
same conditions.   Symbols as in Fig. 1.

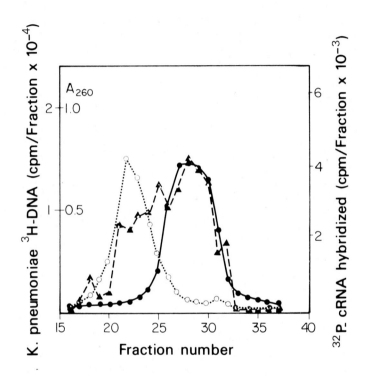

obtained by glycerol gradient centrifugation and ethidium bromide-
caesium chloride density-gradient centrifugation (Lindahl et al.,
1976).   A trailing of hybridization into the cellular DNA region
in caesium chloride gradients was also observed.   Recentrifugation
of DNA in this lighter density range (1.700-1.710 g/cm^3) and hybridization of gradient fractions gave a profile as shown in Fig. 2.

The majority of HVP DNA again banded at a density of 1.700-1.710 g/cm^3 and only a small amount of HVP DNA was detected in the higher density range.

   Similar studies were performed with one HVP-carrying baboon cell line which was antigen-negative in immunofluorescence tests and contained only about two HVP genomes per cell.   HVP DNA appeared to be integrated, as the main hybridization peak from a first caesium chloride gradient was in a density position of 1.706 g/cm^3.

   HVP and EBV are closely related lymphotropic viruses but although they share cross-reacting VCA and EA, EBNA or an analogous nuclear antigen cannot be detected in HVP-carrying baboon LCL by conventional anticomplement immunofluorescence tests.   However, in recent studies employing a newly developed acid-fixed binding technique, a nuclear antigen was identified in HVP-carrying baboon cells which cross-reacts with EBV-specified EBNA (Ohno et al., 1977).

   From these preliminary data, HVP DNA carried in baboon LCL has an approximate density of 1.715-1.716 g/cm^3 corresponding to a guanine + cytosine content of 56-57%;   these values are similar to those reported for EBV.   Producer LCL appear to contain both non-integrated and integrated HVP DNA whereas the non-producer LCL contained only integrated HVP DNA.   Further studies with the latter cell line and the EBV, stably converted cell line, AW-Ramos, which contains only one EBV genome-equivalent, present in integrated form (Andersson-Anvret & Lindahl, 1977[1]), may provide a comparative means for studying integration of herpesvirus DNA in lymphoid cells.

SUMMARY

   Baboon lymphoblastoid cell lines (LCL) transformed with herpes-virus papio were evaluated for the state of HVP DNA in the cells by caesium chloride density-gradient centrifugation and DNA-cRNA filter hybridization.   Five HVP producer cultures and one non-producer culture were studied and non-integrated and integrated HVP DNA were detected in all producer cultures whereas only integrated HVP DNA could be demonstrated in the non-producer LCL.   Non-integrated HVP DNA had a density of 1.715-1.716 g/cm^3 in caesium chloride corresponding to a guanine + cytosine content of 56-57%.

----

[1] Unpublished data

ACKNOWLEDGEMENTS

These studies were supported by grants from the Swedish
Cancer Society and by contracts N01-CP-33316 and
N01-CP-33219 within the Virus Cancer Program of
the National Cancer Institute, and by grant
No. VC-185, American Cancer Society.
L. Falk is a Scholar of the Leukemia
Society of America, Inc.

REFERENCES

Adams, A. & Lindahl, T. (1975)   Epstein-Barr virus genomes with
    properties of circular DNA molecules in carrier cells.   *Proc.
    nat. Acad. Sci. (Wash.)*, *72*, 1477-1481

Deinhardt, F., Falk, L., Wolfe, L.G., Schudel, A., Nonoyama, M.,
    Lai, P., Lapin, B. & Yakovleva, L. (1977)   *Susceptibility of
    marmosets to Epstein-Barr virus-like baboon herpesviruses.*
    In: *Proceedings, Marmosets in Experimental Medicine Conference,
    Oak Ridge, 1977* (in press)

Falk, L., Deinhardt, F., Nonoyama, M., Wolfe, L.G., Bergholz, C.,
    Lapin, B., Yakovleva, L., Agrba, V., Henle, G. & Henle, W. (1976)
    Properties of a baboon lymphotropic herpesvirus related to
    Epstein-Barr virus.   *Int. J. Cancer*, *18*, 798-807

Falk, L.A., Henle, G., Henle, W., Deinhardt, F. & Schudel, A. (1977)
    Transformation of lymphocytes by *Herpesvirus papio*.   *Int. J.
    Cancer*, *20*, 219-226

Lindahl, T., Adams, A., Bjursell, G., Bornkamm, G.W., Kaschka-
    Dierich, C & Jehn, U. (1976)   Covalently closed circular duplex
    DNA of Epstein-Barr virus in a human lymphoid cell line.
    J. molec. Biol., *102*, 511-530

Ohno, S., Luka, J., Falk, L. & Klein, G. (1977)   Detection of a
    nuclear, EBNA-type antigen in apparently EBNA-negative, *Herpes-
    virus papio* (HVP) transformed lymphoid lines by the acid-fixed
    nuclear binding technique.   *Int. J. Cancer*, *20*, 941-946

ANNEALING OF ALKALI-RESISTANT HSV DNA STRANDS AND ISOLATION OF S AND L COMPONENTS

A. FRIEDMANN & M. BROIT

Department of Genetics,
The Hebrew University of Jerusalem,
Jerusalem, Israel

Y. BECKER

Laboratory for Molecular Virology,
Hebrew University-Hadassah Medical School,
Jerusalem, Israel

INTRODUCTION

The relationship of the structure of herpesvirus DNA (Clements et al., 1976; Delius & Clements, 1976; Hayward et al., 1975; Skare & Summers, 1977) to its biological activity is still not clear and the genetic information encoded in the S and L components and their function *in vivo* need to be elucidated. In this study an experimental approach is presented for isolating intact L, S and repeat sequences of herpes simplex virus type 1 (HSV-1) DNA. The rationale of the experimental approach is based on the finding that alkali denaturation of HSV DNA followed by centrifugation in an alkaline sucrose gradient yields intact HSV-1 single-stranded DNA molecules (Gordin et al., 1973; Kieff et al., 1971; Wilkie, 1973). Taking into account the isomeric structure of the viral DNA, renaturation of alkali-denatured intact virus DNA strands will yield molecular structures that are partially double-stranded. Endonuclease digestion of the reannealed molecules followed by centrifugation of the double-stranded DNA fragments in a neutral sucrose gradient results in separation of the S and L components according to their size.

MATERIALS AND METHODS

Cell and virus

Cell and virus growth conditions and purification of virions have been previously described (Becker et al., 1968).

Alkali denaturation of HSV-1 DNA

Purified virus pellets prepared from 6×10^7 infected cells were suspended in 0.5 ml of TBS[1] for five hours and then briefly sonicated to obtain a homogeneous suspension of virus particles. Sodium dodecyl sulfate (SDS) was added to a final concentration of 0.5% and pronase (nuclease free, Calbiochem, San Diego, Calif.) to 1 mg/ml and the mixture was incubated at 37°C for four hours. After this period sodium chloride was added to a final concentration of 1 M and sodium hydroxide to 0.1 N. The total volume of the reaction mixture (usually 1-1.3 ml) was layered on to a linear 5-20% (w/v) alkaline sucrose gradient prepared in TBS containing 0.1 N sodium hydroxide and centrifuged at 25 000 rpm for five hours at 20°C in the SW27 rotor of the Beckman ultracentrifuge. Fractions (1 ml) were collected by puncturing the bottom of the centrifuge tube. The radioactivity (^{3}H-methyl-thymidine) was measured in a Packard scintillation spectrophotometer using 20-μl aliquots after precipitation with 10% trichloroacetic acid (TCA). Samples from the fast-sedimenting peak in the gradient were collected and dialysed against tris-EDTA buffer (TE: 0.01 M tris hydrochloride, pH 8, 0.001 M EDTA) with several changes over a period of 10-12 hours.

Reassociation of fast-sedimenting DNA

The concentration of DNA in the fast-sedimenting peak was measured by absorption at 260 μm in a Gilford spectrophotometer and the concentration was adjusted to 0.1-0.2 μg/ml. The DNA was dialysed for two hours against 70% (w/v) formamide (Fluka, Switzerland) in TE buffer and then for four hours against 50% formamide in 10 × TE buffer at 4°C.

Spreading of reannealed DNA for electron microscopy

This was performed according to Davis et al. (1971).

S$_1$ endonuclease digestion of reannealed DNA

Reannealed DNA solutions were dialysed for 10 hours (with three changes) against a solution containing 0.01 M sodium chloride, 0.3 M sodium acetate, 3×10^{-5} M zinc chloride, pH 4.5. S$_1$ endonuclease prepared from α-amylase according to Sutton (1971) was added, and the

---

[1] TBS: 0.15 M sodium chloride, 0.05 M tris hydrochloride, pH 7.4

mixture was incubated at 37°C for 60 minutes.   The reaction mixture
was then layered on to a linear 5-20% (w/v) sucrose gradient (prepared
in TE buffer) and centrifuged at 25 000 rpm for five hours at 5°C in
the SW27 rotor.   Fractions (1 ml) were collected from the bottom of
the tubes and the radioactivity in 1.0 ml from each fraction was
measured.   Fractions from the heavy and light peaks were pooled (see
results) and dialysed against TE buffer for five hours.

Caesium chloride density-gradient centrifugation of the S₁ endonuclease-digested fractions

The pooled DNA fractions [from the linear 5-20% (w/v) sucrose
gradients] were made up to 1.700 g/cm³ with caesium chloride, and
centrifuged in the 50Ti rotor at 35 000 rpm for 70 hours at 15°C.
Fractions (15 drops) were collected from the bottom of the tubes and
the radioactivity in each fraction was measured.

RESULTS

*Electron microscope analysis of reannealed alkali-resistant HSV DNA
strands*

Analysis of the molecular structures resulting from reannealing
concentrations of HSV DNA resulting in interstrand reassociation
(< 0.1 µg/ml) revealed mainly DNA molecules with internal double-
stranded regions and single-stranded ends.   Length measurements of
the double-stranded regions revealed that some of the DNA molecules
had a double-stranded region ranging in length from 5.0 to 12.5 µm
while other DNA molecules had a double-stranded region of 32-40 µm
(Fig. 1A,B).

A quantitative analysis of the double-stranded sequences in more
than 100 DNA molecules is presented in Figure 2.   Two major types of
annealed DNA molecules can be seen.   One type had a double-stranded
sequence ranging from 5 to 12.5 µm and the other from 32 to 40 µm.
Two additional minor classes had double-stranded sequences of 14-17 µm
and 21-23 µm, respectively.   Electron microscopy of these molecules
also revealed that the single-stranded terminal regions were longer
in the DNA hybrid molecules that had double-stranded sequences of
5.0-12.5 µm than in DNA hybrid molecules that had double-stranded
regions of 32-40 µm.   Many of the double-stranded molecules of length
40 µm had only one short single-stranded end.   In addition, DNA
molecules which are fully double-stranded but have a small single-
stranded DNA circle were also seen.   Reannealed double-stranded (ds)
DNA molecules which have a contour length of 50-52.5 µm resembling
intact HSV-1 DNA molecules were also found (Fig. 2).

It is suggested that the dsDNA molecules were formed by reannealing
of two different intact alkali-resistant strands that resulted from
the denaturation of four DNA isomers present in the virion DNA

FIG. 1.   ELECTRON MICROGRAPH OF REANNEALED HSV-1 DNA
UNDER CONDITIONS ALLOWING INTERSTRAND ANNEALING

HSV-1 DNA at a concentration of 0.1-0.2 µg/ml was annealed.
(A) DNA molecule with a double-stranded central region to which long
     single strands are attached.   The length of the double-stranded
     region is 10.3 µm.
(B) A molecule with a double-stranded central region of 38.8 µm in
     length, and short single-stranded ends.   Arrows indicate the
     borders of the double-stranded regions.   Bars represent 1 µm.

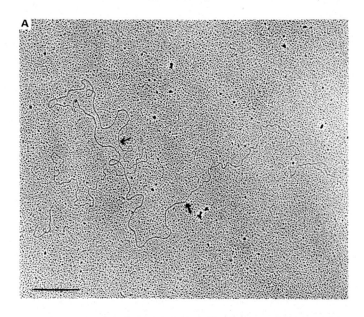

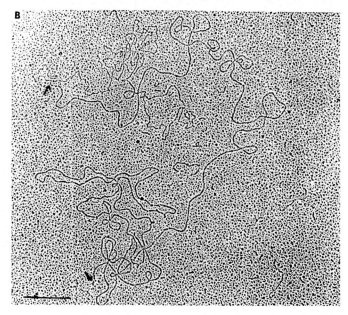

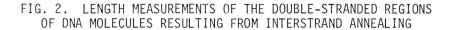

FIG. 2.   LENGTH MEASUREMENTS OF THE DOUBLE-STRANDED REGIONS
OF DNA MOLECULES RESULTING FROM INTERSTRAND ANNEALING

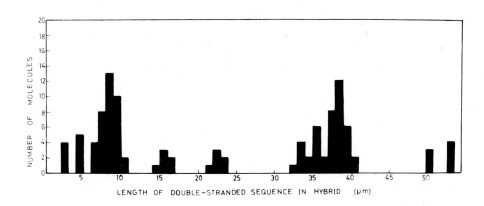

population.   Length measurements of the majority of the molecules
showed a striking resemblance to the contour length of the L and S
components of the HSV-1 DNA described by Sheldrick & Berthelot (1974).

Isolation of reannealed dsDNA sequences

To obtain the L and S components of the viral DNA the ^{3}H-thymidine
labelled reannealed DNA molecules were treated with S_1 endonuclease to
digest the single-stranded sequences present in the hybrid DNA molecules.   The double-stranded sequences were separated by centrifugation
in neutral sucrose gradients.   Two distinct bands of DNA fragments
appeared (Fig. 3).   Calculation of the average S-values of the two
bands relative to the intact double-stranded ^{14}C-thymidine labelled
HSV-1 DNA marker revealed that the average S-value of the lower band
was 48 (corresponding to approximately 75×10^6 daltons) and the upper
band had an S-value of 27 (corresponding to 18×10^6 daltons).   The
molecular weight values of these two bands correspond to the size of
the S and L components of the HSV-1 genome.   The radioactivity at
the position of intact HSV DNA molecules is due to reannealed complete
genomes (Fig. 2).

The 48S and 27S double-stranded DNA preparations (Fig. 3) were
dialysed and centrifuged in separate caesium chloride density gradients.
The mean density of the 48S double-stranded DNA fragments was slightly
less (about 1.714 g/cm[3]) than that of the complete viral DNA molecules
(Fig. 4A).   In contrast, the 27S double-stranded DNA fragments had a
mean density higher (about 1.722 g/cm[3]) than that of the intact virion

FIG. 3. NEUTRAL SUCROSE GRADIENT CENTRIFUGATION OF REANNEALED HSV-1 DENATURED DNA AFTER S_1 ENDONUCLEASE DIGESTION

^{3}H-thymidine labelled HSV-1 DNA from the fast-sedimenting band from the alkaline sucrose gradient was reannealed under conditions allowing interstrand reannealing.   The reannealed DNA was exposed to S_1 endonuclease and centrifuged in a neutral sucrose gradient (5-20%) in the SW27 rotor of the Beckman preparative ultracentrifuge. for five hours at 25 000 rpm at 20°C.   The gradient was collected dropwise and the TCA-precipitable radioactivity in 200 μl of each fraction was determined. ^{14}C-thymidine labelled purified HSV-1 DNA served as size marker.

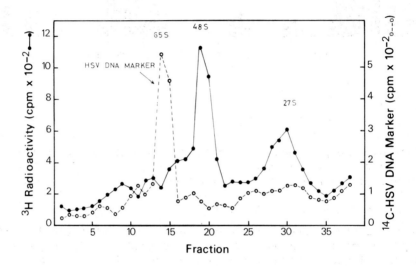

DNA (Fig. 4B) although some of the 27S DNA was lighter in density than the parental viral DNA.   The 27S double-stranded fragments may thus contain both the S region and the repeat sequences.

DISCUSSION

Reannealing of the alkali-resistant intact HSV-1 DNA strands at a concentration of 0.1-0.2 μg/ml resulted in the appearance of hybrid DNA molecules with double- and single-stranded sequences at one or both sides of the molecules.   Most of these hybrids fall into two

FIG. 4.   CAESIUM CHLORIDE EQUILIBRIUM DENSITY CENTRIFUGATION
OF THE 48S AND 27S BANDS FROM THE NEUTRAL SUCROSE GRADIENT
SHOWN IN FIG. 3

Fractions 19-21 and 28-31 of the neutral sucrose gradients were
separately pooled and made up to 1.70 g/cm^3 with caesium chloride.
The DNA was then centrifuged to equilibrium in the 50 Ti rotor
of the Beckman preparative ultracentrifuge for 72 hours at 35 000 rpm
at 20°C.   The gradient was collected dropwise and the radioactivity
in the fractions was determined. ^{14}C-thymidine labelled HSV-1 DNA
was used as density marker.

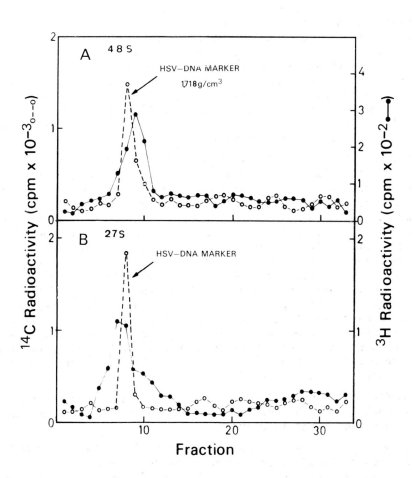

major subgroups: one with a duplex sequence of 2.5-12 μm and the second
of 32-40 μm.   The lengths correspond to the S plus repeat sequences and
to the L plus repeat sequences, respectively.   It is possible to suggest
that hybrids with a duplex of 2.5 μm indicate annealing of the terminal
repeat of the S region.   The hybridized sequences that are longer may
indicate involvement of the S sequence and the adjacent repeat sequences.
Similar hybridization of the L component with or without a repeat
sequence can be proposed.   The above data strongly suggest that the
double-stranded DNA fragments we have isolated are the S and L components
of the HSV-1 genome.   The properties of the isolated L and S components
are yet to be studied.

A possible organization of the virion DNA molecule is presented in
Figure 5A.   The four isomeric HSV DNA forms differ in the relative
arrangement of the S and L regions.   Since the exact mechanism by
which rearrangements of the L and S regions occurs is not known, there
are two possibilities: (a) rearrangement of the L and S components does
not involve any change in the DNA strands, namely the same strands are
ligated; or (b) rearrangement of the L and S regions involves ligation
of one strand to the second strand.   This leaves one component of viral
DNA unchanged while the second component will be ligated to opposite
strands (Fig. 5A).   The DNA strands are designated + and − and the
numbers denote the isomeric forms (Fig. 5A).

Three possibilities exist regarding degradation of the HSV DNA by
alkali: (a) the alkali-resistant strands could consist of all eight
single-stranded forms; (b) only the + strands are resistant to alkali,
and (c) only the − strands are alkali-resistant.   If (a) is true, the
DNA hybrids described in Figure 5B should be formed.   However, forms
B(2) and B(3) in Figure 5 have never been observed.   The only form
observed is B(1) (Fig. 5), namely intact double-stranded molecules.
These molecules constituted about 5% of the molecules measured (Fig. 2).
If (b) and (c) are true, forms C(2), C(3) and C(4) (Fig. 5) should be
seen.   Indeed, these forms did constitute the majority of the hybrid
molecules (Fig. 2 and Fig. 5D).   It is also possible to suggest that
alkali treatment results in degradation of one of the DNA strands.
If this is correct, then the hybrid DNA molecules seen in this study
favour the possibility that rearrangements of the L and S components
involve opposite ligation and suggest that the organization of the
viral DNA proposed in Figure 5 is correct.

An additional possibility is that, in one or two of the viral DNA
isomers, both strands are degraded by alkali but in the other two DNA
isomers only one strand is degraded.

Removal of the single-stranded sequences from the hybrid DNA
molecules was achieved by incubation with S_1 endonuclease which
digests single-stranded but not double-stranded DNA.   Centrifugation
in sucrose gradients yielded DNA molecules the size of the L region

FIG. 5.   HSV DNA MOLECULAR ISOMERS AND HYBRIDS

(A) Schematic illustration of the HSV-1 DNA structure and isomeric organization.   The letters designate base sequences, + and - refer to the two homologous strands of the DNA molecule. The heavy black lines mark the repeat DNA sequences flanking the S and L components (IR_L, TR_L, IR_S, TR_S); (B) Illustration of all the possible structural arrangements which can theoretically result from reannealing of the eight DNA strands resulting from denaturation of the four structural isomers shown in (A). Only +1 × all other + and - strands is shown; (C) Schematic representation of hybrid DNA molecules assuming that the same strand in each isomeric form of DNA is resistant to alkali treatment. In this case all the + strand reanneals with the other three - strands; (D) Observed reannealed structures as interpreted by us: (1) Intact HSV-1 molecule resulting from (+ × -) type reannealing; (2) The S region and its repeats reannealed; (2a) Hybridized sequences longer than the S region and its repeats; (3) Two intact strands reannealed by the L region or L and its repeats; (3a) one intact strand reannealed with a fragmented strand of the L and its repeat sequences; (4) L component reannealed. We interpret these structures as resulting from reannealing of a single intact DNA molecule with an intact L single-stranded region, the repeat sequence TR_S self-annealed to the same strand giving rise to molecules with a terminal single-stranded loop.

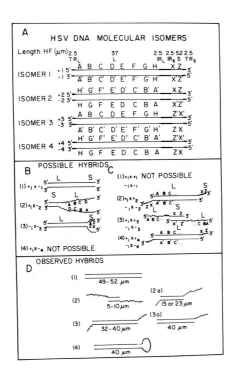

and the size of the S region with or without the repeat sequences, as
well as repeat sequences only.   Analysis in caesium chloride density
gradients revealed that the L component has a density lower than that
of the S component.   This analysis has provided additional information on the base composition of the L and S regions of HSV DNA.   It
is now possible to further study the genetic properties of the isolated
L and S components of HSV DNA.

SUMMARY

   DNA isolated from highly purified virions of herpes simplex virus
type-1 (HF strain) was denatured by centrifugation in alkaline sucrose
gradients.   DNA molecules corresponding to intact single-stranded
virion DNA (50×10^6 daltons) were isolated and adjusted to neutral
pH.   The DNA was annealed under conditions permitting reassociation
of intact single-stranded molecules and studied by electron microscopy.   Three classes of DNA molecules showing double-stranded
sequences were observed: (a) fully double-stranded DNA molecules the
size of the intact HSV DNA genome, namely 52 µm;   (b) DNA hybrids with
a region of partial double-strandedness ranging from 5 to 12 µm, plus
long single strands;   and (c) DNA hybrids with a double-stranded
region of 32-40 µm, plus short single strands.   (These results suggest
that the alkali-resistant single-stranded HSV DNA molecules are
composed of several subclasses that permit annealing of either the
total genome or the S or L components.)   The 5 µm double-stranded
region probably constitutes the S component of HSV DNA and the
sequences longer than 5 µm and shorter than 12 µm represent annealing
of the repeat sequences on either or both sides of the S component.
The double-stranded sequences with a length of 32-40 µm may represent
the L component.   Treatment of the annealed, partially double-stranded
hybrid DNA molecules with S_1 endonuclease to remove the single-stranded
termini and centrifugation in neutral sucrose gradients yielded two
distinct peaks.   Centrifugation of fractions from the two peaks in
caesium chloride density gradients showed that the small DNA component
(possibly the S and the repeat sequences) had a higher buoyant density
and the longer (possibly the L) DNA component had a lower density
than the HSV DNA marker.   Annealing of alkali-resistant viral DNA
strands therefore provides a means of isolating the L, S and repeat
sequence regions of HSV DNA.

ACKNOWLEDGEMENTS

This study was supported by Contract No 1CP 3310 within
the Virus Cancer Program of the National Cancer
Institute, and a grant (to Adam Friedmann) from
the Hebrew University Central Research Fund.

REFERENCES

Becker, Y., Dym, H. & Sarov, I. (1968)   Herpes simplex DNA.
    Virology, 36, 184-192

Clements, J.B., Cortini, R. & Wilkie, N.M. (1976)   Analysis of
    herpes DNA substructure by means of restriction endonucleases.
    J. gen. Virol., 30, 243-256

Davis, R.W., Simon, M. & Davidson, N. (1971)   Electron microscope
    heteroduplex methods for mapping regions of base sequence homology
    in nucleic acids.   *Meth. Enzym., 21*, 413-428

Delius, H. & Clements, J.B. (1976)   A partial denaturation map of
    herpes simplex virus type 1 DNA: evidence for inversion of
    unique DNA regions.   *J. gen. Virol., 33*, 125-133

Gordin, M., Olshevsky, U., Rosenkranz, H.S. & Becker, Y. (1973)
    Studies on herpes simplex virus DNA: denaturation properties.
    Virology, 55, 280-284

Hayward, E.S., Jacob, R.J., Wadsworth, S.C. & Roizman, B. (1975)
    Anatomy of herpes simplex virus DNA: evidence for four popula-
    tions of molecules that differ in relative orientation of their
    long and short components.   *Proc. nat. Acad. Sci. (Wash.), 72*,
    4243-4247

Kieff, E.D., Bachenheimer, S.L. & Roizman, B. (1971)   Size, composi-
    tion and structure of the deoxyribonucleic acid of subtype 1 and
    2 herpes simplex virus.   *J. Virol., 8*, 125-132

Sheldrick, P. & Berthelot, N. (1974)   Inverted repetitions in the
    chromosome of herpes simplex virus.   *Cold Spring Harb. Symp.
    quant. Biol., 39*, 667-678

Skare, J. & Summers, W.C. (1977)   Structure and function of herpes
    virus genomes II. Eco RI, Xba, and HindIII endonuclease cleavage
    sites on herpes simplex virus type 1 DNA.   *Virology, 76,* 581-595

Sutton, W.D. (1971)   A crude nuclease preparation suitable for use in
    DNA reassociation experiments.   *Biochim. Biophys. Acta, 24,* 522-
    531

Wilkie, N.M. (1973)   The synthesis and substructure of herpes virus
    DNA: the distribution of alkali labile single strand interrup-
    tions in HSV-1 DNA.   *J. gen. Virol., 21,* 453-467

DISCUSSION SUMMARY

N.M. WILKIE

Medical Research Council Virology Unit,
Institute of Virology,
Glasgow, UK

The initial reaction to the session might have been one of slight disappointment at the apparent slow rate of progress since the last major herpesvirus meeting at Cold Spring Harbor in 1976. It is evident, however, that this is due to the severe technical problems involved in working with large complex genomes and difficult cell systems.

Firstly, let us consider the viruses best studied at the molecular level; these are herpes simplex virus types 1 and 2 (HSV-1, HSV-2) and pseudorabies virus. The current state of knowledge of the general sequence arrangement in the genomes of a number of herpesviruses was summarized. HSV-1 DNA has now been further characterized using restriction endonucleases. It was reported that there are forms of microheterogeneity close to the joint region in strain KOS DNA as well as unit-length additions of a small sequence to the repetitious regions bounding the L region. However, studies have shown unit-length additions and deletions of a small sequence to the repetitions bounding the S region of strain Angelloti. The reasons for differences in the sequence heterogeneity between different strains remain unclear.

Defective genomes of HSV-1 have also been analysed in more detail. It is now reported that the defective DNA of HSV-1 strain Justin contains at least three types of genome, all being multiple repetitions of a basic unit which contains sequences from the repetition bounding S and from the unique S region. The three forms differ in the amount of the unique S sequence represented. It has been found that defectives from strain Angelloti can contain sequences

from the L region as well as the repetitive regions, and
have a density similar to that of normal HSV DNA, unlike
the Justin defectives.   Evidence to suggest that
"scrambling" of sequences may occur in the generation of
defective genomes has been obtained, and this might
suggest that we are dealing with some form of illegitimate
recombination.   It has also been found that the Justin
defective codes for an early mRNA, but the way in which
defective genomes interfere with the replication cycle is
still not known.

Previous work has provided evidence that virion genomes
of pseudorabies virus can be converted into circles and
concatemeric forms inside infected cells.   In the only
study of DNA replication reported to this session, it
was suggested that, at early times in the replication cycle,
DNA synthesis can be initiated on circular and linear DNA,
leading to the formation of concatemeric complexes of
limited molecular weight.   At later times, replicating
molecules are associated with much larger concatemeric or
aggregated forms.   Single strands from parental genomes
were found to be transferred to progeny molecules in an
intact manner.   This would not be expected if single
strands derived from parental molecules entered freely
into active recombinational processes round the "joint"
region between the L and S segments (this might split
them), although the results would not exclude the possibility
that some progeny DNA might replicate and/or recombine in
such a way as to split S and L.   More information about the
rate of formation of the inverted rearrangements of HSV-1,
HSV-2 and pseudorabies virus DNA is obviously required.

Marker rescue experiments, and the mapping of cross over
points in intertypic recombinants between HSV-1 and HSV-2,
have allowed fairly rapid progress in the physical mapping
of temperature-sensitive (*ts*) mutants, drug-resistant
mutants and virus-specific polypeptides.   These studies
suggest that an immediate early polypeptide, a membrane
polypeptide and a structural polypeptide can be assigned
to the S region.   Two mutants which control the transcriptional programme of the virus also appear to map in the S
sequence, although there is not yet general agreement about
the precise map location of *ts* D.   A tendency for some phosphoproteins to cluster in a region of the L unique sequence
is also noted.

The results do not allow an orientation of the genetic
map with the physical map, but several anomalies are
revealed on comparing the physical studies with the genetics.
These can be divided roughly into three categories:

(1) the recombination frequencies of markers in the
L region do not appear to be very well related to
map distances;   (2) the relative orders of the markers
in the L region are different in the genetic and
physical maps;   (3) mutants which map in the repetitive
regions bounding the S region are genetically linked to
mutants in the L unique region in such a way as to produce a linear map;   this would not be anticipated if
both forms of orientation of the L region entered freely
into recombination events.   One possible explanation of
the observed genetic linkage of mutants in the S
repetitious sequences to those in the L unique region
would be provided if only molecules with one orientation
of L could initiate replicative cycles and/or enter into
recombination events leading to viable progeny.   This
possibility was raised in discussion, and as supporting
evidence the observation was offered that several recombinants between HSV-1 and HSV-2 show the minimum number
of cross overs when drawn with one particular orientation
of the L region.   It is therefore exceedingly important
that we obtain a better understanding of the physical
structure and sequence arrangement of those molecules
involved in recombination and replicative processes.
The various anomalies may not be resolved until much
more genetic and physical mapping is carried out.
Studies were reported on the use of drug-resistance
markers in genetic studies, and when the physical
locations of such markers and the *syn* locus are known
(and we already have evidence for the location of a
phosphonoacetic acid-resistant locus), this class of
mutant will be of great use in the interpretation of
genetic crosses.

Analyses of the genomes of cytomegalovirus (CMV)
and varicella-zoster virus (VZV) continue.   It was
reported that the DNA from field isolates of virus from
patients with shingles (zoster) and chicken pox
(varicella) have identical restriction endonuclease
patterns, suggesting great similarity in genetic content.
Surprisingly, zoster DNA has a slightly different density
from that of varicella.   This would not be predicted
from the restriction endonuclease profile and we await
further developments in this area with great interest.
DNA from CMV can now be isolated as two molecular weight
forms, of 150 and 100×10^6 daltons respectively.   It
was reported that CMV DNA is infectious, although the
infectivity is substantially less than that of other
herpesvirus DNAs studied to date.   It was shown that
the sequences present in the 100×10^6 dalton form are

also present in the 150×10^6 dalton form.   On the
basis of partial denaturation mapping, it was also
suggested that the 150×10^6 dalton molecules show
sequence rearrangements and inversions similar to that
of HSV DNA.   However, the restriction endonuclease
analysis of CMV DNA is not yet sufficiently well
advanced to support the partial denaturation mapping
data.   It was further suggested that CMV might have
an inverted repetitious sequence.   If CMV has a long
and short section both of which can be inverted, we
may expect to find more inverted repetitious sequences
in this molecule.

In a study on the plasmid forms of Epstein-Barr
virus (EBV) DNA in a number of cell lines from patients
suffering from Burkitt's lymphoma, nasopharyngeal
carcinoma and infectious mononucleosis, and from normal
individuals, it was found that circles in the molecular
weight range $101-106 \times 10^6$ daltons were present.   These
values are all close to the molecular weights of linear
virion DNAs.   However, the history of B95-8 suggests
that the original virus, 883L, may have been considerably
smaller until passed through marmoset lines, where it
apparently picked up an additional 10×10^6 daltons or so.
The reason for this, or for the differing performance of
various strains in transformation assays, still remains
unclear.   It is obviously of critical importance to
establish physical maps for EBV DNA to enable detailed
comparative hybridization studies to be carried out.
As was pointed out, the popular strains P3HR-1 and B95-8,
may in fact be atypical.   The call would therefore be
to study more field isolates.

Studies have been carried out on the form of EBV
DNA present in the Ramos B cell line and cord-blood
leukocytes transformed with EBV.   It was reported that
the cord-blood leukocytes contain mainly circular plasmid
DNA whereas the Ramos line contains mainly integrated DNA.
The spectre of the problem of aggregation versus true
integration is not yet laid, as was pointed out in
discussion, but it has been found that prior treatment
of cord-blood leukocytes with the bacterial polysaccharide
B-cell mitogen results in transformed cells in which the
viral DNA now appears to be integrated.   This is a most
intriguing observation, and may offer a useful tool in
the study of EBV transformation.

Studies on herpesvirus papio (HVP), an endogenous
baboon virus, which shares sequence homology with EBV,
were presented.   Lymphoblastoid cell lines may contain

some integrated as well as free HVP DNA and further
studies with this interesting system are awaited.
T-cell lymphocytes transformed by herpesvirus saimiri
contain viral DNA in a non-integrated closed circular
form.   The circles contain two areas of repetitious
sequences which separate a small and a large unique
region.   The unique regions both contain sequences
from the L region of the virion chromosome, but lack
sequences from the left-hand end of the L region.
The plasmid DNA is therefore a kind of "defective"
genome, which may explain why these cells are not
virus producers.

Considering the current state of our knowledge of
the mechanism of transformation by herpesviruses, there
should be no mental block to prevent us examining the
notion that transformed cells, or tumour cells, might
contain only plasmid viral DNA.   However, it has to
be pointed out that solid experimental evidence is still
required, and the current hybridization techniques have
not been sufficiently refined to the point where
insertions of small subgenomic fragments of herpesvirus
DNA into the cell chromosome can be comfortably detected.

It seems likely that both CMV and EBV DNA contain
inverted repetitious sequences and it is obviously of great
importance to fit the sequence arrangement of CMV, EBV and
HPV genomes into the list that has been compiled.   The
most intriguing and obvious questions remain unanswered:
What is the significance of the inverted repetitions so
commonly observed in those herpesviruses studied to date?
Do they have something to do with the replicative
mechanism?   Do they contain control elements?   Do they
contain insertion sequences?   What are the evolutionary
origins of the various regions of the genome?   Hopefully,
the answers to at least some of the questions will be
available by the next International Symposium on Oncogenesis and Herpesviruses.

VIRAL ANTIGENS – STRAIN DIFFERENCES

THE STRUCTURAL PROTEINS AND GLYCOPROTEINS OF HERPESVIRUSES: A REVIEW

P.G. SPEAR & M. SARMIENTO

*University of Chicago,
Chicago, Ill., USA*

R. MANSERVIGI

*Istituto di Microbiologia,
Università degli Studi,
Ferrara, Italy*

INTRODUCTION

In this review attention is focused on the structural proteins and glycoproteins specified by herpesviruses. The objective is to summarize available information about the roles of these proteins in the morphogenesis and function of the virion. An underlying assumption is that certain aspects of virion structure and function should be common to all herpesviruses. Other contributions to this Symposium (Bernhard et al.[1]; Deinhardt[2]; Killington et al.[3]; Ludwig et al.[4]) and published elsewhere (Honess & Watson, 1977; Killington et al., 1977; Roizman & Furlong, 1974; Spear, 1978) have reviewed information about the polypeptide compositions of herpesviruses and about antigenic relationships between different members of the herpesvirus family.

---

[1] See p. 215

[2] See p. 169

[3] See p. 185

[4] See p. 235

THE NUCLEOCAPSID

The nucleocapsids produced by different herpesviruses are remarkably similar not only in morphology but also in certain aspects of polypeptide composition (Dolyniuk et al., 1976b; Gibson & Roizman, 1972;
Killington et al., 1977; Perdue et al., 1974; Pwelll & Watson, 1975;
Stevely, 1975). One common feature of the nucleocapsids that have so
far been characterized is a major polypeptide constituent, probably the
major hexon protein, whose molecular weight falls within the narrow
range of 140 000 - 160 000 daltons. Three to six minor polypeptide
constituents are also reproducibly observed. Although common antigens
have been detected on the nucleocapsids of biologically diverse herpesviruses (Bernhard et al.[1]; Honess et al., 1974; Kirkwood et al., 1972),
the extent to which the constituent polypeptides are similar in structure
and function remains to be determined.

The functions of the nucleocapsid proteins presumably relate to the
assembly and maintenance of this structure but no clear picture has yet
emerged as to their individual roles in nucleocapsid formation. Capsid
shells can form in the absence of viral DNA and, in studies with herpes
simplex virus (HSV), it has been shown that these empty capsids lack two
of the polypeptides normally found in nucleocapsids (Gibson & Roizman,
1972). The possibility exists that the normal pathway of morphogenesis
may require the insertion of viral DNA into preformed capsids. If
this is the case one might predict that certain of the nucleocapsid
proteins will be shown to play an active role in mediating this insertion
of the DNA. It is of interest that some of the HSV nucleocapsid
proteins can be phosphorylated (Gibson & Roizman, 1974) and that poly-
amines have been detected in HSV nucleocapsids (Gibson & Roizman,
1971). The significance of these observations is presently uncertain,
however, and it remains to be determined whether other herpesviruses
are similar in these respects.

THE PROCESS OF ENVELOPMENT

As was originally shown for herpes simplex virus type 1 (HSV-1)
(Spear & Roizman, 1972) and has now been demonstrated for several herpesviruses (Cassai et al., 1975; Dolyniuk et al., 1976a; Fiala et al.,
1976; Killington et al., 1977; Kim et al., 1976 a,b; Perdue et
al., 1974; Stevely, 1975; Stinski, 1976; Strnad & Aurelian, 1976),
virions contain approximately 20-30 polypeptides, most or all of which
appear to be virus-specified. Inasmuch as naked nucleocapsids
contain only four to eight polypeptides, it must be inferred

---

[1] See p. 215

that most of the virion polypeptides are acquired during the process of
envelopment. The acquired polypeptides include some 10-15 non-glycosylated species and about half a dozen glycoproteins, for all herpesviruses that have been analysed to date. Although the precise location
of all these proteins in virions is not known, results obtained with
HSV (Olshevsky & Becker, 1972; Roizman & Furlong, 1974; Sarmiento &
Spear[1]) and our current understanding of membrane organization indicate
that most of the herpesvirus glycoproteins will be found to be integral
membrane proteins whose carbohydrate moieties are exposed to the exterior
surface of the virion and that most of the non-glycosylated proteins
acquired during envelopment probably reside between the nucleocapsid
surface and the inner surface of the lipid bilayer of the envelope.

The primary site of herpesvirus envelopment is clearly the inner
nuclear membrane of the cell although envelopment at cytoplasmic
membranes has apparently been observed (Epstein, 1962; Fong et al.,
1973; Siminoff & Menefee, 1966; Stackpole, 1969). It has been
suggested that cytoplasmic envelopment may be the trivial consequence
of nuclear degeneration and leakage of naked nucleocapsids into the
cytoplasm (Darlington & Moss, 1969) or, alternatively, that cytoplasmic
envelopment may be the final stage of virion maturation, preceeded by
envelopment of nucleocapsids at the inner nuclear membrane and then
de-envelopment of the particles due to fusion with cytoplasmic membranes
(Stackpole, 1969). It could be argued that all the electron micrographs presented as illustrations of cytoplasmic envelopment actually
show instead the de-envelopment of virions from the perinuclear space
or endoplasmic reticulum. It is perhaps significant that most of the
published studies of this phenomenon were done with herpesviruses that
are poor producers of infectious virus in the cell systems used.
Moreover, recent studies to be discussed below raise the possibility
that certain herpesviruses may have evolved a mechanism to prevent the
fusion of progeny virions with altered membranes of the infected cell,
thus preventing the release of naked nucleocapsids into the cytoplasm
of the already infected cell and perhaps promoting the accumulation of
infectious virus.

Because envelopment of nucleocapsids is effected by budding of the
particles through a cellular membrane and because virions appear to be
devoid of normal cellular proteins, it can be inferred that extensive
reorganization of membrane constituents must occur at the site of
envelopment. This process must begin by the migration of the viral
envelope proteins from their sites of synthesis to the inner nuclear
membrane. It seems likely that the two kinds of envelope proteins,
i.e., glycoproteins and non-glycosylated proteins, migrate by different
pathways. The viral glycoproteins probably never exist in soluble
form in the cell but rather become incorporated into membranes as nascent
peptides on membrane-bound polyribosomes. This assertion is based on

---

[1] Unpublished data

earlier studies with HSV (Spear et al., 1970; Spear & Roizman, 1970) and on current ideas of membrane protein biosynthesis. The viral glycoproteins probably migrate through the membrane systems of the cell, acquiring carbohydrate moieties at specific sites along the way, with the net result that these proteins become distributed throughout the cytoplasmic and nuclear membranes of the cell.

Most of the non-glycosylated envelope proteins, on the other hand, are probably not integral membrane proteins but migrate through the cytoplasm from their sites of synthesis to the interior of the nucleus, presumably via the nuclear pores. Although the mechanisms are not understood, it seems likely that these non-glycosylated envelope proteins play key roles in mediating envelopment of the nucleocapsid. One could imagine that some of these proteins have strong affinities for the nucleocapsid surface, some for each other and some for the viral glycoproteins, and that these affinities could explain at least the congregation of proteins and nucleation events that initiate envelopment. In fact, evidence has been obtained in the case of HSV for some of the kinds of intermolecular interactions described above (Gibson & Roizman, 1972; Roizman & Furlong, 1974; Sarmiento & Spear[1]). This simple scheme does not explain, however, certain aspects of envelopment, such as the exclusion of most host proteins from the envelope and the membrane fusion that must occur in order to pinch off the budding nucleocapsid and complete the envelopment process. Moreover, one suspects that envelopment is a more dynamic process than the above description would imply and that enzymatic reactions of various kinds may be required, perhaps to alter the conformation of particular proteins as the budding process proceeds. In fact, evidence has been presented that one of the HSV nucleocapsid proteins is cleaved during envelopment (Gibson & Roizman, 1972, 1974). One could imagine that alteration of nucleocapsid structure during envelopment might be necessary in order for disassembly of the nucleocapsid to proceed efficiently as soon as it is liberated into a new host cell.

It is not yet known which of the many envelope proteins actually play essential roles in the process of envelopment but it appears that at least two of the HSV-1 glycoproteins are not required for virion morphogenesis. This conclusion is based on studies of several viral mutants. One class of mutants, which is typified by altered plaque morphology (polykaryocytes instead of clumped, rounded cells), fails to produce the glycoprotein designated $VP8(C_2)$ but yet is capable of producing infectious virions (Heine et al., 1974; Keller et al., 1970; Manservigi et al., 1977). In addition, a temperature-sensitive mutant designated HSV-1[HFEM]tsB5 fails to accumulate glycoprotein $VP7(B_2)$ at non-permissive temperature but can produce virions even though they are non-infectious (Sarmiento, Haffey & Spear[1]). Other viral mutants, particularly those with lesions in the non-glycosylated envelope

---

[1] Unpublished data

proteins, should be very useful in sorting out the requirements for
envelopment.   The appropriate mutants are apparently not yet available
or have not yet been identified.

FUNCTIONS OF THE VIRION ENVELOPE PROTEINS

It seems clear that the major function of the virion envelope is
to mediate entry of the nucleocapsid into a host cell so that infection
can be initiated.   This assertion is based on findings that naked
nucleocapsids are not infectious (Rubenstein et al., 1972; Stein et
al., 1970), that neutralizing antibodies are directed against envelope
constituents (Cohen et al., 1978; Honess & Watson, 1974; Powell et
al., 1974; Sarmiento & Spear[1]; Spear, 1975) and that absence of a
particular glycoprotein from the virion envelope results in very low
specific infectivity (Sarmiento, Haffey & Spear[1]).   The mode of entry
of virus into a host cell has been the subject of some controversy.
Dales & Silverberg (1969) originally proposed, on the basis of electron
microscopic observations, that the attachment of virions to the host-
cell surface triggered their phagocytosis, which was followed by partial
disruption of the virus and release of the DNA.   On the other hand,
Morgan et al. (1968) proposed that adsorption of the virus was followed
by fusion of the virion envelope with the cell surface membrane,
thereby liberating the nucleocapsid into the cytoplasm.   It seems
likely that the latter hypothesis is the correct one, based on electron
microscopic comparisons of the intracellular distribution of nucleocapsids after exposure of cells to purified infectious virions or to
non-infectious nucleocapsids (Abodeely et al., 1970), on findings that
one of the HSV-1 envelope proteins required for virion infectivity
plays an essential role in HSV-induced cell fusion (Manservigi et al.,
1977), and on other considerations to be discussed below.

The envelope constituents that mediate viral adsorption to and
penetration of the host cell undoubtedly include the glycoproteins,
based on findings that these proteins are exposed at the surfaces of
intact virions (Olshevsky & Becker, 1972; Roizman & Furlong, 1974;
Sarmiento & Spear[1]) and are therefore available for interactions with
cellular constituents, and on the above-mentioned findings that at
least some of the envelope glycoproteins are targets of neutralizing
antibodies.   The identification of specific functions with individual
glycoproteins has not yet been achieved for most herpesviruses and is
just beginning to be done for HSV.   HSV-1 virions contain four antigenically distinct glycoproteins designated VP8(C_2), VP7(B_2), VP8.5(A)
and VP18(D_2), and one or two other glycosylated species that may be
unrelated to the four listed above (Spear, 1976).   The glycoprotein(s)
responsible for adsorption of virions to the host cell have not yet
been identified although it is possible to rule out the participation

---

[1] Unpublished data

of VP8(C_2) and possibly also of VP7(B_2) in adsorption.   This statement
is based on findings that infectious virus can be produced in the
absence of VP8(C_2) (Heine et al., 1974; Keller et al., 1970;
Manservigi et al., 1977) and that virions lacking VP7(B_2) can bind to
cells although they cannot initiate infection (Sarmiento, Haffey &
Spear[1]).   VP18(D_2) appears to be a good candidate for the adsorption
factor, in part because it is apparently one of the targets of neutralizing antibodies (Cohen et al., 1978; Honess & Watson, 1974).

One of the HSV-1 glycoproteins required for viral penetration has
been identified as VP7(B_2).   This identification was based on studies
(Sarmiento, Haffey & Spear[1]) done with a temperature-sensitive mutant,
HSV-1[HFEM]tsB5, which fails to accumulate VP7(B_2) at non-permissive
temperature and which produces non-infectious VP7(B_2)-deficient virions
under these conditions.   It was found that these VP7(B_2)-deficient
virions could bind to cells but could not initiate infection.   The
block in infectivity could be overcome by treatment of cells to which
the virions had adsorbed with polyethylene glycol, an agent known to
promote membrane fusion.   This observation, coupled with the earlier
finding that VP7(B_2) plays an essential role in the promotion of HSV-
induced cell fusion (Manservigi et al., 1977), supports the hypothesis
that the function of virion-associated VP7(B_2) is to promote fusion
between the virion envelope and cell surface membrane.   As would be
predicted from this hypothesis, it was found that VP7(B_2) elicited the
production of neutralizing antibodies in rabbits (Sarmiento & Spear[1]).

The functions of the other HSV-1 virion glycoproteins are not
known although, as mentioned above, we can conclude that VP8(C_2) is not
required for infectivity.   It is of interest that mutants which fail
to produce VP8(C_2) usually cause extensive cell fusion, in contrast to
the clumping of cells caused by most wild-type viruses (Keller et al.,
1970; Manservigi et al., 1977).   Studies of several viral mutants and
wild-type strains have led us to conclude that the HSV fusion-promoting
activity is usually modulated or inhibited in infections with wild-type
viruses and that mutations can abrogate this inhibition, yielding
fusion-inducing variants.   Evidence has been obtained that these
mutations can occur at several genetic loci which affect the production
or properties of at least two different gene products (Ruyechan, Morse,
Knipe & Roizman[1]).   There is reason to believe that one kind of
mutation alters VP7(B_2) so that its fusion-promoting activity is no
longer suppressed whereas another kind of mutation probably eliminates
the fusion modulator.   It should be noted that some of the fusion-
inducing variants express their mutant phenotype only in certain cell
types but not in others, suggesting that cell-dependent differences in
the processing (glycosylation?) of particular viral gene products may
affect their functions.

---

[1] Unpublished data

The exact number of viral gene products that govern the nature of infected cell interactions is not yet known but certain generalizations can be made: (1) Some of the structural glycoproteins, which become incorporated into cell surface membranes as well as into virions, participate in modifying cellular interactions. (2) Cell fusion probably requires an initial adhesion between cells (analogous to virion adsorption?) prior to membrane fusion and thus may require the activities of viral gene products in addition to $VP7(B_2)$. (3) One or more viral gene products can modulate or inhibit HSV-induced cell fusion. Glycoprotein $VP8(C_2)$ seemed initially to be a good candidate for a fusion-modulating protein (Manservigi et al., 1977) but evidence has been presented that its absence does not necessarily result in the fusion-inducing phenotype (Ruyechan, Morse, Knipe & Roizman[1]). The possibility has been raised, however, that a gene which governs the expression of this glycoprotein may be closely linked to a gene for a fusion-modulator. (4) The activities of both the fusion-promoting and fusion-modulating factors may be modified not only by non-lethal mutations but also by the activities of cellular products.

Evidence for the existence of a fusion-modulating factor seems compelling even though its identity has not yet been established. We propose that the role of this factor in replication may be to prevent progeny virions from fusing with the modified membranes of the already infected cell, in order to promote accumulation of progeny virions or, stated another way, to prevent their eclipse. This phenomenon, which should be demonstrable if it exists, is conceived of as being analogous to the interference phenomenon described for retroviruses (Vogt & Ishizaki, 1966).

Although this discussion has ignored the cellular determinants of infectivity, the cellular receptors for herpesviruses will undoubtedly attract much attention in the future.

SUMMARY

The virions of different herpesviruses are similar with respect to the number and kinds of constituent polypeptides, in spite of variability in the structures of individual polypeptides. The total number of virion polypeptides and glycopeptides ranges from 20 to 30 for different viruses and, in general, no more than one-quarter of these polypeptides is detectable in naked nucleocapsids, implying that most of the virion polypeptides are acquired during the process of envelopment. Although the functions of most individual structural proteins

---

[1] Unpublished data

have not been identified, one can predict that the nucleocapsid proteins
serve primarily structural roles or may mediate packaging of the viral
genome, that the non-glycosylated envelope proteins play essential roles
in the process of envelopment and that the glycoproteins, which are
probably all exposed to the virion surface, mediate adsorption to and
penetration of the host cell.   Two of the herpes simplex virus glycoproteins have been identified as targets of neutralizing antibodies and
one of these proteins has been shown to mediate viral penetration,
probably by promoting fusion between the virion envelope and cell
surface membrane.

ACKNOWLEDGEMENTS

Work done by the authors was supported by grants to P.G. Spear
from the American Cancer Society and from the National Cancer
Institute (CA-19264).   M. Sarmiento received support as a
predoctoral fellow from Virology Training Grant
5 T01AI00238-13 and P.G. Spear is the recipient
of USPHS Research Career Development
Award 5 K04 CA 00035.

REFERENCES

Abodeely, R.A., Lawson, L.A. & Randall, C.C. (1970)   Morphology and
    entry of enveloped and deenveloped equine abortion (Herpes) virus.
    J. Virol., 5, 513-523

Cassai, E.N., Sarmiento, M. & Spear, P.G. (1975)   Comparison of the
    virion proteins specified by herpes simplex virus types 1 and 2.
    J. Virol., 16, 1327-1331

Cohen, G.H., Katze, M., Hydrean-Stern, C. & Eisenberg, R.J. (1978)
    Type-common CP-1 antigen of herpes simplex virus is associated
    with a 59,000-molecular-weight envelope glycoprotein.   J. Virol.,
    27, 172-181

Dales, S. & Silverberg, H. (1969)   Viropexis of herpes simplex virus
    by HeLa cells.   Virology, 37, 475-480

Darlington, R.W. & Moss, L.H., III (1969)   The envelope of herpes-
    virus.   Progr. med. Virol., 11, 16-45

Dolyniuk, M., Pritchett, R. & Kieff, E. (1976a)   Proteins of Epstein-
    Barr virus.   I. Analysis of the polypeptides of purified enveloped
    Epstein-Barr virus.   J. Virol., 17, 935-949

Dolyniuk, M., Wolff, E. & Kieff, E. (1976b)   Proteins of Epstein-Barr virus. II. Electrophoretic analysis of the polypeptides of the nucleocapsid and the glucosamine- and polysaccharide-containing components of enveloped virus.   *J. Virol.*, *18*, 289-297

Epstein, M.A. (1962)   Observations on the mode of release of herpes virus from infected HeLa cells.   *J. Cell Biol.*, *12*, 589-597

Fiala, M., Honess, R.W., Heiner, D.C., Heine, J.W., Murnane, J., Wallace, R. & Guze, L.B. (1976)   Cytomegalovirus proteins. I. Polypeptides of virions and dense bodies.   *J. Virol.*, *19*, 243-254

Fong, C.K.Y., Tenser, R.B., Hsiung, G.D. & Gross, P.A. (1973)   Ultrastructural studies of the envelopment and release of guinea pig herpes-like virus in cultured cells.   *Virology*, *52*, 468-477

Gibson, W. & Roizman, B. (1971)   Compartmentalization of spermine and spermidine in herpes simplex virion.   *Proc. nat. Acad. Sci. (Wash.)*, *68*, 2818-2821

Gibson, W. & Roizman, B. (1972)   Proteins specified by herpes simplex virus. VIII. Characterization and composition of multiple capsid forms of subtypes 1 and 2.   *J. Virol.*, *10*, 1044-1052

Gibson, W. & Roizman, B. (1974)   Proteins specified by herpes simplex virus. X. Staining and radiolabeling properties of B-capsid and virion proteins in polyacrylamide gels.   *J. Virol.*, *13*, 155-165

Heine, J.W., Honess, R.W., Cassai, E. & Roizman, B. (1974)   The proteins specified by herpes simplex virus. XII. The virion polypeptides of type 1 strains.   *J. Virol.*, *14*, 640-651

Honess, R.W., Powell, K.L., Robinson, D.J., Sim, C. & Watson, D.H. (1974)   Type specific and type common antigens in cells infected with herpes simplex virus type 1 and on the surfaces of naked and enveloped particles of the virus.   *J. gen. Virol.*, *22*, 159-169

Honess, R.W. & Watson, D.H. (1974)   Herpes simplex virus-specific polypeptides studies by polyacrylamide gel electrophoresis of immune precipitates.   *J. gen. Virol.*, *22*, 171-183

Honess, R.W. & Watson, D.H. (1977)   Unity and diversity in the herpesviruses.   *J. gen. Virol.*, *37*, 15-38

Keller, J.M., Spear, P.G. & Roizman, B. (1970)   The proteins specified by herpes simplex virus. III. Viruses differing in their effects on the social behavior of infected cells specify different membrane glycoproteins.   *Proc. nat. Acad. Sci. (Wash.)*, *65*, 865-871

Killington, R.A., Yeo, J., Honess, R.W., Watson, D.H., Duncan, B.E., Halliburton, I.W. & Mumford, J. (1977)   Comparative analyses of the proteins and antigens of five herpesviruses.   *J. gen. Virol.*, *37*, 297-310

Kim, K.S., Sapienza, V.J., Carp, R.I. & Moon, H.M. (1976a) Analysis of structural proteins of purified murine cytomegalovirus. *J. Virol.*, *17*, 906-915

Kim, K.S., Sapienza, V.J., Carp, R.I. & Moon, H.M. (1976b) Analysis of structural proteins of purified human cytomegalovirus. *J. Virol.*, *20*, 604-611

Kirkwood, J., Geering, G. & Old, L. (1972) *Demonstration of group- and type-specific antigens of herpesviruses.* In: Biggs, P.M., de-Thé, G. & Payne, L.N., eds, *Oncogenesis and Herpesviruses*, Lyon, International Agency for Research on Cancer (*IARC Scientific Publications* No. 2), p. 479

Manservigi, R., Spear, P.G. & Buchan, A. (1977) Cell fusion induced by herpes simplex virus is promoted and suppressed by different viral glycoproteins. *Proc. nat. Acad. Sci. (Wash.)*, *74*, 3913-3917

Morgan, C., Rose, H.M. & Mednis, B. (1968) Electron microscopy of herpes simplex virus. I. Entry. *J. Virol.*, *2*, 507-516

Olshevsky, U. & Becker, Y. (1972) Surface glycopeptides in the envelope of herpes simplex virus. *Virology*, *50*, 277-279

Perdue, M.L., Kemp, M.C., Randall, C.C. & O'Callaghan, D.J. (1974) Studies on the molecular anatomy of the L-M strain of equine herpes virus type 1: Proteins of the nucleocapsid and intact virion. *Virology*, *59*, 201-216

Powell, K.L., Buchan, A., Sim, C. & Watson, D.H. (1974) Type-specific protein in herpes simplex virus envelope reacts with neutralizing antibody. *Nature (Lond.)*, *249*, 360-361

Powell, K.L. & Watson, D.H. (1975) Some structural antigens of herpes simplex virus type 1. *J. gen. Virol.*, *29*, 167-178

Roizman, B. & Furlong, D. (1974) *The replication of herpesviruses.* In: Fraenkel-Conrat, H. & Wagner, R.R., eds, *Comprehensive Virology*, Vol. 3, New York, Plenum Press, pp. 229-403

Rubenstein, D.S., Grave-1, M. & Darlington, R. (1972) Protein kinase in enveloped herpes simplex virions. *Virology*, *50*, 287-290

Siminoff, P. & Menefee, M.G. (1966) Normal and 5-bromo-deoxyuridine-inhibited development of herpes simplex virus. An electron microscope study. *Exp. Cell Res.*, *44*, 241-255

Spear, P.G. (1975) *Glycoproteins specified by herpes simplex virus type 1: their synthesis, processing and antigenic relatedness to HSV-2 glycoproteins.* In: de-Thé, G., Epstein, M.A. & zur Hausen, H., eds, *Oncogenesis and Herpesviruses II, Part 1*, Lyon, International Agency for Research on Cancer (*IARC Scientific Publications* No. 11), pp. 49-61

Spear, P.G. (1976) Membrane proteins specified by herpes simplex viruses. I. Identification of four glycoprotein precursors and their products in type 1-infected cells. *J. Virol.*, *17*, 991-1008

Spear, P.G. (1978) *Herpesvirion envelopes and infected cell membranes.* In: Blough, H.A. & Tiffany, J.M., eds, *Cell Membranes and Viral Envelopes*, New York, Academic Press (in press)

Spear, P.G., Keller, J.M. & Roizman, B (1970) The proteins specified by herpes simplex virus. II. Viral glycoproteins associated with cellular membranes. *J. Virol.*, *5*, 123-131

Spear, P.G. & Roizman, B. (1970) The proteins specified by herpes simplex virus. IV. The site of glycosylation and accumulation of viral membrane proteins. *Proc. nat. Acad. Sci. (Wash.)*, *66*, 730-737

Spear, P.G. & Roizman, B. (1972) Proteins specified by herpes simplex virus. V. Purification and structural proteins of the herpes-virion. *J. Virol.*, *9*, 143-159

Stackpole, C.W. (1969) Herpes-type virus of the frog renal adeno-carcinoma. I. Virus development in tumor transplants maintained at low temperature. *J. Virol.*, *4*, 75-93

Stein, S., Todd, P. & Mahoney, J. (1970) Infectivity of herpes simplex virus particles with and without envelopes. *Canad. J. Microbiol.*, *16*, 953-957

Stevely, W.S. (1975) Virus-induced proteins in pseudorabies-infected cells. II. Proteins of the virion and nucleocapsid. *J. Virol.*, *16*, 944-950

Stinski, M.F. (1976) Human cytomegalovirus; Glycoproteins associated with virions and dense bodies. *J. Virol.*, *19*, 594-609

Strnad, B.C. & Aurelian, L. (1976) Proteins of herpesvirus type 2: 1. Virion, nonvirion, and antigenic polypeptides in infected cells. *Virology*, *69*, 438-452

Vogt, P.K. & Ishizaki, R. (1966) Patterns of viral interference in the avian leukosis and sarcoma complex. *Virology*, *30*, 368-375

SIMILARITIES AND DIFFERENCES BETWEEN VARIOUS HERPESVIRUSES: A REVIEW

F. DEINHARDT & H. WOLF

*Max v. Pettenkofer-Institute of Hygiene and
Medical Microbiology of the
University of Munich,
Munich, Federal Republic of Germany*

VIRUS CLASSIFICATION

Herpesviruses can be divided into four groups, as has been suggested by the Herpesvirus Study Group of the International Committee for the Nomenclature of Viruses. The proposed provisional classification of herpesviruses appears at the back of this present volume (see p. 1079). Some comments on the proposed classification are given below.

Alphaherpesviridae

Primary infections with alphaherpesviridae, such as the prototype, human herpesvirus 1 (herpes simplex type 1), in their natural hosts are usually followed by a self-limited acute, but not fatal disease, whereas transmission to other than their natural host species not infrequently results in a more severe and frequently fatal disease. Generalized fatal diseases also occur if primary infections take place in newborn or very young individuals, e.g., the almost always fatal infection of newborn human babies with herpes simplex virus (herpes neonatorum or Hass disease). Primary infections are usually followed by a lifelong persistence of the virus and reactivations occur not infrequently during the lifetime of the individual. Abortive cycles of virus multiplication may induce or enhance cell transformation at least under experimental conditions and association of some of the members of this group of herpesviruses with naturally occuring carcinoma has been claimed.

Betaherpesviridae

These comprise the group of cytomegaloviruses.   They generally cause a harmless acute disease after primary infection but, like the alphaherpesviridae, often persist for long periods of time and probably throughout the lifetime of the individual; they can become activated during other diseases or as a result of stress and cause severe disease in patients with impaired immune mechanisms.   Some cases of infectious mononucleosis in man, particularly those following blood transfusions, are due to human cytomegalovirus (human herpesvirus 5) and congenital infections can lead to various pathological conditions in the newborn. Cytomegaloviruses, under experimental conditions, have induced a lympho-proliferative disease in monkeys, have been reported to cause transfor-mation of fibroblastoid cells *in vitro* (Deichmann[1];   Geder et al.[2]; Rapp & Shillitoe[3]) and are said to be associated with Kaposi's sarcoma (Glaser et al., 1977;   Giraldo et al., 1972).

Gammaherpesviridae

Epstein-Barr virus (EBV) of man, the Epstein-Barr virus-like agents of non-human primates, Marek's disease virus of chickens and herpes-virus of turkeys are typical representatives of this group.

Gammaherpesviruses are the cause of benign or malignant lymphopro-liferative diseases, such as infectious mononucleosis, and probably some forms of lymphoma (Burkitt's lymphoma) and anaplastic naso-pharyngeal carcinoma (NPC) in man, experimentally induced lymphoblastic leukaemias or lymphomas in non-human primates and neurolymphomatosis or Marek's disease in chickens.   Primary infections are followed by a lifelong carrier state, but reactivations do not seem to occur as fre-quently as with alpha- or bethaherpesviruses.   Reactivations of EBV in man, with a serological response but without recurrent disease, have recently been described.   The exact mechanisms - primary infection, reactivation of a persisting infection or reinfection from the outside - whereby EBV contributes to Burkitt's lymphoma or nasopharyngeal carcinoma are, however, not known.

Unclassified herpesviridae

Other currently unclassifiable herpesviridae, e.g., the herpes-viruses of catfish and frogs, have not been studied as extensively as the mammalian and avian herpesviruses;   the association of the herpes-virus of frogs (Lucké herpesvirus) with kidney carcinomas is, however, of special interest.

----

[1] Personal communication

[2] See p. 591

[3] See p. 431

GENERAL COMPARISON OF THE VARIOUS GROUPS OF HERPESVIRIDAE

Most animal species which have been adequately studied harbour
their own herpesviruses of the alpha, beta and possibly also gamma
groups.   Space does not allow a comparative review of all the characteristics of these various types of herpesviruses.   Information on the
proteins has been provided by Spear et al[1] and specific aspects
of base composition, size, structure and restriction enzyme analysis
of the DNA of different herpesvirus groups have been discussed by zur
Hausen et al[2] and Sheldrick[3].   Only a few general characteristics
require emphasis.   All herpesviruses are transmitted horizontally
and the primary acute infections are usually followed by a lifelong
carrier state.   Reactivations of the viruses occur not infrequently
and may be triggered by other diseases, fever, exposure to UV light,
stress or a decrease in immune surveillance.   Virus isolates of the
same group and from the same animal species are not necessarily identical, but may show biological, biochemical and possibly antigenic
differences, e.g., the differences observed between various EBV
isolates of man or between herpesvirus saimiri (HVS) or herpesvirus
ateles (HVA) isolates of New-World non-human primates.   There is,
however, at least a partial antigenic cross-reactivity and partial
DNA homology among the viruses within individual groups - at least
between the viruses of the same or more closely related animal species -
whereas there are no similar relationships between the viruses of
different groups.

GAMMAHERPESVIRIDAE OF PRIMATES

The remainder of this discussion will be limited to the gammaherpesviridae of primates.   If we compare these viruses, the following
emerges.   Epstein-Barr virus-like agents apparently exist in many Old-
World non-human primate species (Gerber et al., 1976; Falk et al., 1976;
Rabin et al., 1977; Rasheed et al., 1977); they all share some common
antigen among themselves and with EBV of man, they are all associated with
B-lymphocytes, they have not been shown to cause lytic infections in
non-lymphocytic cells, and have a 30-60% homology between their DNAs
and EBV DNA.   Similar agents isolated from New-World monkeys, herpesvirus saimiri (HVS) and herpesvirus ateles (HVA), in contrast, infect
only lymphocytic cells with T-cell markers, cause lytic infections in

---

[1] See p. 157

[2] See p. 3

[3] Unpublished data

non-lymphoid cells, and although they share common antigens and
partial DNA homology among themselves, do not cross-react with the
EBV-like viruses of the Old-World primates and there is no DNA homology between the two types of viruses. Although there is extensive
antigenic overlapping between, for example, HVS and HVA, there is
only a 30% DNA homology and even various isolates of HVA which appear
antigenically identical can be distinguished from each other by
differences in their DNA sequences (Fleckenstein et al., 1978).
The same holds true for the EBV-like viruses of Old-World primates
and EBV of man, which all share very similar or identical viral
capsid and early antigens, but differ in their virus-determined
nuclear antigens (Klein et al., 1978; Ohno et al., 1978) and the
EBV-like agents of chimpanzees (Gerber et al., 1976) or baboons (Falk
et al., 1976) which share only a 40% DNA homology with EBV of man.
In addition, even different EBV isolates of man do not have identical
DNAs; thus the DNA of EBV isolated from an infectious mononucleosis
patient has been reported to lack 12-15% of the sequences present in
EBV isolated from Burkitt's lymphoma (Pritchett et al., 1975).

On the basis of their biological behaviour, we can distinguish
between EBV strains which can lytically infect but not transform and
those which can transform or lytically infect. We recognize the
difference between Marek's disease virus of chickens and the non-
pathogenic, but otherwise very similar herpesvirus of turkeys, and
recently an HVS variant has been isolated which will infect marmosets,
inducing a lifelong carrier state, but will not cause lymphomatous
disease (Schaffer et al., 1975). The antigens of the non-pathogenic
HVS variant seem to be unaltered, if compared to the wild parent
strain of HVS, but the respective DNAs of the oncogenic and non-
oncogenic strains of HVS have not been compared as yet. All of the
EBV-like agents isolated from various baboons suffering from lymphomatous disease and kept at a primate colony in Sukhumi, USSR, as well as
from healthy baboons from colonies kept in the USA, appear to be
antigenically identical; their DNAs have not been compared, but
initial results might indicate a difference in their biological
characteristics. The isolate from a lymphomatous baboon has induced
lymphoproliferative disease in inoculated marmosets, whereas an antigenically very similar or identical isolate from a normal baboon has
not, but both viruses transform lymphocytes *in vitro* (Deinhardt et
al., 1978; Falk et al., 1977). However, these are only preliminary
results obtained in only a few animals, and need extension and confirmation. The disease induced in the inoculated marmosets in these
first experiments is similar to an extremely severe mononucleosis,
rather than a true lymphoma. Some animals succumbed to this disease
during the acute stage, whereas others which survived the early stage
of severe generalized lymphoproliferation, recovered completely without subsequent development of lymphoma or other lymphadenopathies.
They have now been observed for more than a year and are under further
surveillance.

Our knowledge of the pathogenic mechanisms operative in all of
these different virus host-cell or virus host-organism interactions,
however, has not proceeded much beyond the descriptive stage.   We do
not know how to relate differences in the DNAs of individual virus
strains to their biological functions.   We do not know, for example,
why HVA will readily transform lymphocytic cells with T-cell characteristics in cell culture but HVS will not, or only very occasionally
(although both viruses cause T-cell lymphoproliferation *in vivo*), or
what determines the difference in host range between HVS and HVA in
the infection of non-lymphocytic primary and continuous primate cell
cultures.

A discussion of the mechanisms which govern the outcome of EBV
infections, namely subclinical silent infections, infectious mononucleosis, or possibly Burkitt's lymphoma, or nasopharyngeal carcinoma,
cannot be given in this short summary and it can be stated only that
at least part of the pathogenesis of these infections is certainly
host and not virus controlled.   It is not known whether, in addition,
differences in EBV strains by themselves or in conjunction with host
or other influences play a role in determining the course of EBV
infections.   Equally puzzling is the difference between the absolutely
silent primary and subsequent persistent infection of squirrel or spider
monkeys with HVS or HVA and the highly malignant invariably fatal
disease these agents cause in several other non-human primate species.
In this instance it is the same virus, and not different virus strains,
which causes this vastly different response in the infected host.
Differences in the immune responses have been made responsible for
varying clinical results (Klein et al., 1973), but this alone is not
entirely satisfactory.   It might be that the viral DNA is incorporated
into the cell genome in different animal species at different sites or
that expression of episomal genomes is partially and/or differently
restricted in cells of one species but not of others.   The isolation
of a non-pathogenic mutant of HVS, the availability of a number of
HVA isolates which are all highly pathogenic yet differ in their DNA
sequences and the recognition of EBV-like agents with different
characteristics in various non-human primates have given us the tools
which should make it possible to unravel some of the mysteries of
the pathogenesis of the infections caused by this group of herpesviruses, thus giving us a better understanding of the mechanisms of
transformation of lymphoblastoid cells by some members of this group.
Beyond this, it is of interest to note that the interrelationships
of these herpesviruses mirror the phylogenetic relationships of their
natural hosts.   In addition to further studies of the biology and
biochemistry of EBV, it will therefore be of particular importance to
investigate which, if any, benign or malignant diseases are caused by
the non-human primate herpesviruses of both the Old and New World
under natural conditions in their original hosts.

REFERENCES

Deinhardt, F., Falk, L., Wolfe, L.G., Schudel, A., Nonoyama, M.,
    Lai, P. & Yakovleva, L. (1978)   Susceptibility of marmosets to
    Epstein-Barr virus-like baboon herpesviruses.   *Prim. Med., 10,*
    163-170

Falk, L., Deinhardt, F., Nonoyama, M., Wolfe, L., Bergholz, C.,
    Lapin, B., Yakovleva, L., Agrba, V., Henle, G. & Henle, W.
    (1976)   Properties of a baboon lymphotropic herpesvirus related
    to Epstein-Barr virus.   *Int. J. Cancer, 18,* 798-807

Falk, L., Henle, G., Henle, W., Deinhardt, F. & Schudel, A. (1977)
    Transformation of lymphocytes by herpesvirus papio.   *Int. J.
    Cancer, 20,* 219-226

Fleckenstein, B., Bornkamm, G., Werner, F.-J., Daniel, M., Falk, L.,
    Mulder, C. & Delius, H. (1978)   Herpesvirus ateles DNA and its
    homology with herpesvirus saimiri nucleic acid.   *J. Virol., 25*
    361-373

Gerber, P., Pritchett, R. & Kieff, E. (1976)   Antigens and DNA of
    a chimpanzee agent related to Epstein-Barr virus.   *J. Virol.,
    19,* 1090-1099

Giraldo, G., Beth, E., Coeur, P., Vogel, C. & Dhru, D. (1972)
    A new model in the search for viruses associated with human
    malignancies.   *J. nat. Cancer Inst., 49,* 1495-1507

Glaser, R., Geder, L., St. Jeor, S., Michelson-Fiske, S. & Haguenau,
    F. (1977)   Partial characterization of a herpes-type virus (K9V)
    derived from Kaposi's sarcoma.   *J. nat. Cancer Inst., 59,* 55-60

Klein, G., Pearson, G., Rabson, A., Ablashi, D., Falk, L., Wolfe, L.,
    Deinhardt, F. & Rabin, H. (1973)   Antibody reactions to herpes-
    virus saimiri (HVS)-induced early and late antigens (EA and LA)
    in HVS-infected squirrel, marmoset and owl monkeys.   *Int. J.
    Cancer, 12,* 270-289

Klein, G., Falk, L. & Falk, K. (1978)   Antigen-inducing ability
    of herpesvirus papio in human and baboon lymphoma lines, compared
    to Epstein-Barr virus.   *Int. J. Cancer* (in press)

Ohno, S., Luka, J., Falk, L. & Klein, G. (1978)   Detection of a
    nuclear, EBNA-type antigen in apparently EBNA-negative, herpes-
    virus papio (HVP)-transformed lymphoid lines by the acid-fixed
    nuclear binding technique.   *Int. J. Cancer, 20 ,* 941-946

Pritchett, R., Hayward, S. & Kieff, E. (1975)   DNA of Epstein-Barr
    virus. I. Comparative studies of the DNA of Epstein-Barr virus
    from HR-1 and B95-8 cells: size, structure and relatedness.
    J. Virol., *15*, 556-564

Rabin, H., Neubauer, R., Hopkins, R., Dzhikidze, E., Shevtsova, Z.
    & Lapin, B. (1977)   Transforming activity and antigenicity of
    an Epstein-Barr-like virus from lymphoblastoid cell lines of
    baboons with lymphoid disease. *Intervirology*, *8*, 240-249

Rasheed, S., Rongey, R.W., Bruszweski, J., Nelson-Rees, W.A., Rabin,
    H., Neubauer, R.H., Esra, G. & Gardner, M.B. (1977)   Establish-
    ment of a cell line with associated Epstein-Barr-like virus from
    a leukemic orangutan. *Science*, *198*, 407-409

Schaffer, P., Falk, L. & Deinhardt, F. (1975)   Attenuation of
    herpesvirus saimiri for marmosets after successive passage in
    cell culture at 39°C. *J. nat. Cancer Inst.*, *55*, 1243-1254

NEUTRALIZATION KINETIC STUDIES WITH GENITAL CYTOMEGALOVIRUS ISOLATES, AN ANTIGENICALLY VARIABLE GROUP

T.H. WELLER, J.L. WANER, D.R. HOPKINS & E.N. ALLRED

The Department of Tropical Public Health,
Harvard School of Public Health,
Boston, Massachusetts, USA

In 1960, we observed that sera from congenitally infected infants exhibited greater neutralizing activity for homologous strains of cytomegalovirus (CMV) than for heterologous strains (Weller et al., 1960). Although the thesis is not accepted by all, evidence continues to accrue in support of the view that isolates of human cytomegalovirus are antigenically heterogeneous. For example, Andersen (1970) also reported that some patients developed higher neutralizing titres against homologous than against heterologous strains of virus. Various investigators have observed that CMV antigens exhibit a degree of strain specificity in the complement-fixation (CF) reaction (Weller, 1971); indeed, in our longitudinal study of CMV CF seroreactivity in adults wherein sera were examined with antigens representing three strains, antigen prepared from the AD169 strain failed to react with 17% of 321 sera positive on examination with two other antigens (Waner et al., 1973). Chiang et al. (1970) noted strain differences when human sera were used in an immunofluorescence test. The introduction in 1969 of techniques yielding CMV antisera in non-primates (Hampar et al., 1969; Krech & Jung, 1969) eliminated human host-associated problems and opened the way for more refined studies. In the first attempt to apply kinetic neutralization studies with rabbit antisera, Andersen (1972) concluded that four strains shared neutralizing antigens but that there was no antigenic identity. Later, Gönczöl & Andersen (1974) observed even greater variation between strains when the same antisera were used in membrane-fluorescence studies. Recently, Huang et al. (1976) utilized guineapig antisera against twelve strains, including two genital isolates, in complement-fixation tests; a high degree of antigenic heterogeneity was recorded.

The high frequency of CMV infections of the female genital tract, first demonstrated in the pregnant female (Alexander, 1967; Medearis et al., 1970; Numazaki et al., 1970) and then in sexually active women (Jordan et al., 1973; Wentworth et al., 1973), has focused attention on CMV infection as a venereal disease. Venereal transmission of CMV was further indicated by the demonstration of virus in human semen (Lang & Kummer, 1972). Recognition that genital infections were frequent, together with the accumulating evidence that the human cytomegaloviruses exhibit antigenic heterogeneity, has raised the question of the existence of human CMV groupings analogous to those of herpes simplex virus types 1 and 2. We here report kinetic neutralization experiments on genital and non-genital strains addressing this question.

MATERIALS AND METHODS

Strains of virus

Three established CMV strains, Davis (51st passage) and Esp. (53rd passage) from congenital infections (Weller et al., 1957) and an adenoidal isolate, AD169 (82nd passage) (Rowe et al., 1956), were studied. Five cervical isolates, Berg., Jack., Scott, Walsh and Wood at the 6th to the 11th culture passage, constituted the genital strains (Waner et al., 1977). All have been maintained in our laboratory since isolation.

Preparation of antisera

When inoculated cultures of human embryonic lung fibroblasts (maintained on Eagle's minimal essential medium with Hanks' salts, plus 5% inactivated fetal calf serum, 35 mg % sodium bicarbonate, 100 µg/ml penicillin, and 100 µg/ml streptomycin) showed 90% cytopathic involvement, the cells were harvested mechanically, washed twice in glycine-buffered saline (0.15 M, pH 8.5) (GBS), pelleted by centrifugation at 250 g, and the sediment then resuspended in 0.5 M (pH 8.5) GBS for storage at -20°C. For use, the thawed concentrate was disrupted either by sonication or mechanically with a Ten Broeck tissue grinder, and extracted in GBS for 24 hours at 4°C. After clarification by low-speed centrifugation (250 g), the supernatant constituted the immunogen. Mature, white, female New Zealand rabbits received as initial inocula 4-6 ml of equal parts of immunogen emulsified with Freund's complete adjuvant; this was given in equal amounts subscapularly and intramuscularly in the thigh. Two weeks later, 4 ml of immunogen without adjuvant were similarly injected and antisera were harvested 21-30 days, or in one instance 69 days, after the initial injection. In this study we employed antisera against four cervical and two established CMV strains.

Kinetic neutralization assay

The method was an adaptation of that of McBride (1959) for polio-virus. Titrations of cell-free virus and of virus-serum mixtures were done with 0.2 ml samples by a plaque technique using human fibroblast cultures grown in wells (16 mm diameter) in plastic trays (Costar No. 3524), maintained at 36°C in a humidified 5% carbon dioxide atmosphere. Each sample was examined in triplicate. After an absorption period of one hour at 36°C, the cultures were washed once with diluent, and overlaid with maintenance medium containing 2.5% methyl cellulose. One to two weeks later the overlay was removed, and the cultures fixed and stained for subsequent counting of plaques, which was done microscopically. In analysing the results, wells containing more than 175 or fewer than 15 plaques were excluded.

Cell-free virus stocks were diluted for use to a concentration of 10^3-10^5 PFU/ml. Depending on potency, rabbit antisera were used at a final dilution of 1:12.5 - 1:125, and complement was added in the form of non-inactivated 25% guineapig serum. All materials were diluted in tissue culture medium, and prewarmed in a 37°C water bath for 10 minutes before 0.4 ml of the virus, 0.4 ml of the antiserum, and 0.2 ml of the guineapig serum working dilutions were thoroughly mixed in a 13 × 100 mm capped tube. At four minutes after mixing 0.2 ml was withdrawn, rapidly diluted 1:10, 1:100, and 1:1000 in medium, and each dilution then plaque assayed in triplicate, and the counts averaged. Similar dilutions and assays were done at eight minutes and at 12 minutes. As a control in each test, comparable amounts of preimmunization rabbit sera were mixed with diluted virus and complement. This mixture was assayed immediately and again 15 minutes later; non-specific decay of titre in excess of 0.1 log invalidated a test.

The results of assays of surviving virus for each period in a neutralization test were plotted on a logarithmic scale against time on a linear scale. For each temporal point the velocity constant K was calculated after McBride (1959). Mean K-values were determined using those points approaching linearity, usually the four- and eight-minute readings. The results of a test were discarded if there was a non-linear fall in viral titre in excess of 0.15 log in two successive four-minute periods or if the titre rose more than 0.1 log over a four-minute period. Figure 1 illustrates the methodology, and depicts results obtained with an AD169 rabbit antiserum and four CMV strains.

To compare the results obtained with different sera the K-values were normalized. Homologous viral-serum values were expressed as 100, and the proportional rate at which a serum neutralized a heterologous virus calculated, i.e., the *NK*-value.

FIG. 1. REPRESENTATIVE KINETIC NEUTRALIZATION RESULTS
WITH AD169 RABBIT ANTISERUM AND TWO ESTABLISHED ISOLATES
AND TWO GENITAL ISOLATES OF CYTOMEGALOVIRUS

Mean K-values are given with the standard deviation; figures in
parenthesis indicate the number of points used in determination of
the mean.

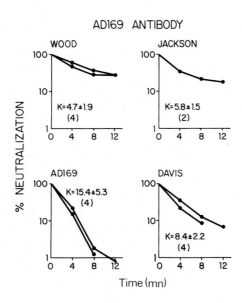

RESULTS AND DISCUSSION

A total of 42 CMV virus-antisera combinations were examined in
the course of performing 151 kinetic neutralization tests that satis-
fied stated criteria, the majority of the pairs being examined two or
three times.   Mean K-values were calculated for each combination and
used to derive the NK-values summarized in Table 1.   The data do not
suggest that genital CMV isolates constitute an antigenically distinct
group.

Unidirectional cross-neutralization patterns, comparable to those
noted by Huang et al. (1976) in their complement-fixation studies with
purified virus provide a confusing picture; for example, Berg. antisera yielded a high NK-value with AD169 virus, whereas AD169 antisera

Table 1. Summary of *NK*-values obtained on examination of eight CMV strains with rabbit antisera prepared against two classical and four genital isolates

CMV virus strain	*NK*-values with CMV rabbit antisera					
	Classical strains		Genital strains			
	AD169	Davis	Berg.	Jack.	Scott	Walsh
AD169	100	63	131	71	60	216
ESP-congenital	60	173	66	91	60	155
Davis-congenital	59	100	64	73	-	-
Wood-genital	31	42	59	30	-	124
Berg.-genital	25	59	100	108	63	110
Jack.-genital	38	51	84	100	45	-
Scott-genital	91	231	82	110	100	226
Walsh-genital	60	-	-	58	50	100

had minimal activity against Berg. virus. However, the data suggest that antisera prepared from selected strains such as Walsh may be broadly reactive and therefore potentially useful as a diagnostic antiserum; however, some reservations are in order, since the Walsh antisera were of comparatively low titre and we have observed that high titred sera are usually more discriminatory in strain differentiation. Conversely, strains such as Scott might be selected as a diagnostic antigen because of breadth of activity in serological tests.

We do not know whether the antigenic mosaic of a CMV strain undergoes alteration on prolonged cultivation *in vitro*. In this study, the genital isolates were used at the 6th to 11th passage level; at the other extreme, the strain of AD169 studied by Huang et al. (1976) was at the 285th passage level. Whether or not analysis of low-passage isolates reflects the situation *in vivo* remains problematic. However, the human CMV appear antigenically complex and heterogeneous with a mosaic of components shared in varying amounts. No grouping is now possible although certain strains are polar, such as Davis and AD169, and are quite distinct. The findings emphasize problems now inherent in preparation of diagnostic reagents and in the contemplation of an effective prophylactic vaccine.

SUMMARY

Antisera were prepared in rabbits against four low-passage genital
isolates, and against two established strains of human cytomegalovirus.
With these sera, and seven strains of virus, 42 virus-antisera combinations were examined by kinetic neutralization procedures, and *NK*-
values derived.   No evidence accrued indicating that the five genital
isolates constituted an antigenically distinct group.   The findings
support the view that the human cytomegaloviruses are antigenically
heterogeneous, with different strains reflecting an antigenic mosaic,
the elements of which are present in varying amounts.

ACKNOWLEDGEMENTS

This work was supported in part by Research Grants
AI-01023 and AI-12381 from the National Institutes
of Health.

REFERENCES

Alexander, E.R. (1967)   Maternal and neonatal infection with cyto-
    megalovirus in Taiwan.   *Pediat. Res., 1*, 210

Andersen, H.K. (1970)   Complement-fixing and virus neutralizing
    antibodies in cytomegalovirus infection as measured against
    homologous and heterologous antigen.   *Acta path. microbiol. scand.,*
    [*B*], *78*, 504-508

Andersen, H.K. (1972)   Studies of human cytomegalovirus strain
    variations by kinetic neutralization tests.   *Arch. ges. Virus-
    forsch., 38*, 297-305

Chiang, W.-T., Wentworth, B.B. & Alexander, E.R. (1970)   The use of
    an immunofluorescence technique for the determination of anti-
    bodies to cytomegalovirus strains in human sera.   *J. Immun.,
    104*, 992-999

Gönczöl, E. & Andersen, H.K. (1974)   Studies on human cytomegalo-virus strain variations by membrane-fluorescence. *Arch. ges. Virusforsch.*, *44*, 147-149

Hampar, B., Martos, L.M., Ablashi, D.V., Siguenza, R.F. & Wells, G.A. (1969)   Differentiation of cross-reacting simian cytomegalovirus strains by late 19S rabbit neutralizing antibodies. *J. Immun.*, *103*, 1155-1156

Huang, E.-S., Kilpatrick, B.A., Huang, Y.-T. & Pagano, J.S. (1976) Detection of human cytomegalovirus and analysis of strain variation. *Yale J. Biol. Med.*, *49*, 29-43

Jordan, M.C., Rosseau, W.E., Noble, G.R., Stewart, J.A. & Chin, T.D. (1973)   Association of cervical cytomegalovirus with venereal disease. *New Engl. J. Med.*, *288*, 932-934

Krech, U. & Jung, M. (1969)   The development of neutralizing anti-bodies in guinea pigs following immunization with human cyto-megalovirus. *Arch. ges. Virusforsch.*, *28*, 248-250

Lang, D.J. & Kummer, J.F. (1972)   Demonstration of cytomegalovirus in semen. *New Engl. J. Med.*, *287*, 756-758

McBride, W.D. (1959)   Antigenic analysis of poliovirus by kinetic studies of serum neutralization. *Virology*, *7*, 45-58

Medearis, D.N., Jr, Montgomery, R. & Youngblood, L. (1970)   Cyto-megalovirus infection of the female genital tract. *Pediat. Res.*, *4*, 461

Numazaki, Y., Yano, N., Morizuka, T., Takai, S. & Ishida, N. (1970) Primary infection with human cytomegalovirus: virus isolation from healthy infants and pregnant women. *Amer. J. Epidem.*, *91*, 410-417

Rowe, W.P., Hartley, J.W., Waterman, S., Turner, H.C. & Huebner, R.J. (1956)   Cytopathic agent resembling human salivary gland virus recovered from tissue cultures of human adenoids. *Proc. Soc. exp. Biol. (N.Y.)*, *92*, 418-424

Waner, J.L., Weller, T.H. & Kevy, S.V. (1973)   Patterns of cytomegalo-viral complement-fixing activity: a longitudinal study of blood donors. *J. infect. Dis.*, *127*, 538-543

Waner, J.L., Hopkins, D.R., Weller, T.H. & Allred, E.N. (1977) Cervical excretion of cytomegalovirus; correlation with secretory and humoral antibody. *J. infect. Dis.*, *136*, 805-809

Weller, T.H. (1971)   The cytomegaloviruses: ubiquitous agents with protean clinical manifestations. *New Engl. J. Med.*, *285*, 203-214, 267-274

Weller, T.H., Macaulay, J.C., Craig, J.M. & Wirth, P. (1957) Isolation of intranuclear inclusion producing agents from infants with illnesses resembling cytomegalic inclusion disease. *Proc. Soc. exp. Biol. (N.Y.)*, *92*, 418-424

Weller, T.H., Hanshaw, J.B. & Scott, D.E. (1960)   Serologic differ-
    entiation of viruses responsible for cytomegalic inclusion disease.
    Virology, 12, 130-132

Wentworth, B.B., Bonin, P., Holmes, K.K., Gutman, L., Wiesner, P. &
    Alexander, E.R. (1973)   Isolation of viruses, bacteria and other
    organisms from venereal disease clinic patients; methodology and
    problems associated with multiple isolations.   *Hlth Lab. Sci.,*
    10, 75-81

OBSERVATIONS ON ANTIGENIC RELATEDNESS BETWEEN VIRUSES OF THE HERPES SIMPLEX "NEUTROSERON"

R.A. KILLINGTON, R.E. RANDALL, J. YEO, R.W. HONESS,
I.W. HALLIBURTON & D.H. WATSON

*Department of Microbiology,
School of Medicine,
University of Leeds,
Leeds, UK*

At least four herpesviruses show significant cross-neutralization with herpes simplex virus type 1 (HSV-1) viz. herpes simplex type 2 (HSV-2), B-virus, SA8 virus and bovine mammillitis virus (BMV), and many other herpesviruses have been linked to herpes simplex virus by other serological means (Honess & Watson, 1977). We have proposed that herpesviruses sharing any common amino-acid sequences as demonstrated by serological means be designated as members of the same "seron" and that viruses which are linked by the more specific reaction of cross-neutralization of virus infectivity be named as members of the same "neutroseron" (Honess & Watson, 1977). Thus HSV-1, HSV-2 and BMV cross-neutralize (Killington et al., 1977; Sterz et al., 1973/74) and therefore form part of a neutroseron.

We are concerned with determining the relationship between conserved and divergent antigenic reactivity of herpesviruses and its molecular basis and we present here further information on the nature of some conserved and divergent antigenic reactivities within a neutroseron, as exemplified by HSV-1, HSV-2 and BMV.

COMMON ANTIGENIC SITES ARE BORNE ON NON-IDENTICAL POLYPEPTIDES

Herpes simplex virus types 1 and 2 share at least six antigenic determinants as demonstrated by gel immunodiffusion and each virus has at least five antigens which are type-specific (Honess et al., 1974). BMV also shares more than four antigens with HSV-1 and HSV-2 and at least some of these antigens are a subset of those shared by HSV-1 and HSV-2 (Killington et al., 1977).

Cells infected with HSV-1 and HSV-2 synthesize some 50 polypeptides which appear to be virus-specific and although viruses of the two types produce a similar number and size range of infected-cell polypeptides (ICP) few of these polypeptides are identical in size (Halliburton et al., 1977; Honess & Roizman, 1973; Powell et al., 1977). We have shown elsewhere that a subset of these infected-cell polypeptides is efficiently precipitated from supernatant fractions of infected cells by homologous antisera (Honess & Watson, 1974).

An experiment in which HSV-1 (strain HFEM) polypeptides are precipitated from infected cells labelled with ^{35}S-methionine is illustrated in Figure 1. In this experiment we also show the changes in the population of polypeptides precipitated at widely differing ratios of immune serum to infected-cell extract. Increasing additions of antiserum to a constant volume of antigen result in increased precipitation until a stable plateau value is achieved (Fig. 1A: *ca* 15% of total incorporated ^{35}S-methionine radioactivity in the experiment illustrated). Washed precipitates formed at different initial ratios of serum to antigen (points marked on Fig. 1A) were solubilized and electrophoresed on a 9.25% polyacrylamide gel slab (illustrated in Fig. 1B). It is apparent that, although there is essentially complete precipitation of a subset of the virus-specific polypeptides available in the supernatant fraction by excess antiserum (slot 5), some polypeptides are efficiently precipitated by very much lower amounts of antibody, resulting in widely different proportions of polypeptides in the precipitates formed at different serum/antigen ratios. The changing proportions of ICP8 to ICP5 and ICP25 to ICP26 provide particularly striking examples (compare slots 1 and 5). We should emphasize that the gel shown in Figure 1B contained approximately equal amounts of radioactivity in each slot and the results should not be interpreted as indicating a decrease in the absolute amount of, e.g., ICP8 precipitated with increasing amounts of antiserum; in no case does the absolute efficiency of precipitation of a polypeptide decrease significantly with increasing addition of antiserum.

Whilst the observation presumably reflects simple differences in antibody titre to different polypeptides and is therefore hardly surprising it is important and useful for two main reasons. Firstly, it provides important evidence that many, if not all, of the polypeptides present in the supernatant fraction are capable of independent precipitation. This, in turn, indicates that most polypeptides are not part of complex aggregates and that independent antigen specificities are involved in precipitating many of the polypeptides. Secondly, while the order of precipitation of different polypeptides might be expected to be a characteristic of a given serum, with few exceptions, this same order is seen with several independently prepared antisera. Thus ICP6 and ICP8 are normally precipitated by the lowest dose of immune serum and presumably, therefore, normally elicit the highest titre antibody response.

FIG. 1. HOMOLOGOUS IMMUNE PRECIPITATES

A. Graphical representation of the percentage counts precipitated for immune precipitates formed after incubation of constant volumes of a ^{35}S-methionine-labelled extract of cells infected with HSV-1 with increasing volumes of homologous general antiserum.   BHK21 cells were labelled with ^{35}S-methionine from 5-18 hours post infection; cells were disrupted by ultrasonic vibration and centrifuged at 38 000 rpm for 60 minutes.   The supernatant fluid (100 µl) was mixed with a range of volumes of general HSV-1 antiserum so as to give the final antiserum ratios of 1:9, 1:3, 1:1, 3:1 and 9:1 (designated 1, 2, 3, 4 and 5) or with preimmune serum at a ratio of 9:1.

B. The immune precipitates formed after overnight incubation were sedimented, washed thoroughly in phosphate-buffered saline, solubilized and separated on polyacrylamide gels in the presence of sodium dodecyl sulfate (SDS) (Honess & Roizman, 1973; Honess & Watson, 1974) together with a sample of the labelled supernatant fluid.(S).   Polypeptides are marked with the appropriate infected-cell polypeptide (ICP) and corresponding virion polypeptide (VP) numbers (Heine et al., 1974; Honess & Roizman, 1973; Spear & Roizman, 1972).   P.I. = Preimmune serum.

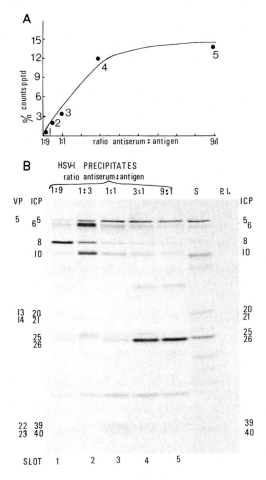

These considerations become more significant when we consider the reactions of supernatant fractions from HSV-1 and HSV-2 (strain 3345) with heterologous as well as homologous antisera. An experiment of this type is illustrated in Fig. 2, which shows ^{35}S-labelled polypeptides separated from immune precipitates formed with an excess of either homologous or heterologous antisera and labelled extracts of cells infected with HSV-1 and HSV-2.   It is obvious that homologous and heterologous antisera react with a virtually identical population of polypeptides within a given antigen sample and that analogous polypeptides are precipitated from cells infected with the two viruses. Moreover, analogous polypeptides are normally precipitated at similar relative antigen/antibody ratios from homologous and heterologous antigens.   Thus antiserum to HSV-1 precipitates ICP8 from either HSV-1 or HSV-2 at low serum/antigen ratios and ICP5 and 26 at high serum/antigen ratios.

We reiterate that almost all these polypeptides have type-characteristic electrophoretic mobility or molecular weight and thus the above experiment shows clearly that common antigenic determinants are possessed by many polypeptides of HSV-1 and HSV-2 which are clearly different in size or conformation and therefore in at least some amino-acid sequences.

By absorption of antisera to HSV-1 or HSV-2 with an excess of cells infected with heterologous virus it has been repeatedly shown that a portion of neutralizing and precipitating antibody is type-specific.   However, whilst it is relatively easy to demonstrate type-common antigenic reactivity on many polypeptides, there are so far few convincing demonstrations of polypeptides which bear exclusively type-specific determinants.   Results from our preliminary experiments suggest that the major glycoprotein region of HSV-1 is precipitated with type 1-specific antiserum.   So far, however, most of our available information on antigenic sites with polypeptides is being obtained both by this approach and by the analysis of polypeptides and antigens of heterotypic recombinant viruses (Halliburton et al., 1977).   The contribution of this subtractive logic to our knowledge of levels of antigenic specificity within the herpes simplex neutroseron is illustrated in the following section.

CROSS NEUTRALIZATION WITHIN A NEUTROSERON IS NOT MEDIATED
BY A SINGLE ANTIGENIC SITE

In this section, which deals with virus neutralization, the term "antigenic site" refers to those sites which have a role in the neutralization of virus infectivity.

It has already been shown that neutralization of HSV-1 and HSV-2 can result from interaction of antibody with either type-specific or type-common antigenic sites (Sim & Watson, 1973).   What is more, Halliburton et al. (1977) in their studies on recombinant viruses

FIG. 2. HETEROLOGOUS IMMUNE PRECIPITATES

Autoradiogram of labelled polypeptides separated on 9.25% polyacrylamide gel slabs from solubilized immune precipitates formed with
supernatant fluids from cells infected with HSV-1 or HSV-2 and an
excess of homologous (hom) or heterologous (het) general antisera.
Supernatant fluids (S) were prepared and precipitated as described
in Figure 1.

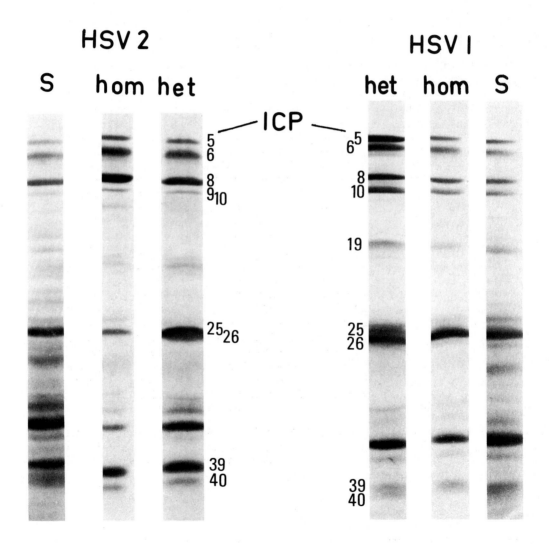

were able to detect a minimum of at least four type 1 and two type 2-specific sites. More recent studies (Killington et al.[1]) on the antigenic differences between a number of different HSV-1 strains have shown that a total of more than four different antigenic sites can be identified on HSV-1 strains but not on HSV-2 strains. Not all of these are possessed by any one HSV-1 strain. However, it seems likely that at least two of these sites are common to the six HSV-1 strains tested, others are present on more than one strain, while at least one site has been found on one strain only.

Cross-neutralization within a neutroseron, however, must be mediated through antibodies to antigenic determinants shared by several viruses. Thus cross-neutralization of HSV-1 and HSV-2 has been related to their common possession of the Band II antigen (Sim & Watson, 1973), since antiserum specific for this antigen (Watson & Wildy, 1969) neutralizes both HSV-1 and HSV-2. BMV has been similarly shown to be neutralized by antiserum to Band II. The possession by BMV of the Band II site has been confirmed by serum absorption experiments. Antiserum to Band II of HSV-1, if absorbed with excess antigen from cells previously infected with BMV, shows substantial loss of neutralizing activity for both HSV-1 and HSV-2. Although it is clear that BMV, HSV-1 and HSV-2 are related by virtue of their common possession of an antigenic site reacting with antiserum to Band II, this cannot be taken to mean that all antibodies in this antiserum which are capable of neutralizing HSV-1 and HSV-2 also neutralize BMV. To investigate this point antisera to both HSV-1 and HSV-2 were absorbed with excess BMV antigen and assayed for residual neutralizing activities against all three viruses. Table 1 shows that BMV is unable to remove all neutralizing activity of antisera to HSV-1 and HSV-2 for the heterologous HSV type. Thus HSV-1 and HSV-2 share at least one antigenic site missing from BMV. Conversely, sites shared by BMV and HSV-1 can be shown to be present on HSV-2 since absorption of antiserum to HSV-1 with excess HSV-2 antigen leaves no residual neutralizing activity for BMV (Table 1). Similarly, sites shared by BMV and HSV-2 are also present on HSV-1 since absorption of antiserum to HSV-2 with excess HSV-1 antigen also removes all neutralizing activity for BMV. Finally, antiserum to VP7/8 (VP: virion polypeptide) of HSV-1, which neutralizes HSV-1 but not HSV-2 (Powell et al., 1974) does not neutralize BMV.

The cross-neutralization which groups these three viruses into a neutroseron is therefore mediated by at least two common antigenic sites, one shared by BMV, HSV-1 and HSV-2 and the other only by HSV-1 and HSV-2.

---

[1] Unpublished data

Table 1. Neutralization of virus infectivity by various antisera[a]

Antiserum to:	Neutralization constant (k) measured against:		
	HSV-1	HSV-2	BMV
HSV-1 absorbed with BMV[b]	$2.8(4.1)$[c]	$0.29(5.9)$[c]	< 0.005[d]
HSV-2 absorbed with BMV	$0.75(1.9)$[c]	$1.4(2.1)$[c]	< 0.005[d]
HSV-1 absorbed with HSV-2	1.4	< 0.005	< 0.005[d]
HSV-2 absorbed with HSV-1	< 0.005	0.40	< 0.005[d]
VP7/8 of HSV-1	0.25	< 0.005	< 0.005[d]

[a] Virus (4×10^4 PFU/ml) was incubated for 3 hours at 25°C with an equal volume of antiserum diluted where necessary. Surviving virus was assayed by the method of Russell (1962). Antisera were inactivated at 56°C before use.

[b] General antisera prepared in RK_{13} cells (Watson et al., 1966) were absorbed with heterologous virus antigen by incubating 1 ml of general antisera with a homogenate of 10^9 infected BHK cells. Absorbed antisera were clarified by sedimentation at 40 000 rpm for 60 minutes and the supernatant fluids concentrated by vacuum dialysis (Sim & Watson, 1973).

[c] Values in parenthesis represent:

$$\frac{k \text{ before absorption}}{k \text{ after absorption}}$$

[d] $k = 0.005$ was the limit of sensitivity in these experiments.

CONCLUSIONS

   Those virus-specific infected-cell polypeptides of HSV-1 and HSV-2 and their structural counterparts which have the presumed same functions and yet have different electrophoretic mobilities (e.g., ICP5/VP5; ICP39,40/VP/22,23) might be considered to possess type-specific antigenicity. However, heterologous immune precipitation has shown these polypeptides to share at least one antigenic site with heterologous virus. As discussed earlier, type-specificity can be demonstrated by virus neutralization, but when such type-specific sera are reacted in immune precipitation experiments preliminary results suggest that in no case is a polypeptide precipitated which is not also precipitated by heterologous general antiserum. Thus although polypeptides which exhibit both type-common and type-specific antigenicity exist, there must be some doubt about the existence of polypeptides carrying only type-specific antigenicity. Similarly, the data suggest that speculation that the HSV genome contains large areas of type-specific gene sequences (Schaffer, 1975), should be treated with caution.

Cross-neutralization between herpesviruses can identify both conserved and divergent gene functions. We can identify antigenic sites at five levels of specificity:

(1) antigenic site(s) common to HSV-1, HSV-2 and BMV;

(2) antigenic site(s) common to HSV-1 and HSV-2 but not possessed by BMV;

(3) antigenic site(s) common to at least six HSV-1 strains;

(4) antigenic site(s) shared by some HSV-1 strains;

(5) antigenic site(s) so far identified only on one HSV-1 strain.

SUMMARY

The antigenic relatedness of three viruses of the herpes simplex type 1 neutroseron - herpes simplex virus types 1 (HSV-1) and 2 (HSV-2) and bovine mammillitis virus (BMV) - has been examined by immune precipitation and virus neutralization tests. Many virus-specific infected-cell polypeptides were shown to possess antigenic sites shared by both HSV-1 and HSV-2. Cross-neutralization between the viruses is mediated through antibodies to at least two antigenic sites, one shared by HSV-1, HSV-2 and BMV and one shared by HSV-1 and HSV-2 but not BMV.

ACKNOWLEDGEMENTS

We would like to thank Dr W.B. Martin for bovine mammillitis virus (the Italian isolate of Castrucci et al., 1972). One of us (R.E. Randall) was in receipt of a Science Research Council Studentship. The work was supported by project grants awarded by the Medical Research Council to D.H. Watson and R.A. Killington.

REFERENCES

Castrucci, C., Pedini, B., Cilli, V. & Arancia, G. (1972)
    Characterization of a viral agent resembling bovine herpes
    mammillitis virus. *Vet. Rec., 90*, 325-335

Halliburton, I.W., Randall, R.E., Killington, R.A. & Watson, D.H.
    (1977)   Some properties of recombinants between type 1 and
    type 2 herpes simplex viruses. *J. gen. Virol.* (in press)

Heine, J.W., Honess, R.W., Cassai, E. & Roizman, B. (1974)   Proteins
    specified by herpes simplex virus.   XII.   The virion polypeptide
    of type 1 strains. *J. Virol., 14*, 640-651.

Honess, R.W. & Roizman, B. (1973)   Proteins specified by herpes
    simplex virus.   XI.   Identification and relative molar rates of
    synthesis of structural and non-structural herpes virus polypep-
    tides in the infected cell. *J. Virol., 12*, 1347-1365

Honess, R.W., Powell, K.L., Robinson, D.J., Sim, C. & Watson, D.H.
    (1974)   Type specific and type common antigens in cells infected
    with herpes simplex virus type 1 and on the surfaces of naked and
    enveloped particles of the virus. *J. gen. Virol., 22*, 159-169

Honess, R.W. & Watson, D.H. (1974)   Herpes simplex virus-specific
    polypeptides studied by polyacrylamide gel electrophoresis of
    immune precipitates. *J. gen. Virol., 22*, 171-185

Honess, R.W. & Watson, D.H. (1977)   Unity and diversity in the herpes-
    viruses. *J. gen. Virol.* (in press)

Killington, R.A., Yeo, J., Honess, R.W., Watson, D.H., Halliburton,
    I.W. & Mumford, J. (1977)   Comparative analyses of the proteins
    and antigens of five herpesviruses. *J. gen. Virol.* (in press)

Powell, K.L., Buchan, A., Sim, C. & Watson, D.H. (1974)   Type specific
    protein in herpes simplex virus envelope reacts with neutralizing
    antibody. *Nature (Lond.), 249*, 360-361

Powell, K.L., Mirkovic, R. & Courtney, R.J. (1977)   Comparative
    analysis of polypeptides induced by type 1 and type 2 strains of
    herpes simplex virus. *Intervirology, 8*, 18-29

Russell, W.C. (1962)   A sensitive and precise plaque assay for herpes
    virus. *Nature (Lond.), 195*, 1028-1029

Schaffer, P.A. (1975)   *Genetics of herpesviruses - a review.*   In:
    de-Thé, G., Epstein, M.A. & zur Hausen, H., eds, *Oncogenesis and
    Herpesviruses II, Part 1*, Lyon, International Agency for Research on
    Cancer (*IARC Scientific Publications* No. 11), pp. 195-217

Sim, C. & Watson, D.H. (1973)   The role of type specific and cross
    reacting structural antigens in the neutralization of herpes
    simplex types 1 and 2.   *J. gen. Virol.*, *19*, 217-233

Spear, P.G. & Roizman, B. (1972)   Proteins specified by herpes
    simplex virus. V. Purification and structural proteins of the
    herpesvirion.   *J. Virol.*, *9*, 143-159

Sterz, H., Ludwig, H. & Rott, R. (1973/74)   Immunologic and genetic
    relationship between herpes simplex virus and bovine herpes
    mammillitis virus.   *Intervirology*, *2*, 1-13

Watson, D.H., Shedden, W.I.H., Elliot, A., Tetsuka, T., Wildy, P.,
    Bourgaux-Ramoisy, D. & Gold, E. (1966)   Virus specific antigens
    in mammalian cells infected with herpes simplex virus.   *Immunology*,
    11, 399-408

Watson, D.H. & Wildy, P. (1969)   The preparation of 'monoprecipitin'
    antisera to herpes virus specific antigens.   *J. gen. Virol.*, *4*,
    163-168

ANALYSIS OF HERPES SIMPLEX VIRUS LOW MOLECULAR-WEIGHT NATIVE PROTEINS BY POLYACRYLAMIDE GEL ELECTROFOCUSING

M.K. O'HARA[1] & R.J. COURTNEY[1]

Department of Virology and Epidemiology,
Baylor College of Medicine,
Houston, Texas, USA

In order to elucidate the role herpes simplex virus type 2 (HSV-2) gene products play in virus replication and transformation, the isolation and eventual characterization of the individual gene products is necessary. To date approximately 50 HSV-specific polypeptides have been detected by sodium dodecyl sulfate polyacrylamide gel electrophoresis (SDS-PAGE), which represents approximately 75% of the coding capacity of the HSV-2 genome (Powell & Courtney, 1975). A similar number of polypeptides has been detected in HSV-1 infected cells (Honess & Roizman, 1973). In an attempt to further characterize the proteins specified by the HSV-2 genome and to identify new proteins, we have used isoelectrofocusing on thin-layer polyacrylamide gels. The use of polyacrylamide gel electrofocus analysis of virus proteins has been recently reported for poliovirus (Hamann et al., 1977) and Newcastle disease virus (Miyakawa et al., 1976). This approach offers several advantages. First, since it allows separation of proteins based on their isoelectric points, proteins can be resolved by a criterion other than molecular weight and this may lead to the identification of proteins not previously defined. A second and significant advantage of this approach is that it enables one to purify virus-specific proteins in their native states. This point is especially significant because protein function can be retained and subsequently studied. The purpose of this communication is to describe the analysis of HSV-2 specific proteins by gel isoelectric focusing and certain characteristics of these virus proteins.

---

[1] Present address: Department of Microbiology, University of Tennessee, Knoxville, Tenn., USA

MATERIALS AND METHODS

The 186 strain of HSV-2 was used in these studies.   For preparation of isotopically labelled proteins, HEp-2 cells were infected with
HSV-2 at a multiplicity of 20 plaque-forming units per cell and were
subsequently pulse-labelled at the indicated times with ^{35}S-methionine
at a concentration of 25 µCi/ml.   After the 1-hour pulse, the whole
cell fractions were harvested, washed, and the cell pellet resuspended
to a concentration of 25×10^6 cells/ml in distilled water.   Prior to
gel electrofocus analysis, the cell extracts were sonicated for 2
minutes.

The procedure described by Vesterberg (1972) for isoelectric
focusing in polyacrylamide gel was followed with minor modifications.
The ampholyte concentration of the gels was 2.4% (w/v) which produced
a pH range of 3.5-9.5.   The concentration of the acrylamide monomer
in the gel was 5% (w/v).   The anode and cathode electrolytes were 1 M
phosphoric acid (H_3PO_4) and 1 M sodium hydroxide, respectively.   For
electrofocusing, approximately 15 µl of the sonicated cell extract was
applied to the anode region of the gel slab and electrofocused for 1
hour at 100 V/cm.   The 5% acrylamide gel concentration selectively
prohibits the migration of high molecular-weight proteins and aggregates.   Therefore, after electrofocusing, approximately 2 cm of gel
at the anode region containing this material was removed.   The electrofocused gel slab was fixed, dried, and then placed on X-ray film
for autoradiography.   The pH gradient of the gel was determined by
placing 1-cm square sections of the electrofocused gel in distilled
water and subsequently measuring the pH.

The SDS-PAGE gel system used has been previously described
(Powell & Courtney, 1975).

RESULTS

*Isoelectric focus analysis of HSV-2 proteins synthesized at various
times after infection*

HEp-2 cells were infected with HSV-2 and pulsed with ^{35}S-
methionine at various times after infection.   At the end of the 1-
hour pulse, the whole cell fractions were harvested and analysed by
gel isoelectrofocusing (Fig. 1).   As seen in the mock-infected lane
(left side), many cell proteins can be resolved by this technique.
At increasing times after infection with HSV-2, the inhibition of
cell protein synthesis, concomitant with the appearance of several
virus-induced proteins, was evident.   Cells which were pulsed 3-4
hours post infection exhibit both cell and virus proteins.   However,
HSV-induced proteins were those predominantly detectable at 5 hours
post infection.   Three proteins appeared to be synthesized primarily

FIG. 1. AUTORADIOGRAM OF A POLYACRYLAMIDE GEL SLAB FOLLOWING
ISOELECTROFOCUSING OF PULSE-LABELLED HSV-2 AND MOCK-INFECTED
CELL EXTRACTS

The cells were pulse-labelled for 1 hour with ^{35}S-methionine at the
time intervals indicated at the top of the gel and were harvested
following the 1-hour pulse.   The approximate isoelectric points for
each of the major bands are indicated at the right of the autoradiogram.

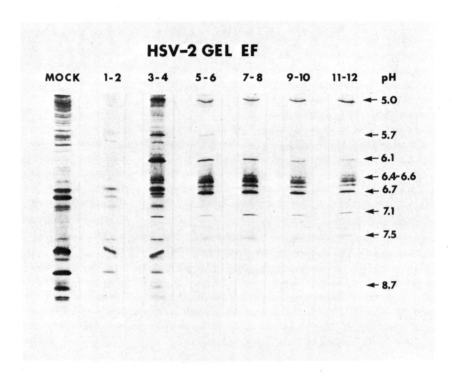

during the early stages of virus replication and had isoelectric
points of 5.7, 6.1 and 7.5.   The other proteins were made in varying
amounts from 4 hours post infection.   The proteins resolved on the
electrofocusing gel were termed virus-specific on the basis of having
an isoelectric point different from that of cellular proteins and
exhibiting increased synthesis at various times after infection.
In addition, direct immunoprecipitation experiments with rabbit anti-
HSV sera have also indicated that the proteins being resolved on the
electrofocusing gel were HSV-specific (data not shown).

Two-dimensional electrophoresis of HSV-2 proteins

In order to obtain information on the molecular weights of the
proteins which were being resolved by isoelectric focusing, two-
dimensional electrophoretic separations were performed.   An HSV-2
infected sample pulsed from 8 to 9 hours post infection was electrofocused as described above to separate the HSV-2 proteins on the basis
of their isoelectric point.   A lane was cut out of the gel, soaked in
a buffer containing 2% sodium dodecyl sulfate (SDS), 0.5 M urea and
1% 2-mercaptoethanol.   After soaking for 1 hour, this electrofocused
gel was then placed on top of a 12% polyacrylamide gel slab containing
SDS.   A second dimension of electrophoresis was then run to separate
the polypeptides on the basis of their respective molecular weights.
An example of such a two-dimensional run is shown in Figure 2.   The
profile of the electrofocused gel is shown at the top of the SDS slab
gel.   A sample of the HSV-2 infected cell extract was applied to the
left portion of the SDS-slab gel.   By co-electrophoresis of standard
molecular-weight marker proteins (bovine serum albumin, 68 000;
ovalbumin, 43 000;   chymotrypsinogen, 25 700;   and myoglobin, 17 200),
estimates of the molecular weights of the proteins electrophoresed in
the second dimension were made (data not shown).   For each of the
protein bands resolved by electrofocusing, corresponding polypeptides
could be resolved in the second dimension on the SDS gel.   For some
protein bands resolved by electrofocusing, one polypeptide was resolved
on the SDS gel, and for other bands, two or more polypeptides were
resolved.

A summary of the HSV-2 specific proteins resolved by polyacrylamide
gel electrofocusing is shown in Figure 3.   The isoelectric points
shown are an average of seven runs and the molecular-weight estimates
are based on four separate analyses by two-dimensional gel electrophoresis.   The molecular weights of the resolved polypeptides range
from 11 750 to 49 250, and the time of synthesis varies from those
which are primarily made early in the virus replication cycle to those
which are made later and throughout the cycle.

                              DISCUSSION

The objective of this communication was to describe the preliminary
results of the analysis of a certain group of HSV-2 specific low
molecular-weight native proteins which could be reproducibly resolved
by polyacrylamide gel isoelectrofocusing.   This technique has also
been used to purify certain of these native proteins.   To date, the
proteins with isoelectric points of 6.4-6.6, 6.7, and 7.1 have been
cut out of the electrofocused gel and recycled through a second gel.
These bands have exhibited nearly total radiochemical purity.   Such
studies are indicative of the potential use of this approach to obtain
purified preparations of HSV-specific native proteins for further biochemical and immunological studies.   Studies have also been initiated

FIG. 2. AN AUTORADIOGRAM OF TWO-DIMENSIONAL GEL
ELECTROPHORESIS OF HSV-2 PROTEINS

HSV-2 infected HEp-2 cells were pulse-labelled with ^{35}S-methionine at
8-9 hours post infection and the whole cell extract was harvested after
the 1-hour pulse. The sample was electrofocused as described in the
text. One lane was cut out of the electrofocused gel and processed
for autoradiography and the autoradiogram is shown on the top of the
SDS-slab gel. Another lane was cut out and soaked in buffer containing
SDS, urea and 2-mercaptoethanol. This electrofocused gel was then
placed on top of the SDS-slab gel and electrophoresed in the second
dimension. For reference, a sample of the infected-cell extract was
placed on the left portion of the SDS-slab gel prior to the electrophoresis of the SDS gel.

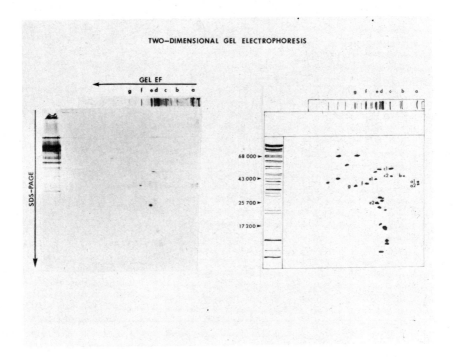

to identify specific proteins which are unique to HSV-1 and HSV-2
transformed hamster cells and cervical cell lines established from
women with cervical cancer. The above studies should provide an
additional approach to the identification and further elucidation of
the role HSV proteins play within the infected and transformed cell.

FIG. 3. SUMMARY OF THE HSV-2 SPECIFIC PROTEINS
RESOLVED BY POLYACRYLAMIDE GEL ELECTROFOCUSING

SUMMARY: HSV-2-SPECIFIC PROTEINS RESOLVED BY
POLYACRYLAMIDE GEL ELECTROFOCUSING

HSV-2 8-9 hr	pI [a]	Time of Synthesis (hr pi)	Precipitation by anti-HSV-2 serum	Molecular Weight [b]
	5.0	3-12	+	39 700 36 900
	5.7	3-4	+	45 250
	6.1	3-8	+	47 300 43 200
	6.4-6.6	5-9	+	49 250 27 400 23 700 22 100 15 000 11 750
	6.7	5-9	+	25 100 40 500
	7.1	3-8	+	37 800
	7.5	3-4	±	36 400

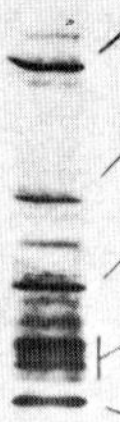

[a] Approximate pI; average of 7 determinations.

[b] Apparent molecular weight values based on second dimension electrophoresis on SDS-PAGE.

SUMMARY

    This communication has demonstrated the potential application of
gel electrofocusing for the isolation and further characterization of
HSV-2 native proteins.   At least eight major HSV-2 specific proteins
with characteristic isoelectric points could be reproducibly resolved
by gel isoelectric focusing.   Their isoelectric points ranged from
5.0 to 7.5 and analysis by two-dimensional electrophoresis on SDS gels
indicated that their molecular weights range from 11 000 to 49 000.

ACKNOWLEDGEMENTS

This investigation was supported by research contract
NO1 CP 53526 within the Virus Cancer Program of the
National Cancer Institute and grant CA 10,893 from
the National Cancer Institute. M.K. O'Hara is the
recipient of a Postdoctoral Fellowship Award
(F1-F32-CA,05889) from the National Cancer
Institute.

REFERENCES

Hamann, A., Wiegers, K.J. & Drzeniek, R. (1977)   Isoelectric focusing
    and 2D-analysis of poliovirus proteins. *Virology, 78*, 359-362

Honess, R.W. & Roizman, B. (1973)   Proteins specified by herpes simplex
    virus. XI. Identification and relative molar rates of synthesis of
    structural and nonstructural herpesvirus polypeptides in the infec-
    ted cell. *J. Virol., 12*, 1347-1365

Miyakawa, T., Takemoto, L.J. & Fox, C.F. (1976) *Supramolecular orga-
    nization of proteins in Newcastle disease virus*. In: Baltimore,
    D., Huang, A.S. & Fox, C.F., eds, *Animal Virology*, Vol. 4, Squaw
    Valley (ICW-UCLA Symposium on Molecular and Cellular Biology),
    pp. 485-497

Powell, K.L. & Courtney, R.J. (1975)   Polypeptides synthesized in
    herpes simplex virus type 2-infected HEp-2 cells. *Virology, 66*,
    217-228

Vesterberg, O. (1972)   Isoelectric focusing of proteins in poly-
    acrylamide gels. *Biochim. Biophys. Acta (Amst.), 257*, 11-19

STUDIES DEMONSTRATING THE IMMUNOLOGICAL IDENTITY OF THE TUMOUR-ASSOCIATED ANTIGEN AG-4 WITH A VIRION ENVELOPE PROTEIN

B.C. STRNAD, M.F. SMITH & L. AURELIAN

*Division of Comparative Medicine,
Department of Biochemistry and Biophysics,
The Johns Hopkins University Schools of
Medicine and Hygiene and Public Health,
Baltimore, Maryland, USA*

Several lines of evidence recently reviewed (Aurelian, 1976) associate herpesvirus type 2 (HSV-2) with carcinoma of the cervix. Consideration of the role of HSV-2 in oncogenesis depends on the understanding of the virus/host-cell interaction, and of the identity and biological function of viral proteins synthesized under productive and abortive conditions.

Forty-seven viral proteins (molecular weights 14 000-260 000) were described in productively infected cells. Of these 24 were present in purified virions, whereas the other 23 were classified as non-structural (Strnad & Aurelian, 1976a). Under abortive conditions resulting from the treatment of cells with cycloheximide added at the time of infection, seven "early" viral proteins ("α") were demonstrated (Strnad & Aurelian, 1976b). However, these studies failed to provide information on the biological function of the viral proteins, and on the role, if any, that they play in oncogenesis.

In this context, it is significant to identify viral antigens that, like AG-4, reflect the progression of the cervical tumour. Only one-third of the early cervical lesions (atypia) and two-thirds of the more advanced ones (*in situ*) progress to invasive cancer (Stern, 1969). This gradation is reflected in the prevalence of seropositivity to AG-4 (Aurelian et al., 1977), an "α" protein (Strnad & Aurelian, 1976b). Furthermore, 86% of invasive cancer patients are AG-4 seropositive prior to treatment; they become negative following tumour removal and seroconvert if cancer recurs (Aurelian, 1976; Aurelian et al., 1977).

The AG-4 antigenic activity has been correlated to infected-cell protein No. 10 (ICP 10) (Strnad & Aurelian, 1976b).   Thus: (i) AG-4 and ICP 10 have similar kinetics of synthesis during productive and abortive infection resulting from treatment of the cells with cycloheximide;   (ii) ICP 10 is precipitated by AG-4 positive but not negative human sera;   (iii) passage history of HSV-2 affects the synthesis of AG-4 and ICP 10 similarly;   and (iv) during fractionation on G-200 and brushite columns, ICP 10 is the only viral protein present in the fraction containing AG-4 activity and absent from those that are AG-4 negative.

Although substantial antigen purification was achieved, the cleanest antigen-containing fraction still had 6-8 proteins as resolved by acrylamide gel electrophoresis.   Two questions pertaining to the identity of AG-4 constitute the focus of this presentation: (i) Does ICP 10 possess the Ag-4 antigenic activity;   and (ii) where on the virion is ICP 10 located?

PURIFICATION OF ICP 10 BY ACRYLAMIDE GEL ELECTROPHORESIS

Courtney & Benyesch-Melnick (1974) described the separation of a high molecular-weight HSV protein by preparative electrophoresis on sodium dodecyl sulfate (SDS)-acrylamide gels without loss of antigenicity.   A modification of this procedure was used.   Briefly, mock-infected or HSV-2 (G) infected HEp-2 cells were labelled with ^{35}S-L-methionine for 4 hours post infection (p.i.).   Extracts were electro-phoresed on 8.5% acrylamide gels in the presence of 0.1% SDS for 15 hours.   This procedure permits the majority of proteins to electro-phorese off the bottom of the gel and results in excellent resolution of the remaining high molecular-weight ones.   Gels were stained, sliced longitudinally, dried and autoradiographed (Strnad & Aurelian, 1976a).   Remaining gels containing infected-cell extracts were stored at -80°C.   Three proteins were resolved in autoradiograms of HSV-2 (G) infected-cell extracts (Fig. 1A).   One of these, absent from uninfected-cell extracts (Fig. 1C), migrated as ICP 10 and its relative mobility was used as a guide for slicing segments out of the remaining gels (Fig. 1B).   The segments were eluted in buffer to obtain ICP 10 or used to prepare antiserum by foot-pad inoculation of rabbits following their homogenization in complete Freund's adjuvant.

Gel segments containing ICP 10 were homogenized and eluted in 0.001 M phosphate buffer, pH 6.4, with 0.1% SDS and 0.001 M dithiothreitol (PSD buffer) at room temperature for one day.   The identity of the eluted protein(s) was determined by electrophoresis on 8.5% SDS-acrylamide gels prior to and after chromatography on SDS-hydroxylapatite (HTP) from which it was eluted with 0.5 M PSD buffer.   Autoradiograms of the gels containing the eluted protein(s) previously dialysed against 0.01 M tris buffer with 0.1% SDS, revealed one protein band

FIG. 1. AUTORADIOGRAMS OF 8.5% SDS-ACRYLAMIDE GELS

(A) HSV-2 (G) infected HEp-2 cell proteins labelled 0-4 hours p.i.
with ^{35}S-L-methionine and electrophoresed for 15 hours; (B) Same
as (A) displaying the ICP-10-containing segment; (C) Mock-infected
HEp-2 cell proteins labelled as in (A).

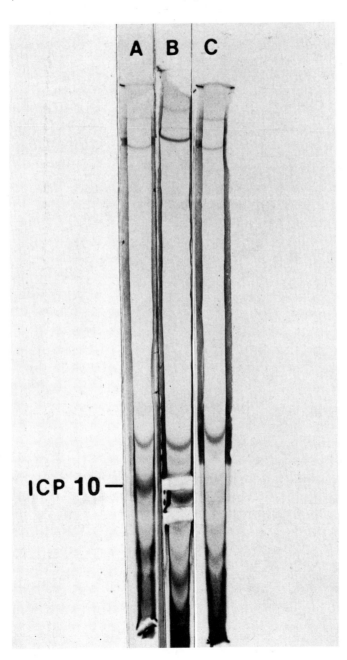

that co-migrates with ICP 10 (Fig. 2).   The eluted protein fixed
complement only with AG-4 positive sera and their IgM (Fig. 3).
AG-4 antibody was previously shown to be IgM whereas antibody to other
viral determinants is IgG (Aurelian et al., 1976a).

FIG. 2. DENSITOMETRIC SCANS OF AUTORADIOGRAMS OF PROTEINS

Proteins were from: (A) HSV-2 (G) infected HEp-2 cells labelled with
^{35}S-L-methionine 0-4 hours p.i.; (B) eluate of SDS-HTP column of
proteins from ICP-10-containing gel segments.

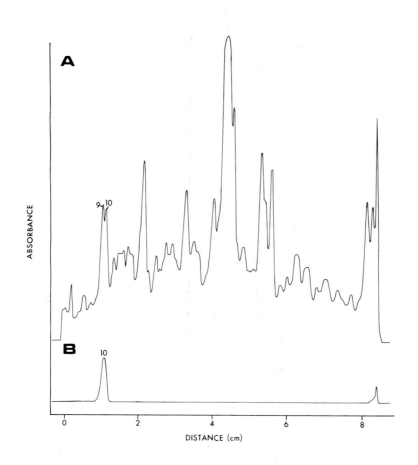

FIG. 3. MICROCOMPLEMENT FIXATION

Microcomplement fixation by AG-4 positive (No. 71 ●——●) and negative (No. 97 ○) sera with ICP 10 eluted from SDS-HTP columns. Percentage fixation is plotted as a function of ICP 10 concentration. Sera were 25×10^{-2} ml/ml. The diluent was veronal buffer.

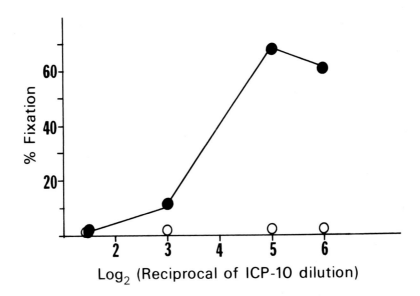

IMMUNOLOGICAL IDENTITY OF ICP 10 AND AG-4

The question that arises from the observation that ICP 10 fixes complement with IgM from AG-4 positive human sera, is whether the same antigen reacts in the two complement-fixation (CF) assays. To inquire into this question, anti-ICP-10 sera were fractionated by sucrose gradient centrifugation (Aurelian et al., 1976a) and the IgG fractions were shown to fix complement with AG-4 (Table 1). Following precipitation with 50% ammonium sulfate, anti-ICP-10 IgG was separated by chromatography on diethylaminoethyl (DEAE) cellulose. Divalent (Fab')$_2$ molecules were produced by pepsin digestion at pH 4.0 and separated from the Fc fragment on G-150 Sephadex. Monovalent Fab' molecules were generated by sequential dialysis against cysteine and iodoacetamide. The results (Table 2) indicate that preincubation of AG-4 antigen with Fab' from anti-ICP 10 completely blocks its ability to fix complement with AG-4 positive human sera. The blocking specificity is evidenced by the observation that anti-ICP-10 Fab' does not block the CF of Visna/anti-Visna and HSV-2/anti-HSV-2 IgG.

The experiment firmly establishes the immunological identity of ICP 10 and Ag-4.

Table 1. Complement-fixing potential of 7S immunoglobulin from anti-ICP-10 sera[a]

Immunoglobulin G (IgG) from:	Complement fixed (%) with		
	Ag-4	AG-H	HSV-2[b]
Preimmune	0	0	0
Preimmune adsorbed with HSV-2[c]	0	0	0
Preimmune adsorbed with HSV-2 lysates[d]	0	0	1.1
Anti-ICP-10 (No. 12-7)	55.6	0	21.6
Anti-ICP-10 (No. 12-21)	93.9	7.8	28.0
Anti-ICP-10 (No. 12-7) adsorbed with HSV-2	0	0	7
Anti-ICP-10 (No. 12-7) adsorbed with HSV-2 lysates	0	0	8.6
Anti-ICP-10 (No. 12-7) adsorbed with pseudovirus[e]	54	0	24.3

[a] A serum is considered positive if, in presence of antigen, it fixes more than 10% complement.

[b] HSV-2 pelleted by centrifugation at 25 000 rpm for 60 minutes in a Spinco SW 27 rotor and resuspended in veronal buffer

[c] HSV-2 pelleted by centrifugation at 25 000 rpm for 60 minutes in a Spinco SW 27 rotor (2100 µg protein) is fixed in 0.1 M sodium acetate, pH 5.0, containing 1% glutaraldehyde for 3 hours at room temperature. Virus is pelleted by centrifugation at 18 000 rpm for 90 minutes and washed twice in 0.2 M potassium phosphate buffer, pH 7.2. The last pellet is used to adsorb 0.1 ml IgG.

[d] HSV-2 pelleted as above or purified by ultracentrifugation on Dextran T-10 gradients is dissociated by exposure to 2% SDS, 5% 2-mercaptoethanol for 15 minutes at 37°C (710 µg protein). Following two cycles of overnight dialysis against veronal buffer, it is incubated for 60 minutes at 37°C with an equal volume of IgG.

[e] Pellets obtained from soluble extracts of uninfected HEp-2 cells prepared as in (c) (2100 µg protein/0.1 ml IgG)

Table 2. Blocking of human AG-4 complement-fixing potential by monovalent Fab'from IgG of anti-ICP-10 serum

Antiserum	Complement fixed (%) with			
	AG-4	Ag-H[a]	HSV-2[b]	Visna[c]
Anti-ICP-10 IgG	93.9	7.8	ND[d]	ND[d]
Fab'	9.5	0	7.7	9
Anti-ICP-10 IgG + Fab'	0	0	ND[d]	ND[d]
Serum 71[e]	51.9	0	76.3	0
Serum 71[e] + Fab'	2.3	0	ND[d]	ND[d]
Serum 350[e]	12	0	ND[d]	ND[d]
Serum 350[e] + Fab'	0	0	ND[d]	ND[d]
Serum 505[e]	28.2	0	ND[d]	ND[d]
Serum 505[e] + Fab'	0	0	ND[d]	ND[d]
Serum 455[e]	0	0	ND[d]	ND[d]
Serum 455[e] + Fab'	0	0	ND[d]	ND[d]
Sheep anti-Visna	0	0	0	77.8
Sheep anti-Visna + Fab'	ND[d]	ND[d]	0	85.4
17[e] IgG	0	0	75.9	0
17[e] IgG + Fab'	0	0	85.8	0

[a] Control for Ag-4 antigen prepared from mock-infected HEp-2 cells

[b] HSV-2 pelleted by centrifugation at 25 000 rpm for 60 minutes in a Spinco SW 27 rotor

[c] Supernatant from infected cells in Eagle's minimum essential medium (MEM)-1% heat-inactivated lamb serum (Dr O. Narayan, Johns Hopkins School of Medicine)

[d] Not done

[e] Human serum

VIRION LOCATION OF ICP 10

Consistent with the conclusion that ICP 10 is a virion protein
(Strnad & Aurelian, 1976b), IgG from anti-ICP-10 sera fix complement
with HSV-2 and their CF potential for Ag-4 is adsorbed with virions
(Table 1).   To determine the location of ICP 10 within the virion,
the protein profile of nucleocapsids and solubilized envelope proteins
was studied.   The latter were prepared from purified ^{35}S-L-methionine
cytoplasmic virions by treatment with 1% Nonidet P-40 (NP-40).
Approximately 30% of the label is solubilized under these conditions.
Capsids free of envelope proteins were prepared from nuclei of
infected cells homogenized with 1% NP-40.   Nuclei were lysed with
0.5% sodium deoxycholate and capsids purified by centrifugation on
10-66% (w/w) sucrose gradients.   Contamination by cellular protein
is less than 1%.   Autoradiograms of SDS-acrylamide gels of these
preparations demonstrate that ICP 10 is an envelope protein (Fig. 4).
Envelope proteins from which NP-40 was extracted with diethyl ether,
fix complement with anti-ICP-10 and AG-4 positive human sera.
Consistent with this observation, anti-ICP-10 sera precipitate purified
HSV-2 virions labelled with ^{125}I (McLellan & August, 1976).   They also
neutralize virus infectivity, but only in the presence of antiglobulin
or complement, indicating that AG-4 occupies on the envelope surface a
site which is sterically removed from those involved in neutralization
and infectivity.   Similar conclusions were reached for Rous sarcoma
virus and Sindbis virus (Schlesinger, 1976).

CONCLUSIONS AND PERSPECTIVES

The salient features of this presentation are the establishment
of the immunological identity of AG-4 as ICP 10 and the demonstration
that it is located on the envelope of the HSV-2 virions.   In view of
the observation that AG-4 antibody reflects the progression of the
cervical tumour (Aurelian et al., 1977), its identity to a viral
structural protein, which most probably is virus-coded, suggests that
the virus plays an active role in tumour growth.

The observation that, in immunized rabbits, unlike in humans
(Aurelian et al., 1976a), AG-4 antibody is IgG must be considered in
the context of immune regulation (Bretscher, 1974), and should counter
the suggestion that cell-mediated immunity (CMI) is involved in
tumour control whereas antibody, if blocking, may play a role in
tumour growth.   Stable IgM synthesis precludes CMI responsiveness.
It is a function of the intrinsic immunogenicity of the antigen
(ICP 10 is highly immunogenic), its presentation (as part of the
cervical tumour) and the generation of IgM feedback, reducing the
level of T-cell help below that required for the IgM to IgG switch.

FIG. 4.   DENSITOMETRIC SCANS OF AUTORADIOGRAMS OF PROTEINS

Proteins were from: (A) cytoplasmic virions labelled with ^{35}S-L-methionine and purified by centrifugation on dextran gradients; (B) envelope proteins solubilized by NP-40 treatment of virions in (A);   (C) ^{35}S-L-methionine labelled nucleocapsids purified by centrifugation on sucrose gradients.

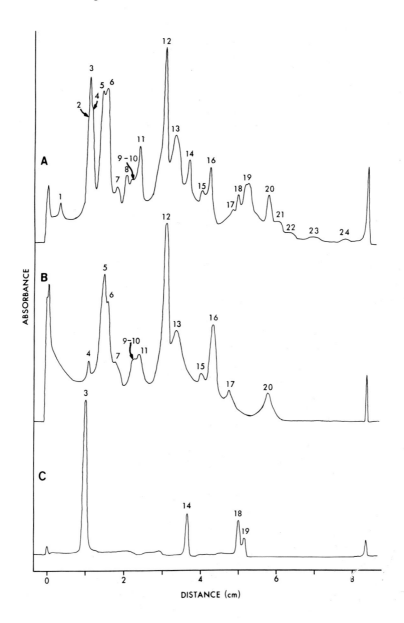

This phenomenon is most probably related to sustained levels of ICP 10 synthesis in the tumour. Significantly, mononuclear cells from patients with cervical cancer do not respond to AG-4 in *in vitro* assays of CMI (Aurelian et al., 1976b).

ACKNOWLEDGEMENTS

This work was supported by Contract No. 1-CP-33345 within the Virus Cancer Program of the National Cancer Institute, and in part by Grant No. CA-16043-01A1 from the National Cancer Institute.

REFERENCES

Aurelian, L. (1976) Coitus and cancer. *Bull. N.Y. Acad. Med., 52*, 910-924

Aurelian, L., Smith, M.F. & Cornish, J.D. (1976a) IgM antibody to a tumor-associated antigen (AG-4) induced by herpes simplex virus type 2: Its use in location of the antigen in infected cells. *J. nat. Cancer Inst., 56*, 471-477

Aurelian, L., Strnad, B.C., Jacobs, R.P., Bell, R.B. & Smith, M.F. (1976b) *Herpesvirus antigens and cell mediated immunity in cervical cancer.* In: Crowell, R.L., Friedman, H. & Prior, J. E., eds, *Tumor Virus Infections and Immunity*, Baltimore, Md, University Park Press, pp. 89-132

Aurelian, L., Strnad, B.C. & Smith, M.F. (1977) Immunodiagnostic potential of a virus-coded tumor-associated antigen (AG-4) in cervical cancer. *Cancer, 39*, 1834-1849

Bretscher, P.A. (1974) On the control between cell-mediated IgM and IgG immunity. *Cell. Immun., 13*, 171-195

Courtney, R.J. & Benyesch-Melnick, M. (1974) Isolation and characterization of a large molecular weight polypeptide of herpes simplex virus type 1. *Virology, 62*, 539-551

McLellan, W.I. & August, J.T. (1976) Analysis of the envelope of Rauscher Murine Oncornavirus: *In vitro* labeling of glycoproteins. *J. Virol., 20*, 627-636

Schlesinger, M.J. (1976)   Formation of an infectious virus-antibody complex with Rous Sarcoma virus and antibodies directed against the major virus glycoproteins.   *J. Virol.*, *17*, 1063-1067

Stern, E. (1969)   *Epidemiology of dysplasia.*   In: Taylor, E.S., Jones, H.W., Jr & Jones, G.S., eds, *Obstetrical and Gynecological Survey*, Baltimore, Md, The Williams Wilkins Co., pp. 711-723

Strnad, B.C. & Aurelian, L. (1976a)   Proteins of herpesvirus type 2: I. Virion, nonvirion, and antigenic polypeptides in infected cells. *Virology*, *69*, 438-452

Strnad, B.C. & Aurelian, L. (1976b)   Proteins of herpesvirus type 2. II. Studies demonstrating a correlation between a tumor associated antigen (AG-4) and a virion protein.   *Virology*, *73*, 244-258

DEFINITION OF AN ANTIGEN SHARED BY HERPESVIRUSES AND ONCORNAVIRUSES

M.I. BERNHARD, L.J. OLD, T. TAKAHASHI & N.H. SARKAR

*Sloan-Kettering Institute for Cancer Research,
New York, NY, USA*

W.C. LAWRENCE

*University of Pennsylvania, School of Veterinary Medicine,
Philadelphia, Penn., USA*

During the past several years we have been analysing antisera to purified herpesvirus nucleocapsids (nc). Ouchterlony analysis indicated that these antisera define a shared antigen present in herpesvirus nc of amphibian, avian, equine and primate origins. More recently, and to our surprise, we have found a serologically identical antigen in avian, reptilian and mammalian oncornaviruses. In this report we summarize the current status of these investigations.

Herpesvirus nc were prepared by the method of Gibson & Roizman (1972) from equine herpesvirus type 1 (EHV-1) grown in mouse L-cells and from herpes simplex virus types 1 and 2 (HSV-1 and HSV-2) grown in Vero and HEp-2 cells. In addition, herpesvirus nc were purified directly from Lucké renal adenocarcinomas of the frog (in collaboration with I. Toplin of Litton Bionetics, Bethesda, Md). EHV-1 nc were also prepared by sedimentation through caesium chloride (CsCl) as a final step. Epstein-Barr virus (EBV) nc, Marek's disease virus (MDV) nc and cytomegalovirus (CMV) nc were prepared by Nonidet P-40 (NP-40) treatment of purified viruses.

Antisera were prepared in (W/Fu × BN)F_1 rats immunized with either EHV-1 nc or HSV-2 nc and a goat immunized with alternate injections of HSV-1 nc and HSV-2 nc. All immunizations were carried out at three-week intervals, the first immunization in complete Freund's adjuvant and all subsequent immunizations in incomplete Freund's adjuvant. Herpesvirus nc used for immunization were first

examined by negative stain electron microscopy and only preparations
free of visible contamination were selected (Fig. 1A,B).   Batches
of nc were also prepared from cells grown in the presence of ^{3}H-amino-
acids or ^{35}S-methionine and were analysed by sodium dodecyl sulfate-
polyacrylamide gel electrophoresis (SDS-PAGE) on 7.5% cylindrical gels
(Weber & Osborn, 1969).   Figure 2 shows typical gel patterns obtained
with EHV-1 nc purified by the method of Gibson & Roizman (1972) and by
sedimentation through caesium chloride.   These gel patterns are in
close agreement with published data (Purdue et al., 1975).

     Table 1 summarizes the immunodiffusion (ID) reactivity of the
antiherpesvirus nc sera in 0.7% agarose gels.   The two rat antisera
and the goat antiserum gave parallel results.   Preimmune sera were
consistently non-reactive.   Nucleocapsid preparations from HSV-1,
HSV-2, EBV, CMV, Lucké tumour herpesvirus and MDV were precipitated
by the antiherpesvirus nc sera and analysis showed reactions of
identity (Fig. 3A).   Extensive specificity testing revealed that
a component present in oncornaviruses of avian, reptilian and mammalian
origins was also precipitated by these antiherpesvirus nc sera.
This oncornavirus antigen showed reactions of identity with herpesvirus nc (Fig. 3B).

     Tests with extracts prepared from feline leukaemia virus (FeLV)-
positive and FeLV-negative cat tissues and murine leukaemia virus
(MuLV)-positive and MuLV-negative mouse tissues revealed a close
relationship between virus infection and antigen expression.   Antigen
was present in a high percentage of virus-infected tissues but was
never found in virus-negative tissues.   The shared herpesvirus-
oncornavirus antigen was not detected in concentrated preparations
of selected viruses belonging to other classes (papovaviruses, pox-
viruses, adenoviruses, myxoviruses, arboviruses, plant viruses and
DNA bacteriophage).

     Considerable effort has gone into excluding trivial explanations
for this cross-reactivity between herpesviruses and oncornaviruses.
Thus far we have ruled out the participation of heterologous sera or
normal cellular components including actin, histones, DNA fragments
and polynucleotides.

     Table 2 summarizes the analysis of the precipitin reaction by
absorption tests.   Absorption of the antiherpesvirus nc sera with
purified herpesvirus nc or oncornaviruses removed all reactivity to
both the herpesviruses and oncornaviruses.   Absorption with a range
of other materials, including extracts of the uninfected cells used
for the production of EHV-1 nc, HSV-1 nc and HSV-2 nc did not
absorb the reactivity of the antisera to the shared herpesvirus-
oncornavirus antigen.

     Immunoelectron microscopy (IEM) showed that the antiherpesvirus
nc sera reacted with a surface component of EHV-1 nc, HSV-1 nc,
HSV-2 nc and Lucké tumour herpesvirus nc (Table 3, Fig. 1C-E).

FIG. 1. HERPESVIRUS PREPARATIONS AND REACTIONS BETWEEN
NC AND ANTISERA

(A) Representative electron micrograph of EHV-1 preparation used for immunization (× 42 000)

(B) High-magnification electron micrograph of HSV-2 nc preparation used for immunization (× 92 500)

(C) EHV-1 nc reacted with rat anti-HSV-2 nc serum.   Nucleocapsids were adsorbed to carbon films, washed four times in distilled water (dH$_2$O), reacted for 30 minutes at room temperature with antiherpesvirus nc serum, washed six times with dH$_2$O, reacted for 30 minutes with antirat/antiferritin hybrid antibody, washed six times with dH$_2$O, reacted for 20 minutes with horse ferritin, washed six times with dH$_2$O and stained for 60 seconds with 2% phosphotungstic acid (PTA), pH 7.0.   Note the heavy accumulation of ferritin surrounding all nc (arrows). (× 42 000)

(D) High-magnification view of HSV-1 nc reacted with anti-EHV-1 nc serum showing specific accumulation of ferritin on the nc surface (× 81 000)

(E) EHV-1 nc reacted with preimmune rat serum. Note the presence of ferritin in the background but not on the nc surface. (× 42 000)

(F) HSV-1 nc reacted with rat anti-EHV-1 nc serum absorbed with FeLV. There is no ferritin labelling of the nc surface. (× 109 000)

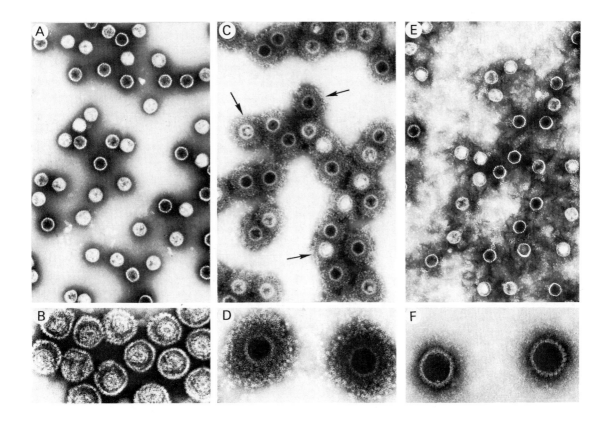

FIG. 2.   TYPICAL GEL PATTERNS OBTAINED BY
SDS-PAGE ANALYSIS OF EHV-1 nc

SDS-PAGE analysis on 7.5% cylindrical gels of EHV-1 nc purified by
the technique of Gibson & Roizman (1972) (sucrose purified) or by
sedimentation through caesium chloride as a final step (CsCl purified).

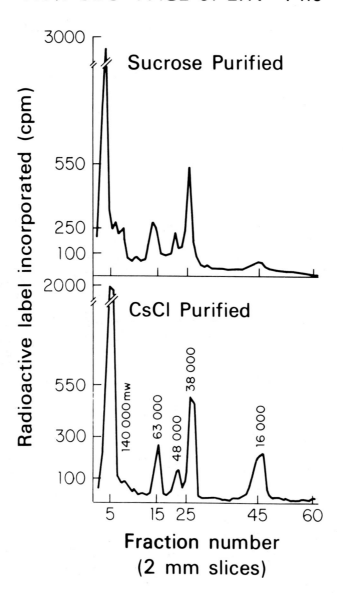

Table 1. Reactivity of antisera to herpesvirus nucleocapsids in immunodiffusion tests[a]

Source of antigen	Rat antisera				Goat antiserum	
	Anti-EHV-1 nc		Anti-HSV-2 nc		Anti-HSV-1 nc & HSV-2 nc	
	Preimmune	Immune	Preimmune	Immune	Preimmune	Immune
A. Herpesvirus preparations[b]						
HSV-1 nc	−	+	−	+	−	+
HSV-2 nc	−	+	−	+	−	+
EHV-1 nc	−	+	−	+	−	+
EBV nc	−	+	−	+	−	+
CMV nc	NT	NT	NT	NT	−	+
MDV nc (strain JMV)	NT	NT	NT	NT	−	+
Lucké tumour herpesvirus nc	−	+	−	+	−	+
B. Oncornavirus preparations[b]						
SSV-1 (simian sarcoma virus)	−	+	−	+	−	+
GaLV (gibbon ape leukaemia virus)	−	+	−	+	−	+
BEV (baboon endogenous virus)	−	+	−	+	−	+
M-7 (baboon endogenous virus)	−	+	−	+	−	+
FeLV (feline leukaemia virus)	−	+	−	+	−	+
HaLV (hamster leukaemia virus)	−	+	−	+	−	+
HaSV (hamster sarcoma virus)	−	+	−	+	−	+
MuLV (Rauscher, Gross and AKR leukaemia viruses)	−	+	−	+	−	+
AMV (avian myeloblastosis virus)	−	+	−	+	−	+
Viper oncornavirus	−	+	−	+	−	+
MuMTV (murine mammary tumour virus, milk-derived)	−	+	−	+	−	+
MPMV (Mason-Pfizer mammary tumour virus)	−	+	−	+	−	+
C. Other virus preparations[b]						
Adenovirus type 5	NT	−	NT	−	NT	−
Human wart virus	NT	−	NT	−	NT	−
SV40	−	−	−	−	NT	−
Vaccinia virus	NT	−	NT	−	NT	−
Influenza virus (WSN)	−	(+)[c]	−	(+)[c]	−	(+)[c]
Influenza virus (Massachusetts B)	−	−	−	−	−	−
Sendai virus	−	(+)[c]	−	(+)[c]	−	(+)[c]
Feline syncytial virus	−	−	−	−	−	−
Semliki Forest virus	−	−	−	−	−	−
Southern bean mosaic virus	−	−	−	−	−	−
IKE δ bacteriophage (DNA)	−	−	−	−	−	−
D. Cellular extracts[d]						
L-M	−	−	−	−	−	−
Vero	−	−	−	−	−	−
WI-38	−	−	−	−	−	−
SK-LMS	−	−	−	−	−	−
HeLa	−	−	−	−	−	−
HEp-2	−	−	−	−	−	−
SA-8 human melanoma	−	−	−	−	−	−
SA-13 human melanoma	−	−	−	−	−	−
SA-14 human melanoma	−	−	−	−	−	−
Pooled normal ovary	−	−	−	−	−	−
Normal frog kidney	−	−	−	−	NT	NT
E. Other antigens						
FCS[e] (100 mg/ml)	−	−	−	−	−	(+)[c]
Histones (100 mg/ml)	−	−	−	−	−	−
Actin (50 mg/ml)	−	−	−	−	−	−
Poly I:C (50 mg/ml)	−	−	−	−	−	−
Poly A:U (50 mg/ml)	−	−	−	−	−	−
C reactive protein (20 mg/ml)	−	−	−	−	−	−

[a] + = Positive precipitin reactions = lines of identity with reference anti-EHV-1 nc serum/HSV-1 nc reactions; − = no precipitin reaction; NT = not tested; nc = nucleocapsids

[b] > 10^{10} herpesvirus nc or virus particles/ml (> 400 µg protein/ml)

[c] Positive precipitin reactions = lines of non-identity with reference anti-EHV-1 nc serum/HSV-1 nc reactions

[d] Cell extracts were prepared by three cycles of freezing and thawing followed by sonication in phosphate-buffered saline (PBS). Soluble antigens were prepared by centrifugation at 80 000 - 100 000 g for 1 hour. The supernatants were concentrated by vacuum dialysis or Millipore immersible molecular separators to 25 - 100 mg/ml.

[e] Fetal calf serum

FIG. 3. IMMUNODIFFUSION REACTIVITY OF ANTIHERPESVIRUS NC SERA

Immunodiffusion reactions in 0.7% agarose gels demonstrating the shared herpesvirus nc - oncornavirus antigen.   (A) The centre well contained rat anti-EHV-1 nc serum.   Note the precipitin reaction of identity among the herpesvirus nc of amphibian, equine and primate origins;   (B) the centre well contained rat anti-HSV-2 nc serum. Note the precipitin reaction of identity among EHV-1 nc and representative oncornaviruses.

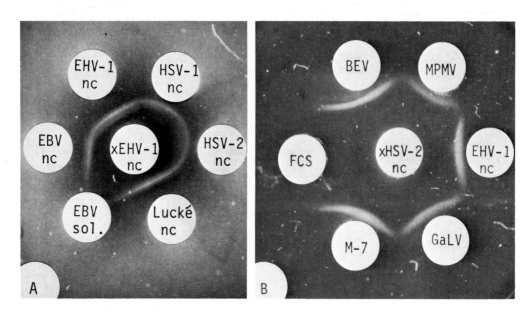

Preimmune sera were consistently negative.   IEM absorption analysis (Table 4) confirmed these observations: purified herpesvirus nc and FeLV, as a representative oncornavirus, absorbed nc reactivity whereas absorption with two viruses that were negative for the shared antigen in ID, feline syncytial virus and Semliki Forest virus, did not absorb IEM reactivity.

Our present objective is to identify the viral component(s) in herpesviruses and oncornaviruses that carries the shared antigen. Because herpesvirus nc are difficult to dissociate while maintaining native antigenicity of the proteins, we have concentrated on identify-- ing the cross-reactive component in oncornaviruses.   Table 5 summarizes ID tests with purified components from Rauscher MuLV,

Table 2. Immunodiffusion absorption analysis of herpesvirus nc antisera[a]

Absorbing antigen	Test antigen					
	EHV-1 nc	HSV-1 nc	HSV-2 nc	EBV nc	Lucké nc	Oncornaviruses
EHV-1 nc	+	+	+	+	+	+
HSV-1 nc	+	+	+	+	+	+
HSV-2 nc	+	+	+	+	+	+
EBV (NP-40 treated)	+	+	+	+	+	+
EBV (intact)	-	-	-	+	NT	NT
Lucké tumour herpesvirus nc	+	+	+	+	+	+
Oncornaviruses[b]	+	+	+	+	+	+
Influenza virus (WSN)	-	-	-	-	NT	-
Sendai virus	-	-	-	-	NT	-
Semliki Forest virus	-	-	-	-	NT	-
Feline syncytial virus	-	-	-	-	NT	-
SV40	-	-	-	-	NT	-
L-M cells	-	-	-	-	NT	-
Vero cells	-	-	-	-	NT	-
HeLa cells	-	-	-	-	NT	-
SK-LMS cells	-	-	-	-	NT	-
Normal ovary extract	-	-	-	-	NT	-
Ovarian tumour extract	-	-	-	-	NT	-
SA-8 human melanoma cells	-	-	-	-	NT	-
SA-13 human melanoma cells	-	-	-	-	NT	-
Sa-14 human melanoma cells	-	-	-	-	NT	-
FCS[c] (100 mg/ml)	-	-	-	-	-	-
Sheep red blood corpuscles	-	-	-	-	NT	-
C reactive protein (20 mg/ml)	-	-	-	-	NT	-
Histones (100 mg/ml)	-	-	-	-	NT	-
Actin (50 mg/ml)	-	-	-	-	NT	-
Poly I:C (50 mg/ml)	-	-	-	-	NT	-
Poly A:U (50 mg/ml)	-	-	-	-	NT	-

[a] + = Absorption of reactivity of antiherpesvirus nc sera to herpesvirus nc or oncornaviruses;
- = No absorption of reactivity of antiherpesvirus nc sera to herpesvirus nc or oncornaviruses;
NT = Not tested.
Absorption technique: Rat antisera to EHV-1 nc and HSV-2 nc were diluted with PBS to approximately two doubling dilutions below the end-point of reactivity and were absorbed with an equal volume of antigen (> 10^10 herpesvirus nc or virus particles/ml or 50-100 mg/ml for cellular antigens). Absorption was carried out at 4°C for 18 hours. The absorbed antisera were centrifuged at approximately 6500 g for 10 minutes before testing. Undiluted goat antiserum was similarly absorbed.

[b] Antiherpesvirus nc sera were absorbed with representative avian, reptilian and mammalian oncornaviruses (see Table 1).

[c] Fetal calf serum

Gross MuLV, baboon endogenous virus (BEV) and simian sarcoma virus (SSV-1). Antigen was demonstrated in the void volume eluates of Rauscher MuLV fractionated by guanidine hydrochloride column chromatography; this fraction contains the MuLV envelope protein p15E as well as other high molecular-weight components. SSV-1 gp70 was the only other purified viral component that reacted with the anti-herpesvirus nc sera. Thus far it has not been possible to determine whether this reaction is related to the shared herpesvirus-oncornavirus antigen.

Table 3. Immunoelectron microscopic analysis of rat antiherpesvirus nc sera[a]

Virus	Sera	
	Preimmune	Immune
HSV-1 intact virions	−	−
HSV-1 nc	−	+
HSV-2 nc	−	+
EHV-1 nc	−	+
Lucké tumour herpesvirus nc	−	+

[a] Both anti-EHV-1 nc and anti-HSV-2 nc sera produced identical results; + = specific ferritin labelling of herpesvirus nc; − = no ferritin labelling of herpesvirus nc

Table 4. Immunoelectron microscopic absorption analysis of rat anti-EHV-1 nc serum[a]

Absorbing antigen	Test antigen			
	EHV-1 nc	HSV-1 nc	HSV-2 nc	Lucké nc
EHV-1 nc	+	+	+	+
HSV-1 nc	+	+	+	+
HSV-2 nc	+	+	+	+
Lucké tumour herpesvirus nc	+	+	+	+
EBV (NP-40 treated)	+	+	+	+
FeLV	+	+	+	NT
Semliki Forest virus	−	−	−	−
Feline syncytial virus	−	−	−	−
FCS[b] (100 mg/ml)	−	−	−	NT

[a] + = Absorption of IEM reaction; − = No absorption of IEM reaction; NT = Not tested

[b] Fetal calf serum

Table 5.   Immunodiffusion tests with purified oncornavirus components

Antigen	Preimmune goat serum	Goat antiserum to HSV-1 nc and HSV-2 nc	Quantity of protein[a] (μg)
Rauscher MuLV[b]			
p15E	-	+	2.2
gp70		-	3.5
p30		-	2.8
p15		-	1.8
p12		-	1.2
p10		-	0.8
Gross MuLV[b]			
p30		-	2.5
BEV[c]			
gp70		-	ND[d]
p30		-	14.5
SSV-1[c]			
gp70	-	+[e]	ND[d]
p30		-	8.3

[a] Approximate quantity (μg) of protein plated;   0.4 μg EHV-1 nc is sufficient to produce a precipitin reaction.

[b] Obtained from Dr E. Fleissner

[c] Obtained from Dr J. Stephenson

[d] Protein concentration not determined

[e] Characteristics of precipitin line did not allow identity to be established with reference antiherpesvirus nc/herpesvirus nc-oncornavirus reactions.

Radioimmunoprecipitations (RIP) with goat or rat antiherpesvirus nc sera and ^{3}H, ^{14}C and ^{125}I-labelled oncornaviruses showed precipitates with low counts in tests with FeLV, AKR-MuLV and BEV.   With FeLV and MuLV, SDS-PAGE analysis revealed that the precipitated component was in the molecular weight range 50-55 000 daltons.   With BEV the precipitated component was 10-15 000 daltons.   These components were not precipitated by preimmune sera.   Dr J. Stephenson of the National Cancer Institute has tested the goat antiherpesvirus nc serum in RIP with purified p30 and gp85 from Rauscher MuLV, FeLV, the endogenous feline oncornavirus RD-114, Mason-Pfizer mammary tumour virus (MPMV), SSV-1 and baboon endogenous virus M-7 and detected no reactivity.   There are several ways to account for these negative

results: low avidity of the antiherpesvirus nc sera for the shared
oncornavirus component, or poor labelling or low concentration of
the antigen.

In view of the unexpected pattern of reactivity that we have
observed with the antiherpesvirus nc sera in immunodiffusion tests
and immunoelectron microscopy, we have been reluctant to draw any
conclusions about the nature of the shared antigen linking herpesviruses and oncornaviruses.   At this stage in the analysis we cannot
exclude the possibility that the antigen may be host-derived rather than
a virus-coded component.   For this reason, the significance of our
observations must await the isolation and characterization of the
molecule carrying this intriguing antigen.

ACKNOWLEDGEMENTS

We wish to thank the following individuals for their most
valuable contributions to this study: M. Eisinger,
E. Fleissner, J. Gruber, U. Hämmerling, C. Lopez,
J. Lemp, S. Palchaudhuri, B. Roizman, H. Snyder,
P. Spear and J. Stephenson.   We also wish to
thank S. Arpadi and R. Casola for their technical assistance. This work was supported in
part by HRC grants No. 167 and No. 690 from
the New York State Health Planning Commission,
National Cancer Institute grant No. CA-19765
and a grant from the Richard Molin Memorial
Foundation for Cancer Research.

REFERENCES

Gibson, W. & Roizman, B. (1972)   Proteins specified by herpes
    simplex virus VIII. Characterization and composition of multiple
    capsid forms of subtypes 1 and 2.   *J. Virol.*, *10*, 1044-1052

Purdue, M.L., Cohen, J.C., Kemp, M.C., Randall, C.C. & O'Callaghan, D.J.
    (1975)   Characterization of three species of nucleocapsids of
    equine herpesvirus type-1 (EHV-1).   *Virology*, *64*, 187-204

Weber, K. & Osborn, M. (1969)   The reliability of molecular weight
    determinates by dodecyl sulfate-polyacrylamide gel electrophoresis.
    J. biol. Chem., *244*, 4406-4412

CROSSED IMMUNOELECTROPHORETIC ANALYSIS AND VIRAL NEUTRALIZING ACTIVITY OF FIVE MONOSPECIFIC ANTISERA AGAINST FIVE DIFFERENT HERPES SIMPLEX VIRUS GLYCOPROTEINS

B.F. VESTERGAARD

Department of Clinical Virology,
Institute of Medical Microbiology,
Copenhagen, Denmark

B. NORRILD

Department of Pediatrics,
Emory University School of Medicine,
Atlanta, Georgia, USA

INTRODUCTION

The envelope antigens of herpes simplex virus (HSV) play an important immunological role in the infected host.   Lesso et al. (1976) demonstrated that rabbits inoculated with a membrane preparation from HSV developed neutralizing antibodies in high titres, and Cappel (1976) found that two injections of HSV envelope proteins solubilized with the non-ionic detergent Nonidet NP-40 (NP-40), induced both a humoral and a cellular immune response against HSV in rabbits.

The non-ionic detergents are effective solubilizers of biological membranes capable of preserving the complex biochemical structure and immunological reactivity of the solubilized proteins (Bjerrum, 1977).

We have shown that HSV glycoproteins can be solubilized from infected cells with the non-ionic detergent Triton X-100 and give rise to well-defined immunoprecipitates by crossed immunoelectrophoresis in Triton X-100 containing agarose gel (Vestergaard, 1973; Vestergaard & Bøg-

Hansen, 1975).   The five immunoprecipitates used in the present study
represent membrane-bound glycoprotein entities of HSV (Vestergaard,
1977), each one composed of several polypeptides (Norrild & Vestergaard,
1977).

MATERIALS AND METHODS

Virus, cell cultures, reference antigens and antibodies

HSV type 1 (F) and type 2 (G) were propagated in a rabbit cornea
cell line.   The cells were harvested 24 hours after a high-multiplicity
infection and solubilized in 5% (v/v) Triton X-100, as described earlier
(Vestergaard et al., 1977).   This crude antigenic preparation had a
protein content of approximately 10 mg/ml and is referred to subsequently as the reference antigen.   Antisera against HSV type 1 or type 2
were raised in infected rabbits as described earlier (Vestergaard,
1973), and purified immunoglobulins were made from pools of whole
sera by the method of Harboe & Ingild (1973).   This preparation is
referred to as polyspecific HSV antibodies.

Crossed immunoelectrophoresis

This technique has been described previously (Vestergaard, 1973).
Technical details are given in legends to figures.   The monospecific
antisera were tested by the intermediate-gel method developed by
Axelsen (1973).   The antiserum to be tested is incorporated in an
intermediate gel introduced between the first and second dimensions
of electrophoresis.   If specific antibodies are present, only the
corresponding precipitate in the crossed immunoelectrophoretic precipitating profile will be lowered.

Titration of immunoprecipitating activity by countercurrent immuno-electroosmophoresis

The electrophoresis was done according to Grauballe et al. (1975).
Each two-fold dilution of antiserum was electrophoresed against three
different dilutions of antigen, in order to ensure optimal ratios of
antibody to antigen.   Precipitates were stained with Coomassie
Brilliant Blue.

Production of monospecific antisera

By manipulating the crossed immunoelectrophoretic precipitating
profile of HSV type 1 and type 2 reference antigens (i.e., by varying
the concentrations of antigen and antibodies and using intermediate
gels) it was possible to obtain separable precipitates of Ag6, Ag8,
Ag9 and Ag11.   Precipitates of Ag4 were obtained by rocket immunoelectrophoresis of purified Ag4 into gel containing polyspecific HSV

type 2 antibodies (Norrild & Vestergaard[1]).   All precipitates were
cut out of the unstained wet gel, disrupted by sonication, mixed with
incomplete Freund's adjuvant and injected intracutaneously into
rabbits, as described earlier (Vestergaard, 1975).

Neutralization

Plaque reduction multiplicity analysis was done by mixing equal
volumes of two-fold dilutions of antisera and approximately 500
plaque-forming units (PFU) of either HSV type 1 or type 2.   After 30
minutes' incubation at 37°C, surviving virus was assayed on rabbit
cornea cells, as described earlier (Vestergaard et al., 1972).

RESULTS

Figure 1A shows the precipitating profile of HSV type 1 reference
antigen with normal rabbit serum in the intermediate gel.   The
antigens are numbered in accordance with previously published papers
(Vestergaard, 1973; Vestergaard & Bøg-Hansen, 1975).   Figure 1B
shows the precipitating profile with anti-Ag11 in the intermediate
gel.   It can be seen that the precipitate of Ag11 has been lowered.
Figure 1C shows the strong reactivity of anti-Ag8, and Figure 1D
demonstrates the lowering of the Ag6 precipitate when anti-Ag6 is
incorporated in the intermediate gel.

Figure 2A shows the precipitating profile of HSV type 2 reference
antigen with normal rabbit serum in the intermediate gel.   The number-
ing is in accordance with earlier papers (Vestergaard, 1973;
Vestergaard & Bøg-Hansen, 1975).   Figure 2B shows the lowering of the
Ag9 precipitate when anti-Ag9 is incorporated in the intermediate gel
and Figure 2C the retention of the Ag4 precipitate in the anti-Ag4
containing intermediate gel.

Table 1 lists the neutralizing titres of the five monospecific
antisera.   Table 2 shows the immunoprecipitating activity of the
same five antisera.   In Table 3, the antisera have been equalized in
respect of immunoprecipitating activity in order to make a direct
comparison of neutralizing potency.

DISCUSSION

Our results clearly show that antibodies directed against a
single HSV glycoprotein were able to neutralize the virus particle.
We have further tried to elucidate the immunological importance of

---

[1] Unpublished data

FIG. 1.   CROSSED IMMUNOELECTROPHORESIS OF HSV TYPE 1
REFERENCE ANTIGEN

Gel: 1% (w/v) agarose (HSB, Mr= - 0.10, Litex, Denmark) dissolved in
0.180 M tris, 0.060 M Barbital, pH 8.6 at 16°C, containing 1% (v/v)
Triton X-100.   First-dimension electrophoresis: 15 μl HSV type 1
reference antigen electrophoresed in 1.5 mm thick gel at 10 V/cm for
90 minutes at 16°C.   Second-dimension electrophoresis: Performed on
7 × 7 cm glass plates for 16 hours at 1.5 V/cm in 1-mm thick gel
containing 10 μl/cm² polyspecific anti-HSV type 1 antibodies.   Intermediate gel: 7 × 1.5 cm gel slab, 1.25 mm thick, containing 15 μl/cm²
normal rabbit immunoglobulin or monoprecipitin.
(A) Normal rabbit immunoglobulin;   (B) Anti-Ag11;   (C) Anti-Ag8;
(D) Anti-Ag6.

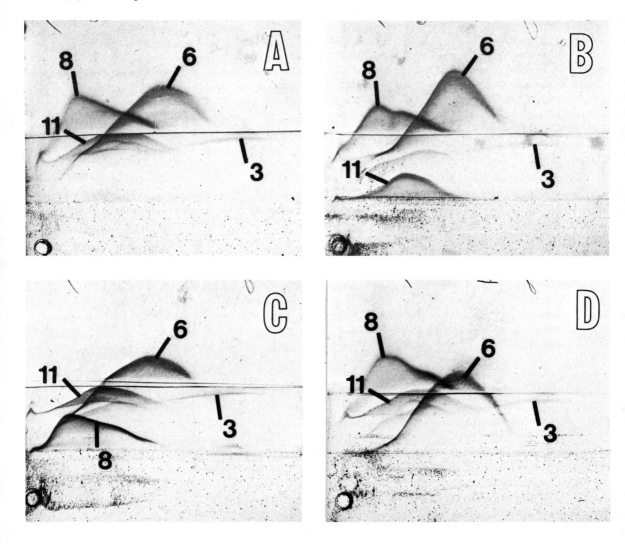

FIG. 2. CROSSED IMMUNOELECTROPHORESIS OF HSV TYPE 2 REFERENCE ANTIGEN

Technique as described in legend to Figure 1. (A) Normal rabbit immunoglobulin; (B) Anti-Ag9; (C) Anti-Ag4.

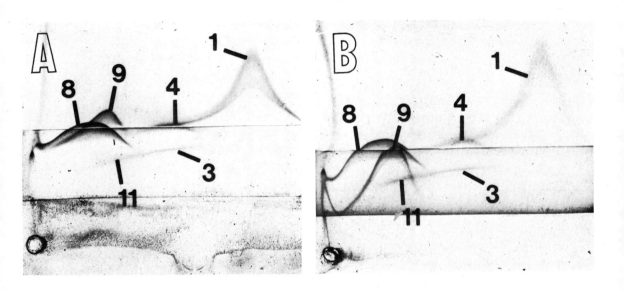

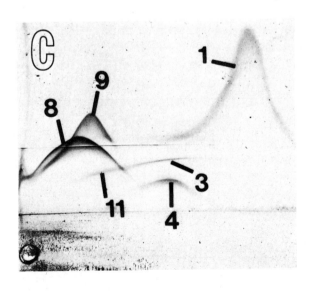

Table 1. Titration of neutralizing potency as measured by plaque reduction multiplicity analysis[a]

Monoprecipitins	HSV-1	HSV-2
Anti-Ag11	60	20
Anti-Ag8	200	60
Anti-Ag6	80	5
Anti-Ag4	15	40
Anti-Ag9	5	20

[a] Titres are expressed as the reciprocal of the serum dilution causing a 50% plaque reduction.

Table 2. Titration of immunoprecipitating activity as measured by countercurrent immunoelectroosmophoresis[a]

Monoprecipitins	Antiserum (microlitres)	Titre
Anti-Ag11	5	0.2
Anti-Ag8	5	0.2
Anti-Ag6	2	0.5
Anti-Ag4	4	0.25
Anti-Ag9	15	0.07

[a] Titres are expressed as the reciprocal of the minimum amount of antiserum (microlitres) capable of producing a visible precipitate after Coomassie Brilliant Blue staining.

each of the five glycoproteins in respect of their representation on the outer virion envelope as targets for neutralizing antibodies.

For that purpose it was necessary to adjust the five monospecific antisera to some kind of equal immunoreactivity, as it would have been meaningless to consider the neutralizing titre alone because the amount and avidity of specific antibodies in the antisera were different.

Table 3. Neutralizing potency of monoprecipitins equalized with respect to immunoprecipitating activity[a]

Monoprecipitins	Neutralizing potency	
	HSV-1	HSV-2
Anti-Ag11	300	100
Anti-Ag8	1000	300
Anti-Ag6	160	10
Anti-Ag4	60	160
Anti-Ag9	75	300

[a] Neutralizing potency = $\dfrac{\text{neutralizing titre}}{\text{immunoprecipitating titre}}$

Titration of immunoprecipitating activity may be too simple a method for the exact measurement of immunoreactive molecules in an antibody preparation but does reflect the amount and avidity of specifically reacting antibodies.

The interpretation of the results presented in Table 3 is difficult, because qualitative factors such as the avidity of the different anti-bodies and the association of certain antigenic sites on the virion with virus/cell attachment sites are not known.   However, one explana-tion might be that the differences in neutralizing potency of the five monoprecipitins reflect quantitative differences in the representation of the corresponding glycoproteins on the outer envelope of the virion. Such an interpretation is supported by our finding that Ag11 and Ag8 are found in larger quantities in HSV-1 infected cells than in HSV-2 infected cells.

Immunoelectrophoretic studies have shown that Ag6 is HSV-1 specific while Ag4 and Ag9 are HSV-2 specific (Norrild & Vestergaard[1]; Vester-gaard, 1973).   Figure 3 demonstrates that anti-Ag6 gives strong immunoprecipitates with four different HSV-1 strains but no precipitates with four different HSV-2 strains.   The reversed patterns are seen when the eight HSV strains are electrophoresed into anti-Ag4-containing gel. The results from the neutralization studies are not as clear-cut.   There may be at least two reasons for this discrepancy.   Firstly, the antigens are complex proteins and may, apart from major type-specific antigenic

---

[1] Unpublished data

FIG. 3.   ROCKET IMMUNOELECTROPHORESIS OF EIGHT DIFFERENT
STRAINS OF HSV

5 μl antigen (prepared as described for reference HSV antigens) were
applied to each well and electrophoresed for 16 hours at 1.5 V/cm into
1% (w/v) agarose (HSA, Mr = - 0.13, Litex, Denmark) containing either
anti-Ag6 or anti-Ag4 at a concentration of 15 μl/cm^2.   HSV strains:
(1) MacIntyre;   (2) MS;   (3) F;   (4) G;   (5) Justin;   (6) Benefield;
(7) A-833 (Nahmias);   and (8) Savage.

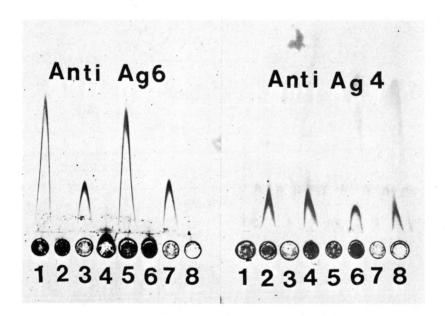

determinants, also possess minor type-common sites.   Secondly, neutralization is a more sensitive method for antibody detection than immunoelectrophoresis (Vestergaard et al., 1977).

In the present work, we have shown that some HSV glycoproteins are
capable of eliciting the production of viral neutralizing antibodies
better than others, and such a finding is important from the point of
view of the development of effective HSV subviral vaccines (Hilleman,
1976).

SUMMARY

Crossed immunoelectrophoresis of Triton X-100 solubilized HSV-infected cells has identified several major HSV glycoprotein antigens in the precipitating profile. Immunization of rabbits with the corresponding precipitates resulted in the production of monospecific antisera against the antigen part of the precipitate. The immunological importance of five different HSV glycoproteins in respect of their representation on the outer virion envelope as targets for neutralizing antibodies was evaluated by comparison of immunoprecipitating activity and neutralizing potency of the corresponding monospecific antisera.

REFERENCES

Axelsen, N.H. (1973)   Intermediate gel in crossed and in fused rocket immunoelectrophoresis. *Scand. J. Immunol.*, *2*, Suppl. 1, pp. 71-77

Bjerrum, O.J. (1977)   Immunochemical investigation of membrane proteins. A methodological survey with emphasis placed on immuno-precipitation in gels. *Biochim. biophys. Acta (Amst.)* (in press)

Cappel, R. (1976)   Comparison of the humoral and cellular immune-responses after immunization with live, UV inactivated herpes simplex virus and a subunit vaccine and efficacy of these immunizations. *Arch. Virol.*, *52*, 29-35

Grauballe, P.C., Vestergaard, B.F., Hornsleth, A., Leerhøy, J. & Johnsson, T. (1975)   Demonstration by immunoelectroosmophoresis of precipitating antibodies to a purified rubella virus antigen. *Infect. Immun.*, *12*, 55-61

Harboe, N. & Ingild, A. (1973)   Immunization, isolation of immuno-globulins, estimation of antibody titres. *Scand. J. Immunol.*, *2*, Suppl. 1, 161-164

Hilleman, M.R. (1976)   Herpes simplex vaccines. *Cancer Res.*, *36*, 857-858

Lesso, J., Hána, L. & Matis, J. (1976)   Reactions of immune sera against the nucleocapsid, envelope and whole herpes simplex virus type 1. *Acta Virol.*, *20*, 48-52

Norrild, B. & Vestergaard, B.F. (1977)   Polyacrylamide gel electro-
    phoretic analysis of herpes simplex virus type 1 immunoprecipitates
    obtained by quantitative immunoelectrophoresis in antibody-
    containing agarose gel.   *J. Virol.*, *22*, 113-117

Vestergaard, B.F. (1973)   Crossed immunoelectrophoretic characteriza-
    tion of herpesvirus hominis type 1 and 2 antigens.   *Acta path.*
    microbiol. scand., *Sect. B, 81*, 808-310·

Vestergaard, B.F. (1975)   Production of antiserum against a specific
    herpes simplex virus type 2 antigen.   *Scand. J. Immunol.*, *4*,
    Suppl. 2, pp. 203-206

Vestergaard, B.F. & Bøg-Hansen, T.C. (1975)   Detection of concanavalin
    A-binding herpes simplex virus type 1 and type 2 antigens by crossed
    immuno-affinoelectrophoresis.   *Scand. J. Immunol.*, *4*, Suppl. 2,
    pp. 211-215

Vestergaard, B.F., Hornsleth, A. & Pedersen, S.N. (1972)   Occurrence
    of herpes- and adenovirus antibodies in patients with carcinoma
    of the cervix uteri.   Measurement of antibodies to herpesvirus
    hominis (types 1 and 2), cytomegalovirus, EB-virus and adenovirus.
    Cancer, 30, 68-74

Vestergaard, B.F., Bjerrum, O.J., Norrild, B. & Grauballe, P.C. (1977)
    Crossed immunoelectrophoretic studies of the solubility and immuno-
    geneticity of herpes simplex virus antigens.   *J. Virol.*, *24*, 82-90

IMMUNOLOGICAL CHARACTERIZATION OF A COMMON ANTIGEN PRESENT IN HERPES SIMPLEX VIRUS, BOVINE MAMMILLITIS VIRUS AND HERPESVIRUS SIMIAE (B VIRUS)

H. LUDWIG & G. PAULI

Institute of Virology, Justus-Liebig-University,
Giessen, Federal Republic of Germany

B. NORRILD & B.F. VESTERGAARD

Institute of Medical Microbiology,
University of Copenhagen,
Copenhagen, Denmark

M.D. DANIEL

New England Regional Primate Research Center,
Harvard Medical School,
Boston, Mass., USA

Herpesviruses have a very complex structure compared to other animal viruses. It is therefore obvious that the different biologically active components cannot easily be separated and characterized. The serological relationship found between herpes simplex virus types 1 and 2 (HSV-1, HSV-2), B virus and bovine mammilitis virus (BMV) (Killington et al.[1]; Sterz et al., 1973) offers a useful tool for analysing the viral components responsible for the cross-reactivity. This is of particular interest since the common antigens induce the production of cross-neutralizing antibodies in the organism and are therefore at least one of the immunogenic components of these viruses.

------

[1] See p. 185

The cross-neutralizing activity of the different strain-specific antisera is shown in Figure 1.   The varying degree of reaction of the different virus strains with each of the heterologous antisera indicates, however, that the common antigenic determinants still have a strain-characteristic profile.   It was therefore of interest to characterize these common antigens.   Antigen preparations were made from infected whole cells or purified virus by Triton X-100 or Nonidet P-40/sodium deoxycholate (NP-40/DOC) treatment (Norrild & Vestergaard, 1977; Pauli & Ludwig, 1977).   Using immunoelectrophoretic methods, such as fused rocket or line electrophoresis (Axelsen et al., 1975), only one common antigen could be detected in all preparations when the various homologous or heterologous antisera were applied in the second dimension gels (Fig. 2).   The presence of only one common

FIG. 1.   CROSS-NEUTRALIZING ACTIVITY OF STRAIN-SPECIFIC ANTISERA

Neutralization tests with HSV-1 (strain Kos), HSV-2 (strain 196) or BMV and homologous as well as heterologous antisera were directed against these viruses (A) and B virus (B). V/V_0 is the fractional reduction in plaque counts: approximately 200 plaques (V_0) were treated with different dilutions of serum; V is the number of plaques obtained.   Bovine sera were taken after infection with BMV (AS-2) and after the first booster inoculation (AS-4).   The human pool serum was derived from 10 individual sera selected for high titres against HSV-1. Serum (B-neg) was derived from rhesus monkeys (specific pathogen-free animals; see Fig. 3); α-B serum (No. 3) was an individual rhesus monkey antiserum to B virus, and α-B serum (pool) a pool of rhesus monkey antisera to B virus.

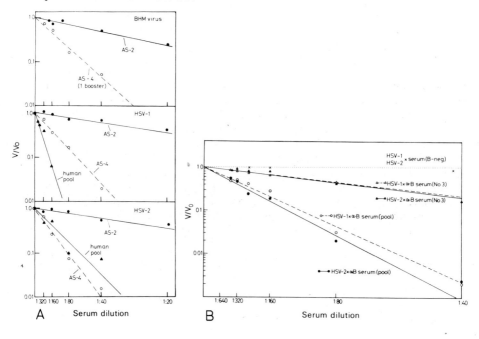

FIG. 2. FUSED-ROCKET IMMUNOELECTROPHORESIS OF TRITON X-100
SOLUBILIZED ANTIGENS OF HERPESVIRUS-INFECTED CELLS
IN DIFFERENT ANTISERA

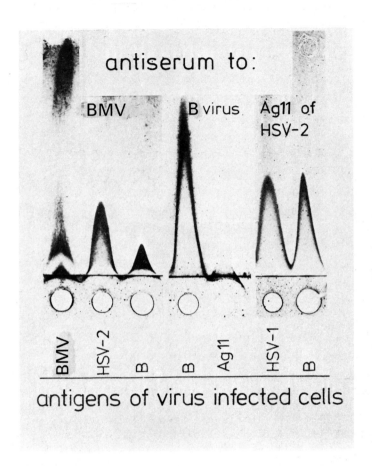

antigen in all four herpesviruses is also shown in crossed immunoelectrophoretic analyses.   Using the intermediate-gel technique,
strain-specific antisera, when incorporated into the intermediate
gel, reacted with only one precipitation arc in the HSV system
(Fig. 3).   This immunoprecipitate corresponds to antigen 11 (Ag11)
defined in the HSV system (Norrild & Vestergaard, 1977).   To support
this finding, monospecific antiserum against Ag11 (Vestergaard &
Norrild,[1]) was applied in the tests.   In fused rocket (Fig. 2)

------

[1] See p. 225

FIG. 3. CROSSED IMMUNOELECTROPHORESIS OF HSV-1 ANTIGEN
WITH INTERMEDIATE GELS

Crossed immunoelectrophoresis of HSV-1 antigen in HSV-1 polyspecific
rabbit serum with intermediate gels containing rhesus monkey serum
from specific pathogen-free animals (NORMAL) or B virus-infected
animals (ANTI-B). The Ag11 is selectively lowered. The autoradiogram is shown.

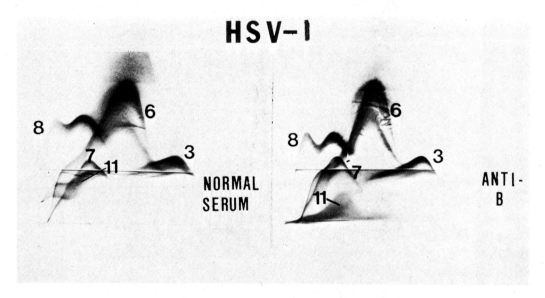

as well as in crossed immunoelectrophoresis this antiserum was able
to pick up the common antigen from different viral preparations. It
may therefore be concluded that Ag11 is the carrier of the cross-
reacting antigen. The characterization of the common antigen by
polyacrylamide gel electrophoresis (PAGE) after labelling with radioactive amino-acids gave the surprising result that this complex
differs in composition in the four viruses. The data are summarized
in Table 1. It is obvious, however, that the Ag11 complex includes
a polypeptide with an apparent molecular weight of 126 000 in all
the different viral preparations. This polypeptide is glycosylated,
as shown by radioactive glucosamine incorporation. From these
findings it is suggested that the common antigenic determinant(s) is
carried by this glycoprotein.

Evidence that the common antigenic sites are exposed on the
surface of the particles can also be obtained by cross-protection
experiments (Table 2). Mice immunized with BMV survived an otherwise fatal HSV-1 or HSV-2 induced encephalitis after intracerebral
challenge (Ludwig & Rott[1]).

---

[1] Unpublished data

Table 1. Polypeptides of the common antigen (AgII complex)[a]

Antigen from cells infected with:	Polypeptides: apparent MW $\times 10^{-3}$
HSV-1	126 (gp)
	111 (gp)
	94
HSV-2	126 (gp)
B virus	126 (gp)
	111 (gp)
	94
	90
BMV	150 (?)
	126 (gp)
	60 (?)

[a] These data were obtained by PAGE in slab gels of precipitates from crossed immunoelectrophoresis in the different heterologous antisera or anti-AgII serum (Norrild et al., unpublished data) or by indirect immunoprecipitation and PAGE analysis in Lämmli-round gels (Pauli & Ludwig, 1977); gp - glycoprotein; ? indicates that only faint bands were detected in the gels. HSV-1 and HSV-2 were propagated in human cells (Norrild & Vestergaard, 1977) or rabbit kidney cells (Ludwig et al., 1974), B virus in either of these cells (Daniel et al., 1975) and BMV in bovine cells (Sterz et al., 1973).

Table 2. Protection of mice with BMV against a lethal encephalitis induced by HSV[a]

Preimmunization with:	LD_{50} determination after challenge with:	
	HSV-1	HSV-2
Cell-free BMV	5×10^{0}	1×10^{-2}
Cell medium	1×10^{-3}	5×10^{-3}

[a] Preimmunization was by subcutaneous and intraperitoneal inoculation; challenge virus was inoculated intracerebrally.

In summary, it has been shown that herpesviruses which are only distantly related in their genetic material, like HSV-1, HSV-2 and BMV (Sterz et al., 1973) and which cause diseases in different natural hosts, share a common glycoprotein antigen, which is exposed on the virus surface.   This holds true even for HSV and B virus, which are clearly distinct in their DNA G+C content.   Antigen analysis shows that the latter virus is certainly not a variant of HSV (Ludwig et al.[1]).   It can be assumed that the shared antigen of the four herpesviruses represents a vestige of a common ancestor.

ACKNOWLEDGEMENTS

We gratefully acknowledge the stimulating discussions with Dr R. Rott.   This work was supported by the Sonderforschungsbereich 47 and the Danish Cancer Society.

REFERENCES

Axelsen, N.H., Krøll, J. & Weeke, B. (1975)   *A Manual of Quantitative Immunoelectrophoresis*.   Oslo, Bergen, Tromsø, Universitetsforlaget

Daniel, M.D., Garcia, F.G., Melendez, L.V., Hunt, R.D., O'Connor, J. & Silva, D. (1975)   Multiple herpesvirus simiae isolation from a rhesus monkey which died of cerebral infarction.   *Lab. Anim. Sci.*, *25*, 303-308

Ludwig, H., Becht, H. & Rott, R. (1974)   Inhibition of herpesvirus-induced cell fusion by Concanavalin A, antisera and 2-Deoxy-D-glucose.   *J. Virol.*, *14*, 307-314

Norrild, B. & Vestergaard, B.F. (1977)   Polyacrylamide gel electrophoretic analysis of herpes simplex virus type 1 immunoprecipitates obtained by quantitative immunoelectrophoresis in antibody-containing agarose gel.   *J. Virol.*, *22*, 113-117

---

[1] Unpublished data

Pauli, G. & Ludwig, H. (1977)   Immunoprecipitation of herpes
    simplex virus type 1 antigens with different antisera and human
    cerebrospinal fluids.   *Arch. Virol.*, *53*, 139-155

Sterz, H., Ludwig, H. & Rott, R. (1973)   Immunologic and genetic
    relationship between herpes simplex virus and bovine herpes
    mammillitis virus.   *Intervirology*, *2*, 1-13

ISOLATION OF THE EPSTEIN-BARR VIRUS NUCLEAR ANTIGEN FROM CHROMATIN PREPARATIONS

G.M. PIKLER[1], G.R. PEARSON & T.C. SPELSBERG

*Mayo Clinic/Foundation,
Rochester, Minn., USA*

The Epstein-Barr virus (EBV)-determined nuclear antigen (EBNA) is associated with the chromatin of lymphoblastoid cells which carry the viral genome (Bahr et al., 1975).   It has been suggested that EBNA represents an EBV-coded or viral-modified chromosomal protein that may participate in the regulation of EBV-induced transformation.   Most of the work on the purification of this EBV antigen has been carried out with the complement-fixing (CF) soluble (S) antigen.   We have been interested in the isolation and characterization of EBNA from the chromatin of EBV-positive lymphoblastoid cells in order to determine its chemical nature, its relationship to the soluble antigen, and finally its biological function in the nucleus.

Using anti-EBNA-positive sera, EBNA was shown to be associated with the chromatin of both NC37 and Raji non-producer cell lines by the anti-complement immunofluorescence assay (ACIF) (Reedman & Klein, 1973) and the ^{51}Cr-labelled microcomplement fixation assay (^{51}Cr-CF) (Cikes, 1975). Chromatin preparations were tested with several agents to determine their ability to dissociate EBNA from the chromatin.   Since chemical agents known to dissociate proteins from the chromatin DNA are also known to denature proteins, studies of the effects of protein denaturing agents on the antigenicity of the CF soluble and nuclear antigens of EBV were performed.   The antigenic activity of both antigens was not destroyed by a variety of denaturing conditions and solvents including heat (> 90°C), low (< pH 1) and high (> pH 12) pH, high levels of sodium chloride and guanidine hydrochloride as well as by RNase and trypsin. Thus, the antigenic activity appeared to be based on the primary structure of a protein.

---

[1] Present address: Developmental Therapeutics, M.D. Anderson Hospital and Tumor Institute, Houston, Texas, USA

   Initial studies of EBNA purification involved the sequential extraction of chromatin proteins with increasing concentrations of sodium
chloride to determine whether EBNA could be selectively dissociated at
certain salt concentrations which did not dissociate much of the aggre-
gating acidic chromatin proteins.   Figure 1A demonstrates that with
0.5 M salt treatment about 60-70% of the initial antigenic activity as
determined by ACIF and ^{51}Cr-CF was extracted.

      FIG. 1.   EXTRACTION OF PROTEIN AND EBNA FROM CHROMATIN:
         RESIDUAL LEVELS IN TREATED CHROMATIN AND EVIDENCE FOR
             TWO CLASSES OF CHROMATIN-ANTIGEN INTERACTIONS

NC37 chromatin was isolated according to Spelsberg & Hnilica (1971),
omitting the 0.35 M sodium chloride extraction.   Protein was determined according to Lowry et al. (1951).   DNA was measured by the
diphenylamine method of Burton (1956).   ACIF was done according to
Reedman & Klein (1973), with Huang's modification (Huang et al., 1974).
^{51}Cr-labelled micro CF was done according to Cikes (1975).   Chromatin
was incubated at 4°C for 90 minutes with a 10 mM tris hydrochloride,
pH 7.4, 1 mM EDTA, 1 mM phenylmethylsulfonyl fluoride (PMSF) buffer with
increasing sodium chloride concentrations in a 20:1 buffer to chromatin
ratio.   After incubation, it was spun at 27 000 rpm ($\approx$ 100 000 g) in a
Spinco SW27 rotor for 40 hours.   Extracts and pellets were dialysed for
24 hours and lyophilized (Pikler et al., unpublished data).   EBNA
concentrations are shown in (A) both for nuclei and for chromatin
(broken and continuous lines, respectively).

A. Salt dissociation of protein and EBNA from NC37 cell chromatin:
residual levels in treated chromatin

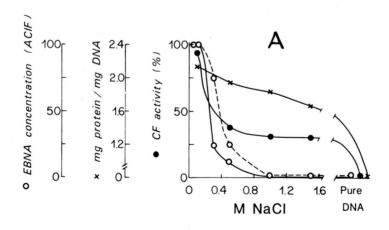

FIG. 1. (Continued)

B. Extracted protein and EBNA from NC37 cell chromatin: evidence for
two classes of chromatin-antigen interactions

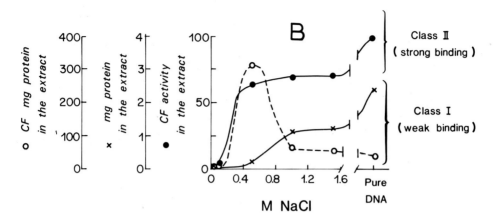

However, only minimal amounts of chromosomal proteins were dissociated.
Extractions with higher salt levels (up to 1.5 M sodium chloride) removed
a major portion of the chromosomal proteins without further dissociation
of the antigenic activity.   Complete removal of all chromosomal proteins,
however, successfully removed the residual antigenic activity from the
DNA.   Figure 1B shows the plots of the CF activity, the amount of
protein and the specific activity of the EBNA (antigenicity per mass of
proteins) in the extracts versus the salt concentrations as calculated
from the data in Figure 1A.   The data show that a multi-fold purification of the EBNA is achieved by its selective extraction using 0.5 sodium
chloride.   They also suggest the existence of two classes of chromatin-
EBNA interactions: a weak binding class representing about 70% of the
total EBNA (class I) which is extracted by 0.5 M sodium chloride and a
high affinity class (about 30% of the total EBNA) (class II) which can
only be removed using conditions which strip all of the protein from the
DNA.

     Further studies utilized only the class I chromatin extracts.   The
CF S-antigen was included for comparative purposes.   Several procedures,
e.g., ion exchange, molecular sieve chromatography, and preparative isoelectric focusing, were applied to these samples.   The last-named proved
far superior to the first two in terms of fractionation and recovery.
Preparative isoelectric focusing employing a Sephadex G-75 superfine
resin and 6 M urea to maintain the chromatin protein fraction in a
solubilized form demonstrated a pI of 4.6 for both EBNA and CF S-antigen
(Fig. 2).   Their location was determined by indirect single radial
immunodiffusion (ISRD) as described by Matsuo et al. (1977), who reported

a pI of 4.8 for the CF S-antigen.   The proteins focusing at pH 4.6
were extracted from the resin and portions subjected to sodium dodecyl
sulfate (SDS)-polyacrylamide gel electrophoresis.   Three major and
three minor bands were observed.   Further purification of EBNA and
comparisons with the CF S-antigen are in progress.

FIG. 2.   ISRD ACTIVITY AFTER ISOELECTRIC FOCUSING WITH
SEPHADEX G-75 IN 6.0 M UREA

Isoelectric focusing was carried out on a LKB Multiphor 2117 using a
urea-Sephadex G-75 superfine resin.   Both CF S-antigen and class I
chromatin extracts were lyophilized and resuspended in 6.0 M urea and
run for 16 hours at 8 watts.   The proteins were eluted in short columns
using 6.0 M guanidine hydrochloride, extensively dialysed and lyophilized.   ISRD was carried out with each fraction according to Matsuo et
al. (1977).   (Pikler et al., unpublished data).

──●─   NC37 CF S-antigen
--○-- NC37 Class I EBNA

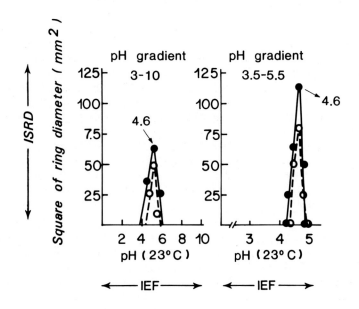

REFERENCES

Bahr, G.F., Mikel, U. & Klein, G. (1975)   Localization and quanti-
    tation of EBV-associated nuclear antigen (EBNA) in Raji cells.
    Beitr. Path., *155*, 72-78

Burton, K. (1956)   A study of the conditions and mechanism of the
    diphenylamine reaction for the colorimetric estimation of deoxy-
    ribonucleic acid.   *Biochem. J.*, *62*, 315-323

Cikes, M. (1975)   An improved quantitative micro-complement fixation
    test.   *J. immun. Meth.*, *8*, 89-100

Huang, D.P., Ho, J.H.C., Henle, W. & Henle, G. (1974)   Demonstration
    of Epstein-Barr virus-associated nuclear antigen in nasopharyngeal
    carcinoma cells from fresh biopsies.   *Int. J. Cancer*, *14*, 580-588

Lowry, O.H., Rosebrough, N.J., Lewis Farr, A. & Randall, R.J. (1951)
    Protein measurement with the folin phenol reagent.   *J. biol.
    Chem.*, *193*, 265-275

Matsuo, T., Nishi, S., Hirai, H. & Osato, T. (1977)   Studies on
    Epstein-Barr virus-related antigens. II. Biochemical properties
    of soluble antigen in Raji Burkitt lymphoma cells.   *Int. J.
    Cancer*, *19*, 364-370

Reedman, B.M. & Klein, G. (1973)   Cellular localization of an
    Epstein-Barr virus (EBV)-associated complement-fixing antigen
    in producer and non-producer lymphoblastoid cell lines.   *Int.
    J. Cancer*, *11*, 499-520

Spelsberg, T.C. & Hnilica, L.S. (1971)   Proteins of chromatin in
    template restriction. I. RNA synthesis *in vitro*.   *Biochim.
    Biophys. Acta (Amst.)*, *228*, 202-211

A NOVEL SURFACE ANTIGEN ON LYMPHOID CELLS TRANSFORMED BY EPSTEIN-BARR VIRUS

Y. HINUMA & K. SAKAMOTO

Department of Microbiology,
Kumamoto University Medical School,
Kumamoto, Japan

We have found a new surface antigen(s), which is distinct from the known Epstein-Barr virus (EBV)-associated membrane antigen (MA) (Klein et al., 1966, 1972), on EBV genome-carrying lymphoid cell lines, as revealed by indirect membrane immunofluorescence with serum from rabbits immunized with the EBV-carrying cells.

Rabbits were immunized with live Raji cells. The antiserum against Raji cells was extensively absorbed with normal human peripheral blood and tonsil cells. The absorbed anti-Raji serum was reactive with the surface of Raji cells but not with that of normal lymphocytes. A number of EBV-carrying lymphoid cell lines other than Raji cells also possessed surface antigen (SA) stainable by the anti-Raji serum, although the percentages of SA-positive cells varied greatly from one cell line to another (from less than 1% to 90%). In contrast, all of the EBV-determined nuclear antigen (EBNA)-negative cell lines tested were not stained with the antiserum. Umbilical cord-blood lymphocytes, as well as adult peripheral blood and tonsil lymphocytes were all negative for SA. However, when the lymphoid cell lines obtained from cord lymphocytes transformed by EBV *in vitro* were examined, they showed about 30-50% of SA-positive cells.

To ensure the specificity of anti-SA antibody, the anti-Raji serum was absorbed with the SA-positive cell line, P3HR-1 (non-producer; NP) or normal lymphocytes. Absorption with the former but not with the latter completely abolished anti-SA reactivity.

The P3HR-1 (NP) cell line was positive for SA but negative for MA, in contrast to the HeHR-1 (producer) line, which was negative for SA but positive for MA. This also suggests that SA is different from MA. The fact that there were several other either SA+MA- or SA-MA+

cell lines further strengthens the distinction between SA and MA.
When absorbed with the P3HR-1 cell line (NP), anti-Raji serum lost
anti-SA reactivity but anti-MA reactivity in a human serum was not
affected.   On the other hand, absorption with HeHR-1 cells removed
anti-MA reactivity but not anti-SA reactivity.   This result again
suggests a distinction between SA and MA.

We then examined the homology or difference in SA between Raji
cells and P3HR-1 (NP) cells.   Anti-P3HR-1 cell rabbit serum was
prepared in the same way as for anti-Raji serum.   The anti-Raji and
anti-P3HR-1 sera were differentially absorbed with each cell line.
The results showed a homology in SA between Raji and P3HR-1 cells,
since, in the majority of absorption tests with homologous and heterologous systems, the result was the complete abolition of the anti-SA
reactivity of these two sera.   However, there was one important
exception: there was only partial reduction of reactivity with the
SA of Raji cells in the anti-Raji serum after absorption with P3HR-1
cells.   This strongly suggests that Raji cells bear an additional SA
other than that on P3HR-1 cells.   It can therefore be assumed that
SA is not a single but a complex antigen.

In conclusion, we have demonstrated an antigen on the surface of
EBV-carrying cells, which is distinct from known MA.   Studies of the
relationship between SA and an antigen responsible for the development
of heterophil antibodies in humans infected with EBV are in progress.

SUMMARY

A surface antigen (SA) was detected on EBV-carrying lymphoid cell
lines by an indirect membrane immunofluorescence test with serum from
rabbits immunized with Raji cells;   the antiserum had been extensively
absorbed with normal human blood and tonsil cells.   The SA was not
detected on normal human umbilical-cord and adult peripheral blood
lymphocytes or EBV-negative cell lines.   The incidences of the SA
and EBV-determined membrane antigen (MA) on certain EBV-carrying cell
lines were not compatible.   Antibody against SA or MA was differentially abolished by absorption with the SA-positive but MA-negative
cell line or the MA-positive but SA-negative cell line, respectively.
The results of cross-absorption tests of antisera against either
Raji cells or P3HR-1 cells suggested that SA is not a single but a
complex antigen.

ACKNOWLEDGEMENTS

This work was supported in part by Grants-in-Aid for
Cancer Research from the Ministry of Education,
Science and Culture and the Ministry
of Health and Welfare, Japan.

REFERENCES

Klein, G., Clifford, P., Klein, E. & Stjernswärd, J. (1966)   Search
     for tumor-specific immune reactions in Burkitt lymphoma patients
     by the membrane immunofluorescence reaction.   *Proc. nat. Acad.
     Sci. (Wash.)*, *55*, 1628-1635

Klein, G., Dombos, L. & Gothoskar, B. (1972)   Sensitivity of
     Epstein-Barr virus (EBV) producer and non-producer human lympho-
     blastoid cell lines to superinfection with EB virus.   *Int. J.
     Cancer*, *10*, 44-57

ALTERED BIOLOGICAL AND BIOCHEMICAL PROPERTIES OF A PHOSPHONOACETATE-RESISTANT MUTANT OF HERPESVIRUS OF TURKEYS

L.F. LEE, K. NAZERIAN & R.L. WITTER

*Science and Education Administration-Federal Research
United States Department of Agriculture,
Regional Poultry Research Laboratory,
East Lansing, Mich., USA*

S.S. LEINBACH & J.A. BOEZI

*Department of Biochemistry,
Michigan State University,
East Lansing, Mich., USA*

We previously reported that phosphonoacetate (PA) inhibited Marek's disease virus (MDV) and herpesvirus of turkeys (HVT) replication and viral DNA synthesis in productively infected duck embryo fibroblasts (DEF) and in non-productively infected chicken lymphoblastoid cells (Lee et al., 1976; Nazerian & Lee, 1976). Steady-state enzyme kinetic analysis (Leinbach et al., 1976) showed that PA interacts with the HVT-induced DNA polymerase at the pyrophosphate binding site and that this interaction causes an inhibition in DNA synthesis. Interest in the mechanism of PA inhibition prompted us to search for and develop HVT and MDV mutants that are resistant to PA. We now report the altered biological and biochemical properties of such an HVT mutant, designated as HVT_{pa}.

Primary and secondary DEF cultures were prepared according to published procedures (Solomon et al., 1971). The GA and JM strains of MDV were propagated in roller bottles and in 150 mm petri plates (Lee, 1971). A preparation of the FC 126 strain of HVT cloned once as cell-free virus was designated as wild-type HVT (HVT_{wt}) (Witter et al., 1970). The methods for determining the effectiveness of PA on

in vitro and *in vivo* replication of viruses are as previously reported
(Lee et al., 1976).

Growth rates of HVT$_{pa}$ and HVT$_{wt}$ were measured in replicate DEF
cultures inoculated with 500 or 2000 plaque-forming units (PFU) of the
appropriate virus and incubated at 37°C or 41°C in a 5% carbon dioxide
atmosphere.   At various times after inoculation, triplicate plates of
infected DEF cultures were harvested and assayed on secondary DEF
cultures at 37°C.   Plaques were counted four days after each assay,
and the number of PFU per culture was compared with the number of PFU
inoculated.

The purification of DNA polymerase from HVT-infected DEF and the
assay conditions were as previously described (Boezi et al., 1974;
Leinbach et al., 1976).   In brief, nuclear extracts were fractionated
by phosphocellulose chromatography and the fractions containing the
virus-induced DNA polymerase activity were pooled, adjusted to a final
concentration of 2 mg/ml bovine serum albumin, 0.5 mM dithiothreitol,
and 50% (v/v) glycerol, and stored at -20°C.   This pooled phosphocellulose fraction was used for all DNA polymerase characterizations.
Steady-state enzyme kinetic analysis was as previously described
(Leinbach et al., 1976).   For thermal inactivation of DNA polymerase,
aliquots of the pooled phosphocellulose fractions containing HVT-
induced DNA polymerase were incubated at 52°C.   Incubation buffer
contained 2 mg/ml bovine serum albumin, 0.5 mM dithiothreitol, 15 mM
tris hydrochloride (pH 8), 200 mM potassium chloride, and 50% glycerol
(v/v).   At appropriate times after incubation, 10-µl aliquots were
transferred to test-tubes on ice.   After 2 minutes on ice, DNA
polymerase activity was assayed by addition of warmed reaction
components to the test-tube and incubation at 37°C for 30 minutes.

GROWTH CHARACTERISTICS OF HVT$_{pa}$ IN CELL CULTURE

The effect of PA on the replication of HVT$_{pa}$ and HVT$_{wt}$ is shown in
Figure 1.   As shown, PA at 35 µg/ml caused a 50% reduction in the
number of plaques produced by HVT$_{wt}$, whereas PA at as much as 300 µg/ml
caused little reduction in the number of plaques produced by HVT$_{pa}$.
The growth characteristics were essentially the same for HVT$_{pa}$ and
HVT$_{wt}$ at 37°C.   At 41°C, HVT$_{wt}$ grew slightly more slowly than it did
at 37°C.   However, HVT$_{pa}$ grew poorly at 41°C;   its 37°C/41°C efficiency
of replication was about 5 (Fig. 2).

REPLICATION OF HVT$_{pa}$ IN CHICKENS

Compared with HVT$_{wt}$, HVT$_{pa}$ replicates poorly in chickens (Table 1).
Viraemia and antibody levels were markedly lower in chickens inoculated
with HVT$_{pa}$ than in those inoculated with HVT$_{wt}$.   Furthermore, chickens

FIG. 1. PHOSPHONOACETATE (PA) SENSITIVITY OF HERPESVIRUS OF TURKEYS (HVT)

Both wild-type (HVT$_{wt}$) and mutant (HVT$_{pa}$) were grown in duck embryo fibroblasts with medium containing different concentrations of PA. Plaques were counted 5 days post inoculation.   (O) - HVT$_{pa}$; (●) - HVT$_{wt}$.

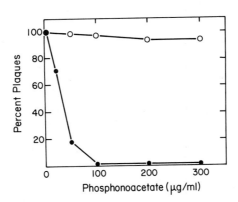

FIG. 2. GROWTH OF WILD-TYPE AND MUTANT HVT

Both wild-type (HVT$_{wt}$) and mutant (HVT$_{pa}$) herpesvirus of turkeys were grown in duck embryo fibroblast culture at 41°C and 37°C and growth measured in PFU.   (O) - HVT$_{pa}$ at 37°C;   (△) - HVT$_{wt}$ at 37°C; (●) - HVT$_{pa}$ at 41°C;   (▲) - HVT$_{wt}$ at 41°C.

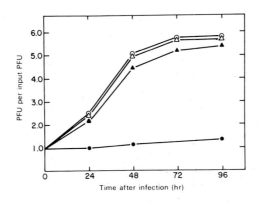

Table 1.   Replication of wild-type (HVT_{wt}) and mutant (HVT_{pa}) herpes-virus of turkeys in chickens and their ability to protect against virulent challenge with Marek's disease virus (MDV)[a]

Vaccine virus	Vaccine dose (PFU)	Virus isolation		Fluorescent antibody		Protective index[a]
		No. chickens positive/No. tested	Mean PFU/ 10^7 buffy coat cells	No. chickens positive/No. tested	Reciprocal titre (range)	
HVT_{wt}	510–2425	14/14	56.1	6/6	160 (80–360)	100
HVT_{pa}	490–49 000	1/26[b]	0.04	5/6	40 (0–80)	51
None	–	0/11	–	0/11	–	–

[a] Vaccination, MDV challenge and terminal evaluation were at 1, 14 and 70 days old, respectively.

[b] The reisolated virus was resistant to PA.

[c] Protective index = $\dfrac{\text{No. of MD (non-vaccinated)} - \text{No. of MD (vaccinated)}}{\text{No. of MD (non-vaccinated)}} \times 100$

vaccinated with HVT_{pa} were less resistant to MDV challenge than those vaccinated with HVT_{wt}.   Virus reisolated from the HVT_{pa}-inoculated chickens remained resistant to PA, indicating that no back mutation had occurred.

PROPERTIES OF THE HVT_{pa}-INDUCED DNA POLYMERASE

The HVT_{pa}-induced DNA polymerase was strongly resistant to PA (Fig. 3).   Addition of 17 µM of PA to the standard reaction mixture inhibited the activity of HVT_{pa}-induced DNA polymerase by 50% whereas only 1.2 µM was sufficient to inhibit the activity of the HVT_{wt}-induced DNA polymerase to the same extent.   The apparent inhibition constant (K_{ipa}) for PA of HVT_{pa}-induced DNA polymerase was about 10 times the K_{ipa} of HVT_{wt}-induced DNA polymerase (Table 2).

We have previously presented evidence that PA inhibits the activity of herpesvirus-induced DNA polymerase by binding at the pyrophosphate binding site of the enzyme (Leinbach et al., 1976).   Accordingly, we determined the apparent inhibition constant for pyrophosphate (K_{ipp}) of the HVT_{pa}-induced DNA polymerase;   it was about twice that of the HVT_{wt}-induced DNA polymerase (Table 2), so the HVT_{pa}-induced DNA polymerase has a decreased affinity for pyrophosphate.   The apparent Michaelis constants of the two enzymes for activated DNA (K_{DNA}) and dCTP (K_{dCTP}) were also determined (Table 2).   No difference in K_{DNA} was seen, but the K_{dCTP} of HVT_{pa}-induced DNA polymerase was about 2.5 times that of the HVT_{wt}-induced DNA polymerase.

FIG. 3. INHIBITION BY PHOSPHONOACETATE (PA) OF DNA POLYMERASES
INDUCED BY MUTANT AND WILD-TYPE HERPESVIRUS OF TURKEYS

V pmol of ^{3}H-dTMP were incorporated into DNA in 30 minutes at 37°C in
the absence of PA, and V_i pmol in the presence of PA. Thus, the PA
concentration that inhibits the enzyme activity by 50% is the
concentration for which V/V_i is 2.   (O) - mutant; (●) - wild type.

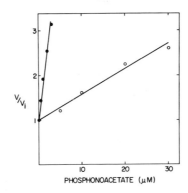

Table 2. Kinetic constants of DNA polymerases induced by mutant
(HVT$_{pa}$) and wild-type (HVT$_{wt}$) herpesvirus of turkeys

Kinetic constant[a]	HVT$_{pa}$-induced DNA polymerase	HVT$_{wt}$-induced DNA polymerase
K_{ipa}	18.0 ± 2.0 μM	1.4 ± 0.6 μM
K_{ipp}	2.5 ± 0.5 mM	1.3 ± 0.2 mM
K_{DNA}	7.2 ± 0.2 μg/ml	7.3 ± 0.2 μg/ml
K_{dCTP}	5.5 ± 0.6 μM	2.1 ± 0.5 μM

[a] The K_i values for phosphonoacetate, K_{ipa} and for pyrophosphate,
K_{ipp} were determined as K_{ii}, as described by Leinbach et al. (1976),
with deoxynucleoside triphosphate as the variable substrate and with
activated DNA at a concentration of 200 μg/ml.

The decreased affinity of HVT_{pa}-induced DNA polymerase for PA suggested a structural change in the enzyme. A change in structure might cause a change in temperature sensitivity of the enzyme. Consequently, the thermal inactivation of HVT_{pa}-induced DNA polymerase and HVT_{wt}-induced DNA polymerase was studied. As shown in Figure 4, the thermal inactivation of both enzymes followed first-order reaction kinetics. The thermal decay of HVT_{pa}-induced DNA polymerase proceeded with a half-life of about 10 minutes and that of the HVT_{wt}-induced DNA polymerase with a half-life of about 17 minutes. The greater temperature sensitivity of the HVT_{pa}-induced enzyme was also demonstrated in crude nuclear extracts.

FIG. 4.   THERMAL INACTIVATION OF DNA POLYMERASE INDUCED BY MUTANT
          AND WILD-TYPE HERPESVIRUS OF TURKEYS AT 52°C

(O) - mutant;   (●) - wild type.

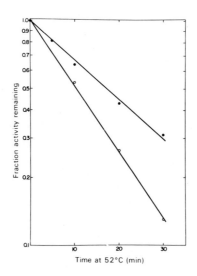

Recently, Hay & Subak-Sharpe (1976) described mutants of HSV types 1 and 2 that are resistant to PA. They also reported that the DNA polymerase activity from mutant-infected cells was more resistant to PA than the DNA polymerase activity from wild type-infected cells. Using partially purified HVT_{pa}- and HVT_{wt}-induced DNA polymerases, we have determined the apparent inhibition constant of HVT_{pa}-induced DNA polymerase to be about 10 times that of HVT_{wt}-induced enzyme. This finding suggests that a mutation in HVT_{pa} DNA polymerase has occurred resulting in its decreased apparent affinity for PA. We found that the affinity of HVT_{pa}-induced DNA polymerase for dCTP has also changed, so that the apparent Michaelis constant for dCTP is about 2.5 times higher than that for the HVT_{wt}-induced enzyme. Also, HVT_{pa}-induced DNA polymerase seemed more temperature sensitive than the HVT_{wt}-induced enzyme.

The failure of HVT_{pa} to confer complete protection against MDV challenge in our experimental chickens was unexpected. The extent to which this property may have been influenced by failure to replicate efficiently *in vivo* is not clear. HVT_{pa} did not replicate as well as the HVT_{wt} *in vitro* at 41°C. Also, thermal inactivation studies showed that HVT_{pa}-induced DNA polymerase was more thermolabile than the HVT_{wt}-induced enzyme. Because normal chicken body temperature ranges between 41°C and 43°C, the low effectiveness of HVT_{pa} as a vaccine virus against MDV challenge may be due to its poor growth at 41°C.

The data in this paper suggest that, as a result of mutation at the level of PA resistance, HVT DNA polymerase may have changed structurally. The data support the hypothesis that inhibition of virus replication is due to a direct effect of PA on DNA polymerase, as well as the hypothesis that virus-induced DNA polymerase may in part be coded for by the HVT DNA.

SUMMARY

A phosphonoacetate (PA)-resistant mutant of the herpesvirus of turkeys (HVT) was isolated and characterized. The mutant (HVT_{pa}) replicates in growth medium containing 300 μg/ml of PA and shows *in vitro* temperature sensitivity at 41°C (its 37°C/41°C efficiency of replication is about 5). HVT_{pa} replicates poorly in chickens and fails to provide complete protection against MDV challenge. The HVT_{pa}-induced DNA polymerase has an apparent inhibition constant for PA 10 times as great, an apparent inhibition constant for pyrophosphate, twice as great, and an apparent Michaelis constant for dCTP 2.5 times as great as the respective figures for the HVT_{wt}-induced enzyme. The HVT_{pa}-induced enzyme is also more thermolabile.

ACKNOWLEDGEMENTS

We should like to thank Mss Mary Cleland, Linda Offenbecker,
and Maiga Gailitis for excellent technical assistance.
This investigation was supported in part by
Grant Number R01CA17554-02 awarded by the
National Cancer Institute.

REFERENCES

Boezi, J.A., Lee, L.F., Blakesley, R.W., Koenig, M. & Towle, H.C.
(1974)   Marek's disease herpesvirus-induced DNA polymerase.
J. Virol., *14*, 1209-1219

Hay, J. & Subak-Sharpe, J.H. (1976)   Mutants of herpes simplex virus
types 1 and 2 that are resistant to phosphonoacetic acid induce
altered DNA polymerase activities in infected cells.   *J. gen.
Virol.*, *31*, 145-148

Lee, L.F. (1971)   Large-scale production of Marek's disease virus.
Avian Dis., *15*, 565-571

Lee, L.F., Nazerian, K., Leinbach, S.S., Reno, J.M. & Boezi, J.A.
(1976)   Effect of phosphonoacetate on Marek's disease virus
replication.   *J. nat. Cancer Inst.*, *56*, 823-827

Leinbach, S.S., Reno, J.M., Lee, L.F., Isbell, A.F. & Boezi, J.A.
(1976)   Mechanism of phosphonoacetate inhibition of herpesvirus-
induced DNA polymerase.   *Biochemistry*, *15*, 426-430

Nazerian, K. & Lee, L.F. (1976)   Selective inhibition by phosphonoacetic acid of MDV DNA replication in a lymphoblastoid cell line.
Virology, *74*, 188-193

Solomon, J.J., Long, P.A. & Okazaki, W. (1971)   *Procedures for the
in vitro assay of viruses and antibody of avian lymphoid leukosis
and Marek's disease*.   United States Department of Agriculture,
Agricultural Research Service (*Agriculture Handbook*, No. 404)

Witter, R.L., Nazerian, K., Purchase, H.G. & Burgoyne, G.H. (1970)
Isolation from turkeys of a cell-associated herpesvirus antigenically related to Marek's disease virus.   *Amer. J. vet. Res.*,
31, 525-538

DISCUSSION SUMMARY

N. FRENKEL

*University of Chicago,
Chicago, Ill., USA*

The studies presented in this session concerned herpes-virus-specific antigens, and will be summarized under four headings as follows: (1) antigenic relatedness of herpesviruses; (2) purification of individual viral antigens; (3) tumour-associated viral antigens; and (4) functional studies of virus-specified polypeptides.

(1) *Antigenic relatedness of herpesviruses*

The wide range of interactions between herpesviruses and their corresponding hosts was reviewed by grouping herpesviruses into four classes according to host range, type of infected cells, disease pattern, structural and immunological properties, and genetic relatedness. By these criteria the α subfamily contains both HSV-1 and HSV-2, the β subfamily contains cytomegalovirus (CMV), and the γ subfamily consists of the lymphocyte-associated viruses, including Marek's disease virus (MDV), herpes-virus of turkeys (HVT), Epstein-Barr virus (EBV) and EBV-like herpesviruses of Old- and New-World primates. Finally, the δ subfamily contains the primitive herpes-viruses including the catfish and frog herpesviruses. A number of reports dealt with the antigenic relatedness of various herpesviruses. The hierarchy of relatedness between HSV-1, HSV-2, bovine herpes mammilitis virus (BHMV), equine herpesvirus (EHV) and pseudorabies virus (PRV), all of which share a common antigenic determinant, was described. Data from cross-neutralization and immuno-absorption assays, immunodiffusion tests and sodium dodecyl sulfate (SDS)-polyacrylamide gel electrophoresis of virion polypeptides all indicate that HSV-1 is closely related to HSV-2, less closely to BHMV and even less closely to EHV and PRV. Furthermore, PRV is more closely related to EHV

than to either BHMV or HSV.   An antigen common to
HSV-1, HSV-2, BHMV and B virus was purified by
crossed immunoelectrophoresis.   The purified cross-
reacting antigens from these viruses share a glycoprotein 126 000 in molecular weight and induce antibodies with cross-neutralizing activities.   Of
interest was the suggestion that the common antigen
might be involved in the capacity of BHMV immunization to protect mice against HSV-induced fatal
encephalitis.   The antigenic relatedness of various
human cytomegalovirus isolates was discussed.
Immunofluorescence tests and analyses of the kinetics
of cross-neutralization, using rabbit sera raised
against the various isolates, showed that there
exists a large antigenic diversity amongst naturally
occurring human CMV isolates, and that the genital
isolates do not fall into a separate class by these
criteria.   The problematic implications of this
heterogeneity on diagnostic testing for CMV as
regards assays of anti-CMV titres was noted, and
the need to CMV strains with a broad spectrum of
antigenic determinants in both diagnostic testing
and immunization was stressed.

It was reported that, by using immunodiffusion tests,
nucleocapsids of HSV-1, HSV-2, EBV, EHV and Lucké herpesvirus could be shown to share a common antigen.   The
surprising finding was also reported that an antigen present
in mammalian oncorna virions displayed a line of identity in
immunodiffusion tests with the herpesvirus group-specific
capsid antigen.   This antigenic determinant could not be
demonstrated in avian oncornaviruses, or in a variety of
other viruses including papova, influenza, Sendai and
vaccinia.   The tests employed sera prepared against
purified HSV nucleocapsids.   The possibility was noted
that small amounts of oncornavirus antigens could have been
induced in the herpesvirus-infected cells, resulting in
the contamination of the HSV capsid preparations, and
that, therefore, future studies will employ sera prepared
against purified oncorna virions which are less likely to
be contaminated with HSV-specific antigens.   Initial
studies have indicated that oncornaviruses p30 and gp85
do not participate in this cross-reactivity.

(2) *Purification of viral antigens for molecular and functional
    characterization*

The use of two-dimensional polyacrylamide gel electrophoresis for the analyses of polypeptides of HSV-1 and HSV-2
infected cells was reported.   The system involves the

electrofocusing of native proteins in the first
dimension, followed by SDS-polyacrylamide gel
electrophoresis in the second dimension.   This
coupled electrophoresis has the advantage of
allowing better resolution of low molecular-weight
polypeptides.   In addition, the electrofocusing
in the first dimension allows the recovery of
native polypeptides for use in enzymatic and
functional studies.

The elegant application of crossed-immuno-
electrophoresis to the analysis of HSV-1 and HSV-2
antigens was described, and the separation of three
type-common and two type-specific HSV glycoproteins
reported.   Antisera prepared against these antigens
display their corresponding type specificity for
neutralization, and when incorporated into an
intermediate gel showed reaction only with their
corresponding antigens.   This technique should
prove to be extremely useful in providing the pure
viral antigens needed to produce monospecific antisera.   As mentioned above a similar approach was
used in the purification of an antigen common to
several herpesviruses.

(3) *Tumour-associated viral antigens*

Studies correlating HSV-2 induced AG-4 with the
HSV-2 infected-cell protein designated as ICP 10 were
described.   The correlation is based on the following:
(i) AG-4 and ICP 10 exhibit similar kinetics of synthesis
in productively infected cells;   (ii) ICP 10 and AG-4 co-
purify during the fractionation of productively infected
cell proteins by various chromatographic steps;   (iii)
human sera containing antibodies to AG-4 also precipitate
ICP 10;   (iv) AG-4 positive human sera fix complement in
the presence of ICP 10 which has been purified in SDS-
polyacrylamide gels;   (v) antisera made against ICP 10
which was purified in polyacrylamide gels fix complement
in the presence of AG-4;   and (vi) both AG-4 and ICP 10
seem to be components of the virion envelope but are
not involved in virus neutralization.   The hypothesis
that virion envelope components could be tumour-associated antigens is not surprising, since herpesviruses,
unlike papova and adenoviruses, derive their envelope
from modified cellular membranes.   Therefore, it can
be expected that HSV tumour-associated membrane
antigens, similar to the TSTA and U antigens of SV40,
might be incorporated into the viral envelope.

Several reports dealt with EBV-specific tumour-associated antigens. Thus it was reported that: (i) the amount of EBV-determined nuclear antigen (EBNA) in various EBV-containing cell lines is directly proportional to the number of EBV genomes in these cells; (ii) in primary infections of cord-blood cells, EBNA is made prior to the synthesis of DNA; however, its synthesis is sensitive to cytosine arabinoside (ara-C); (iii) the identity of the soluble complement-fixing (CF) antigen with EBNA was further established by showing that the soluble CF antigen is capable of blocking EBNA staining in anti-complement fluorescence tests. Of particular interest was the report of a novel and more sensitive assay for EBNA, employing reconstitution of EBNA staining by adding solubilized extracts from chromatin of cells suspected of containing EBNA to cells (e.g., chick red blood cells) which have been fixed with methanol/acetic acid. This assay should be most useful in following EBNA through various purification steps. as well as in diagnostic testing. In addition, the assay has already revealed the presence of EBNA-like antigenic activity associated with other lymphotropic herpesvirus systems. Attempts to purify EBNA by differential salt extractions were reported. These experiments revealed two classes of EBNA which differ in their susceptibility to elution with 0.5 N sodium chloride. Further studies should elucidate the full meaning of this observation. Of interest was the suggestion that EBNA might be a DNA-protein antigenic complex, as EBNA staining is sensitive to DNase treatment. Finally, several possible roles for EBNA were discussed, as either a positive regulator for transcription and/or for DNA synthesis, or a negative repressor type protein.

A new surface(s) antigen present in lymphoid cells transformed by EBV, as evidenced by immunofluorescence (IF) tests with rabbit serum raised against Raji cells and adsorbed extensively with normal cells, was reported. The new surface antigen is distinct from the membrane antigen which has been described previously. Evidence suggests that this S determinant is a virus-induced host-coded antigen.

(4) *Functional studies of virus-specified polypeptides*

Experiments designed to elucidate viral functions involved in HSV-induced cell fusion were described. Briefly, analyses of glycoproteins synthesized by two plaque-morphology mutants of HSV-1 and recombinants of these mutants revealed the involvement of two glyco-

proteins, B2 and C2, in virus-induced cell fusion.
B2 promotes cell fusion and mutants of this gene are
unable to induce cell fusion.   C2 normally suppresses
fusion and mutants in this gene will form syncytial
plaques provided they have a functional B2.   In cells
infected with virus capable of expressing both the B2
and C2 functions the fusion-suppression function is
dominant, with the resultant non-syncytial wild-type
plaque morphology.   Of interest was the suggestion
that the glycoproteins B2 and C2 are involved not only
in cell-cell fusion but also in virus-cell fusion
during adsorption and penetration.   In line with this
are the observations that both B2 and C2 are components
of the virion envelope, and the observation that a
temperature-sensitive mutation in the fusion-promotor
protein B2 is lethal at the non-permissive temperature.

A second viral function which was discussed in this
session was the virus-coded DNA polymerase.   The isolation of a set of phosphonoacetic acid (PAA)-resistant
mutants of MDV and HVT, whose DNA polymerases displayed
altered kinetics, was described.   Chickens infected
with HVT PAA-resistant virus showed lower viraemia and
had reduced antibody levels than those infected with
the PAA-susceptible virus.   In addition, HVT PAA-
resistant virus showed decreased capacity to protect
chickens against subsequent MDV challenge.

CELL-VIRUS INTERACTION: MOLECULAR EVENTS IN PERMISSIVE AND SEMI-PERMISSIVE CYCLES

HUMAN HERPESVIRUS 1 AS A MODEL OF REGULATION OF HERPESVIRUS MACROMOLECULAR METABOLISM: A REVIEW

B. ROIZMAN & L.S. MORSE

*Marjorie B. Kovler Viral Oncology Laboratories,
The University of Chicago,
Chicago, Ill., USA*

Toute création est à l'origine,
la lutte d'une forme en puis-
sance contre une forme imitée.

ANDRE MALRAUX, La Création Artistique

INTRODUCTION

This review again is a brief statement of the current knowledge concerning the replication of herpesviruses, particularly as it evolved in the past three years, since the Second Symposium on Herpesviruses and Oncogenesis. As its predecessor (Roizman et al., 1975a), this review suffers from two constrictive limitations. First, it deals primarily with human herpesvirus 1 (herpes simplex 1, HSV-1) and its close relative, HSV-2. Although HSV-1 and HSV-2 remain useful models against which to pit the expanding knowledge of the herpesvirus universe, our future knowledge of herpesviruses depends on recognition and exploitation of diversity. Second, limitation of space precludes detailed documentation of every facet discussed in the text; the documentation for many of the diagrams presented in the text in most instances will be found in the citations.

A characteristic of biological systems, and herpesviruses are no
exception, is that their replication is highly reproducible.   The
herpesvirus-infected cell is, superficially at least, a magnificent
copy machine.   The work of the past decade has led to a partial
uncovering of its innards, and pursuing further the allusion to the
copy machine, the replication of herpesvirus can be divided into
three series of events.   First, the original - the parent virus -
becomes disaggregated during and immediately after penetration into
the cell (Fig. 1).   Ultimately, viral DNA enters the nucleus and
becomes the focus of most subsequent events (Roizman & Furlong, 1974).

FIG. 1.   SCHEMATIC DESCRIPTION OF THE GENERAL REPLICATIVE
AND METABOLIC EVENTS IN A HERPES SIMPLEX VIRUS-INFECTED CELL

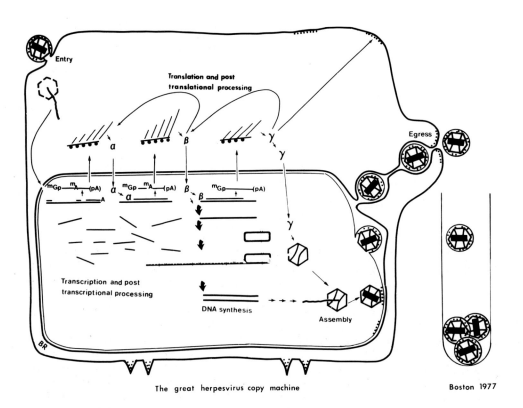

We have always thought that viral DNA is all that is required for multiplication because "naked" DNA, i.e., DNA digestible by nuclease, is infectious (Lando & Ryhiner, 1969; Sheldrick et al., 1973). Alas, intact, "naked" DNA on a mole per mole basis has but a small fraction (10^{-5}) of the specific infectivity of virions; we cannot exclude the possibility that DNA that is infectious carries essential "impurities" in the form of viral proteins bound to it.

The second series of events involves the synthesis of viral components and assembly of viral progeny. Characteristically, the components are made in three alternating waves of transcription and translation. These waves are regulated; current evidence indicates that the final products form at least three groups designated as α, β and γ whose synthesis is co-ordinately regulated and sequentially ordered (Honess & Roizman, 1974; Roizman et al., 1975a,b). Viral DNA synthesis takes place in the nucleus. The DNA is packaged into capsids in the nucleus; these become enveloped at the nuclear membrane and egress through the cysternae of the endoplasmic reticulum (Roizman & Furlong, 1974). The third series of events concerns the fate of the infected cells. Unlike the mechanical copier, the infected cell makes only one set of replicas before its irreversible demise. The cause of cell death is not understood although there are abundant clues. Condensation and margination of chromosomes, disaggregation of the nucleolus, cessation of host RNA, DNA and protein synthesis, alteration in the structure and immunological specificity of the plasma membrane and alteration in the social behaviour of infected cells are the most striking phenomena heralding cell death (Roizman & Furlong, 1974).

In this review, we shall be concerned primarily with the regulation of synthesis of viral gene products. it is convenient to begin with a review of the polypeptides specified by HSV-1 and HSV-2.

THE SYNTHESIS OF VIRAL POLYPEPTIDES

With respect to the objectives of this review, virus-specific polypeptides represent the terminal gene products whose synthesis is regulated. We shall be concerned in this section with three aspects of viral polypeptides, i.e., their identification, enumeration of their properties and analyses of the requirements for their synthesis.

Identification

The identification of infected-cell polypeptides (ICP) that are virus-specific is indirect. It is based primarily on the observation that the rate of synthesis of host polypeptides decays very rapidly after infection. Hence, the major criterion for defining

polypeptides as virus-specific is that their rate of synthesis
increases after infection (Honess & Roizman, 1973; Powell &
Courtney, 1975).   Adjunct criteria, such as the demonstration that
the polypeptides react with sera prepared against infected cells
in isologous hosts and that the properties of the polypeptides are
genetically determined by the virus, have also been used (Honess &
Roizman, 1973; Powell & Courtney, 1975) but their applicability is
more limited.   Thus, a large number of viral polypeptides are
insoluble in solutions useful for radioimmune precipitation tests
(Honess & Roizman, 1973; Powell & Courtney, 1975), only a small
number of viral polypeptides have been shown to be over-produced, or
under-produced, by certain virus strains (Honess & Rʳ'zman, 1973;
Powell & Courtney, 1975), and only approximately hʳ ɾ of the HSV-1
and HSV-2 ICPs differ in electrophoretic mobility (Morse et al.,
1978).   At this time, *in vitro* protein synthesis directed by a
viral transcript has not been applied extensively to determine the
genetic origin of ICPs.

Enumeration and properties

The HSV-1 and HSV-2 genomes each contain 1.6×10^5 base pairs
of which 10% are reiterated twice (Roizman et al., 1975a; Wadsworth
et al., 1975).   The maximum asymmetric coding capacity of the DNA
excluding possible regions of high-density encoding as a result of
frameshifts, etc., is therefore approximately 44 000 amino-acids.
The polypeptides identified in the first round as virus-specific
numbered about 50 in both HSV-1 (Honess & Roizman, 1973) and HSV-2
(Powell & Courtney, 1975) infected cells, and these ranged from about
20 000 to > 250 000 in molecular weight.   Marsden et al. (1976)
reported several additional virus-specific polypeptides of smaller
molecular weight in HSV-1 infected cells, but these did not appre-
ciably increase the requirement for coding the sequence of circa
41 000 amino-acids that would require approximately 90% of the
calculated coding capacity of the DNA.   In the second round (Morse
et al., 1978), the number of virus-specific polypeptides in the
20 000 - > 250 000 molecular weight range decreased to approximately
44 with a slightly smaller coding requirement (Table 1).

The decrease in the number of probable virus-specific polypeptides
recognized at this time reflects the realization that a majority of
viral polypeptides undergo rapid structural changes such that the
product differs in the electrophoretic mobility from the precursor.
It is noteworthy that the change in electrophoretic mobility (Fig. 2,
Table 1) is to a higher apparent molecular weight (Honess & Roizman,
1975a; Morse et al., 1978; Pereira et al., 1977; Powell & Courtney,
1975).   The most common modifications are those that result in
phosphorylation and glycosylation of viral polypeptides although
sulfation has also been reported (Erickson & Kaplan, 1973).   The
most striking feature of both of these modifications is that they
appear to occur in discrete steps.   In the case of glycosylation,

Table 1. Electrophoretic properties of HSV infected-cell polypeptides[a]

Polypeptide No.	Form	Molecular weight (×10⁻³) HSV-1 (F)	HSV-2 (G)	Group	Polypeptide No.	Form	Molecular weight (×10⁻³) HSV-1 (F)	HSV-2 (G)	Group
1	b	> 221	221	γ	20	-	77·	78·	γ
	a				21	-	72.5	73.5·	-
2	b	205	> 205	γ	23	-	71	72	γ
	a	196	198	-	24	b	68	68	β/γ
3	-	194	191	γ		a	67.5	67	-
4	c	170·	180·	α	25	b	64	63	γ
	b	165	177	-		a	63	62.5	-
	a	163	172	-	26	b	61.5·	62	β
5	b	151	153	γ		a	60	60	-
	a	149	151	-	27	b	58	59	α
6	b	146	146·	β		a	56.5	58	-
	a	143	143	-	28	-	56	57	-
7	-	139·	138·	-	29	b	55	54.5	β
7.5	b	132·	135	-		a	54.5	53	-
	a	130	131	-	31	-	52	52	-
8	-	128	127	β	32	-	51.5	50.5	γ
9	b	122	121	γ	33	-	50	49	γ
	a	119	119	-	34	-	49.5	48	-
10	-	117·	122·	β/γ	35	b	46.5	45·	γ
11	-	114	114·	γ		a	45	-	-
12	-	111	113	-	36	-	42.5	42.5	β
13	-	109	112	-	37	b	39	39.5·	γ
14	-	106	107	-		a	-	38.5	-
15	-	103·	101·	γ	38	-	37	35.5	-
16	-	101	100	-	39	b	36	35	β
17	-	92	91·	β		a	35	-	-
18	b	88·	85·	γ	40	-	33.7	34	β
	a	85	-	-	41	-	32	33.5	β
19	-	78	79	γ	43	-	26.5	26	γ
					44	-	24.5	25	γ

[a] The polypeptides are numbered in order of decreasing molecular weight. The table also identifies those polypeptides which undergo changes in their electrophoretic mobility and are designated as a, b, or c forms. Polypeptides which show intratypic variability are marked with a solid black dot (·). (Data from Morse et al., 1978)

the data strongly argue for stepwise addition of oligosaccharide chains to the glycoprotein precursor (Honess & Roizman, 1975b; Spear, 1976). In the case of several phosphorylated polypeptides (e.g., ICP 4), the decrease in electrophoretic mobility is in discrete steps (Pereira et al., 1977).

The data presented in Table 1 are significant from several points of view: (i) The stagewise modification of non-glycosylated polypeptides to *lower* electrophoretic mobilities has many implications. One possibility is that the modifications enable the polypeptide to function at the "site" of action. The stagewise modifications might imply that each stage is required for translocation or for binding to a particular site. We cannot exclude the possibility that each processed form of the polypeptide (e.g., ICP 4 a, b, c) may have a different function and that the abundance of polypeptide in each form is regulated. (ii) There is intertypic variability in the molecular weights of non-structural polypeptides in addition to that reported previously for the structural polypeptides (Pereira et al., 1976).

FIG. 2. THE ESSENTIAL FEATURES OF REGULATION
OF HSV PROTEIN SYNTHESIS

(A) The synthesis of polypeptides representative of α (ICP 4), β (ICP 6) and γ (ICP 5) polypeptide groups in untreated cells pulse-labelled with ^{14}C-amino-acids at different times after infection.   The synthesis of these three sets of polypeptides is co-ordinately regulated and sequentially ordered in a cascade fashion (Honess & Roizman, 1974); (B) Cycloheximide was added to infected cultures at the time indicated by the first arrow and washed out at the time interval indicated by the second arrow.   Polypeptides of the α group were synthesized immediately after removal of cycloheximide added at the time of infection (Honess & Roizman, 1974);   (C) Addition of the amino-acid analogue, canavanine, to cell cultures at the time of infection allowed α polypeptide synthesis but prevented the synthesis of β polypeptides (Honess & Roizman, 1975);   (D) The addition of actinomycin D to infected cell cultures simultaneously with the removal of a cycloheximide block prevented the synthesis of the β polypeptide group (Honess & Roizman, 1974).   The enucleation of infected cells after removal of a cycloheximide block shows a similar inhibition of β polypeptide synthesis; (E) The addition of canavanine to infected cell cultures after α polypeptide synthesis but before maximum synthesis of β polypeptides greatly reduced the synthesis of γ polypeptides and normal shut-off of α polypeptides (Honess & Roizman, 1975);   (F) Cycloheximide was removed from infected cell cultures and the synthesis of β polypeptides was allowed.   After two hours, cells were either enucleated or treated with actinomycin D.   Under those conditions, the synthesis of γ polypeptides was greatly reduced (Honess & Roizman, 1974).

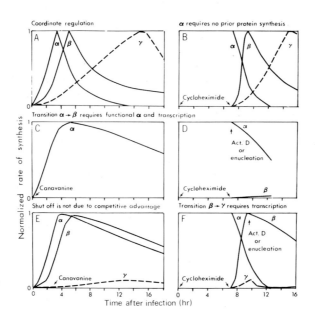

The intratypic variability in the molecular weight of the polypeptides
as well as the formation of multiple forms of the same polypeptide as
a consequence of processing reinforce our conclusion that the polypeptides should not be designated by their apparent molecular weights.

The regulation of the synthesis of viral polypeptides

Current evidence indicates that viral polypeptides form at least
three groups whose synthesis is co-ordinately regulated and sequentially ordered in a cascade fashion.   Before we describe what is known
about these groups and especially our understanding of the mechanism
underlying the transition of synthesis from one group to the next, a
more precise definition of this tautologized description is necessary.
Thus, the emphasis on a *minimum* of three polypeptide groups is more
descriptive than speculative;   the operational definitions employed
in the initial studies revealed three groups (Honess & Roizman, 1974;
Roizman et al., 1975b).   However, even then and more so now, it was
evident that β and perhaps γ are not homogeneous groups and that at
least with respect to some properties it is convenient to subdivide β
polypeptides into β_1 and β_2 groups (Honess & Roizman, 1974, 1975a;
Pereira et al., 1977).   Co-ordinate regulation implies that the polypeptide synthesis begins, reaches peak rates and declines synchronously.
A characteristic of herpesvirus polypeptide synthesis is that an abundance control is superimposed on top of the co-ordinate regulation
(Honess & Roizman, 1973).   In simple terms, viral polypeptides within
a co-ordinately regulated group are not all made at the same rate.
Sequential ordering implies that in the infected cells viral protein
synthesis undergoes at least two transitions as the cells shift from
production of α to β to γ polypeptides.   Each transition involves
initiation of synthesis of one group and termination of synthesis of
the preceding group of viral polypeptides.

α Polypeptides

α Polypeptides by definition require no prior infected-cell protein
synthesis in order to be made.   Operationally, they are defined as the
virus-specific polypeptides made immediately after withdrawal of puro-
mycin or of cycloheximide present in the culture medium during
infection and for several (2-15) hours thereafter (Honess & Roizman,
1974).   From the time of their discovery, a total of four, i.e., ICP
4, 0, 22 and 27, were designated as α.   Of these, only ICP 4 and 27
have been clearly mapped and recognized as virus-specific in both HSV-1
and HSV-2 infected cells (Morse et al., 1978).   ICP 22 is most likely
a host polypeptide induced by virus infection since it is also induced
by heat treatment in uninfected cells (Honess & Roizman, 1975a).
With respect to ICP 0, its electrophoretic mobility varies depending
on the polyacrylamide gel concentration.   Most recently, the detection of ICP 0 varied considerably from preparation to preparation.
ICP 4 of HSV-1 maps in S, partially in the reiterated *ac* sequences
(Frenkel et al., 1975, 1976; Morse et al., 1978).   The results of

studies on intratypic recombinants formed in cells infected with HSV-1 and HSV-2 (Morse et al., 1978) virions or transfected with HSV-1 DNA and fragments of HSV-2 DNA, are readily interpretable as indicating that there are two copies of ICP 4 templates per DNA molecule and that both copies are expressed (Knipe et al., 1978; Morse et al., 1978). ICP 27 was mapped at the right end of L entirely in the reiterated sequences (b'a') (Morse et al., 1978). In untreated infected cells, α polypeptides reach peak rates of synthesis between two and four hours post infection and decline thereafter (Honess & Roizman, 1974). Some α polypeptides are overproduced in cells infected with certain *ts* mutants or with HSV-1 virus populations containing defective DNA (Courtney et al., 1976; Frenkel et al., 1975; Marsden et al., 1976).

β *Polypeptides*

β Polypeptides require the presence in the infected cells of functional α polypeptides in order to be made (Honess & Roizman, 1975a). Operationally, they are also defined as reaching peak rates of synthesis between five and seven hours post infection (Honess & Roizman, 1974). Some of the β polypeptides are listed in Table 1. The functions currently ascribed to β polypeptides are viral DNA polymerase, thymidine kinase, and inhibition of host macromolecular metabolism (Garfinkle & McAuslan, 1974; Honess & Roizman, 1974, 1975; Leiden et al., 1976; Powell & Purifoy, 1977).

γ *Polypeptides*

The structural (virion) polypeptides comprise the largest and perhaps the only component of the γ group. The synthesis of γ polypeptides requires the presence of functional polypeptides belonging to the prior groups. HSV-1 γ polypeptides are characteristically made at increasing rates of synthesis until 15-18 hours post infection (Honess & Roizman, 1974).

Requirements for the synthesis of α polypeptides

Several lines of evidence indicate that HSV DNA is transcribed by a host transcriptase. Among the evidence are the observations that the synthesis of viral polypeptides (α, β or γ) is blocked by α-amanitin in cells sensitive to the drug, but not in cells containing an α-amanitin-resistant RNA polymerase (Costanzo et al., 1977). Another, less compelling observation cited earlier in the text is that "naked" HSV is infectious. If this is in fact the case, it would be expected that α polypeptide synthesis requires only the presence of DNA capable of initiating infection in permissive cells, i.e., that there should be no temperature-sensitive mutants which at non-permissive temperature preclude the synthesis of α polypeptides unless these be mutants defective in uncoating of the DNA.

Transition from α *to* β *polypeptide synthesis*

When infected-cell protein synthesis is "synchronized" by exposure to inhibitors of protein synthesis (Fig. 2) during and for several hours after infection, β polypeptide synthesis follows soon after and rapidly replaces the synthesis of α polypeptides.   Addition of actinomycin D in appropriate concentrations to these cultures just prior to the withdrawal of inhibitors of protein synthesis resulted in continued synthesis of HSV-1 α polypeptides and in either gross reduction or absence of synthesis of β polypeptides (Honess & Roizman, 1974). In a similar fashion (Fig. 2), infection and maintenance of HSV-1 infected cells in the presence of amino-acid analogues (canavanine or azetidine) resulted in a continued synthesis of α polypeptides concurrently with grossly reduced amounts of most, but not all β polypeptides (Honess & Roizman, 1975a; Pereira et al., 1977).   It is convenient to designate the β polypeptides made in the presence of the analogues as β_1.   Lastly, enucleation of cells just prior to withdrawal of inhibitors of protein synthesis resulted in the synthesis of only α polypeptides (Fig. 2).   Enucleation of cells while both α and β polypeptides were being made resulted in a relatively rapid disappearance of α polypeptide synthesis.   These experiments indicate the following: (i) Functional α mRNA accumulates in the cytoplasm in the presence of inhibitors of protein synthesis.   (ii) The transition from α to β polypeptide synthesis requires *de novo* transcription of viral DNA in the presence or with the participation of functional α polypeptides. (iii) The cessation of α polypeptide synthesis is effected in the cytoplasm and requires the presence or participation of functional β polypeptides. (iv) α and β mRNA do not compete for a common cytoplasmic factor since the synthesis of corresponding polypeptides is not mutually exclusive.

Central to understanding the transition from α to β polypeptide synthesis is the function of α polypeptides.   The data are fragmentary but several observations appear to be significant.   First, both ICP 4 and 27 are processed and translocated into the nucleus (Pereira et al., 1977).   The evidence that the site of "action" of these polypeptides is in the nucleus is based on the observations that *ts* mutations that map in the S component and might conceivably be in ICP 4 [HSV-1(17 *tsD*) and HSV-1(HFEM *tsLB2*)] appear to block at non-permissive temperatures the normal processing and translocation of ICP 4.   Processing and translocation of ICP 4 are also reduced or delayed in the presence of amino-acid analogues (Pereira et al., 1977).   Second, at non-permissive temperatures, cells infected with *tsD* produce only α polypeptides in higher than usual amounts whereas *tsLB2* make β_1 polypeptides as well as excess amounts of α polypeptides.   Marker rescue experiments suggest that both *tsD* and *tsLB2* map in the reitereated *a'c'* and *ca* sequences (Knipe et al., 1978).   If both *tsLB2* and *tsD* are mutations in the gene

specifying ICP4, it follows that: (1) ICP 4 acts at multiple sites of
the genome; and (2) different regions of ICP 4 are DNA site-specific.

Transition from β to γ polypeptide synthesis

Several lines of evidence have led to the conclusion that the
transition from β to γ polypeptide synthesis requires the transcription
of viral DNA in the presence or with the participation of β polypeptides,
and that, in many respects, the requirements for this transition are
similar to those of α to β (Honess & Roizman, 1974; Roizman et al.,
1975a,b).

Perhaps the most significant question that must be answered is the
role of viral DNA synthesis in the transition from β to γ polypeptide
synthesis. Elsewhere in these proceedings, Wolf & Roizman[1] reaffirmed
observations reported in this and other laboratories (Honess & Watson,
1977; Powell et al., 1975) that, even though the transition from β to
γ polypeptide synthesis is not affected by inhibitors of DNA synthesis,
the amounts of β polypeptides made are grossly diminished relative to
the yield in untreated infected cells (Fig. 3). Two points should be
made in connection with these observations.

First, DNA synthesis can play two functions in affecting the transition from β to γ polypeptide synthesis. Thus, DNA synthesis may
simply augment the amount of viral DNA available for transcription.
Alternatively, the effects of DNA synthesis could be the consequences
of primer synthesis, endonucleolytic cleavage, or of other changes in
the structure of DNA such as to enable transcription of sequences
specifying γ polypeptides.

In examining the experiments done so far, it is clear that the
increase in the size of the DNA pool available for transcription is
the only function of viral DNA synthesis that was evaluated to date.
Indeed, the drugs used in these experiments - hydroxyurea, cytosine
arabinoside, and phosphonoacetate (Honess & Roizman, 1974; Honess &
Watson, 1977; Powell et al., 1975; Wolf & Roizman[1]) - at appropriate
concentrations could be expected to reduce viral DNA synthesis below
detectable levels but would not block the events associated with initiation of DNA synthesis. We must conclude, therefore, that while we
do not know whether initiation of DNA synthesis plays a role in the
transition from β to γ polypeptide synthesis, the amount of viral DNA
in the cells does play a role in defining the rate of γ polypeptide
synthesis. In retrospect, the notion that the γ polypeptide synthesis
is tied in some fashion to the amount of viral DNA present in the cells
should have been expected since for optimum progeny size it would be
necessary to control the amount of viral DNA that is withdrawn for
assembly into virions.

---

[1] See p. 327

FIG. 3.   REGULATION OF THE TRANSITION FROM β
TO γ POLYPEPTIDE SYNTHESIS

Hydroxyurea (HU) or phosphonoacetic acid (PAA) was added at the time
of infection and maintained in cell cultures at concentrations sufficient
to inhibit viral DNA synthesis.   The infected cells were then pulse-
labelled with ^{14}C-amino-acids at various times post infection to label α,
β, or γ polypeptides.   In contrast to normal rates of synthesis of α and
β polypeptides, γ polypeptide synthesis was markedly reduced.   In the
two righ-hand panels, actinomycin D or cordycepin was added to cell
cultures eight hours post infection and washed out after 90 minutes.
Cells were pulse-labelled with ^{14}C-amino-acids at 30-minute intervals
and the normalized rates of synthesis of representative β and γ polypeptides were plotted as indicated.   These experiments show that γ mRNA
has a short half-life in contrast to the functional stability of β mRNA.
(Data from Honess & Roizman, 1975;   see also Wolf & Roizman, p. 327).

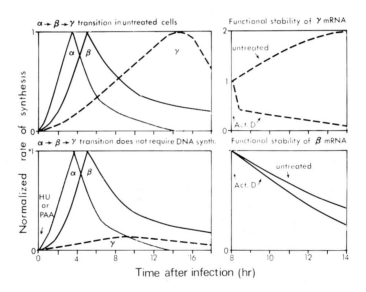

The second and perhaps more interesting point concerns the mechanism
by which the rate of production of γ polypeptides is tied to the pool
size of viral DNA.   Data detailed elsewhere (Honess & Roizman, 1974;
Wolf & Roizman[1]) indicate that the functional half-life of γ mRNA is

---

[1] See p. 327

very much shorter relative to that of α or β RNA (Fig. 3).   The
discriminatory mechanism is not known.   A putative structural feature
of the RNAs that might underline the differences in the functional
half-life of these mRNAs is described in the next section.

TRANSCRIPTION AND POST-TRANSCRIPTIONAL REGULATION

The central and salient conclusion of the studies on viral protein
synthesis described in the preceding section is that whereas *cessation*
of synthesis of a particular group of polypeptides follows a cytoplasmic event, the *initiation* of synthesis of a new group of polypeptides
requires that a competent viral mRNA molecule present itself to the
cytoplasmic protein synthesizing machinery.   In order for this to
occur, the DNA must be transcribed, the transcript must be processed,
and the resulting mRNA molecule must be translocated into the cytoplasm.   Considering the amount of work that was already put in to
elucidate this sequence, the results of studies done to date project
a woefully inadequate picture.

The genetic source of the enzyme that transcribes viral DNA

All of the available data are in accord with the hypothesis that
viral DNA is transcribed principally by host RNA polymerase II.   For
reasons noted earlier in the text, the least significant evidence is
the fact that denuded viral DNA is infectious (Lando & Ryhiner, 1969;
Sheldrick et al., 1973).   The most significant observation is that
the synthesis of all groups of viral polypeptides is inhibited by α-
amanitinin-sensitive cells but not in cells containing an RNA polymerase resistant to that drug (Costanzo et al., 1977).   The observation
that the appearance of viral RNA in isolated nuclei is similarly
inhibited by this drug (Ben-Zeev & Becker, 1977) does not carry the
same weight because only a fraction of viral RNA species accumulating
in the nucleus carry genetic information.

Evidence that transcription is regulated

The evidence avidly sought by many laboratories is that: (a) the
extent of transcription is under some temporal control;   (b) the
abundance of transcripts generated from different regions of viral DNA
is also controlled (Clements et al., 1977;   Frenkel & Roizman, 1972;
Frenkel et al., 1973;   Jones et al., 1977;   Kozak & Roizman, 1974;
Roizman et al., 1975a;   Swanstrom et al., 1975).   There is universal
agreement that transcription is regulated but the foundations of this
universal belief are somewhat weak because of several cumulative
problems.   First, viral RNA like all eukaryotic RNA species is
"processed" after synthesis;   in simplistic terms processing involves
cleavage (Jacquemont & Roizman, 1975a;   Wagner & Roizman, 1969),
adenylation (Bachenheimer & Roizman, 1976;   Silverstein et al., 1973,
1976) and methylation (Bartkoski & Roizman, 1976, 1978;   Moss et al.,

1977).   Therefore, the RNA labelled in the cell during the shortest
labelling interval may not correspond exactly to the primary transcript either in size or in sequence complexity defined as the fraction
of the DNA from which it is derived.   Second, viral RNA accumulates
in the infected cell even after it has ceased to direct protein
synthesis (Clements et al., 1977; Kozak & Roizman, 1974).   The
consequences of processing and accumulation are very significant.
Let us examine the example of a primary transcript consisting of
sequences ABCDE that is processed in such a way that only sequences B,
C and D are conserved.   Hybridization of labelled DNA to excess of
unlabelled RNA should reveal a scarcity of RNA sequences derived from
A and E relative to the more abundant B, C and D RNA sequences.   However, hybridization of the short pulse-labelled RNA to DNA fragments
blotted on to nitrocellulose filters should make A and E sequences
appear more abundant for the simple reason that, because B, C and D
sequences are conserved, the labelled RNA from these regions is diluted
with unlabelled sequences that accumulated prior to the labelling
interval.   In consequence, B, C, and D sequences would appear to be of
a lower specific activity than those arising from A and E.   Third, there
is ample documentation that transcription is largely symmetrical
(Fig. 4; Jacquemont & Roizman, 1975b).   Therefore, estimations of
both complexity and abundance of the RNA suffer from the fact that,
in addition to the desirable DNA-RNA hybrids and the less desirable
DNA-DNA hybrids, there form the least desirable RNA-RNA hybrids.
Lastly, measurements of RNA sequence complexity by liquid-phase hybridization require that viral RNA be in vast excess.   This is not always
easy to attain; consider, for example, the significance of tests
showing that RNA made in the presence of inhibitors of DNA synthesis
is transcribed from a smaller portion of the DNA than RNA extracted
from untreated infected cells (Swanstrom et al., 1975) in light of the
fact that treated and untreated infected cells make exactly the same
proteins but in different relative ratios (Honess & Roizman, 1974;
Powell et al., 1975; Wolf & Roizman[1]).   Although most of these
problems and limitations can be dealt with, they have not.   We wish
to under-score the real possibility that technical problems might
give us erroneous measures of sequence complexity and abundance of
accumulated RNA [see for example, the data of Kozak & Roizman (1974)
on the relationship between the multiplicities of infection and
sequence complexity of early (2-3 hour) RNA] and that the accumulated
RNA might be confused for primary transcripts.

Notwithstanding these limitations, two lines of evidence sustain
the hypothesis that there exists a temporal control of transcription.
First, the transition from α to β to γ polypeptide synthesis requires
de novo transcription of viral DNA (Clements et al., 1977; Honess &

---

[1] See p. 327

FIG. 4. HSV-1 DOUBLE-STRANDED (DS) RNA

The two left-hand panels show the sequence complexity and abundance
classes of double-stranded RNA as analysed by two different methods
described by Jacquemont & Roizman (1975b).   Hybridizations were performed with excess double-stranded RNA to *in vitro* labelled, sheared,
and denatured DNA as shown.   Purified viral double-stranded RNA is
homologous to > 70% of viral DNA and forms at least two abundance
classes.   The right-hand panel shows the thermal transition of self-
annealed labelled RNA from HSV-1 infected cells.   The thermal transition was measured by sensitivity to RNase A and by hybridization of
viral DNA fixed to filters.   The T_m of the RNA is consistent with that
expected for a double-stranded RNA of 68 moles % - slightly higher than
the average G + C content of HSV DNA.

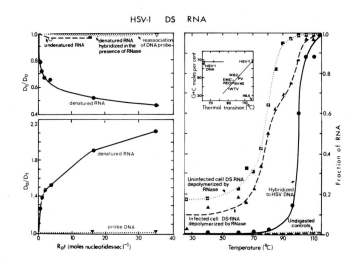

Roizman, 1974, Jones et al., 1977; Roizman et al., 1975b).   This
observation merely indicates that transcripts made in the absence
of α polypeptides do not give rise to mRNA specifying subsequent
polypeptide groups either because these sequences are not among
those transcribed or because the transcripts are not suitable.   In
the first instance, the appropriate sequences in the DNA would have
to be transcribed.   In the second instance, the DNA is transcribed,
but the resulting transcripts cannot be processed to yield the appropriate mRNA.   The second observation (Fig. 5) is that the complexity

FIG. 5. ACCUMULATION OF VIRAL RNA

All panels represent the hybridization of labelled herpesvirus DNA
with excess RNA from fractionated infected cells as described by
Frenkel & Roizman (1972) and Kozak & Roizman (1974).   The three left
panels show that the sequence complexity of viral RNA in the *cytoplasm*
reaches 43% of viral DNA late in infection (Kozak & Roizman, 1974;
Silverstein et al., 1976).   This is also the total DNA represented in
polysomes throughout infection.   Most mRNA appears to be adenylated
(Silverstein et al., 1976; Stringer et al., 1977).   The RNA consists
of at least two classes differing in abundance (Frenkel & Roizman,
1972).   The most abundant class binds to nitrocellulose filters
(Silverstein et al., 1976).   When the cells are restricted to making
α polypeptides only, such as during cycloheximide or canavanine treatment (Frenkel, unpublished data), only 12% of the DNA is represented
in the polysomes (Jones et al., 1977; Kozak & Roizman, 1974).   αRNA
and late RNA are not additive in summation tests.   Further, cytoplasmic RNA does not self-anneal.   *Nuclear* RNA from cells making α only
or β and γ, contains sequences that arise from a larger fraction of
the genome than that represented in polyribosomes (Frenkel & Roizman,
1972; Kozak & Roizman, 1974).   This indicates that translocation is
regulated.   The extent of total transcription is unclear because
the symmetrical transcripts in nuclei are not present in a uniform
abundance (Jacquemont & Roizman, 1975b; Kozak & Roizman, 1975).

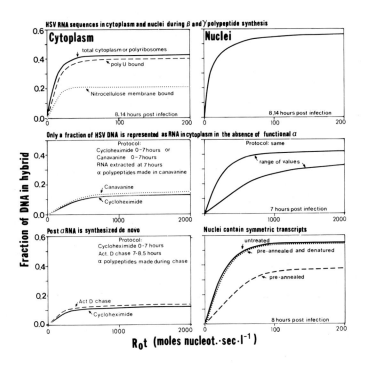

of viral RNA accumulating in cells infected and maintained in the
presence of cycloheximide is less than that accumulating in the
absence of inhibitors (Clements et al., 1977;   Kozak & Roizman, 1974).
The exact complexity of cycloheximide RNA appears to be in disagreement.   In this laboratory, the untreated infected cells contain
transcripts homologous to more than 60% of the viral DNA.   The viral
transcripts accumulating in nuclei of cells infected and maintained in
the presence of cycloheximide were found to be homologous to as much as
45% of total DNA in contrast to cytoplasmic RNA from the same cells
which is homologous to 10-12% of viral DNA (Fig. 5;   Jones & Roizman[1];
Jones et al., 1977;   Kozak & Roizman, 1974).   Clements et al. (1977),
on the basis of hybridization of labelled RNA to restriction endonu-
clease-generated DNA fragments blotted to nitrocellulose filter by
the technique of Southern (1975), concluded that the complexities of
RNA accumulating in the nucleus and cytoplasm of cells infected and
maintained in the presence of cycloheximide were identical.   However,
because the procedure used by Clements et al. (1977) does not measure
the fraction of each DNA fragment saturated by this RNA, the conclusion
on identity of the complexities of nuclear and cytoplasmic RNAs might
not be accurate.   Nonetheless, there is no disagreement that the
complexity of the RNA made in the absence of infected-cell protein
synthesis is significantly lower than that of RNA made in untreated
infected cells.

This and the preceding sections made painfully evident the following: (i) the initiation and termination of transcription are most
likely regulated;   (ii) transcriptional regulation is most evident in
the transition for α and β protein synthesis, or, in operational terms,
during the shift from transcription in the absence of infected-cell
protein synthesis to transcription in the presence of newly made viral
polypeptides;   and (iii) host RNA polymerase II participates in the
transcription of the virus.   The inevitable conclusion that must be
made is that viral polypeptides probably modify the transcription by
interacting with the template-polymerase complex.   Identification of
the viral polypeptides specifying this function will probably emerge
from genetic and biochemical studies.

Evidence that processing and translocation of RNA are regulated

We have repeatedly emphasized that the transition from α to β to
γ RNA synthesis involves two events, i.e., the appearance in the cytoplasm of RNA suitable for translation of polypeptides comprising the
next group and a cytoplasmic event that terminates the synthesis of
the prior polypeptide group.   The accumulation of translatable RNA
in the cytoplasm requires processing and translocation of RNA in
addition to transcription.   There is reasonable evidence that, in
addition to transcription, both processing and translocation of RNA
are regulated.

---

[1] Unpublished data

Two lines of evidence indicate that the translocation of RNA is regulated. First, the complexity of the viral RNA accumulating in the cytoplasm does not exceed 50% of the DNA, both because it drives less than 50% of the DNA (Fig. 5) into DNA-RNA hybrid, and because the RNA does not self-anneal (Jacquemont & Roizman, 1975b; Kozak & Roizman, 1974, 1975; Silverstein et al., 1973). By contrast, nuclear RNA drives more than 60% of viral DNA into hybrid (Fig. 5) and does self-anneal (Jacquemont & Roizman, 1975a,b; Kozak & Roizman, 1974). This clearly establishes that translocation is regulated. The actual amount of DNA driven into hybrid by excess viral RNA appears to be approximately 43% (Kozak & Roizman, 1974; Silverstein et al., 1973, 1976). This is only 2% less than the sequence complexity in one strand (45%). However, because some of the RNA most likely arises from reiterated ca and ab sequences, it is likely that the true complexity of the RNA might be significantly lower. Second, as noted earlier in the text, in our studies, the RNA sequences accumulating in the cytoplasm of cells infected and maintained in the presence of cycloheximide are homologous to only 10-12% of the DNA in contrast to nuclear RNA which is homologous to a larger fraction of viral DNA (Fig. 5). The discriminating signals in the RNA that determine whether the RNA will be translocated into the cytoplasm are as yet unknown. As cited earlier in the text, current evidence indicates that, following synthesis, viral RNA is cleaved, methylated, and adenylated. However, it does not seem likely that in HSV-1 infected cells translocation is determined by the extent of adenylation because non-adenylated or poorly adenylated viral RNA molecules are readily detected in the cytoplasm (Silverstein et al., 1976; Stringer et al., 1977). Furthermore, because the non-adenylated molecules were larger than the adenylated molecules, the RNA was not degraded during extraction. In the same vein, although caps with sequences $7^mG(5')ppp(5')X^mpY^mpNP$ or $7^mG(5')ppp(5')X^mpNp$ and N^6-methyladenosine ($6mA$) are present in cytoplasmic RNA, there is no evidence that they constitute signals for translocation.

There is evidence that cleavage of RNA and methylation are also regulated. For example, the observation that high molecular-weight viral RNA (> 45S) was found to contain two sets of sequences differing 5000-fold in abundance whereas the sequences present in smaller size molecules differed considerably less in abundance (Jacquemont & Roizman, 1975a), suggests that processing is at least selective and almost certainly regulated. Another example of regulation of processing concerns internal methylation of viral mRNA. Whereas viral mRNAs made during first few hours after infection and especially α mRNAs are capped at the 5' end, internally methylated (predominantly $6mA$), and adenylated at the 3' end, the mRNAs entering the cytoplasmic pool and polyribosomes 11-15 hours post infection are capped and methylated but lack $6mA$ (Fig. 6; Bartkoski & Roizman, 1976). As illustrated in Table 2, this observation is significant for three reasons (Bartkoski & Roizman, 1978). First, the lack of internal methylation cannot be attributed

FIG. 6.   ELUTION PROFILES OF HSV-1 SPECIFIC RNA
OR INFECTED-CELL RNA ON DEAE-SEPHADEX COLUMNS

The RNA was labelled with ^{3}H-methylmethionine from 0-7 hours in the
presence of cycloheximide (panels A and C) or from 11-14 hours post
infection in untreated cells (B and D).   RNA translocated into the
cytoplasm during the synthesis of α and β polypeptides is adenylated
as well as methylated at the 5' terminus and internally.   RNA translocated into the cytoplasm during the synthesis of γ polypeptides
(11-14 hours post infection) lacks internal methylation.   Both host
and viral RNA are affected (Bartkoski & Roizman, 1976, 1978).

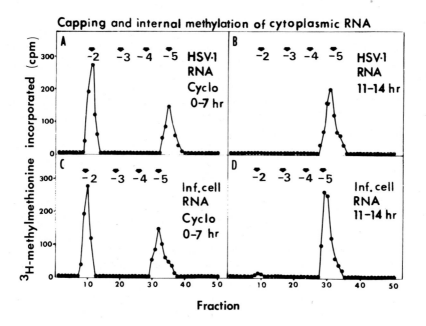

to rapid decay of a host methylase unreplenished because of the host
shut-off following infection.   The basis of this conclusion is that
the internal methylation of α RNA labelled 11-15 hours post infection
and maintainance in the presence of cycloheximide (50 µg/ml) cannot
be differentiated from that of early RNA from untreated infected cells
and from uninfected untreated cells.   Second, the argument that γ mRNA
lacks internal methylation sites is weakened considerably by the
observation that $6mA$ is absent not only from viral mRNA but also from
host RNA entering the cytoplasm 11-15 hours post infection.   Lastly,

Table 2. Distribution of methyl label in cytoplasmic poly(A) RNA from HSV-1 infected cells[a]

Genetic origin of RNA	Treatment		Labelling interval[b] (hours)	% cpm		Class of polypeptide (or RNA) made during labelling interval
	Drug	Interval[b] (hours)		Cap	Internal methylation	
Poly(A) - RNA late in infection lacks internal methylation						
Viral[c]	None	-	0 - 14	63	37	α, β, γ
Viral	Cycloheximide	0 - 8	0 - 8	45	55	(α, RNA)
Viral	None	-	11 - 14	95	5	<β, ≫γ
Viral and cell	None	-	11 - 14	99	1	<β, ≫γ
Lack of internal methylation is not due to decay of methylating enzyme						
Viral and cell	Cycloheximide	0 - 15	0 - 5	48	52	(host and α RNA)
Viral and cell	Cycloheximide	0 - 15	5 - 10	43	57	(host and >α RNA)
Viral and cell	Cycloheximide	0 - 15	10 - 15	49	51	(host and ≫α RNA)
Loss of internal methylation of viral and cell RNA coincides with peak synthesis of functional β polypeptides						
Viral	Canavanine	0 - 14	11 - 14	42	58	>α [nf]^d
	Canavanine	2.8 - 14	11 - 14	57	43	α [f], >β [nf], <γ [nf]^d
	Canavanine	5 - 14	11 - 14	76	24	<α [f], >β [f, nf], >γ [nf]^d
	Canavanine	7.5 - 14	11 - 14	83	16	>γ [f, nf]^d
	None	-		90	10	<β, ≫γ
Cell[c]	Canavanine	0 - 14	11 - 14	53	47	-
	Canavanine	2.8 - 14	11 - 14	48	52	-
	Canavanine	5 - 14	11 - 14	66	34	-
	Canavanine	7.5 - 14	11 - 14	73	27	-
	None	-	11 - 14	88	12	-
Loss of internal methylation occurs under conditions of markedly reduced γ polypeptide synthesis						
Viral (PAA^s)	PAA	0 - 14	11 - 14	100	0	<α, >β, ≪γ
Viral (PAA^r)	PAA	0 - 14	11 - 14	92	8	<β, ≫γ

[a] This table summarizes the data which show that RNA late in infection lacks internal methylation. The lack of internal methylation is not due to the rapid turnover of the enzyme as shown by the stability of methylation in RNA made in the presence of cycloheximide up to 15 hours post infection. The addition of canavanine as late as five hours post infection blocks the shut-off of internal methylation and suggests that the shut-off of internal methylation is a viral function specified by β polypeptides. The inhibition of internal methylation also occurs in cells treated with phosphonoacetic acid, which blocks viral DNA synthesis and reduces the amount of γ polypeptides made (Bartkoski & Roizman, 1978).

[b] Time after infection

[c] Purified by hybridization to DNA

[d] f - functional; nf - non-functional

6mA is present in both viral and host mRNA late in infection of cells treated with the amino-acid analogue canavanine as late as five hours post infection. At this time, canavanine no longer affects the transition from β to γ polypeptide synthesis yet it does preclude the loss of internal methylation of both host and viral DNA. It would seem, therefore, that the change in the structure of mRNA late in infection is a function determined by the virus and that it affects all RNA made at that time. Whether lack of internal methylation is the structural characteristic responsible for the relatively short half-life of γ mRNA remains to be seen.

The interesting question is the fate and function of the missing methyl groups. One non-trivial hypothesis is that some viral poly-

peptides inhibit all internal methylation of all RNA synthesized late
in infection.   Another ascribes to viral polypeptides actuation of
some mechanism that causes cleavage of all RNA molecules at the site
of methylation.   The hypothesis is especially attractive because one
could readily envision that early in infection and especially during
α polypeptide synthesis the mRNA contains sequences specifying both
β and γ polypeptides but that β sequences only are translated, and
that cleavage of the RNA at a methylated site followed by capping
could then render the putative β sequences available for translation.
This hypothesis envisions that *6mA* is a punctuation mark signalling
sites for cleavage of RNA.   Alas, the real reason for the absence of
6mA remains a mystery.

GENE ARRANGEMENT IN HSV DNA

The approximate location of templates specifying known viral markers
and polypeptides in HSV DNA is beginning to emerge from several studies.
Previous studies have shown by a classical recombination analysis that
temperature-sensitive mutations can be arranged in a linear array both
for markers within and between the L and S components (Benyesh-Melnick
et al., 1975;   Schaffer, 1975;   Subak-Sharpe et al., 1975).   Recently
the use of marker rescue analysis (Knipe et al., 1978;   Wilkie et al.,
1975), marker transfer studies (Ruyechan et al.[1]), and analysis of
HSV-1 × HSV-2 intertypic recombinants (morse et al., 1978) have been
employed to investigate the viral gene organization (Fig. 7).

Several aspects of the arrangement of HSV gene templates bear
upon the regulation of macromolecular synthesis.   First, there appears
to be a clear segregation of templates specifying α polypeptides in
that ICP 27 and ICP 4 map at the termini of the L and S components at
least partly within the reiterated regions.   As Figure 7 shows, the
positions of α templates and mutants presumably mapping within the
genes for ICP 4 and ICP 27, coincide with the map positions of some α
RNA sequences as previously reported (Jones et al., 1977).   Taken
together, the data strongly suggest that the *b'a'*, *a'c'* and *ac*
reiterated sequences contain at least a portion of genes specifying
structural information.   The proximity of α templates near the termini
of the L and S components also suggests the possibility that the promoter for transcription of these functions is at the termini.   Second,
although no β or γ polypeptides were unambiguously mapped in the S
component, those in the L component appear to be intermixed.   It is
also of interest to note that viral functions most likely involving
β polypeptides (e.g., TK, resistance to phosphonoacetate, and accelerated shut-off of host macromolecular synthesis) were intermixed with
γ functions (syncytial plaque morphology).

---

[1] Unpublished data

FIG. 7. LOCATION OF TEMPLATES SPECIFYING HSV MARKERS AND POLYPEPTIDES

The location of templates specifying HSV markers and polypeptides was
determined from analysis of HSV-1 X HSV-2 intertypic recombinants
(Morse et al., 1978) and from marker transfer and marker rescue studies
(Knipe et al., 1978; Ruyechan et al., unpublished data).
The template location of α RNA represents data from Jones et al. (1977),
while the origin of defective DNA represents data from Frenkel et al.
(1975, 1976, personal communication).

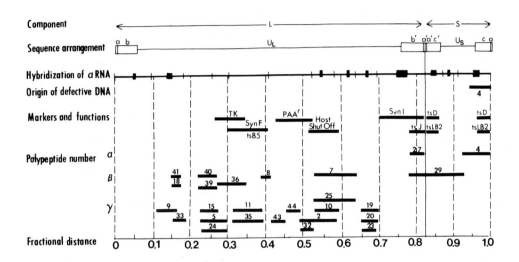

The apparent random distribution of templates for β and γ polypeptides is of special interest in view of the evidence cited earlier
in the text indicating that the sequential switch-on of the co-ordinately regulated β and γ polypeptide synthesis is determined at the
transcriptional and post-transcriptional levels (Honess & Roizman,
1974, 1975; Roizman et al., 1975a, b). One possible explanation
consistent with all of the available data is that β and γ templates
are segregated on opposite strands. In support of this hypothesis
are the following data: (i) Trace amounts of α RNA hybridize to
sequences occupied by β and γ templates. Consistent with this finding, in many experiments in which attempts were made to restrict viral
protein synthesis to α polypeptides, trace amounts of a subset of β
polypeptides designated as β_1 (ICP 6, 8, 17, 29, 39, 41) were also

made (Pereira et al., 1977).   Normal synthesis of β_1 polypeptides,
however, required transcription in the presence of functional α polypeptides (Pereira et al., 1977).   One possible explanation is that
the trace amounts of β_1 polypeptides and corresponding RNA represent
read-through from right to left through a putative β_1 promoter.
(ii) The hypothesis predicts nuclear transcripts considerably greater
in length than the polyribosomal mRNA as well as the accumulation of
large amounts of RNA transcribed from both strands and capable of
annealing to form double-stranded RNA.   As cited earlier in the text,
clear transcripts are larger than polyribosomal viral RNA (Jacquemont
& Roizman, 1975;   Wagner & Roizman, 1969) and a very large fraction of
the DNA is transcribed symmetrically (Jacquemont & Roizman, 1975b;
Kozak & Roizman, 1975).

CONCLUSION

> The effort to understand the universe
> is one of the very few things that
> lifts human life a little above the
> level of farce and gives it some of
> the grace of tragedy.
>
> *STEVE WEINBERG, The First Three Minutes*

The central question that this Symposium has attempted to answer
is the demarcation of the unity and diversity among herpesviruses.
The painstaking dissection of the infected cell into its component
macromolecules is carried out in many laboratories based on the belief
and conviction but hopefully not on the illusion that every change in
the structure, accumulation, and function of macromolecules plays an
eventual role in the multiplication of the virus.   Obviously in
addition to the question whether detailed examination of the 5' cap
structure on viral mRNA will elucidate the regulation of viral gene
expression, there is the added question whether HSV-1 or, in fact, any
herpesvirus is a useful model of the herpesvirus universe.

In point of fact, there is considerable unity among herpesviruses.
It encompasses not only the superficial aspects of structure but also
the general pattern of replication.   Thus, pseudorabies virus DNA
synthesis is inhibited by 5'-fluorouracil (Kaplan & Ben-Porat, 1961)
and yet the drug does not inhibit the synthesis and assembly of
capsids (Reissig & Kaplan, 1962).   A sequential ordering of events
similar to that seen in HSV-infected cells has been seen in several

quite diverse herpesviruses. The resemblance of pseudorabies replication with that of HSV is very striking (Ben-Porat et al., 1971, 1974, 1975; Jean et al., 1974; Rakusanova et al., 1971, 1972) but even Epstein-Barr virus (EBV) and HSV share many features (Roizman & Kieff, 1975; Roizman et al., 1977). Thus the EBV-determined nuclear antigen (EBNA), early antigen (EA) and viral capsid antigen (VCA) correspond in many respects to α, β and γ polypeptides of HSV. EBNA, EA and VCA are sequentially ordered and the decrease in the rate of synthesis of VCA following exposure of cells to inhibitors of DNA synthesis is in many respects similar to that observed in HSV-infected cells. A minor difference, and perhaps the only one noted so far, is that, in lymphoblasts restringently infected with EBV, adenylation does play a role in translocation of viral RNA from the nucleus to the cytoplasm (Orellana & Kieff, 1977).

The unity will, ultimately and irresistibly, yield to diversity as the focus of our attention. Already intratypic differences between HSV-1 isolates with respect to sequences in DNA, polypeptide structure, etc., have become apparent and these cannot help but become more commonplace as we begin to examine the many herpesviruses infecting the animal kingdom. The most striking and perhaps significant evidence of diversity among herpesviruses concerns the extent to which the expression of the viral genome is *perceptibly* regulated by the host genome. The brief review of the regulation of HSV protein synthesis totally ignored any regulatory participation in the process by the host genome for the simple reason that it is in most instances imperceptible.

The function of the host in directing and regulating viral multiplication does become apparent in studies of EBV and cytomegalovirus infections. Host functions do play an important role in the transition from EBNA to EA to VCA and probably in similar events in cytomegalovirus infection as well. The reason why host function is less readily demonstrable in the course of replication of HSV than that of EBV or of cytomegaloviruses is not clear; that it exists there is no doubt because in every sense, latent human HSV infections fit the definition of virus replication under a tight host control. There is no doubt that defining the host functions that determine the course and outcome of herpesvirus infection is a major challenge and will be a prominent direction of research in the foreseeable future.

ACKNOWLEDGEMENTS

The studies conducted at the University of Chicago were aided
by grants from the National Cancer Institute (CA 08494 and
CA 19264), the American Cancer Society (VC 103L), and
the National Science Foundation (PCM 76-06254).
L.S. Morse is a US Public Health Service
predoctoral trainee (5-T32 GM 07183).

REFERENCES

Bachenheimer, S.L. & Roizman, B. (1972)   Ribonucleic acid synthesis
in cells infected with herpes simplex virus. VI. Polyadenylic
acid sequences in viral messenger ribonucleic acid.   *J. Virol.,*
10, 875-879

Bartkoski, M. & Roizman, B. (1976)   RNA synthesis in cells infected
with herpes simplex virus.   XIII. Differences in the methylation
patterns of viral RNA during the reproductive cycle.   *J. Virol.,*
20, 583-588

Bartkoski, M. & Roizman, B. (1978)   Regulation of herpesvirus macromolecular synthesis. VII. Inhibition of internal methylation of
mRNA late in infection.   *Virology, 85*, 146-156

Ben-Porat, T., Rakusanova, T. & Kaplan, A.S. (1971)   Early functions
of the genome of herpesvirus.   II. Inhibition of the formation of
cell-specific polysomes.   *Virology, 46*, 890-899

Ben-Porat, T., Jean, J.-H. & Kaplan, A.S. (1974)   Early functions of
the genome of herpesvirus.   IV. Fate and translation of immediate
early viral RNA.   *Virology, 59*, 524-531

Ben-Porat, T., Kervina, M. & Kaplan, A.S. (1975)   Early functions of
the genome of herpesvirus.   V. Serological analysis of "immediate-
early" proteins.   *Virology, 65*, 355-362

Benyesh-Melnick, M., Schaffer, P.A., Courtney, R.J., Esparza, T. &
Kimura, S. (1975)   Viral gene functions expressed and detected
by temperature sensitive mutants of herpes simplex virus.   *Cold*
Spring Harb. Symp. quant. Biol., 39, 731-746

Ben-Zeev, A. & Becker, Y. (1977)   Requirement of host cell RNA polymerase II in the replication of herpes simplex virus in α-amanitin-sensitive and -resistant cell lines. *Virology,* *76,* 246-254

Clements, J.B., Watson, R.J. & Wilkin, N.M. (1977)   Temporal regulation of herpes simplex virus type 1 transcription: location of transcripts on the viral genome. *Cell, 12,* 275-286

Costanzo, F., Campadelli-Fiume, G., Foa-Tomas, L. & Cassai, E. (1977)   Evidence that herpes simplex virus DNA is transcribed by cellular RNA polymerase II. *J. Virol., 21,* 996-1001

Courtney, R.J., Schaffer, P.A. & Powell, K. (1976)   Synthesis of virus specific polypeptides by temperature-sensitive mutants of herpes simplex type 1. *Virology, 75,* 306-318

Erickson, J.S. & Kaplan, A.S. (1973)   Synthesis of proteins in cells infected with herpesvirus. IX. Sulfated proteins. *Virology, 55,* 94-102

Frenkel, N. & Roizman, B. (1972)   Ribonucleic acid synthesis in cells infected with herpes simplex virus: Control of transcription and of RNA abundance. *Proc. nat. Acad. Sci. (Wash.), 69,* 2654-2658

Frenkel, N., Silverstein, S., Cassai, E. & Roizman, B. (1973)   RNA synthesis in cells infected with herpes simplex virus. VI. Control of transcription and of transcript abundances of unique and common sequences of herpes simplex 1 and 2. *J. Virol., 11,* 886-892

Frenkel, N., Jacob, R.J., Honess, R.W., Hayward, G.S., Locker, H. & Roizman, B. (1975)   The anatomy of herpes simplex virus DNA. III. Characterization of defective DNA molecules and biologic properties of virus populations containing them. *J. Virol., 16,* 153-167

Frenkel, N., Locker, H., Batterson, W., Hayward, G. & Roizman, B. (1976)   Anatomy of herpes simplex DNA. VI. Defective DNA originates from the S component. *J. Virol., 20,* 527-531

Garfinkle, B. & McAuslan, B. (1974)   Regulation of herpes simplex virus induced thymidine kinase. *Biochem. biophys. Res. Commun., 58,* 822-829

Honess, R.W. & Roizman, B. (1973)   Proteins specified by herpes simplex virus. XI. Identification and relative molar rates of synthesis of structural and non structural herpesvirus polypeptides in the infected cell. *J. Virol., 12,* 1347-1365

Honess, R.W. & Roizman, B. (1974)   Regulation of herpesvirus macromolecular synthesis. I. Cascade regulation of the synthesis of three groups of viral proteins. *J. Virol., 14,* 8-19

Honess, R.W. & Roizman, B. (1975a)   Regulation of herpesvirus macro-
    molecular synthesis: Sequential transition of polypeptide syn-
    thesis requires functional viral polypeptides. *Proc. nat. Acad.
    Sci. (Wash.), 72*, 1276-1280

Honess, R.W. & Roizman, B. (1975b)   Proteins specified by herpes
    simplex virus. XIII. Glycosylation of viral polypeptides.
    J. Virol., 16, 1308-1326

Honess, R.W. & Watson, D.H. (1974)   Herpes simplex virus-specific
    polypeptides studied by polyacrylamide gel electrophoresis of
    immune precipitates. *J. gen. Virol., 22*, 171-185

Honess, R.W. & Watson, D.H. (1977)   Herpes simplex virus resistance
    and sensitivity to phosphonoacetic acid. *J. Virol., 21*, 584-600

Jacquemont, B. & Roizman, B. (1975a)   Ribonucleic acid synthesis in
    cells infected with herpes simplex virus: Characterization of viral
    high molecular weight nuclear RNA. *J. gen. Virol., 29*, 155-165

Jacquemont, B. & Roizman, B. (1975b)   Ribonucleic acid synthesis in
    cells infected with herpes simplex virus. X. Properties of viral
    symmetric transcripts and double stranded RNA prepared from them.
    J. Virol., 15, 707-713

Jean, J.H., Ben-Porat, T. & Kaplan, A.S. (1974)   Early functions of
    the genome of herpesvirus. III. Inhibition of the transcription of
    the viral genome in cells treated with cycloheximide early during
    the infective process. *Virology, 59*, 516-523

Jones, P.C., Hayward, G.S. & Roizman, B. (1977)   Anatomy of herpes
    simplex virus DNA. VI. α RNA is homologous to non-continuous sites
    in both L and S components of viral DNA. *J. Virol., 21*, 268-276

Kaplan, A.S. & Ben-Porat, T. (1961)   The action of 5-fluorouracil on
    the nucleic acid metabolism of pseudorabies virus-infected and non-
    infected rabbit kidney cells. *Virology, 13*, 78-92

Knipe, D.M., Ruyechan, W.T., Roizman, B. & Halliburton, I.W. (1978)
    Molecular genetics of herpes simplex virus: Demonstration of
    regions of obligatory and non-obligatory identity within diploïd
    regions of the genome by sequence replacement and insertion.
    Proc. nat. Acad. Sci. (Wash.) (in press)

Kozak, M. & Roizman, B. (1974)   Regulation of herpesvirus macromolecular
    synthesis: nuclear retention of non translated viral RNA sequences.
    Proc. nat. Acad. Sci. (Wash.), 71, 4322-4326

Kozak, M. & Roizman, B. (1975)   RNA synthesis in cells infected with
    herpes simplex virus. IX. Evidence for accumulation of abundant
    symmetric transcripts in nuclei. *J. Virol., 15*, 36-40

Lando, D. & Ryhiner, M.L. (1969)   Pouvoir infectieux du DNA d'herpes-
    virus hominis en culture cellulaire. *C.R. Acad. Sci. (Paris),
    269*, 527-530

Leiden, J., Buttyan, R. & Spear, P.G. (1976)   Herpes simplex virus
    gene expression in transformed cells.   I. Regulation of the viral
    thymidine kinase gene in transformed L cells by products of super-
    infecting virus.   *J. Virol.*, *20*, 413-424

Marsden, H.S., Crombie, I.K. & Subak-Sharpe, J.H. (1976)   Control of
    protein synthesis in herpesvirus-infected cells: Analysis of
    the polypeptides induced by wild type and sixteen temperature-
    sensitive mutants of HSV strain 17.   *J. gen. Virol.*, *31*, 347-372

Morse, L.S., Buchman, T.G., Roizman, B. & Schaffer, P.A. (1977)
    Anatomy of herpes simplex virus DNA.   IX. Apparent exclusion of
    some parental DNA arrangements in the generation of intertypic
    (HSV-1 X HSV-2) recombinants.   *J. Virol.*, *24*, 231-248

Morse, L.S., Pereira, L., Roizman, B. & Schaffer, P. (1978)   Anatomy
    of HSV DNA.   XI. Mapping of viral genes by analysis of polypeptides
    and functions specified by HSV-1 X HSV-2 recombinants.   *J. Virol.*,
    26, 384-410

Moss, B., Gershowitz, A., Stringer, J., Holland, L. & Wagner, E. (1977)
    5'-terminal and internal methylated nucleosides in herpes simplex
    virus type 1 mRNA.   *J. Virol.*, *23*, 234-239

Orellana, T. & Kieff, E. (1977)   Epstein-Barr virus-specific RNA.
    II. Analysis of polyadenylated viral RNA in restringent, abortive,
    and productive infections.   *J. Virol.*, *22*, 321-330

Pereira, L., Cassai, E., Honess, R.W., Roizman, B., Terni, M. &
    Nahmias, A. (1976)   Variability in the structural polypeptides
    of herpes simplex virus 1 strains: potential application in mole-
    cular epidemiology.   *Infect. Immun.*, *13*, 211-220

Pereira, L., Wolff, M., Fenwick, M. & Roizman, B. (1977)   Regulation of
    herpesvirus synthesis.   V. Properties of α polypeptides specified
    by HSV-1 and HSV-2.   *Virology*, *77*, 733-749

Powell, K. & Courtney, R. (1975)   Polypeptides synthesized in herpes
    simplex virus type 2 infected HEp-2 cells.   *Virology*, *66*, 217-
    228

Powell, K.L., Purifoy, D.J.M. & Courney, R.J. (1975)   The synthesis
    of herpes simplex virus proteins in the absence of virus DNA syn-
    thesis.   *Biochem. biophys. Res. Commun.*, *66*, 262-271

Powell, K. & Purifoy, D. (1977)   Nonstructural proteins of herpes
    simplex virus.   I. Purification of the induced DNA polymerase.
    J. Virol., *24*, 618-626

Rakusanova, T., Ben-Porat, T., Himeno, M. & Kaplan, A.S. (1971)
    Early functions of the genome of herpesvirus.   I. Characterization
    of the RNA synthesized in cycloheximide-treated, infected cells.
    Virology, *46*, 877-889

Rakusanova, T., Ben-Porat, T. & Kaplan, A.S. (1972)   Effect of herpes-
    virus infection on the synthesis of cell-specific RNA.   *Virology*,
    49, 537-548

Reissig, M. & Kaplan, A.S. (1962)   The morphology of noninfective
    pseudorabies virus produced by cells treated with 5-fluorouracil.
    Virology, *16*, 1-8

Roizman, B. & Furlong, D. (1974)   *The replication of herpesviruses.*
    In: Fraenkel-Conrat, H. & Wagner, R.R., eds, *Comprehensive
    Virology*, *Vol. 3*, New York, Plenum Press, pp. 229-403

Roizman, B., Hayward, G., Jacob, R., Wadsworth, S.W. & Honess, R.W.
    (1974)   Human herpesvirus 1: A model for molecular organization
    of herpesvirus virions and their DNA.   *Chem. virol. Carcinogen.*,
    2, 188-198

Roizman, B., Hayward, G., Jacob, R., Wadsworth, S.W., Frenkel, N.,
    Honess, R.W. & Kozak, M. (1975a)   *Human herpesviruses 1: A model
    for molecular organization and regulation of herpesviruses -
    A review.*   In: de-Thé, G., Epstein, M.A. & zur Hausen, H., eds,
    Oncogenesis and Herpesviruses II, Part 1, Lyon, International
    Agency for Research on Cancer (*IARC Scientific Publications* No. 11),
    pp. 3-38

Roizman, B., Kozak, M., Honess, R.W. & Hayward, G. (1975b)   Regulation
    of herpesvirus macromolecular synthesis: Evidence for multilevel
    regulation of herpes simplex 1 RNA and protein synthesis.   *Cold
    Spring Harb. Symp. quant. Biol.*, *39*, 687-701

Roizman, B. & Kieff, E.D. (1975)   *Herpes simplex and Epstein-Barr
    viruses in human cells and tissues: A study in contrasts.*   In:
    Becker, F.F., ed., *Cancer: A Comprehensive Treatise, Vol. 2*,
    New York, Plenum Press, pp. 241-322

Roizman, B., Frenkel, N., Kieff, E.D. & Spear, P.G. (1977)   *The
    structure and expression of human herpesvirus DNA in productive
    infection and in transformed cells.*   In: Watson, J.D. & Hyatt,
    H., eds, *Origins of Human Cancer*, Cold Spring Harbor, N.Y.,
    Cold Spring Harbor Laboratory, pp. 1064-1111

Schaffer, P.A. (1975)   Temperature-sensitive mutants of herpesviruses.
    Curr. Top. Microbiol. Immunol., *70*, 51-100

Sheldrick, P., Laithier, M. & Ryhiner, M. (1973)   Infectious DNA
    from herpes simplex virus: Infectivity of double-stranded and
    single-stranded molecules.   *Proc. nat. Acad. Sci. (Wash.)*, *70*,
    3621-3625

Silverstein, S., Bachenheimer, S.L., Frenkel, N. & Roizman, B. (1973)
    The relationship between post transcriptional adenylation of
    herpesvirus RNA and mRNA abundance.   *Proc. nat. Acad. Sci. (Wash.)*,
    70, 2101-2104

Silverstein, S., Millette, R., Hones, P. & Roizman, B. (1976)   RNA synthesis in cells infected with herpes simplex virus. XII. Sequence complexity and properties of RNA differing in extent of adenylation. *J. Virol.*, *18*, 977-991

Southern, E.M. (1975)   Detection of specific sequences among DNA fragments separated by gel electrophoresis. *J. molec. Biol.*, *98*, 503-512

Spear, P.G. (1976)   Membrane proteins specified by herpes simplex viruses. I. Identification of four glycoprotein precursors and their products in type-1 infected cells. *J. Virol.*, *17*, 941-1008

Stringer, J.R., Holland, L.E., Swanstrom, R.I., Pivo, K. & Wagner, E.K. (1977)   Quantitation of herpes simplex virus type 1 RNA in infected HeLa cells. *J. Virol.*, *21*, 889-901

Subak-Sharpe, J.H., Brown, J.M., Ritchie, D.A., Timbury, M.C., Macnab, J.C.M., Marsden, H.S. & Hay, J. (1974)   Genetic and bio-chemical studies with herpesvirus. *Cold Spring Harb. Symp. quant. Biol.*, *39*, 717-730

Swanstrom, R., Pivo, K. & Wagner, E. (1975)   Restricted transcription of the herpes simplex virus genome occurring early after infection and in the presence of metabolic inhibitors. *Virology*, *66*, 140-150

Wadsworth, S., Jacob, R. & Roizman, B. (1975)   Anatomy of herpes simplex virus DNA. II. Size, composition and arrangement of inverted terminal repetitions. *J. Virol.*, *15*, 1487-1497

Wagner, E.K. & Roizman, B. (1969)   RNA synthesis in cells infected with herpes simplex virus. II. Evidence that a class of viral mRNA is derived from a high molecular weight precursor synthesized in the nucleus. *Proc. nat. Acad. Sci. (Wash.)*, *64*, 626-633

Wilkie, N.M., Clements, J.B., Macnab, J.C.M. & Subak-Sharpe, J.H. (1975)   The structure and biological properties of herpes simplex virus DNA. *Cold Spring Harb. Symp. quant. Biol.*, *39*, 657-666

REGULATION OF HERPES SIMPLEX VIRUS TYPE 1 DNA SYNTHESIS: TEMPERATURE-SHIFT STUDIES WITH DNA-NEGATIVE TEMPERATURE-SENSITIVE MUTANTS

D.S. PARRIS & P.A. SCHAFFER

Division of Basic Sciences,
Sidney Farber Cancer Institute,
Harvard Medical School,
Boston, Mass., USA

R.J. COURTNEY

Department of Virology and Epidemiology,
Baylor College of Medicine,
Houston, Texas, USA

INTRODUCTION

Investigations with temperature-sensitive (*ts*) mutants of herpes simplex virus (HSV) types 1 and 2 conducted in several laboratories have demonstrated that mutants in approximately one-half of the HSV cistrons identified to date are defective in the synthesis of viral DNA at the non-permissive temperature (Schaffer, 1975). Efforts are currently in progress to identify the function of selected HSV genes in the viral DNA synthetic process.

On the genetic map of HSV-1 strain KOS, mutants which fail to synthesize viral DNA are located in two regions of the genome (Fig. 1). DNA⁻ mutants in groups A, D, and C map in a tight cluster spanning about three recombination units. Group-B mutants are located 24 units to the right of A, D, and C on the genetic map (Jofre et al.[1]; Schaffer et al., 1974). Marker rescue studies have placed the A, D,

---

[1] Unpublished data

FIG. 1. LINKAGE MAP OF HSV-1 STRAIN KOS CISTRONS

DNA⁻ *ts* mutants (□), DNA± *ts* mutants (▤), and DNA⁺ *ts* mutants (■) are
included.

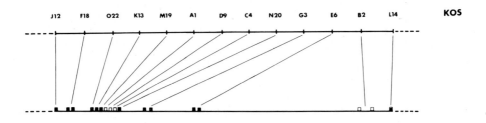

and C groups in the L region and the B group in the S region of the
viral DNA molecule (J. Bookout[1]; Parsis et al.[2]).   Temperature shift-
up studies of mutants in DNA⁻ complementation groups A, B, C, and D
conducted previously demonstrated that, for the synthesis of viral DNA,
the product of the B gene is required only transiently during the early
stages of infection while the products of the A, C, and D genes are
required continuously (Schaffer et al., 1976).

    When mutants in the four groups were tested for their ability to
induce functional viral DNA polymerase (DP) at the non-permissive
temperature, DP activity of mutants in the C and D groups was found to
be temperature-sensitive *in vivo* (Aron et al., 1975).   Viral DP
activity in cells infected with group-A mutants was normal while group-
B mutants induced reduced levels of the enzyme at the non-permissive
temperature.   Although these studies have implicated the C and D
genes in the induction of viral DP activity and have suggested other
roles for group-A and group-B mutants, it was not known whether the
block in viral DNA synthesis exhibited by these mutants occurred at
the level of transcription or translation.

---

[1] Personal communication

[2] Unpublished data

METHODS AND RESULTS

In order to investigate this problem, cells infected with the wild-type virus (strain KOS) or with mutants in DNA⁻ groups B, C and D (*ts* B2, *ts* C4, *ts* D9) were shifted from the non-permissive temperature (39°C) to the permissive temperature (34°C) in the presence of inhibitors of protein and RNA synthesis. Mutant *ts* E5 was included as a control. Phenotypically, group-E mutants are DNA⁺ and DP⁺ (Aron et al., 1975); they are located between mutants in groups B and C on the genetic map (Fig. 1).

Briefly, human embryonic lung fibroblasts were infected with 10-15 plaque-forming units of each virus per cell. Infected cells were incubated at 37°C for one hour, overlaid with medium, and incubated in water baths at 34°C or 39°C until nine hours post infection. At this time actinomycin D (Act D; Calbiochem, La Jolla, Calif.) was added to half the cultures at a final concentration of 1 μg/ml, all cultures were labelled with 10 μCi of ³H-thymidine (Schwarz/Mann, Orangeburg, N.Y.) per millilitre, and half the cultures with and without Act D were shifted-down to the permissive temperature. All cultures were harvested at 18 hours post infection and DNA determinations were conducted by the method of Aron et al. (1975).

Polypeptide synthesis was monitored in parallel cultures incubated from 0 to 9 hours in methionine-free medium and from 9 to 18 hours in medium containing ³⁵S-methionine (10 μCi/ml; New England Nuclear, Boston, Mass.). Polyacrylamide slab gel electrophoresis of total cellular extracts was performed as previously described (Courtney et al., 1976). Polypeptides were designated by their molecular weight according to the terminology proposed by Bone & Courtney (1974) and classified as α, β, or γ, as reported by Honess & Roizman (1974).

Figure 2 illustrates the synthesis of viral (density 1.725 g/cm³) and cellular (density 1.700 g/cm³) DNA in infected cells labelled from 9 to 18 hours post infection and maintained at 39°C (a) and at 34°C (b). Efficient inhibition of cellular DNA synthesis occurred with all viruses tested. Inhibition was approximately equal at both temperatures for each virus except in the case of *ts* B2 in which it was greater at 39°C than at 34°C. As previously reported (Aron et al., 1975), no viral DNA was synthesized at the non-permissive temperature by cells infected with mutants in groups B, C, or D, while viral DNA was synthesized in cells infected with *ts* E5, albeit at a reduced level, compared with the wild-type virus at this temperature. While cells infected with each mutant synthesized viral DNA at 34°C, *ts* C4-infected cells synthesized less viral DNA than the wild-type virus; in cells infected with *ts* B2 and *ts* D9, significantly more viral DNA was synthesized than in cells infected with the wild-type virus.

FIG. 2. CAESIUM CHLORIDE EQUILIBRIUM SEDIMENTATION
OF VIRAL AND CELLULAR DNA FROM INFECTED CELLS

Cells were maintained continuously at 39°C (a) or at 34°C (b) and
were labelled with ^{3}H-thymidine (10 μCi/ml) from 9 to 18 hours post
infection.   Centrifugation was in a Beckman 50 Ti rotor at 40 000
rpm for 68 hours at 23°C.   The direction of sedimentation is from
right to left.   The results presented are representative of two or
three separate determinations.   Density of viral DNA: 1.725 g/cm^3;
density of cellular DNA: 1.700 g/cm^3.

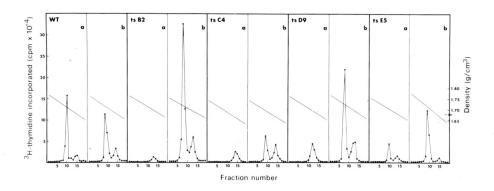

In previous studies the increased levels of DNA synthesized by *ts* B2
and *ts* D9 from 9 to 18 hours were shown to result from a delay in the
time of maximum viral DNA synthesis[1].   Although the maximum rate of
viral DNA synthesis occurs at 4-6 hours in cells infected with the
wild-type virus, nine hours was selected as the time of temperature
shift-down to enable *ts* B2 and *ts* D9 to direct the synthesis of all
the gene products required for DNA synthesis to the point at which
DNA synthesis was blocked.

When infected cultures were shifted from the non-permissive to
the permissive temperature at nine hours post infection in the absence
of inhibitor (Fig. 3a), viral DNA was synthesized in all cases.   However, the absolute levels of DNA synthesized by DNA⁻ mutants following
shift-down were significantly lower compared with those observed when
cultures were maintained at 34°C and labelled during the same period
(cf. Fig. 2b).   Therefore, only minimal reversibility of the *ts*
defects occurred in DNA⁻ mutant-infected cells.   In contrast, viral
DNA synthesis following shift-down in cells infected with *ts* E5 and
the wild-type virus exceeded that produced in infected cells maintained
at 34°C (Fig. 2b).

---

[1] Unpublished data

FIG. 3.   CAESIUM CHLORIDE EQUILIBRIUM SEDIMENTATION
OF VIRAL AND CELLULAR DNA FROM INFECTED CELLS (SHIFT-DOWN)

Cells were maintained at 39°C until 9 hours post infection.   At this
time, ³H-thymidine (10 μCi/ml) was added and cultures were incubated
at 34°C (shift-down) in the absence (a) or in the presence (b) of Act
D (1 μg/ml).   Gradients were centrifuged as described in the legend
to Figure 2.

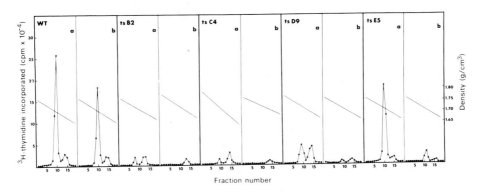

Following temperature shift-down in the presence of Act D (Fig. 3b),
no viral DNA was synthesized in cells infected with *ts* B2 or *ts* C4.
Cells infected with *ts* D9, on the other hand, synthesized low but
reproducible levels of viral DNA in the presence of Act D following
shift-down, as did the DNA⁺ mutant *ts* E5.   The presence of Act D in
wild-type virus-infected cultures following shift-down reduced the
level of viral DNA synthesis only slightly.   Thus, after initial
screening, *de novo* transcription appeared to be required for viral DNA
synthesis following shift-down in the case of *ts* B2 and *ts* C4 but not
in the case of *ts* D9.

The time required for the synthesis of functional transcripts in
ts B2- and *ts* C4-infected cells following shift-down was next determined.
Mutant-infected cultures incubated at 39°C were shifted-down to 34°C at
9 hours.   At intervals following shift-down, Act D and ³H-thymidine
were added and incubation was continued at 34°C until 18 hours.   In
ts B2- and *ts* C4-infected cells, no viral DNA was synthesized following
temperature shift-down when transcription was inhibited prior to 2
hours after shift (Fig. 4a,b,c).   If cultures were incubated for 2 or
3 hours before the addition of Act D (Fig. 4d,e),small but reproducible
amounts of viral DNA were synthesized.   The low levels of viral DNA
synthesis observed probably reflect the instability of the mRNA species
transcribed and the lateness in the replicative cycle.   Thus, the

FIG. 4. CAESIUM CHLORIDE EQUILIBRIUM SEDIMENTATION
OF DNA FROM CELLS INFECTED WITH *ts* B2 AND *ts* C4

Cells were incubated at 39°C until 9 hours post infection at which
time they were shifted-down to 34°C.   At 15 minutes (a), 30 minutes
(b), 1 hour (c), 2 hours (d), or 3 hours (e) following shift-down,
Act D (1 μg/ml) and ^{3}H-thymidine (10 μCi/ml) were added to the cultures
and incubation was continued at 34°C until 18 hours post infection,
when all cultures were harvested.   Centrifugation of gradients was
carried out as described in the legend to Figure 2.

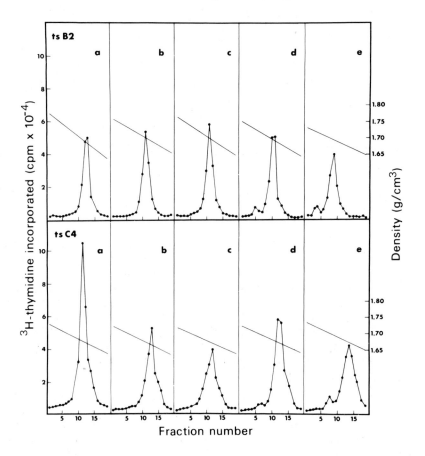

synthesis of new mRNA and protein species was required for at least
two hours following temperature shift-down in order to recover partial
DNA synthetic capability in *ts* B2- and *ts* C4-infected cells.

Since *de novo* transcription was not required for viral DNA synthesis following shift-down of *ts* D9-infected cells, experiments were performed to determine the time at which the transcripts encoding the D gene product were synthesized. For this purpose, *ts* D9-infected cultures were incubated at 39°C and shifted-down to 34°C at selected intervals. Act D and ^{3}H-thymidine were added at the time of shift-down as described above. Figure 5 shows that *ts* D9-infected cells shifted-down as early as two hours post infection in the presence of Act D synthesized viral DNA. The amount of viral DNA synthesized increased as the time of incubation at 39°C increased reaching maximum levels at six hours post infection. The pattern of viral DNA synthesis in wild-type virus-infected cells was similar to that in *ts* D9-infected cells except that less viral DNA was synthesized following shift-down at two hours. The reduced amounts of viral DNA synthesized when both wild-type and *ts* D9-infected cells were shifted-down at eight hours in the presence of Act D probably reflects the lateness in the replicative cycle and the reduced labelling period. These experiments demonstrate that functional mRNA species required for viral DNA synthesis are made at the non-permissive temperature in *ts* D9-infected cells and that these species are synthesized as early as two hours post infection. Thus, the block in viral DNA synthesis exhibited by *ts* D9 can be by-passed by shifting to the permissive temperature at this time in the absence of transcription.

In an effort to determine whether the *ts* D9 block occurs at the translational or post-translational level, *ts* D9-infected cells were: (*a*) incubated at 34°C from 0-18 hours; and (*b*) incubated at 39°C for nine hours and shifted-down to 34°C at this time. Cycloheximide (50 µg/ml; Calbiochem, La Jolla, Calif.) and ^{3}H-thymidine were added to both sets of cultures at nine hours. No detectable viral DNA was synthesized in either case demonstrating that cycloheximide treatment effectively inhibited at least one function essential for viral DNA synthesis even at the permissive temperature. Therefore, whether the *ts* block in viral DNA synthesis was translational or post-translational could not be ascertained in this manner.

Having demonstrated that *ts* B2 and *ts* C4 were blocked at the level of transcription but that *ts* D9 was not, the effect of each *ts* lesion on viral polypeptide synthesis following shift-down was examined. Figure 6 illustrates the polypeptide profiles of mutant and wild-type virus-infected cells maintained continuously at the permissive or non-permissive temperature and labelled with ^{35}S-methionine from 9 to 13 hours post infection (Fig. 6a) and of cells shifted-down from 39°C to 34°C at nine hours post infection in the presence of label with or without Act D (Fig. 6b). In general, polypeptide synthesis following temperature shift-down in the presence of Act D was qualitatively similar to that observed at the non-permissive temperature although the relative quantities of some polypeptides were altered.

FIG. 5. CAESIUM CHLORIDE EQUILIBRIUM SEDIMENTATION
OF VIRAL AND CELLULAR DNA IN *ts* D9-INFECTED CELLS

Cultures were incubated at 39°C and shifted-down to 34°C at 2 hours
(a), 4 hours (b), 6 hours (c), or 8 hours (d).   At the time of shift-
down, Act D (1 μg/ml) and ^{3}H-thymidine (10 μCi/ml) were added.
Cultures were then incubated at 34°C until 18 hours post infection and
harvested.   Centrifugation was carried out as described in the legend
to Figure 2.

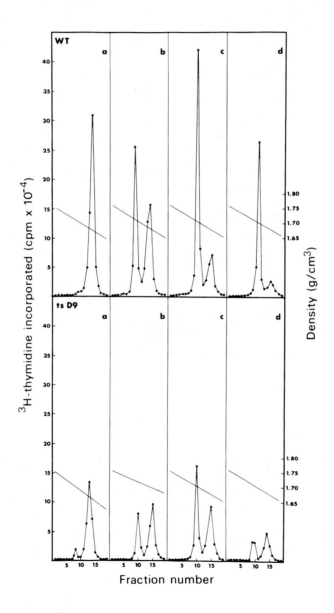

FIG. 6. POLYACRYLAMIDE (7%) SLAB GEL ELECTROPHORETOGRAMS
OF TOTAL CELLULAR EXTRACTS OF INFECTED CELLS

Cells were grown from 0 to 9 hours in methionine-free medium and labelled from 9 to 18 hours in medium containing ^{35}S-methionine (10 μCi/ml). Cells were maintained at 39°C or at 34°C throughout the course of the experiment (a) or were grown from 0 to 9 hours at 39°C and shifted-down at nine hours post infection in the presence or absence of 1 μg Act D/ml (b).

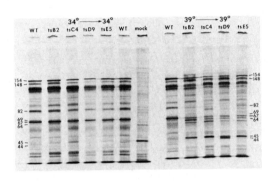

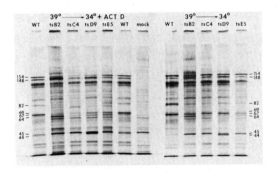

Compared with wild-type virus-infected cells, cells infected
with *ts* B2 synthesized moderately elevated levels of the non-
structural α polypeptide, VP175, at the non-permissive temperature
and following shift-down in the presence and absence of Act D.
Moderate increases in β polypeptides VP148 and VP64 were evident at
39°C and following shift-down in the presence but not in the absence
of Act D.   With regard to γ polypeptides, VP154, the major capsid
polypeptide, and VP82, VP69, and VP67 were under-produced relative
to wild-type virus-infected cells at 39°C.   The synthesis of VP154
and VP67 was further reduced in cells shifted down to 34°C in the
presence of Act D while only a slight reduction occurred in the
absence of inhibitor.   Other changes observed following shift-down in
the absence of inhibitor included slight under-production of VP82,
VP67, and VP44, and moderate over-production of VP64 and VP45.

No alterations in the synthesis of the α polypeptide VP175 or
in the β polypeptide VP148 were observed in *ts* C4-infected cells at
39°C or following shift-down in the presence or absence of inhibitor.
The levels of β polypeptides VP64 and VP47 were only slightly
elevated at 39°C and following shift-down in the presence of Act D,
while wild-type levels were observed following shift-down in the
absence of inhibitor.   VP45 was over-produced and VP44 was under-
produced at 39°C and following shift to 34°C in the presence and
absence of Act D.   Cells infected with *ts* C4 under-produced γ polypeptides VP154, VP82, VP69, VP67 at 39°C and following shift-down in
the presence of Act D.   The decrease in VP 154 following shift-down in
the presence of inhibitor was particularly marked.   In contrast,
wild-type levels of these polypeptides were produced following
shift-down in the absence of inhibitor.

The synthesis of α polypeptides in *ts* D9-infected cells was
similar to that observed in wild-type virus-infected cells.   The β
polypeptide VP148 was over-produced slightly at 39°C and following
shift-down in the presence of Act D, while it was synthesized in
wild-type amounts following shift-down in the absence of Act D.   In
addition, β polypeptide VP44 was greatly over-produced at 39°C as well
as following shift-down in the presence and absence of inhibitor.
The over-production of VP44 by *ts* D9, regardless of the conditions of
incubation, compared with its under-production by all other mutants
tested, was a distinct characteristic of this mutant.   Although the
γ polypeptide VP154 was under-produced by cells infected with *ts* D9
at 39°C and following temperature shift-down in the presence of Act D,
its level was greater than in *ts* B2 or *ts* C4 virus-infected cells.

The DNA$^+$ mutant *ts* E5 exhibited qualitative polypeptide defects
similar to those of *ts* C4.   However, γ polypeptides VP154 and VP82
were only slightly under-produced at 39°C and following shift-down
in the presence of Act D.

These studies show that the recovery of synthesis to normal levels of a variety of α, β and γ polypeptides, as well as of DNA synthesis, following temperature shift-down in the absence of transcription, although not completely reversible for any of the DNA⁻ mutants examined, was greatest for *ts* D9.   Those mutants blocked at the level of transcription, *ts* B2 and *ts* C4, not surprisingly showed minimal recovery of viral protein synthesis following shift-down.   Specifically, inhibition of transcription of the DNA⁻ mutants reduced the synthesis of many γ polypeptides while it allowed the accumulation of higher than normal levels of some β species.   This was not the case, however, for the α polypeptide VP175 whose synthesis was constant, if aberrant, in *ts* B2-infected cells.

DISCUSSION

The use of *ts* mutants of HSV-1 defective in the synthesis of viral DNA at the non-permissive temperature has facilitated the characterization of functions essential for viral DNA synthesis. These studies have suggested that the role of the B gene product is regulatory because it is required only transiently and because the B lesion blocks viral DNA synthesis at the level of transcription. In addition, the severe defects in polypeptide synthesis of this mutant relative to those of the other DNA⁻ mutants examined provides evidence that the *ts* B gene is expressed prior to the C and D genes.   Although the C gene product is required continuously, a property characteristic of structural genes directly involved in DNA synthesis, the block in viral DNA synthesis occurs at the level of transcription.   Further, the production of *ts* DP activity *in vivo* suggests that the C gene function involves the regulation of viral DP production, although the experiments described herein cannot establish whether the C gene is regulatory or structural in nature.

As previously reported (Courtney et al., 1976) and as further established in these studies, the defects in polypeptide synthesis produced by *ts* D9 were the least severe of all the DNA⁻ mutants tested.   It was shown recently in this laboratory that *ts* D9, alone among the DNA⁻ mutants, is resistant to phosphonoacetic acid (PAA). Spontaneous revertants of *ts* D9 were no longer *ts*, were sensitive to PAA, and induced viral DP activity which resembled that of the wild-type virus (Jofre et al., 1977).   Together with the present results showing that the *ts* D gene blocks replication at the post-transcriptional level, these results strongly indicate that the D gene encodes viral DP or a modifier of viral DP.

SUMMARY

     The regulation of expression of viral genes involved in the
synthesis of herpes simplex virus type 1 DNA was studied using
three DNA⁻ temperature-sensitive (*ts*) mutants (B, C, and D).   These
mutants were examined for their ability to synthesize viral DNA and
polypeptides following temperature shift-down in the presence or
absence of the transcription inhibitor actinomycin D.   The results
demonstrated that the B gene product is required transiently early
in infection and apparently controls a transcriptional step required
for HSV DNA synthesis.   The C gene product is required continuously
during infection and also controls a transcriptional step needed for
viral DNA synthesis.   In contrast, the product of the D gene does
not directly control a transcriptional step, is required continuously,
appears to be directly involved in HSV DNA synthesis, and is probably
the gene for viral DNA polymerase.   The results further showed that
recovery of viral DNA and polypeptide synthesis following temperature
shift-down in the absence of inhibitor was greater for the D mutant
than for the mutants blocked in viral DNA synthesis at the level of
transcription.

ACKNOWLEDGEMENTS

     This research was supported by Contract No. NO1 CP 53,526
   within the Virus Cancer Program of the National Cancer
  Institute and Research Grants Nos CA 05,465, CA 20,260,
       and CA 10,893 from the National Cancer Institute.
       The authors wish to acknowledge the excellent
           technical assistance of Ms Joyce Burek.

REFERENCES

Aron, G.M., Purifoy, D.J.M. & Schaffer, P.A. (1975)   DNA synthesis
and DNA polymerase activity of herpes simplex virus type 1
temperature-sensitive mutants.   *J. Virol.*, *16*, 498-507

Bone, D.R. & Courtney, R.J. (1974)   A temperature-sensitive mutant
of herpes simplex virus type 1 defective in the synthesis of the
major capsid polypeptide.   *J. gen. Virol.*, *24*, 17-27

Courtney, R.J., Schaffer, P.A. & Powell, K.L. (1976)   Synthesis of
virus-specific polypeptides by temperature-sensitive mutants of
herpes simplex virus type 1.   *Virology*, *75*, 306-318

Honess, R.W. & Roizman, B. (1974)   Regulation of herpesvirus macromolecular synthesis.   I. Cascade regulation of the synthesis of
three groups of viral proteins.   *J. Virol.*, *14*, 8-19

Jofre, J.T., Schaffer, P.A. & Parris, D.S. (1977)   Genetics of
resistance to phosphonoacetic acid in strain KOS of herpes simplex
virus type 1.   *J. Virol.*, *23*, 833-836

Schaffer, P.A. (1975)   Temperature-sensitive mutants of herpesviruses.   *Curr. Top. Microbiol. Immunol.*, *70*, 51-100

Schaffer, P.A., Tevethia, M.J. & Benyesh-Melnick, M. (1974)
Recombination between temperature-sensitive mutants of herpes
simplex virus type 1.   *Virology*, *58*, 219-228

Schaffer, P.A., Bone, D.R. & Courtney, R.J. (1976)   DNA-negative
temperature-sensitive mutants of herpes simplex virus type 1:
Patterns of viral DNA synthesis after temperature shift-up.
J. Virol., *17*, 1043-1048

VIRUS TRANSCRIPT MAPPING STUDIES IN CELLS INFECTED WITH TEMPERATURE-SENSITIVE MUTANTS OF HERPES SIMPLES VIRUS TYPE 1

R.J. WATSON & J.B. CLEMENTS

Institute of Virology,
University of Glasgow,
Glasgow, UK

The temporal regulation of herpes simplex virus type 1 (HSV-1) transcription has been studied previously by hybridization, in liquid phase, of radiolabelled viral DNA probes to excess unlabelled RNA from infected cells (Frenkel & Roizman, 1972; Swanstrom & Wagner, 1974). These studies have indicated that much of the viral genome is expressed both before (early) and after (late) the onset of viral DNA replication. By contrast, cytoplasmic RNA isolated from cells infected and maintained in the presence of the protein synthesis inhibitor cycloheximide was complementary to only 10% of the viral DNA (Kozak & Roizman, 1974). These authors reported that RNA accumulating in the nucleus during a cycloheximide block was homologous to 50% of the viral DNA.

Estimates of the proportion of viral DNA represented as stable RNA transcripts provide no information concerning the genome location of the homologous DNA. Hybridization of radiolabelled RNA to HSV-1 DNA fragments, generated by restriction endonucleases and immobilized on to nitrocellulose membranes by the method of Southern (1975), has allowed this information to be obtained for transcripts isolated from cells productively infected with HSV-1, at early and late times post infection, and from cells infected and maintained in the presence of DNA- or protein-synthesis inhibitors (Clements et al., 1977).

The patterns of hybridization obtained for late and early RNA were found to be quantitatively dissimilar, although both early and late nuclear and cytoplasmic RNAs hybridized to every fragment of DNA generated by the enzyme digests used for analysis. RNA labelled in the continuous presence of the DNA-synthesis inhibitor cytosine arabinoside was found to give a similar hybridization pattern to early, but not late, RNA (Clements et al., 1977). In contrast, RNA labelled

in the continuous presence of cycloheximide, termed immediate early
RNA, was found to hybridize only to certain DNA fragments (Clements
et al., 1977), notably to those fragments containing the repeats
flanking the short unique (U$_S$) region, part of the repeats flanking
the long unique (U$_L$) region and to certain fragments which map in both
unique regions. Few viral RNA sequences could be detected in the
nucleus which were not present in the cytoplasm.

The use of temperature-sensitive (*ts*)mutants of HSV-1 at the non-
permissive temperature (*T*np) has allowed a greater definition of virus
genes controlling the synthesis of viral polypeptides (Marsden et al.,
1976) and the expression of viral functions (Schaffer et al., 1973;
Subak-Sharpe et al., 1974).   The purpose of this study is to report
on the use of the blot hybridization technique to examine transcripts
synthesized in BHK C13 cells infected at *T*np with several DNA-negative
ts mutants of HSV-1.

The six *ts* mutants of HSV-1 strain 17 examined here (*ts* K, *ts* D,
ts T, *ts* B, *ts* E and *ts* S) fall into four complementation groups
(Brown et al., 1973; Crombie, 1975) as *ts* D and *ts* T and also *ts* B
and *ts* E do not complement.   A spontaneous revertant of *ts* D, *ts* DR/4
(Taylor, 1976) has also been examined.   Unless stated to the contrary,
in these experiments virus was adsorbed and the RNA labelled at *T*np
(38.5°C).

Cells grown in 90-mm petri dishes were infected at multiplicities of
50-200 plaque-forming units per cell.   After one hour unadsorbed virus
was removed by washing, then low-phosphate medium containing 1 mCi/ml
$^{32}PO_4$ was added and the cells were labelled for a further seven hours.
After labelling, cells were fractionated into nucleus and cytoplasm
and RNA was extracted as described previously (Clements et al., 1977).
Labelled RNA was incubated with blot strips containing the denatured,
unlabelled fragments of HSV-1 DNA, generated by single and double
digests with the *Hin*dIII, *Bgl*II and *Hpa*I restriction endonucleases
and hybridization was visualized by autoradiography.   Physical maps
for the DNA fragments generated by the enzyme digests used were those
obtained by Wilkie (1976) and Wilkie et al. (1977).

Figures 1 and 2 show RNA from cells infected at *T*np with *ts* K,
ts T, *ts* D and *ts* DR/4 hybridized to the DNA fragments generated by
*Hpa*I and *Hin*dIII digestion, respectively.   Also shown is immediate
early (IE) RNA, labelled in cells infected with wild-type HSV-1 in the
continuous presence of 200 μg/ml cycloheximide.   Since cycloheximide
inhibits viral protein synthesis it is probable that IE RNA is transcribed by an unmodified, preexisting host-cell RNA polymerase.

IE RNA and RNA from *ts* K, *ts* D and *ts* T-infected cells contains an
abundance of material which hybridizes to *Hpa*I *a*, *cde*, *gh*, *m* and *s*.
In addition there is readily detectable hybridization to *Hpa*I *f* and *l*.
*Hpa*I *a*, *cde*, *gh* and *m* each contain either one or both of the inverted
repeats while *Hpa*I *s*, *f* and *l* map within the U$_L$ region (Fig. 3).

FIG. 1. AUTORADIOGRAPHS OF *Hpa*I BLOTS

Cytoplasmic (C) and nuclear (N) RNA from cells infected with wild-type HSV-1 in the presence of cycloheximide (immediate early; IE) and with mutants *ts* T, *ts* K, *ts* D and the revertant *ts* DR/4 at *T*np, were hybridized to unlabelled fragments of DNA generated by restriction endonuclease *Hpa*I.

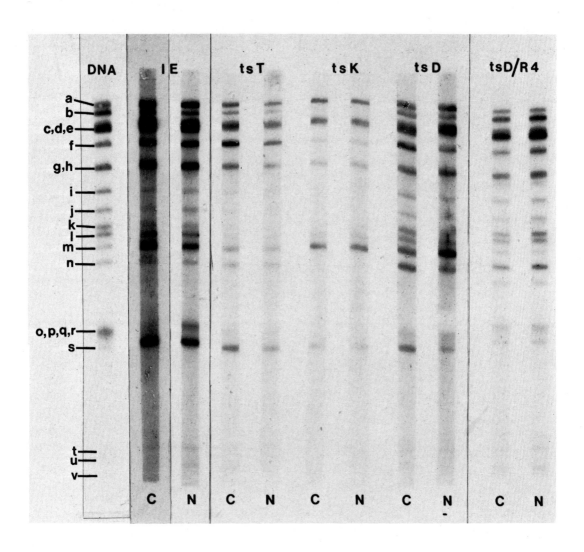

FIG. 2. AUTORADIOGRAPHS OF *Hind*III BLOTS

Cytoplasmic RNA from cells infected with various *ts* mutants of HSV-1, and with the wild type in the continuous presence of cycloheximide (IE), cytosine arabinoside (ara-C) and after virus DNA replication (late) were hybridized to *Hind*III blot strips.

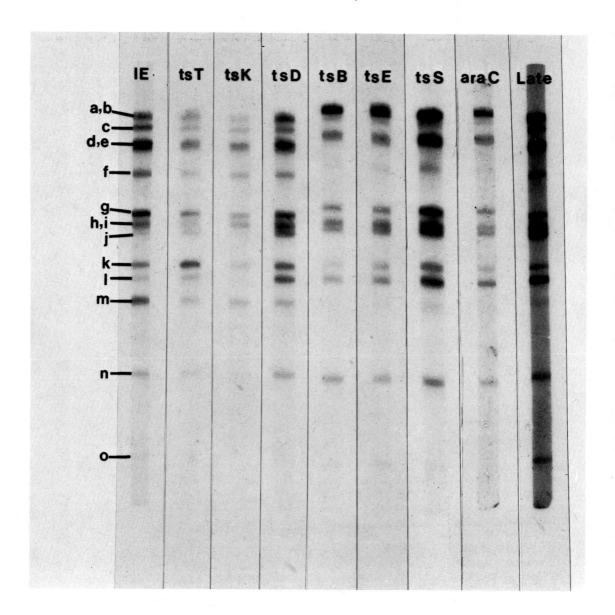

The *Hin*dIII digest (Fig. 2) shows essentially the same result, with an abundance of RNA which hybridizes to *Hin*dIII *m*, a fragment which contains the short repeat (Fig. 3).

FIG. 3. PHYSICAL MAPS FOR HSV-1 DNA FRAGMENTS

Physical maps for the DNA fragments generated by *Hin*dIII, *Bgl*II and *Hpa*I digestion are represented for one genome arrangement. Fragments which span the joint region are not shown, but are represented as "fusion fragments" of the terminal fragments generated by inversion of the unique DNA regions (e.g., *Hin*dIII fragment c = d + m).

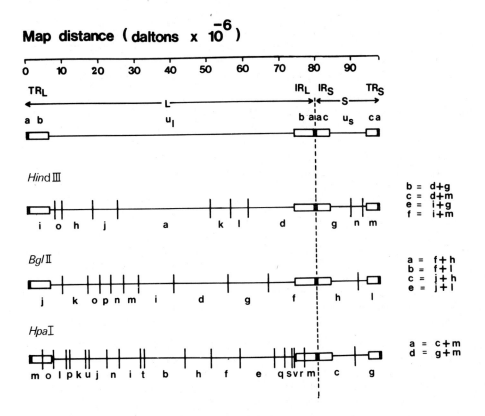

IE RNA, *ts* D and *ts* T RNA, but not *ts* K RNA, all show additional hybridization to *Hpa*I *n* and *b* and (at low levels) to the remaining *Hpa*I fragments. Quantitatively, there is relatively greater hybridization of RNA from *ts* D-infected cells to *Hpa*I *b*, *i*, *j* and *k* and *Hin*dIII *hi* and *j* compared with RNA from *ts* T-infected cells or IE RNA. As *ts* D and *ts* T are in the same complementation group (Crombie, 1975)

the reason for this quantitative difference is unclear, but may indicate limited functionality (since neither mutant is "leaky") of the
defective polypeptide synthesized by one or both of these mutants.

In contrast to these restricted patterns, RNA from cells infected
with the spontaneous revertant of ts D (ts DR/4), shows a pattern which
resembles that of the wild type (Fig. 4).   There is little hybridization to HpaI m and relatively less to HpaI a.   It has been shown that
the polypeptides specified by this revertant at Tnp are qualitatively
identical and quantitatively almost identical to those specified by
the wild type (Taylor, 1976).

Transcripts labelled at Tnp in cells infected with ts B, ts E and
ts S were hybridized to the HpaI (Fig. 4) and HindIII (Fig. 2) fragments.   For comparison, the hybridization patterns of RNA labelled in
cells infected with wild-type HSV-1 early (0-1 hour post infection),
late (0-7 hours post infection) and for 0-7 hours in the continuous
presence of 50 µg/ml cytosine arabinoside (ara-C) are shown.

RNA labelled under these various conditions hybridizes to all
the DNA fragments generated by HpaI, BglII and HindIII digests.   As
the differences observed here are quantitative rather than qualitative,
autoradiographs were scanned using a microdensitometer to estimate the
relative hybridization to each DNA fragment.   The microdensitometer
traces for cytoplasmic RNA labelled in ts B, ts E and ts S-infected
cells and in cells infected with the wild type in the presence of
cytosine arabinoside are shown for HpaI (Fig. 5) and HindIII (Fig. 6).

RNA from cells infected in the presence of cytosine arabinoside and
also from ts B, ts E and ts S-infected cells contains a low concentration of sequences complementary to HpaI m, a fragment to which an
abundance of IE RNA hybridizes.   The hybridization patterns obtained
with ts B and ts E, which do not complement, are almost identical, but
differ in some respect to those obtained with ts S or cytosine arabinoside, for example, in the relative hybridization to HpaI b (Fig. 5) and
HindIII l (Fig. 6).

Our RNA mapping data, obtained using the enzyme digests described
here, and also with BglII and HpaI/HindIII in double digest, are summarized in Figure 7.   It can be seen that certain regions of HSV-1
DNA are represented in IE RNA which are not expressed in ts K-infected
cells.   This is probably due to breakthrough of protein synthesis,
even at the high concentrations of cycloheximide used (200 µg/ml),
since IE RNA labelled in subsequent experiments has shown a similar
hybridization pattern to that of ts K RNA (Watson & Clements[1]).   It
is of interest that virus proteins synthesized in ts K-infected cells
at Tnp are predominantly, though perhaps not entirely, α-polypeptides

---

[1] Unpublished data

FIG. 4. AUTORADIOGRAPHS OF *Hpa*I BLOTS

Cytoplasmic (C) and nuclear (N) RNA from cells infected with *ts* B, *ts* S and *ts* E and from cells infected with the wild-type HSV-1 before virus DNA replication (early), after virus DNA replication (late) and in the continuous presence of cytosine arabinoside (ara-C) were hybridized to *Hpa*I blot strips.

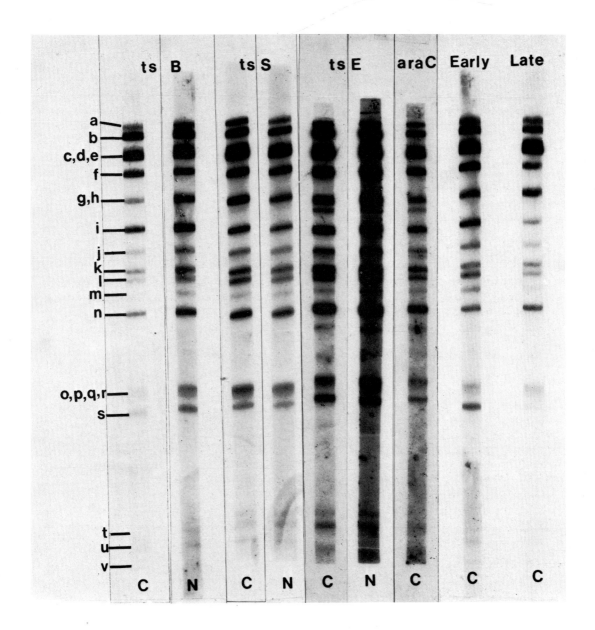

FIG. 5. MICRODENSITOMETER TRACES OF *Hpa*I AUTORADIOGRAPHS

Microdensitometer traces of autoradiographs of cytoplasmic RNA from cells infected with *ts* B, *ts* E and *ts* S, and with wild-type HSV-1 in the presence of ara-C, hybridized to *Hpa*I blot strips.

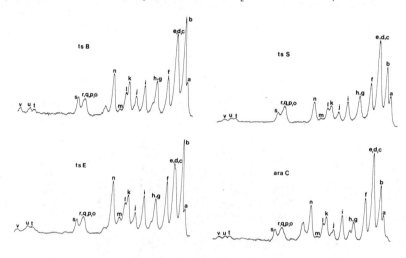

FIG. 6. MICRODENSITOMETER TRACES OF *Hin*dIII AUTORADIOGRAPHS

Autoradiographs of cytoplasmic RNA from cells infected with *ts* B, *ts* E, *ts* S and with wild-type HSV-1 in the presence of ara-C, hybridized to *Hin*dIII blot strips were scanned with a microdensitometer

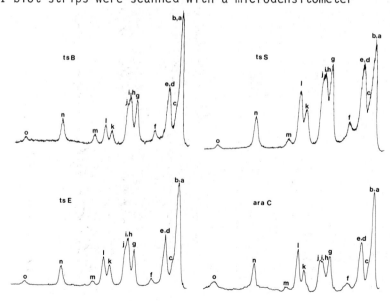

FIG. 7.   SUMMARY OF TRANSCRIPT MAPPING DATA

Mapping data for cytoplasmic immediate early RNA and RNA from cells infected with *ts* K, *ts* T, *ts* D and *ts* B are summarized, using the following criteria: (*a*) undetectable hybridization to a fragment is not indicated; (*b*) low levels of hybridization are indicated by a broken line; (*c*) clearly detectable hybridization to a region is represented by a single line; (*d*) fragments to which an abundance of material hybridized are indicated by a double continuous line.

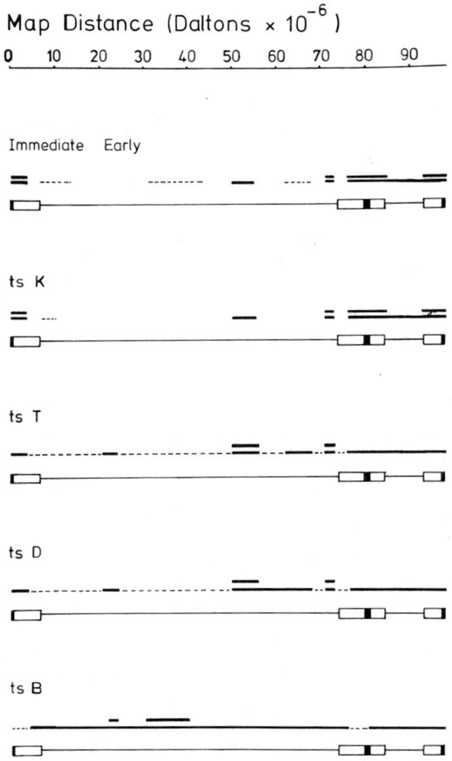

(Marsden[1]), i.e., proteins which are translated on release of a cyclo-heximide block in the presence of actinomycin D (Honess & Roizman, 1974).   α-Polypeptides also accumulate in *ts* D and *ts* T-infected cells (Marsden et al., 1976).

---

[1] Personal communication

RNA from *ts* K and *ts* T (and *ts* D)-infected cells hybridizes predominantly to those regions expressed immediately early. This indicates that at least two viral products are required for the switch-on of regions transcribed early in the replicative cycle. The region which maps between 51 and 56 (Fig. 7) is transcribed at greater relative abundance in *ts* T (and *ts* D)-infected cells than in *ts* K-infected cells. This may represent a region which is expressed very early in the replicative cycle. It is of interest that the polypeptide Vmw 136, an early polypeptide which is synthesized in *ts* K, *ts* D and *ts* T-infected cells at *T*np, and sometimes on release of a cycloheximide block in the presence of actinomycin D (Marsden[1]), has tentatively been mapped in this area by an examination of polypeptides expressed by intertypic recombinants between HSV-1 and HSV-2 (Preston et al.[2]). This technique has also been used to map the polypeptide Vmw 175 (an α-polypeptide) in the S region (Preston et al.[2]), a region which is represented by IE transcripts.

The evidence presented above suggest that *ts* K is blocked at the immediate early stage of the replicative cycle. It was therefore of interest to determine whether the polypeptides which accumulate in *ts* K-infected cells at *T*np are sufficient, on down-shift to the permissive temperature, to allow expression of additional regions of the genome.

Cells infected with *ts* K were incubated at *T*np for three hours and then either maintained at *T*np or shifted-down to the permissive temperature (31°C) in the presence or absence of 200 µg/ml cyclo-heximide. The infected cells were then incubated with $^{32}PO_4$ for five hours and the RNA labelled under these various treatments was extracted and hybridized to blot strips containing the *Hpa*I fragments.

The results (Fig. 8) indicate that the defective polypeptide regains activity on down-shift and allows the transcription of additional DNA sequences which map throughout the genome. It is not clear whether all these additional transcripts are functional: they have, however, been found to direct the synthesis of virus-specific thymidine-kinase activity in a cell-free translation system (Preston[2]).

In summary, the experiments presented here suggest that at least two viral products, namely those temperature-sensitive in *ts* K and *ts* T (and *ts* D)-infected cells, are required for the progression from immediate early transcription to a more advanced transcriptional pattern. The temperature-sensitive *ts* K product appears to be an absolute requirement for this progression. In *ts* T (or *ts* D)-infected cells, however, additional regions of the genome are expressed at *T*np, albeit at low abundance. This suggests that either the defective

---

[1] Personal communication

[2] Unpublished data

ts T product may retain some limited function under non-permissive
conditions or, alternatively, this additional transcription is mediated
by the regulatory protein defective in *ts* K-infected cells at *T*np.

FIG. 8. *Ts* K DOWN-SHIFT

Cells infected with *ts* K at *T*np (38.5°C) were shifted down to the
permissive temperature (31°C) either in the presence (+CH) or absence
(-CH) of cycloheximide.   The hybridization patterns of RNA labelled
after down-shift were compared to that of RNA labelled at *T*np by
hybridization of cytoplasmic (C) or nuclear (N) RNA to *Hpa*I blot strips.

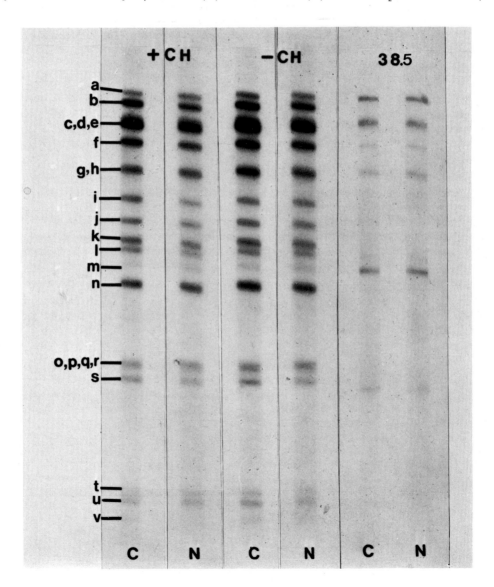

None of the DNA-negative mutants of HSV-1 so far examined show a late pattern of transcription. This is consistent with the view that viral DNA replication is required for late gene expression.

SUMMARY

Nuclear and cytoplasmic transcripts, synthesized in cells infected with six DNA-negative temperature-sensitive (*ts*) mutants of HSV-1 (*ts* B, *ts* D, *ts* E, *ts* K, *ts* S and *ts* T) under non-permissive conditions, were isolated and hybridized to unlabelled fragments of HSV-1 DNA, generated by restriction endonuclease digestion and immobilized on to nitrocellulose membranes by the method of Southern (1975).

In this way it has been possible to map those regions of the HSV-1 genome represented by stable transcripts in cells infected with these mutants and compare them with those regions transcribed in cells infected with the wild-type virus at early and late times post infection (before and after viral DNA replication) and in the presence of DNA- and protein-synthesis inhibitors.

Viral transcription in *ts* D, *ts* T and *ts* K-infected cells is restricted, the patterns of hybridization being similar, but not identical to that observed with immediate early RNA. Since these three mutants fall into two complementation groups, these experiments suggest that at least two viral products are required for the switch-on of early transcripts.

In contrast, transcript mapping with the other early mutants (*ts* B, *ts* E and *ts* S) has shown a much less restricted transcriptional pattern, the pattern obtained resembling that with early, rather than late RNA.

ACKNOWLEDGEMENTS

We wish to thank Professor J.H. Subak-Sharpe for his continued interest in this work and Dr N.M. Wilkie for providing us with physical maps for the DNA fragments. R.J. Watson is the recipient of a Medical Research Council grant for training in research techniques.

REFERENCES

Brown, S.M., Ritchie, D.A. & Subak-Sharpe, J.H. (1973)   Genetic studies with herpes simplex virus type 1.   The isolation of temperature-sensitive mutants, their arrangement into complementation groups and recombination analysis leading to a linkage map. *J. gen. Virol.*, *18*, 329-346

Clements, J.B., Watson, R.J. & Wilkie, N.M. (1977)   Temporal regulation of herpes simplex virus type 1 transcription: location of transcripts on the viral genome.   *Cell*, *12*, 275-285

Crombie, I.K. (1975)   *Genetic and biochemical studies with herpes simplex virus type 1.*   Thesis, Glasgow

Frenkel, N. & Roizman, B. (1972)   Ribonucleic acid synthesis in cells infected with herpes simplex virus: controls of transcription and of RNA abundance.   *Proc. nat. Acad. Sci. (Wash.)*, *69*, 2654-2658

Honess, R.W. & Roizman, B. (1974)   Regulation of herpesvirus macromolecular synthesis.   I. Cascade regulation of the synthesis of three groups of viral proteins.   *J. Virol.*, *14*, 8-19

Kozak, M. & Roizman, B. (1974)   Regulation of herpesvirus macromolecular synthesis: nuclear retention of non-translated viral RNA sequences.   *Proc. nat. Acad. Sci. (Wash.)*, *71*, 4322-4326

Marsden, H.S., Crombie, I.K. & Subak-Sharpe, J.H. (1976)   Control of protein synthesis in herpesvirus-infected cells: analysis of the polypeptides induced by wild-type and sixteen temperature-sensitive mutants of HSV-1 strain 17.   *J. gen. Virol.*, *31*, 347-372

Schaffer, P.A., Aron, G.M., Biswal, N. & Benyesh-Melnick, M. (1973)   Temperature-sensitive mutants of herpes simplex virus type 1: isolation, complementation and partial characterisation. *Virology*, *52*, 57-71

Southern, E.M. (1975)   Detection of specific sequences among DNA fragments separated by gel electrophoresis.   *J. molec. Biol.*, *98*, 503-533

Subak-Sharpe, J.H., Brown, S.M., Ritchie, D.A., Timbury, M.C., Macnab, J.C.M., Marsden, H.S. & Hay, J. (1974)   Genetic and biochemical studies with herpesvirus.   *Cold Spring Harb. Symp. quant. Biol.*, *39*, 717-730

Swanstrom, R.I. & Wagner, E.K. (1974)   Regulation of synthesis of
    herpes simplex type 1 virus mRNA during productive infection.
    Virology, 60, 522-533

Taylor, A.F. (1976)   *Quantitative genetic studies with herpes
    simplex virus type 1.* Thesis, Glasgow

Wilkie, N.M. (1976)   Physical maps for HSV-1 DNA for restriction
    endonucleases Hind III, Hpa I and Xba.   *J. Virol., 20,* 222-233

Wilkie, N.M., Cortini, R. & Clements, J.B. (1977)   Structural studies
    and physical maps for the herpes simplex virus genome. *J. Anti-
    microb. Chemother., 3,* Suppl. A, pp. 47-62

THE REGULATIONS OF γ (STRUCTURAL) POLYPEPTIDE SYNTHESIS IN HERPES SIMPLEX VIRUS TYPES 1 AND 2 INFECTED CELLS

H. WOLF & B. ROIZMAN

Marjorie B. Kovler Viral Oncology Laboratories,
University of Chicago,
Chicago, Ill., USA

It has been reported by this (Fenwick & Roizman, 1977; Honess & Roizman, 1973, 1974, 1975) and other laboratories (Marsden et al., 1976; Powell & Courtney, 1975; Powell et al., 1975) that the synthesis of the polypeptides specified by herpes simplex virus types 1 and 2 (human herpesvirus types 1 and 2, HSV-1 and HSV-2) is tightly regulated. Specifically, the data show that the polypeptides form at least three groups designated as α, β and γ whose synthesis is co-ordinately regulated and sequentially ordered in a cascade fashion (Honess & Roizman, 1974). Although several α polypeptides have been identified, their function is unknown. The β polypeptides include several enzymes involved in viral DNA metabolism. The γ polypeptides comprise largely structural (virion) polypeptides (Honess & Roizman, 1973, 1974; Roizman et al., 1975). Previous studies have also shown that the sequential transition from α to β polypeptide synthesis required transcription of viral DNA in the presence of functional α polypeptides and was independent of viral DNA synthesis. The transition from β polypeptide synthesis was also found to be independent of viral DNA synthesis although in the presence of inhibitors there was a reduction in the amounts of γ polypeptides made (Honess & Roizman, 1974; Honess & Watson, 1977; Powell et al., 1975). The objectives of the studies described in this report were to identify the factors regulating the synthesis of γ polypeptides, and we are reporting the results of two series of experiments.

The first series of experiments was designed to study the synthesis of viral proteins under conditions in which the synthesis of viral progeny DNA was inhibited. In this series, the cells were infected at different multiplicities and incubated in the presence of phosphonoacetate (100 µg/ml) or hydroxyurea (4 mg/ml). One set of replicate

cultures was exposed to the drugs continuously and the synthesis of
viral polypeptides measured at intervals after infection (Fig. 1).

FIG. 1.   AUTORADIOGRAMS OF ELECTROPHORETICALLY SEPARATED
POLYPEPTIDES MADE IN HEp-2 CELLS INFECTED WITH 1 PFU
OF HSV-1 (STRAIN F) PER CELL

The cultures were labelled with L(U-^{14}C)-leucine, L(U-^{14}C)-isoleucine
and L(U-^{14}C)-valine (2 μCi/ml, 300 mCi/mmol, from New England Nuclear,
Cambridge, Mass., USA) 13.5-14 hours post infection and harvested
immediately after labelling.   The procedures for labelling, collection
and solubilization of infected cells as well as for the electrophoresis
of the solubilized polypeptides, autoradiography and quantitation of
the polypeptides were the same as described previously (Honess &
Roizman, 1973, 1974, 1975).   (A) Infected, untreated cells; (B) the
cells were infected and maintained in the presence of 100 μg of phosphonoacetate per ml of medium; (C) the cells were infected and maintained in the presence of phosphonoacetate until five hours post
infection.   At that time, the drug was withdrawn.   The enumeration
of infected-cell polypeptides is as described by Morse et al.
(see p. 41).

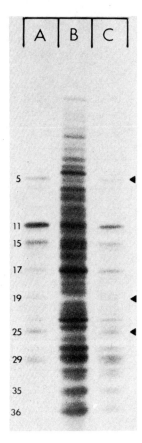

In another set, the drug was withdrawn at five hours post infection
and again the synthesis of viral polypeptides was measured as described in the legend to Figure 1.   The results of these experiments
were as follows: (i) In HSV-1 infected cells, at low multiplicities
of infection (1 PFU per cell, Fig. 1) some γ proteins (e.g., 5, 19,
25) were not made or were made in highly reduced amounts. At high
multiplicities of infection (25 PFU per cell, not shown; 500 PFU per
cell, Fig. 2) these polypeptides were made and formed a significant
fraction of the viral polypeptides made in the presence of inhibitors
of DNA synthesis.   (ii) In HSV-2 infected cells, the results were
essentially the same except that polypeptides Nos 11 and 12 were
barely detected at all multiplicities tested (1 and 25 PFU per cell not
shown, 500 PFU per cell, as shown in Figure 3) in the presence of
inhibitors of DNA synthesis.

FIG. 2.   AUTORADIOGRAMS OF ELECTROPHORETICALLY SEPARATED
POLYPEPTIDES MADE IN HEp-2 CELLS INFECTED WITH 500 PFU OF
HSV-1(F) PER CELL AND PULSE-LABELLED WITH ^{14}C-AMINO-ACIDS
AT TIME INTERVALS (IN HOURS) POST INFECTION SHOWN

The cells were harvested immediately after the 30-minute labelling
interval.   PAA: phosphonoacetate; "0" hours was defined as the
time of exposure of cells to virus.

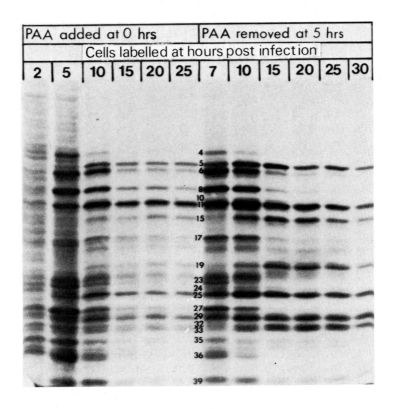

FIG. 3.   AUTORADIOGRAMS OF ELECTROPHORETICALLY SEPARATED
POLYPEPTIDES MADE IN HEp-2 CELLS INFECTED WITH 500 PFU OF
HSV-2(G) PER CELL

The experimental procedures were the same as those described in the
legends to Figures 1 and 2 except that hydroxyurea (HU) (4 mg/ml)
was used in place of phosphonoacetate.

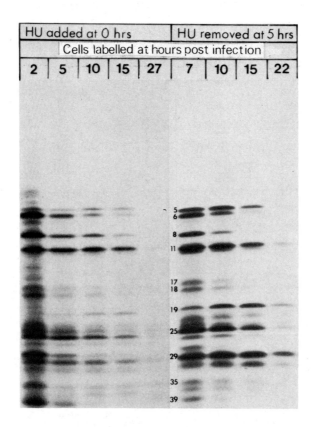

In the second series of experiments, we studied the functional
half-life of viral mRNA.   In this series the cells were exposed to
actinomycin D (4 µg/ml) several hours after infection and the rates
of synthesis of viral polypeptides were measured at intervals thereafter as described below and in the legend to Figure 4.   The choice
of the drug was predicated on the observation that it affects the
transcription of DNA (Egyhazi, 1974).   Figure 4 shows some of the
autoradiograms of electrophoretically separated polypeptides extracted
17 hours after infection, i.e., five hours after the inhibitors were
added.   At that, rather late, time after infection, the rate of
synthesis of most proteins was declining and the drug hastened the

FIG. 4. AUTORADIOGRAMS, AND SCANS OF THE AUTORADIOGRAPHIC IMAGES, OF ELECTROPHORETICALLY SEPARATED POLYPEPTIDES MADE IN HEp-2 CELLS INFECTED WITH 50 PFU OF HSV-1(F) PER CELL

(A) Untreated infected cells; (B) Cells treated with actinomycin D (4 μg/ml) from 12 hours post infection; (C) Cells treated with cordycepin (50 μg/ml) from 12 hours post infection. The cultures were pulse-labelled at 16.5 hours post infection for 15 minutes with ^{14}C-amino-acids, then harvested. The figure shows the autoradiographic images and the corresponding densitometric scans.

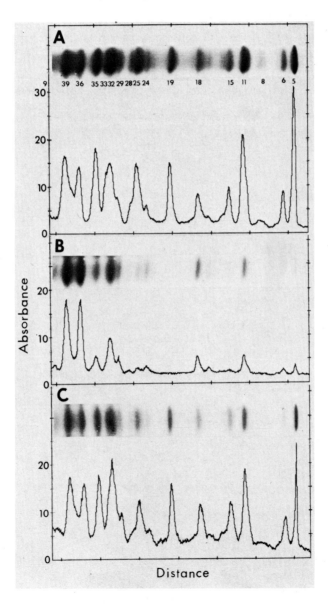

overall decline in viral protein synthesis.   In order to measure the
relative rates of synthesis of the various proteins, the autoradiograms were scanned with a laser densitometer linked to a computer and
the relative rates of synthesis were computed as described by Honess
& Roizman (1973, 1974, 1975).   The data (Fig. 5) show that the polypeptides form at least two classes differing in the rates at which their
synthesis decays in the presence of actinomycin D.   Panel A is representative for polypeptides Nos 5, 11, 15 and 19;   panel B represents
polypeptides Nos 32, 35, 29, 18, 8 and 6 and panel C is representative
for Nos 23, 36 and 35.

FIG. 5.   RELATIVE RATES OF SYNTHESIS OF VIRAL POLYPEPTIDES
MADE IN HEp-2 CELLS INFECTED WITH 50 PFU OF HSV-1 PER CELL
AND EXPOSED TO ACTINOMYCIN D AT 12 HOURS POST INFECTION

The experimental design was the same as that described in the legend
to Figure 4.   The relative rates of synthesis were calculated from
computer-aided planimetry of the densitometric measurements as described by Honess & Roizman (1973, 1975).   (A) Polypeptides Nos 5, 11,
15 and 19;   (B) Polypeptides Nos 32, 35, 29, 18, 8 and 6;   (C) Polypeptides Nos 23, 36 and 35.

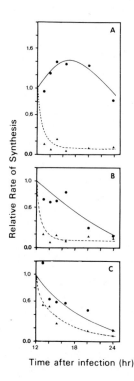

The significance of the data stems from two observations. First, the synthesis of polypeptides represented in panel C decays only slightly more rapidly in the presence of the drug than in its absence. The synthesis of polypeptides represented in panel A decays very rapidly in the presence of actinomycin D, i.e., considerably faster in the presence of the drug than in its absence. The observation that, between 12 and 18 hours after infection, the rate of synthesis of polypeptides represented in panel A actually increases suggests a continued flow of mRNA from the nucleus into the cytoplasm. In the light of this conclusion, the rapid decline in the synthesis of these polypeptides in the presence of the drug suggests a relatively short half-life.

The relationship between the two series of experiments is illustrated in Figure 6. The data presented in this figure show that those proteins whose messenger RNAs have a relatively short functional half-life are also the ones which are not synthesized at low multiplicities of infection when progeny DNA synthesis is blocked. Furthermore, the figure shows that the effect of cordycepin, which affects processing of transcripts (Darnell et al., 1971), differs from that of actinomycin D. These observations will be discussed elsewhere (Wolf[1]).

From the data presented in this report, we conclude the following:

(1) The transition from α to β to γ polypeptide synthesis is in most cases independent of viral DNA synthesis.

(2) Because many γ messenger RNAs have a short functional half-life, γ polypeptide synthesis is especially dependent on replenishment of polyribosomal RNA with fresh messenger RNA.

(3) The rates of γ polypeptide synthesis reflect the amount of viral DNA templates available for transcription. The functional half-life of α and β messenger RNA is considerably longer (Fenwick & Roizman, 1977) and the synthesis of these proteins is therefore less dependent on amplification of viral DNA templates available for transcription.

The conclusions presented in this paper are significant from two points of view. First, they may well account for the observation that, in cells infected with some human herpesviruses, the inhibition of DNA synthesis results in the disappearance of viral structural components. This is especially noteworthy in the case of cells infected with cytomegalovirus or with Epstein-Barr virus because the viral DNA pool available for transcription is generally low and therefore the production of mRNA specifying structural polypeptides would also be low. Second, they suggest a very simple and effective pattern for regulation of viral assembly in infected cells. Thus, at the outset of synthesis of viral DNA, the amount of functional γ mRNA would be expected to be low, the synthesis of structural proteins would be relatively low, and in consequence, there would be little assembly.

---

[1] Unpublished data

FIG. 6.   AUTORADIOGRAMS OF ELECTROPHORETICALLY SEPARATED
POLYPEPTIDES MADE IN HEp-2 CELLS INFECTED WITH HSV-1(F)

From left to right: Slot 1: untreated infected cells; slot 2: infected
cells were exposed to actinomycin·D (act D) (4 μg/ml) 5 hours post
infection; slot 3: infected cells were exposed to cordycepin (cord)
(50 μg/ml) at 5 hours post infection; slot 4: untreated infected
cells; slot 5: cells infected and maintained in the presence of
phosphonoacetate (PAA) (100 μg/ml).

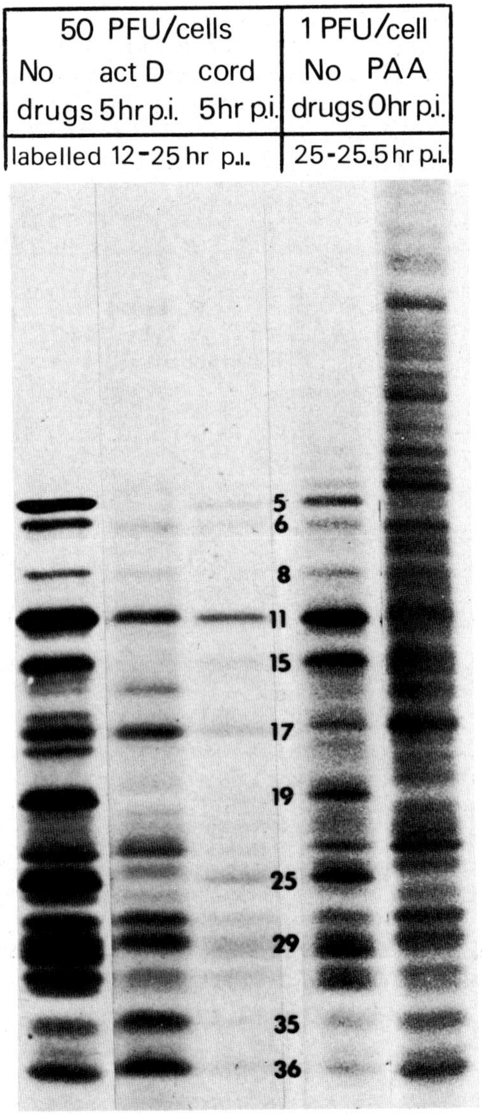

As the pool of DNA increases, the rate of synthesis of γ polypeptides would increase and in consequence, the rate of assembly would also go up. This apparent regulatory mechanism would preclude premature assembly when the size of the viral DNA pool is low and would ensure a high rate of assembly when the viral DNA pool attained the appropriate size.

SUMMARY

The polypeptides specified by herpes simplex viruses types 1 and 2 form at least three groups designated as α, β and γ. The structural polypeptides are largely contained in the γ polypeptide group. In this study, we investigated the transition from β to γ polypeptide synthesis. Our data show the following: (i) γ polypeptide synthesis in the presence of inhibitors of DNA synthesis is multiplicity-dependent. Some γ polypeptides are not detectable in cells infected with 1 PFU per cell but form a significant fraction of viral polypeptides in cells infected with 25-500 PFU per cell. (ii) The mRNAs specifying these polypeptides have a relatively short half-life as measured by the relative rate of decay of γ polypeptide synthesis in infected cells following exposure to actinomycin D. Our data thus suggest that: (i) the transition from β to γ polypeptide synthesis does not require the synthesis of viral DNA; and (ii) the rate of synthesis of viral structural (γ) polypeptides is linked to the size of the viral DNA pool as a consequence of a relatively short-lived mRNA.

ACKNOWLEDGEMENTS

These studies were aided by grants from the National Cancer Institute (CA 08494 and CA 19264), the American Cancer Society (ACS VC 103L), and the National Science Foundation (PCM 76-06254). H. Wolf was a fellow of the Deutsche Forschungsgemeinschaft (DFG).

REFERENCES

Egyhazi, E. (1974)   Actinomycin D and RNA synthesis.   *Nature (Lond.),*
    250, 221-222

Darnell, J.E., Philipson, L., Wall, R. & Adesnik, M. (1971)   Poly-
    adenylic acid sequences: Role in conversion of nuclear RNA into
    messenger RNA. *Science, 174,* 507-510

Fenwick, M. & Roizman, B. (1977)   Regulation of herpesvirus macro-
    molecular synthesis. VI. Synthesis and modification of viral
    polypeptides in enucleated cells. *J. Virol., 22,* 720-725

Honess, R.W. & Roizman, B. (1973)   Proteins specified by herpes
    simplex virus. XI. Identification and relative molar rates of
    synthesis of structural and non-structural herpes virus poly-
    peptides in the infected cell. *J. Virol., 12,* 1247-1365

Honess, R.W. & Roizman, B. (1974)   Regulation of herpesvirus macro-
    molecular synthesis. I. Cascade regulation of the synthesis of
    three groups of viral proteins. *J. Virol., 14,* 8-19

Honess, R.W. & Roizman, B. (1975)   Regulation of herpesvirus macro-
    molecular synthesis: Sequential transition of polypeptide
    synthesis requires functional viral polypeptides. *Proc. nat.*
    Acad. Sci. (Wash.), 72, 1276-1280

Honess, R.W. & Watson, D.H. (1977)   Herpes simplex virus resistance
    and sensitivity to phosphonoacetic acid. *J. Virol., 21,* 589-600

Marsden, H.S., Crombie, I.K. & Subak-Sharpe, J.H. (1976)   Control
    of protein synthesis in herpesvirus infected cells: Analysis of
    polypeptides induced by wild type and sixteen temperature sensi-
    tive mutants of HSV strain 17. *J. gen. Virol., 31,* 347-372

Powell, K.L. & Courtney, R.J. (1975)   Polypeptides synthesized in
    herpes simplex virus type 2 infected HEp-2 cells. *Virology, 66,*
    217-228

Powell, K.L., Purifoy, D.J.M. & Courtney, R.J. (1975)   The synthesis
    of herpes simplex virus proteins in the absence of virus DNA
    synthesis. *Biochem. biophys. Res. Commun., 66,* 262-271

Roizman, B., Kozak, M., Honess, R.W. & Hayward, G. (1975)   Regulation
    of herpesvirus macromolecular synthesis: Evidence for multilevel
    regulation of herpes simplex virus 1 RNA and protein synthesis.
    Cold Spring Harb. Symp. quant. Biol., 39, 687-702

THE THYMIDINE KINASE GENE OF HERPES SIMPLEX VIRUS TYPE 1: CELL-FREE PROTEIN SYNTHESIS AND SUBSTRATE SPECIFICITY STUDIES

K.J. CREMER, W.P. SUMMERS & W.C. SUMMERS

Departments of Therapeutic Radiology,
Molecular Biophysics and Biochemistry,
and Human Genetics,
Yale University Medical School,
New Haven, Conn., USA

The thymidine kinase (TK) gene of herpes simplex virus (HSV) provides a very useful experimental tool with which to study the genetics of the virus as well as the host. Since the genetic marker resides on the viral chromosome, it can be introduced into a variety of host cells to study the genetic properties of the host. It was this feature that attracted us to the HSV TK experimental system in our work aimed at developing translation suppressors in mammalian cell lines.

As a consequence of there being two independent pathways to supply thymidylate (Fig. 1), mutants lacking one of these (i.e., the TK pathway) can be isolated easily. Since the analogue bromodeoxyuridine (BUDR) is toxic when incorporated by the TK pathway, mutation resistance to this drug is most commonly the result of loss of the TK activity. Thus, TK-negative (TK⁻) virus mutants can be isolated by picking surviving plaques in the presence of BUDR (a TK⁻ host cell simplified this selection). Kit and his co-workers first demonstrated this selection in a series of classic papers (Dubbs & Kit, 1964; Kit & Dubbs, 1977). In order to select for recovery of the TK activity, it is necessary to block *de novo* thymidylate synthesis with an antifolate drug (amethopterin) and require the virus to grow using thymidine (Fig. 1). Only viruses which have intact TK can phosphorylate thymidine to thymidylate. Thus, both forward mutations (TK$^+\rightarrow$TK$^-$) and revertant mutations (TK$^- \rightarrow$ TK$^+$) can be selected.

FIG. 1. BIOSYNTHETIC PATHWAYS LEADING TO DEOXYTHYMIDYLATE

THFA: tetrahydrofolic acid

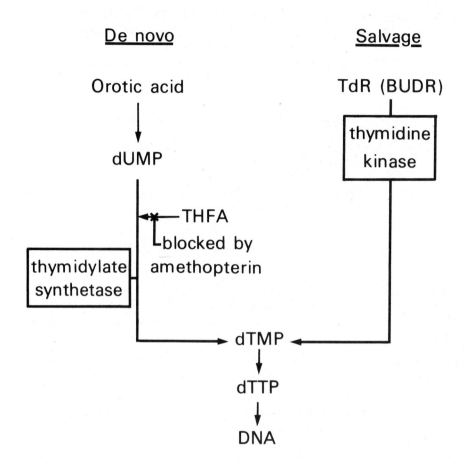

In this paper we shall discuss the characterization of a number of independently isolated TK mutants of HSV-1.   We have used specific substrate properties of the HSV TK to distinguish it from the host-cell TK, and have used an *in vitro* mRNA-dependent protein synthesis system to study some of the TK⁻ mutants.

ISOLATION AND CHARACTERIZATION OF HSV-TK MUTANTS

Since our initial report on independently isolated HSV-TK⁻ mutants (Summers et al., 1975), we have isolated another eleven mutants. These are described in Table 1.   It is important to note that each mutant was isolated from a different freshly cloned stock of HSV-TK⁺ (strain Cl 101).   In this way, all isolates are independent and unique.

Table 1. Properties of mutant strains of herpesvirus[a]

Strain	Phenotype	Intact TK peptide	Fragment peptide
Cl 101	S	+	-
B2006	R	-	-
TK 41	R	+	-
TK 42	R	+	-
TK 42 *syn*	R	-	+[b]
TK 43	R	-	+
TK 44	R	+	-
TK 45	R	-	-
TK 46	R	-	-
TK 47	R	-	+[b]
TK 48	R	+	-
TK 49	R	-	-
TK 50	R	-	+

[a] Phenotype indicates sensitivity (S) or resistance (R) to growth in BUDR.   All mutants were selected following growth in 100 μg/ml BUDR. The ability to detect the presence of the intact TK peptide or a shorter peptide by gel electrophoresis is indicated. All mutants induced less than 1% (limit of detection) of wild-type TK activity.

[b] Size of new protein fragment: 26 000 daltons

In our first report (Summers et al., 1975), we used mutagens in an attempt to induce specific types of mutations.   We have no evidence indicating any specific mutagenicity.   Indeed, recent quantitative studies of TK⁺ → TK⁻ mutation frequencies suggest that there was no significant difference between the number of mutants obtained, with

or without mutagen.   It should be noted, however, that the selection
for TK⁻ is carried out in the presence of 100 μg/ml of BUDR, so all
stocks may have been exposed to BUDR mutagenesis.

Each mutant was assayed for its ability to induce virus-specific
TK activity after infection, and for its ability to synthesize the
40 000 molecular weight protein which is the HSV-TK polypeptide.
Some mutants induce the synthesis of a shorter polypeptide and have
lost the ability to induce TK activity.

The data on 30 mutants (Summers et al., 1975; Table 1) are
summarized in Table 2.   It is interesting to note that, of the eight
mutants which give short fragments, four seem to be indistinguishable.
We shall discuss this situation below.   The spectrum of mutants
revealed by this study is similar, at least on the face of it, to
that of other genetic systems.   About one-third (12/30) of the
mutants have intact protein molecules, but have inactive or very weak
enzymatic properties, as would be expected of missense mutants.   The
rest have shortened or absent polypeptides.   These are expected to
be deletion mutants, chain termination mutants, internal start mutations, or some sort of protein or mRNA processing mutants.

Table 2.   Spectrum of HSV-TK mutants

Phenotype	Proportion of mutants
No intact TK protein	18/30
Short fragment	8/18
Intact TK protein	12/30
Partial activity (1%, 3%, 25%)	3/12

USE OF ^{125}I-DEOXYCYTIDINE TO ASSAY HSV TK

In our study of the genetics of HSV TK, we have often needed a
simple, rapid test for the HSV-TK function which could be carried out
even in the presence of an active cell TK.   Thus, we wished to screen
isolates on Vero or BHK cells (TK⁺), rather than having to use exclusively the few TK⁻ cell lines available.   By extending the work of
Cooper (1973), we have been able to achieve such an assay (Summers &
Summers, 1977).   A number of workers (e.g., Cheng, 1976; Jamieson
& Subak-Sharpe, 1974) have noted that the substrate specificity of
the viral enzyme is much broader than that of the cell TK.   The HSV
TK is a general deoxypyrimidine kinase and will use, for example

deoxycytidine analogues.   We have synthesized high specific-activity ^{125}I-deoxycytidine (IdC) and find that its incorporation into acid-insoluble material is dependent on infection of cells (TK$^+$ or TK$^-$) with HSV-TK$^+$ virus.   In some cell lines, e.g., BHK, a cell deoxy-cytidine deaminase must be blocked with tetrahydrouridine (Camiener, 1968).

Since ^{125}IdC can be obtained at very high specific activities, and since it is not a substrate for cell TK, it should prove of advantage in studies on the *in vitro* synthesis of active viral thymidine kinase in the cell-free systems.   In these cases, where synthesis may be low and reconstitution of the dimeric enzyme may be inefficient, it is crucial to have the endogenous activity as low as possible.

IN VITRO PROTEIN SYNTHESIS IN RESPONSE TO HSV-TK$^+$ AND TK$^-$ mRNA

One question arising from the analysis of the TK$^-$ mutants of HSV is whether the mutation gives the same phenotype *in vitro* as it does *in vivo*.   For example, mutants which are altered in some step in post-translation modification may not display the same phenotype *in vitro* as *in vivo*.   Furthermore, *in vitro*, one has the opportunity to test the effects on the TK mutants of suppressor tRNAs isolated from other sources such as *E. coli* or yeast.

Our initial step was to develop an *in vitro* system which was programmed with polysomes from HSV-infected cells.   While this system faithfully reproduced the *in vivo* phenotype of the mutants tested (Cremer et al., 1977), it was only partly purified from infected cells.   Thus, the possibility of post-translational modification could not be excluded in this polysome-directed system.

Recently, we have used purified cytoplasmic RNA from HSV-infected cells to programme an *in vitro* protein-synthesizing system derived from rabbit reticulocytes following the method of Pelham & Jackson (1976).   This system directs the synthesis of most of the major HSV polypeptides, including those with molecular weights greater than 100 000 daltons, and synthesizes a substantial amount of the 40 000 protein identified as the HSV TK.   Figure 2 shows an autoradiograph of a sodium dodecyl sulfate (SDS)-polyacrylamide gel electrophoreto-gram of several *in vitro* reactions programmed with RNA prepared from wild-type or mutant HSV-infected cells.   While some differences are seen between the various mutants, most of these are related to the quality of the individual RNA preparations.   A more constant feature, however, is the appearance of polypeptides at the exact positions expected for the "fragments" of the TK polypeptide with molecular weights of 35 000, 31 000 and 26 000 daltons.   Thus, these mutants are producing the same polypeptide products *in vitro* as those seen *in vivo*.   The only component in this system from the infected cell is the purified mRNA.   If any protein processing or modification of the mutant protein is occurring *in vitro*, it must be nearly complete as very little intact protein is left. Furthermore, it must be carried out by rabbit reticulocyte factors.

ON THE NATURE OF THE TK MUTANTS

On the basis of their reasonable reversion frequency (10^{-5} – 10^{-6}), and of the synthesis *in vitro* in a totally heterologous system of the expected mutant polypeptides, it is tempting to conclude that at least the four mutants shown in Figure 2 are not deletions, but rather are chain termination mutants. Other possibilities have not been excluded, however. Consider the case of protein processing mutants. It is known from bacterial systems that proteolytic systems exist which degrade "abnormal" polypeptides, e.g., short-chain mutants, and non-functional missense mutants. Thus, these mutants may have an altered amino-acid sequence which creates a new site for protease action. Such a protease might proceed until some limit, or "core" structure is produced. This would result in a number of independent mutants showing the same final "core" peptide, as is the case with four of the mutants in Table 2. This model requires that this processing be efficiently carried out *in vitro* as well as *in vivo*. Until more is known about the details of the protein degradation pathways, we can only keep this problem in mind.

Another possibility to consider is that the mutation has its effect at the level of post-transcription RNA processing. The mRNA, as it is used to programme the cell-free system, may be aberrant or modified as the result of some *in vivo* processing such as ligation (Sambrook, 1977) or cleavage. Testing this hypothesis will require a more detailed knowledge of the TK mRNA molecule than we now possess.

SUMMARY

The HSV thymidine kinase genetic system has a number of advantages for the study of virus and cell genetics. Both forward and reverse mutants are readily selected. The enzyme can be assayed directly in the presence of the cell TK by the choice of the appropriate substrate, for example, ^{125}IdC. The gene product, HSV TK, can be identified by SDS-polyacrylamide gel electrophoresis and mutants can be found with alterations in the electrophoretogram. The *in vitro* synthesis of HSV TK in response to HSV mRNA has been achieved and can be used to analyse specific mutant virus.

FIG. 2.   SDS-POLYACRYLAMIDE GEL AUTORADIOGRAM OF ^{35}S-METHIONINE-
LABELLED PRODUCTS OF CELL-FREE PROTEIN SYNTHESIS AND
^{35}S-METHIONINE *IN VIVO* LABELLED CELL EXTRACTS

The gel was a 7-15% acrylamide slab gel, using the discontinuous
buffer system with sodium dodecyl sulfate (SDS) as described by
Laemmli (1970).   Each cell-free reaction contained 10 µl of micrococcal nuclease-treated reticulocyte lysate as described by Pelham &
Jackson (1976), 10 µCi of ^{35}S-methionine (specific activity, 500-1000
Ci/mmol), and 5-15 µg of cytoplasmic RNA from HSV-infected LMTK⁻ cells.
Cytoplasmic RNA was prepared, as described by Anderson et al. (1974),
from cells infected for 9 or 11 hours with wild-type or TK⁻ mutant
virus.   Vero cells infected with HSV were labelled from 5 to 7 hours
after infection with ^{35}S-methionine (25 µCi/ml).   Samples (a - k) are
products of cell-free translations programmed with cytoplasmic RNA
prepared from cells infected with the following viruses: (a, f, g)
21 TK⁺; (b, h) 38 TK⁻; (c, k) 20 TK⁻; (d, i) 21 TK⁻; (e, j) 37 TK⁻.
Samples (l - p) are Vero cells infected with the following viruses:
(l, m) 21 TK⁺; (n) 20 TK⁻; (o) 21 TK⁻; (p) 37 TK⁻.   The dots and
lines indicate the positions of the fragment polypeptides.   Their
respective apparent molecular weights are: 21 TK⁺, 40 000 daltons;
38 TK⁻, 35 000 daltons; 20 TK⁻, 31 000 daltons; 21 TK⁻, 37 TK⁻,
26 000 daltons.

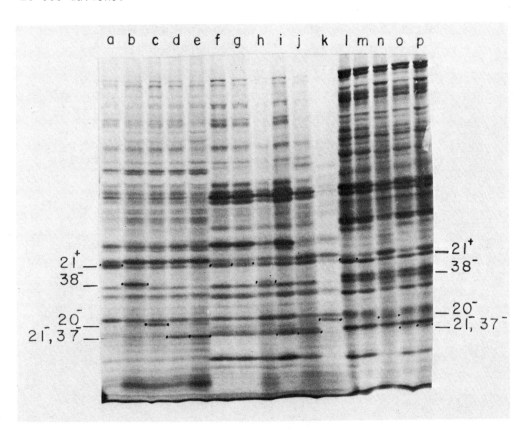

ACKNOWLEDGEMENTS

We thank Dr R.F. Gesteland for much help with the cell-free
synthesis experiments, and for the hospitality of his
laboratory for some phases of this work. This effort
was supported by grants CA 06519, CA 13515 from
the US Public Health Service and VC 60F from
the American Cancer Society.

REFERENCES

Anderson, C.W., Lewis, J.B., Atkins, J.F. & Gesteland, R.F. (1974)
Cell-free synthesis of adenovirus 2 proteins programmed by
fractionated messenger RNA: a comparison of polypeptide products
and messenger RNA lengths. *Proc. nat. Acad. Sci. (Wash.)*, *71*,
2756-2760

Camiener, G.W. (1968)   Studies of the enzymatic deamination of
aracytidine. V. Inhibition *in vitro* and *in vivo* by tetrahydrouridine and other induced pyrimidine nucleosides. *Biochem.
Pharmacol.*, *17*, 1981-1991

Cheng, Y.C. (1976)   Deoxythymidine kinase induced in HeLa TK⁻ cells
by herpes simplex virus type 1 and type 2. *Biochim. Biophys.
Acta (Amst.)*, *452*, 370-381

Cooper, G.M. (1973)   Phosphorylation of 5-bromodeoxycytidine in
cells infected with herpes simplex virus. *Proc. nat. Acad.
Sci. (Wash.)*, *70*, 3788-3792

Cremer, K.J., Gesteland, R.F. & Summers, W.C. (1977)   Cell-free
synthesis of herpes simplex virus proteins. *J. Virol.*, *22*,
750-757

Dubbs, D.R. & Kit, S. (1964)   Mutant strains of herpes simplex
deficient in thymidine kinase-inducing activity. *Virology*, *22*,
493-505

Jamieson, A.T. & Subak-Sharpe, J.H. (1974)   Biochemical studies on
the herpes virus-specified deoxypyrimidine kinase activity.
J. gen. Virol., *24*, 481-492

Kit, S. & Dubbs, D.R. (1977)   Regulation of herpesvirus thymidine
    kinase activity in LM (TK⁻) cells transformed by ultraviolet
    light-irradiated herpes simplex virus.   *Virology, 76*, 331-340

Laemmli, U.K. (1970)   Cleavage of structural proteins during the
    assembly of the head of bacteriophage T4.   *Nature (Lond.), 227*,
    680-685

Pelham, R.B. & Jackson, R.J. (1976)   An efficient mRNA-dependent
    translation system from reticulocyte lysates.   *Europ. J. Biochem.,
    67*, 247-256

Sambrook, J. (1977)   Adenovirus amazes at Cold Spring Harbor.
    Nature (Lond.), 268, 101-104

Summers, W.C. & Summers, W.P. (1977)   [^{125}I]deoxycytidine used in a
    rapid, sensitive, and specific assay for herpes simplex virus
    type I thymidine kinase.   *J. Virol., 24*, 314-318

Summers, W.P., Wagner, M. & Summers, W.C. (1975)   Possible peptide
    chain termination mutants in thymidine kinase gene of a mammalian
    virus, herpes simplex virus.   *Proc. nat. Acad. Sci. (Wash.), 72*,
    4081-4084

CELL-FREE SYSTEMS FOR *IN VITRO* TRANSLATION OF HERPES SIMPLEX VIRUS MESSENGER RNA

C.M. PRESTON

Medical Research Council,
Institute of Virology,
Glasgow, UK

This communication deals with techniques currently available for *in vitro* translation of herpes simplex virus (HSV) mRNA. Three basic considerations are important in establishing a cell-free system for mRNA-dependent synthesis of viral polypeptides:

(1) The system should possess a high efficiency of initiation of protein synthesis.

(2) The reaction should represent accurate translation of added mRNA.

(3) Endogenous protein synthesis should provide only a very low background in the system.

Translation *in vitro* of HSV mRNA poses additional problems, since the pattern of protein synthesis in infected cells is complex (Honess & Roizman, 1974; Marsden et al., 1976) and the mRNA is not of the high efficiency *in vivo* that has been demonstrated in other virus systems (Hay[1]; Nuss et al., 1975; Preston[2]). In view of these factors, the reticulocyte lysate was chosen as the starting material in the development of a suitable cell-free system, as it has low nuclease levels, initiates protein synthesis efficiently and elongates polypeptides accurately. The background of reticulocyte protein synthesis, however, is so high as to mask all but the major products made in response to added mRNA.

---

[1] Personal communication

[2] Unpublished data

Initial attempts to reduce the background protein synthesis were performed using vesicular stomatitis virus (VSV) mRNA, since this was a well-defined system.   It was found that reticulocyte polysomes engaged in protein synthesis could be effectively removed from the lysate by a rapid centrifugation step.   The supernatant from this procedure contained ribosomal subunits and monomers, which could be concentrated by precipitation at pH 5.   Addition of ribosomal salt-wash fraction, containing initiation factors, to the "pH 5 fraction" resulted in a system which retained the activity and accuracy of the complete lysate but provided only a low background (mainly globin) of reticulocyte protein synthesis (Preston & Szilagyi, 1977).

When RNA from HSV-infected cells was added to this cell-free system, distinct virus-induced polypeptides could be detected, but the efficiency of translation was much lower than that of VSV mRNA. Activity was increased, however, by addition of reticulocyte high-speed supernatant (S100).   This cell-free system showed a partial dependence on ribosomal salt-wash proteins, and it was found that the fraction from uninfected BHK cells was most effective in stimulating protein synthesis.   Seventeen virus-induced polypeptides could be detected when cytoplasmic RNA from HSV-infected cells was added, whilst the background of reticulocyte protein synthesis was low (Preston, 1977).

Recently, an alternative method for removing the background of protein synthesis from reticulocytes whilst retaining the high activity has been described (Pelham & Jackson, 1976).   This involves pre-incubation of the cell-free system with micrococcal nuclease, which is dependent upon the presence of Ca^{2+} ions for activity, followed by addition of EGTA to inactivate the enzyme.   This provided a means of removing all traces of endogenous protein synthesis from cell-free systems, and was therefore tested with the fractionated reticulocyte system.   As shown in Table 1, reticulocyte protein synthesis (i.e., in the presence of *E. coli* rRNA) was severely inhibited by preincubation with concentrations of nuclease greater than 25 units/ml, whereas translation of infected-cell mRNA was unaffected until the concentration was raised to 750 units/ml.

The polypeptides synthesised *in vitro* in response to cytoplasmic RNA from infected or uninfected BHK cells with or without preincubation with micrococcal nuclease are shown in Figure 1.   For comparison, the polypeptides synthesized by the nuclease-treated unfractionated reticulocyte lysate are also shown.   It is clear that preincubation with the enzyme has removed essentially all the background of endogenous protein synthesis without affecting the efficiency of translation of added mRNA or the nature of the reaction products.   Furthermore, translation in the complete lysate gives very similar results.

It is clear, therefore, that preincubation with micrococcal nuclease can be used in the fractionated reticulocyte cell-free system to eliminate endogenous mRNA, and that HSV mRNA is translated as

FIG. 1.   EFFECT OF PREINCUBATION WITH MICROCOCCAL NUCLEASE
ON POLYPEPTIDES SYNTHESIZED BY CELL-FREE SYSTEMS

Reactions were carried out as described in Table 1.   Tracks 1-3 show
the polypeptides synthesized by the unfractionated reticulocyte lysate,
pretreated with micrococcal nuclease (100 units/ml) (Pelham & Jackson,
1976);   tracks 6-8 show the polypeptides synthesized by the fractionated
reticulocyte system (Preston, 1977) after pretreatment with micrococcal
nuclease (100 units/ml);   tracks 9-11 show the polypeptides synthesised
in the untreated fractionated reticulocyte cell-free system.   The added
RNA (final concentration 240 µg per ml) was *E. coli* rRNA (tracks 1, 6
and 9), uninfected BHK cell cytoplasmic RNA (tracks 2, 7 and 10) or
HSV-1 infected BHK cell cytoplasmic RNA, extracted at eight hours after
infection at 31°C (tracks 3, 8 and 11).   The ^{35}S-methionyl polypeptides
synthesized *in vivo* in a one-hour labelling period by BHK cells (labelled
6.5-7.5 hours after infection at 37°C, track 4) and uninfected BHK cells
(track 5) are included.   The designation of virus-induced polypeptides
synthesised *in vitro* shown on the right of track 11 follows that of
Preston (1977).

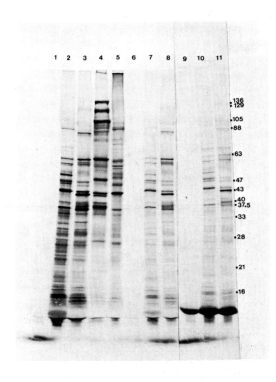

Table 1. Effects of micrococcal nuclease on the fractionated
reticulocyte cell-free system[a]

Nuclease concentration (units/ml)	^{35}S-methionine incorporation (cpm $\times$ 10^{-3})	
	+ Infected-cell RNA	+ *E. coli* rRNA
0	43	30
7.5	35	28
25	38	24
75	35	12
250	28	7
750	6	2

[a] The components of the fractionated reticulocyte cell-free system
(Preston, 1977), minus ^{35}S-methionine and added RNA, were incubated
at 20°C with 1 mM calcium chloride and various concentrations of
micrococcal nuclease (P-L biochemicals) for 10 minutes. EGTA was
then added at 2.5 mM, followed by ^{35}S-methionine and *E. coli* rRNA
or cytoplasmic RNA from HSV-1 infected cells. Incubation was
continued for 90 minutes at 30°C, and ^{35}S-methionine incorporation
into protein determined.

efficiently as in the unfractionated reticulocyte lysate. Whilst the
unfractionated lysate is easier to prepare, the fractionated system is
more useful for studies on the individual components of protein
synthesis. The choice of cell-free system depends on the nature of
the problem to be investigated.

SUMMARY

     A cell-free system active in translation of HSV mRNA was obtained
by fractionation of reticulocyte lysates. Endogenous protein synthesis
was further reduced by preincubation with micrococcal nuclease, although
this treatment did not affect the translation of infected (or uninfected)
BHK cell RNA. Polypeptides synthesized by the fractionated reticulocyte
cell-free system were very similar to those produced by unfractionated
reticulocyte lysates.

ACKNOWLEDGEMENTS

The author is grateful to M. Dunlop
for technical assistance.

REFERENCES

Honess, R.W. & Roizman, B. (1974)   Regulation of herpesvirus macro-
    molecular synthesis. *J. Virol., 14*, 8-19

Marsden, H.S., Crombie, I.K. & Subak-Sharpe, J.H. (1976)   Control of
    protein synthesis in herpesvirus-infected cells: analysis of the
    polypeptides induced by wild type and sixteen temperature-sensitive
    mutants of HSV strain 17. *J. gen. Virol., 31*, 347-372

Nuss, D.L., Oppermann, H. & Koch, G. (1975)   Selective blockage of
    initiation of host protein synthesis in RNA-virus-infected cells.
    Proc. nat. Acad. Sci. (Wash.), 72, 1258-1262

Pelham, H.R.B. & Jackson, R.J. (1976)   An efficient mRNA-dependent
    translation system from reticulocyte lysates. *Europ. J. Biochem.,
    67*, 247-256

Preston, C.M. (1977)   The cell-free synthesis of herpesvirus-induced
    polypeptides. *Virology, 78*, 349-353

Preston, C.M. & Szilagyi, J.F. (1977)   Cell-free translation of RNA
    synthesized *in vitro* by a transcribing nucleoprotein complex pre-
    pared from purified vesicular stomatitis virus. *J. Virol., 21*,
    1002-1009

EARLY VIRUS-SPECIFIC PROTEINS SYNTHESIZED IN HUMAN CYTOMEGALOVIRUS INFECTED CELLS

M.F. STINSKI

Department of Microbiology,
College of Medicine,
University of Iowa,
Iowa City, Iowa, USA

In cytomegalovirus (CMV)-infected cells there is an induction of host-cell protein synthesis concomitant with an overall stimulation of macromolecular synthesis by the virus (Stinski, 1977; Tanaka et al., 1975). The detection of virus-specific proteins, referred to as infected cell-specific polypeptides (ICSP), by radioisotope pulse-labelling and subsequent slab sodium dodecyl sulfate (SDS)-poly-acrylamide gel electrophoresis (PAGE) is hindered by this high back-ground of host-cell protein synthesis. To enhance the synthesis of viral proteins relative to that of the host cell so that early ICSP are clearly identifiable, CMV-infected cells were treated with cyclo-heximide (CH) for various intervals and then radioisotope pulse-labelling was done in hypertonic medium. These procedures have been shown to reduce host protein synthesis in several virus/cell systems (England et al., 1975; Harter et al., 1976; Nuss et al., 1975).

This report describes the synthesis of at least 15 ICSP that are referred to as early ICSP because they are made prior to viral DNA replication. Early ICSP were detected in permissive cells treated with an inhibitor of viral DNA synthesis and also in cells that are non-permissive for viral DNA replication. The early virus-specific proteins synthesized during CMV replication are crucial for the process of lytic infection and may also play a role in persistent infection and cellular transformation by CMV.

The Towne strain of human CMV and human fibroblast (HF) and guineapig embryo fibroblast (GPEF) cells were employed for this study. Cell cultures were infected at a multiplicity of 10-20 plaque-forming units (PFU)/cell. Cycloheximide, at a concentration of 50 µg/ml, was added 2 hours post infection (p.i.) in order to inhibit the translation of viral messenger RNA (mRNA). After the removal of CH, the cells were washed four times with minimal essential medium containing 5% of the normal concentration of methionine. The proteins were labelled with ^{35}S-methionine (20 µCi/ml) for 2-hour periods in either isotonic (110 mM sodium chloride) or hypertonic (210 mM sodium chloride) medium containing 5% of the normal concentration of methionine and 5 µg/ml of actinomycin D to inhibit further transcription of the viral DNA during the pulse period. Cells were harvested, the samples were solubilized in 1.0% SDS and 1.0% 2-mercapto-ethanol, and then an equal volume of each sample was analysed by slab SDS-PAGE in 9% gels as previously described (Stinski, 1977). After electrophoresis, the gels were stained, dried, and analysed by auto-radiography according to the method of Fairbanks et al. (1971).

Early ICSP synthesis was analysed by adding CH at 2 hours p.i. and then removing CH at various intervals up to 18 hours p.i.. Cells were pulsed with ^{35}S-methionine in isotonic medium. Under these conditions, early ICSP were first detected at 6-8 hours p.i., and, subsequently detected in increasing relative molar ratio until 14-16 hours p.i. (Fig. 1A). Synthesis of early ICSP with an apparent molecular weight of 71 000 was detected as early as 2-4 hours p.i. when cells were pulsed with ^{35}S-methionine in hypertonic medium (data not shown). When CH was removed at 18 hours p.i. and cells were pulsed at various intervals, the synthesis of early ICSP decreased in relative molar ratio with time.

Although early ICSP were detected up to 12-14 hours after the removal of CH, they could not be detected at approximately 16-18 hours (Fig. 1A). Figure 1B is from the same experiment as illustrated in Figure 1A, except that twice the concentration of protein was analysed to detect early ICSP present in low molar ratios. At least 12 early ICSP with electrophoretic mobilities different from those of host-cell polypeptides were detected when cells were radioactively pulsed in isotonic medium at 18-20 hours p.i. (Fig. 1B). Treatment of cells with CH prior to radioisotope pulse-labelling enhanced CMV-induced protein synthesis relative to host. The early ICSP represent the translation products of the early viral mRNAs. Synthesis of early viral mRNA must be by a preexisting cellular enzyme or by one present in the virion, because early mRNA accumulates in the presence of CH. The early viral mRNAs were stable for approximately 12-14 hours after the removal of CH, as determined by the translation of early ICSP.

The profile of early ICSP, synthesized in cells after treatment with CH for 2-10 hours p.i., was compared with that of late ICSP, synthesized after viral DNA synthesis. To further reduce host protein synthesis, the medium used for radioisotope pulse-labelling was made hypertonic by adding sodium chloride to a final concentration of 210 mM. Hypertonic medium was used for the remainder of the radio-isotope pulse-labelling experiments to be described. Under these conditions, at least 15 early ICSP and 22 late ICSP were detected and they are identified according to their apparent molecular weight

FIG. 1. AUTORADIOGRAM OF SDS-POLYACRYLAMIDE GEL SLAB
CONTAINING ELECTROPHORETICALLY SEPARATED POLYPEPTIDES
SYNTHESIZED IN CMV-INFECTED CELLS DURING THE EARLY
PHASE OF INFECTION

Infected (I) and uninfected (U) cells were treated with cycloheximide
(CH) at 2 hours p.i. until 18 hours p.i. CH was removed at various
intervals prior to pulse-labelling for 2 hours with ^{35}S-methionine
in isotonic medium as indicated above. ICSP are denoted by their
apparent molecular weight ($\times 10^3$). Twice the concentration of protein
was applied to the gel in B as compared to A.

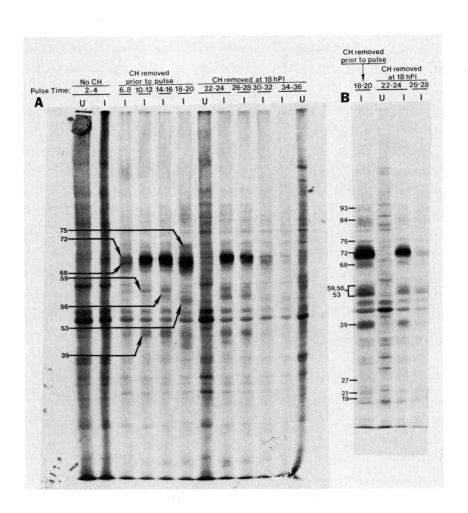

($\times 10^3$) (Fig. 2).   A majority of early ICSP have apparent molecular
weights which differ from those of late ICSP with the exception of
ICSP 115, 110, 68, and 27.   Whether the latter ICSP represent viral
proteins synthesized before and after viral DNA replication will
require further investigation.   The majority of the late ICSP have
been identified as structural components of virions and dense bodies
of CMV (Stinski, 1977).   Since a specific class of ICSP are synthesized
early but not late in infection, the synthesis of CMV proteins appears
to be subjected to a control system delineated by the synthesis of
viral DNA.

FIG. 2.   COMPARISON OF ELECTROPHORETICALLY SEPARATED
POLYPEPTIDES SYNTHESIZED BEFORE AND AFTER VIRAL
DNA REPLICATION IN CMV-INFECTED CELLS

Infected (I) and uninfected (U) cells were either treated or not
treated with cycloheximide (CH) at 2 hours p.i. for various intervals.
The CH was removed prior to pulse-labelling for 2 hours with ^{35}S-
methionine in hypertonic medium as indicated above.   ICSP are denoted
by their apparent molecular weight ($\times 10^3$).   Host-cell polypeptides
are either labelled with the letter (h) or not labelled at all.

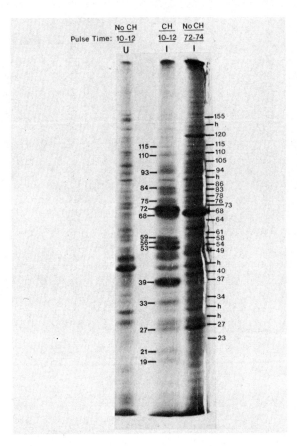

Phosphonoacetic acid (PAA) inhibits the replication of CMV DNA (Huang, 1975) and indirectly prevents the synthesis of the late ICSP of CMV (Stinski, 1977).   If the early ICSP of CMV represent the translation products of mRNA which is synthesized prior to viral DNA, then PAA should have no effect on early ICSP synthesis.   To test this, infected cells were treated with CH from 2-10 or 2-14 hours p.i. and either treated with PAA (100 µg/ml) or left untreated.   After the removal of CH, cells were pulsed for 2 hours with ^{35}S-methionine. Early ICSP synthesis was detected in cells treated with PAA, whereas late ICSP synthesis was inhibited by treatment with PAA (Fig. 3).

FIG. 3. EFFECT OF AN INHIBITOR OF CMV DNA SYNTHESIS ON EARLY AND LATE INFECTED CELL-SPECIFIC POLYPEPTIDE SYNTHESIS

Infected (I) and uninfected (U) cells were either treated or not treated with phosphonoacetic acid (PAA).   For early pulse periods, cells were treated with cycloheximide (CH) at 2 hours p.i..   CH was removed prior to pulse-labelling for 2 hours with ^{35}S-methionine in hypertonic medium as indicated above.   Polypeptides associated with purified virions plus dense bodies were electrophoresed in parallel to infected cells pulsed at late periods.   Apparent molecular weights ($\times$ 10^3) of viral structural polypeptides and ICSP are indicated.

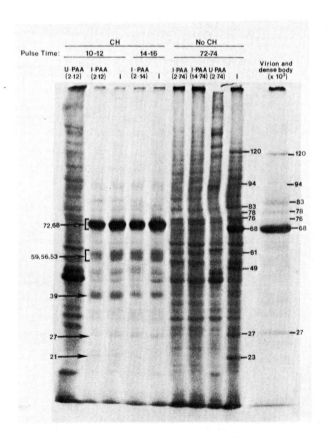

Even when PAA was added at 14 hours p.i., after the synthesis of the early ICSP, late ICSP were still not detected at 72-74 hours p.i. (Fig. 3). In the absence of PAA, late ICSP with the same electrophoretic mobilities as the polypeptides associated with virions and dense bodies of CMV were synthesized (Fig. 3). Hence, early CMV ICSP represent the translation products of mRNA that is transcribed prior to or in the absence of viral DNA synthesis.

Infection of non-permissive GPEF cells with CMV results in the development of a cytopathic effect (Fioretti et al., 1973) and the induction of a unique virus-induced DNA polymerase (Hirai et al., 1976). However, non-permissive cells do not permit the synthesis of CMV DNA (St. Jeor et al., 1974) or the production of infectious virus (Fioretti et al., 1973). To determine whether CMV early ICSP are synthesized in non-permissive cells, GPEF cells were infected with CMV and treated with CH from 2-10 and 2-14 hours p.i.. After removal of the CH, the cells were pulsed with ^{35}S-methionine. The permissive HF cells were treated in a similar manner for comparison. Lysates of infected HF and GPEF cells were electrophoresed in parallel. The early ICSP detected in non-permissive cells had the same electrophoretic mobilities as those detected in permissive cells and there were no ICSP in GPEF that were not also detected in infected HF cells (Fig. 4). The molecular weights of the early ICSP detected in CMV-infected HF and GPEF cells are presented in Table 1. Host-cell protein synthesis was higher in infected GPEF cells than in HF cells and, consequently, some polypeptides with low levels of incorporated radioactivity could not be identified with certainty in the infected GPEF cells. Nevertheless, the majority of the CMV early ICSP synthesized in permissive cells are also synthesized in non-permissive GPEF cells. Hence, early ICSP of CMV are synthesized in cells derived from different genotypes. These observations suggest that the early ICSP represent viral genome products rather than host-induced proteins.

To determine whether late ICSP of CMV were synthesized in non-permissive GPEF cells, infected cells were pulsed with ^{35}S-methionine at 72-74 hours p.i.. Cell lysates were electrophoresed in parallel with purified virions and dense bodies of CMV and with infected HF cells pulsed at 72-74 hours p.i.. Even though early ICSP were synthesized in both HF and GPEF cells, late ICSP were not detected in the non-permissive GPEF cells (Fig. 5). Since non-permissive cells do not allow for the synthesis of CMV DNA (St. Jeor et al., 1974), these observations confirm that CMV DNA synthesis is required for late CMV genome expression.

In CMV-infected cells, viral DNA synthesis is initiated at approximately 20 hours p.i. and reaches maximum levels at approximately 80 hours p.i.[1]. The synthesis of the early CMV proteins begins at

---

[1] Unpublished data

FIG. 4. AUTORADIOGRAM OF ELECTROPHORETICALLY SEPARATED
POLYPEPTIDES SYNTHESIZED IN CMV-INFECTED PERMISSIVE
HUMAN FIBROBLAST (HF) CELLS AND NON-PERMISSIVE
GUINEAPIG EMBRYO FIBROBLAST (GPEF) CELLS
AT EARLY TIMES AFTER INFECTION

Infected (I) and uninfected (U) cells were treated with cycloheximide
(CH) at 2 hours p.i. for various intervals.   CH was removed prior to
pulse-labelling for 2 hours with ^{35}S-methionine in hypertonic medium
as indicated above.   ICSP are denoted by their apparent molecular
weight ($\times 10^3$).

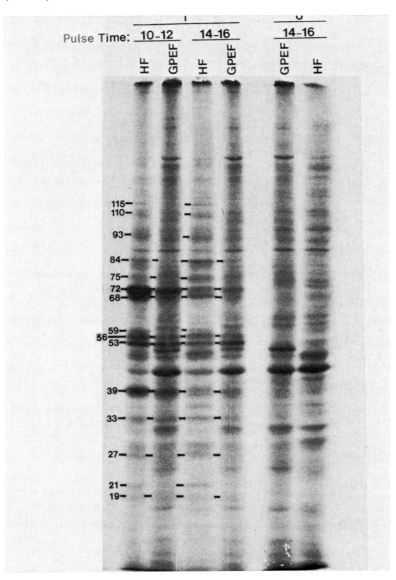

Table 1. Molecular weights of early CMV-infected cell-specific polypeptides in permissive human fibroblast and non-permissive guineapig embryo fibroblast cells[a]

Human fibroblast cells ($\times 10^3$)[b]	Guineapig embryo fibroblast cells ($\times 10^3$)[b]
115[c]	115[c]
110[c]	ND[d]
93[c]	93[c]
84[c]	84[c]
75	75
72	72
68	68
59	59[c]
56	56
53	53
39	39
33[c]	33
27	27
21	ND[d]
19	19

[a] Infected cells were treated with cycloheximide (50 μg/ml) 2-10 hours p.i. and pulsed for 2 hours with ^{35}S-methionine in hypertonic medium

[b] Apparent molecular weights were determined from a 9% SDS-polyacrylamide gel using the following standards: thyroglobulin (160 000), phosphorylase a (94 000), bovine serum albumin (68 000), ovalbumin (43 000) and cytochrome c (11 700).

[c] Additional work is needed to establish their identity with certainty since these polypeptides have low levels of incorporated radioactivity.

[d] ND - Not detected

2-4 hours p.i. and reaches maximum levels at approximately 14-16 hours p.i.. In addition, the early viral mRNA appears to remain translatable for approximately 12-14 hours after the removal of CH. These

FIG. 5. AUTORADIOGRAM OF ELECTROPHORETICALLY SEPARATED
POLYPEPTIDES FROM CMV-INFECTED PERMISSIVE HUMAN
FIBROBLAST (HF) CELLS AND NON-PERMISSIVE
GUINEAPIG EMBRYO FIBROBLAST (GPEF) CELLS
SYNTHESIZED EARLY AND LATE AFTER INFECTION

Cells were either treated or not treated with cycloheximide (CH) at
2 hours p.i.. The CH was removed prior to pulse-labelling for 2
hours with ^{35}S-methionine in hypertonic medium as indicated above.
Polypeptides associated with purified virions plus dense bodies
were electrophoresed in parallel to infected HF cells pulsed from
72 to 74 hours p.i. Structural viral polypeptides and ICSP are
indicated according to their apparent molecular weight ($\times 10^3$).

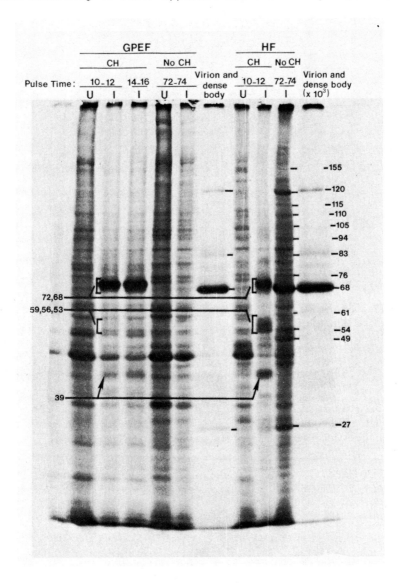

observations suggest that the synthesis of early CMV viral mRNA and proteins is completed in the infected cell within approximately 14 hours p.i. and that this process is transient.   The reasons why CMV DNA synthesis is not initiated until approximately 20 hours p.i. and why the viral DNA synthesis is a relatively slow process in HF cells and not detectable in non-permissive cells remain to be investigated. Since the early CMV genome expression stimulates host-cell macromolecular synthesis, it is tempting to postulate that CMV requires a host-cell function(s) for viral DNA replication and that this function(s) is species-specific.

ACKNOWLEDGEMENTS

My sincere thanks to Darrell R. Thomsen for expert assistance. This investigation was supported by US Public Health Service grant 1-01AI13562-01VR from the National Institute of Allergy and Infectious Diseases.

REFERENCES

England, J.M., Howett, M.K. & Tan, K.B. (1975)   Effect of hypertonic conditions on protein synthesis in cells productively infected with simian virus 40.   *J. Virol.*, *16*, 1101-1107

Fairbanks, G., Steck, T.L. & Wallach, D.F.H. (1971)   Electrophoretic analysis of the major polypeptides of the human erythrocyte membrane.   *Biochemistry*, *10*, 2606-2617

Fioretti, A., Furukawa, T., Santoli, D. & Plotkin, S.A. (1973)   Nonproductive infection of guinea pig cells with human cytomegalovirus. *J. Virol.*, *11*, 998-1003

Harter, M.L., Shanmugam, G., Wold, W.S.M. & Green, M. (1976)   Detection of adenovirus type 2-induced early polypeptides using cycloheximide pretreatment to enhance viral protein synthesis.   *J. Virol.*, *19*, 232-242

Hirai, K., Furukawa, T. & Plotkin, S.A. (1976)   Induction of DNA polymerase in WI-38 and guinea pig cells infected with human CMV.   *Virology*, *70*, 251-255

Huang, E.S., Chen, S.T. & Pagano, J.S. (1973)   Human cytomegalovirus.
    I. Purification and characterization of viral DNA.   *J. Virol.*, *12*,
    1473-1481

Huang, E.S. (1975)   Human cytomegalovirus.   IV. Specific inhibition
    of virus-induced DNA polymerase activity and viral DNA replication
    by phosphonoacetic acid.   *J. Virol.*, *16*, 1560-1565

Nuss, D.L., Oppermann, H. & Koch, G. (1975)   Selective blockage
    of initiation of host protein synthesis in RNA-virus infected
    cells.   *Proc. nat. Acad. Sci. (Wash.)*, *72*, 1258-1262

Stinski, M.F. (1977)   Synthesis of proteins and glycoproteins in
    cells infected with human cytomegalovirus.   *J. Virol.*, *23*, 751-767

St. Jeor, S.C., Albrecht, T.B., Funk, F.D. & Rapp, F. (1974)
    Stimulation of cellular DNA synthesis by human cytomegalovirus.
    J. Virol., *13*, 353-362

Tanaka, S., Furukawa, T. & Plotkin, S.A. (1975)   Human cytomegalo-
    virus stimulated host cell DNA synthesis.   *J. Virol.*, *15*,
    297-304

ANALYSIS OF VIRAL GENE FUNCTIONS BY MEANS OF EARLY TEMPERATURE-SENSITIVE MUTANTS OF HUMAN CYTOMEGALOVIRUS

S. IHARA, K. HIRAI & Y. WATANABE

*Department of Molecular Biology,
Tokai University School of Medicine,
Tokai, Japan*

Human cytomegalovirus (CMV) is unique among herpesviruses in that viral replication requires an exceptionally long eclipse period of 2-3 days (Plummer et al., 1969), during which period several virus-mediated events are known to occur, such as early cell rounding (Furukawa et al., 1973), the induction of virus-specific antigens (The et al., 1974) and a virus-specific DNA polymerase (Hirai & Watanabe, 1976; Hirai et al., 1976; Huang, 1975a,b), and the stimulation of cellular DNA and RNA synthesis (DeMarchi & Kaplan, 1976; Hirai & Watanabe, 1976; St. Jeor et al., 1974; Tanaka et al., 1975). In order to explore the significance of these events in the replication of CMV, we have undertaken a study of early temperature-sensitive (*ts*) mutants of CMV. The present paper summarizes the information on: (i) the isolation of *ts* mutants of CMV; (ii) division into DNA$^+$ and DNA$^-$ mutants; and (iii) characterization of DNA$^-$ mutants in respect of several viral functions.

ISOLATION AND GROWTH PROPERTIES OF *ts* MUTANTS OF CMV

Wild-type CMV (Towne strain) was triply plaque-purified on human embryo lung (HEL) cells to obtain genetically homogeneous virus populations. Temperature-sensitive mutants which form plaques at 34°C but not at 39°C were sought after UV-irradiation of wild-type virus at a dose which reduced virus titre to 1-0.5% of the original value, and 15 mutants were obtained out of 528 plaque isolates, as summarized in Table 1. Some mutants exhibited temperature sensitivity at 36°C. The plaque isolate used as wild-type virus in the mutant derivation seemed to be relatively heat-stable; infectivity was reduced at 43°C in 0.8% sodium chloride, 0.05 M tris hydrochloride, pH 7.4, at a rate of

Table 1. Growth properties of *ts* mutants of CMV[a]

Virus	Plaques formed at 34°C (PFU/ml)	Plating efficiency	
		36°C/34°C	39°C/34°C
Wild-type	2.6×10^6	1.4	1.9
ts 197	4.4×10^4	2.3×10^{-4}	1.8×10^{-4}
ts 380	1.1×10^5	1.8	9.1×10^{-5}
ts 589	6.0×10^5	2.2×10^{-3}	1.7×10^{-5}
ts 614	1.6×10^5	1.3	6.3×10^{-5}
ts 256	1.5×10^6	2.2	6.7×10^{-6}
ts 71	5.4×10^4	1.4	1.8×10^{-4}
ts 212	3.4×10^5	1.3	2.9×10^{-5}
ts 442	6.0×10^5	1.0	1.7×10^{-5}
ts 526	5.2×10^4	2.1	1.2×10^{-1}[b]
ts 567	1.6×10^5	0.9[b]	6.3×10^{-5}
ts 569	4.4×10^6	1.1	9.1×10^{-5}[b]
ts 633	3.0×10^5	1.1	3.3×10^{-5}
ts 637	1.0×10^6	1.2	1.0×10^{-5}
ts 664	2.3×10^5	1.3	4.3×10^{-5}
ts 676	1.7×10^6	1.4	5.9×10^{-6}

[a] Each strain was propagated at 34°C and the virus produced was assayed at 34°C, 36°C and 39°C and the results expressed in PFU/ml. Incubation periods for plaque assay were three weeks at 34°C, two weeks at 36°C, and 10 days at 39°C.

[b] Abnormal plaques (tiny aggregates of several rounded cells) formed at 36°C or 39°C and were scored as plaques.

one power of 10 in 5 hours. Although the unpredictable lability of CMV has been frequently reported (Weller, 1971), we have not encountered to date any difficulties in the preservation of stocks of wild-type virus and mutants at −80°C without preservatives.

SEARCH FOR EARLY *ts* MUTANTS OF CMV

Mutants were examined for their ability to synthesize viral DNA in the infected HEL cells at 39°C.   The viral DNA synthesized was determined by hybridization of DNA from the infected cells to a tritiated complementary RNA (^{3}H-cRNA) essentially as described by Hirai et al. (1974).   An example of such an experiment is shown in Figure 1. Five mutants out of 15 failed to produce detectable amounts of viral DNA at 39°C (Table 2).   At present we classify these five mutants as DNA$^-$ and the rest of the mutants as DNA$^+$.

FIG. 1. SYNTHESIS OF VIRAL DNA BY TEMPERATURE-SENSITIVE MUTANTS

Monolayers of infected HEL cells (5 × 10^6) cultured at either 34°C or 39°C were harvested at the indicated times.   DNA was extracted and immobilized on a membrane filter (10 µg DNA/filter), and then hybridized to ^{3}H-cRNA (5 × 10^5 cpm) in 6 × SSC (standard saline citrate) at 68°C for 24 hours.   Membrane-bound ^{3}H was counted.   wt = wild-type virus.

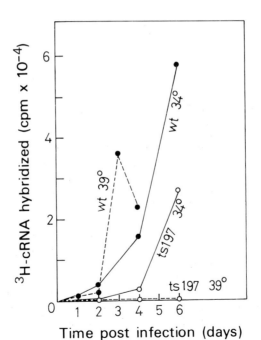

Table 2. Phenotypic characteristics of DNA⁻ mutants of CMV at the non-permissive temperature in comparison with a representative DNA⁺ mutant and wild-type virus

Virus	Complementation group	Viral DNA	Viral DNA polymerase	Early cell rounding	Induction of		Viral antigens		Nuclear[b] inclusion	Capsids in nuclei	
					Cell DNA synthesis	Cell RNA synthesis	EA[a]	LA[a]		Empty	Cored
ts 197	A	−	+	+	+	+	+	−	−	−	−
ts 380	A	−	+	+	+	+	+	−	±	−	−
ts 589	A	−	+	+	+	+	+	−	−	−	−
ts 614	A	−	+	+	+	+	+	−	−	−	−
ts 256	B	−	−	+	+	+	+	±	(+)[c]	+	±
ts 442	−	+	+	+	+	+	+	+	+	+	+
wild-type	−	+	+	+	+	+	+	+	+	+	+

[a] Indirect immunofluorescence patterns observed eight days after infection at 39°C. EA represents a fine granular fluorescence pattern in a nucleus similar to that observed in wild-type virus-infected cells cultured in the presence of 200 µl/ml of phosphonoacetate. LA represents large inclusion-type granules in a nucleus similar to those observed in wild-type virus-infected cells at late stages of infection.

[b] A skein-like structure observed electron microscopically after staining with uranyl acetate and lead citrate (Smith & De Harven, 1973)

[c] Smaller in size than those observed in wild-type virus-infected cells

CAPACITY TO INDUCE CMV-SPECIFIC DNA POLYMERASE

DNA⁻ mutants were tested for their ability to induce virus-specific DNA polymerase which was characterized by both the dependency of its activity on ammonium sulfate and by sensitivity to phosphonoacetic acid in the reaction mixture for polymerase assay (Hirai & Watanabe, 1976; Hirai et al., 1976; Huang, 1975a,b). Among the mutants, ts 256 seemed to have a defect in the induction of DNA polymerase that can be stimulated by ammonium sulfate (Table 3). One interesting feature that emerged was that the activity of DNA polymerase in cells infected with the mutant at 39°C was significantly sensitive to phosphonoacetic acid despite the failure of stimulation by ammonium sulfate. An alternative possibility may be that CMV induces a single species of DNA polymerase which responds to both the effectors, and that the ts 256-induced, altered polymerase is unable to respond only to ammonium sulfate.   Whichever is correct, the results support the concept that the ammonium sulfate-dependent polymerase is a virus-mediated entity and responsible for the replication of CMV DNA.

Table 3. Induction of viral DNA polymerase[a]

Virus	Additions[b]	³H-TMP incorporated							
		Cultured at 34°C				Cultured at 39°C			
		Assayed at 34°C (cpm/50 μg protein)	(% of control)	Assayed at 39°C (cpm/50 μg protein)	(% of control)	Assayed at 34°C (cpm/50 μg protein)	(% of control)	Assayed at 39°C (cpm/50 μg protein)	(% of control)
Mock-infected	-	24 192	100	20 743	100	11 497	100	10 589	100
	AS	5 467	23	4 964	24	2 751	24	1 874	18
	PAA	22 411	93	20 741	100	11 335	99	10 252	98
Wild-type	-	16 993	100	21 587	100	7 165	100	9 710	100
	AS	54 384	320	80 566	373	18 132	253	25 717	265
	PAA	8 603	51	8 631	40	2 827	40	2 049	21
ts 256	-	19 384	100	21 013	100	10 118	100	8 048	100
	AS	35 451	183	59 393	283	2 563	25	2 425	30
	PAA	10 678	54	10 615	51	6 127	60	4 802	60

[a] Virus-infected cells were cultured for 3.5 days at either 34°C or 39°C, and the DNA polymerase activity in the nuclear fraction was determined as described previously (Hirai & Watanabe, 1976), except that the reaction pH was 7.5 and the temperature as indicated. Figures are mean values for duplicate assays.

[b] The concentrations of ammonium sulfate (AS) and phosphonoacetate (PAA) in the reaction mixture were 0.1 M and 25 μg/ml, respectively. Results with other DNA⁻ mutants were essentially similar to those with wild-type virus.

OTHER PHENOTYPIC CHARACTERISTICS OF DNA⁻ MUTANTS

Table 2 gives a summary of the data available to date on the phenotypes of DNA⁻ mutants at the non-permissive temperature. The indirect immunofluorescent (IF) test using sera from hospital patients showed that all the mutants are able to induce virus-specific antigens in infected-cell nuclei at either 34°C or 39°C. Four DNA⁻ mutants showed, however, a fine granular IF pattern which was indistinguishable from an early antigen pattern observed in wild-type virus-infected cells in which viral DNA replication was arrested by phosphonoacetic acid (Hirai et al.[1]), the result further supporting the early defectiveness of these mutants at 39°C. One mutant, ts 256, produced a small inclusion-type fluorescent pattern. A large block of inclusion-type fluorescence which appeared at late stages of wild-type virus infection (no phosphonoacetic acid) was observed with most of the DNA⁺ mutant tested at 39°C.

In accordance with the results of the IF test, electron microscopy (performed by Miss F. Maeda) showed that DNA⁻ mutants, except for ts 256, neither induced noticeable morphological changes in the infected-cell nuclei nor any structure related to virions at 39°C, while ts 256 induced empty capsids in a considerable population of infected cells.

---

[1] Unpublished data

Cellular DNA synthesis, as determined by ^{3}H-thymidine incorporation, was stimulated by all the mutants tested at either 34°C or 39°C.   It follows, therefore, that the induction of cellular DNA synthesis does not require viral DNA replication

COMPLEMENTATION GROUP

Complementation between pairs of DNA$^-$ mutants was carried out by an infectious centre assay essentially according to Brown et al. (1973), and DNA$^-$ mutants were divided into two groups (Table 2), group A corresponding to the DNA polymerase-positive members and group B to the DNA polymerase-negative member.   All the DNA$^-$ mutants complemented well with the DNA$^+$ mutants tested.   Although the infectious centre method cannot distinguish between complementation and recombination, several lines of evidence summarized in Table 2 suggest that groups A and B may be defective in different cistrons.

SUMMARY

Fifteen *ts* mutants of CMV, which are unable to form normal plaques at 39°C on HEL cells but do form plaques at 34°C, have been isolated following mutagenesis by ultraviolet light.   Five mutants defective in viral DNA synthesis at 39°C were divided into two different complementation groups and examined for various phenotypic characteristics.

REFERENCES

Brown, S.M., Ritchie, D.A. & Subak-Sharpe, J.H. (1973)   Genetic studies with herpes simplex virus type 1. The isolation of temperature-sensitive mutants, their arrangement into complementation groups and recombination analysis leading to a linkage map. *J. gen. Virol.*, *18*, 329-346

DeMarchi, J.M. & Kaplan, A.S. (1976)   Replication of human cytomegalovirus DNA: lack of dependence on cell DNA synthesis. *J. Virol.*, *18*, 1063-1070

Furukawa, T., Floretti, A. & Plotkin, S. (1973)   Growth characteristic of cytomegalovirus in human fibroblasts with demonstration of protein synthesis early in viral replication.   *J. Virol.*, *11*, 991-997

Hirai, K., Robb, J.A. & Defendi, V. (1974)   Integration of SV40 and induction of cellular DNA synthesis after a ts SV40 infection. *Virology*, *59*, 266-274

Hirai, K., Furukawa, T. & Plotkin, S.A. (1976)   Induction of DNA polymerase in WI-38 and guinea pig cells infected with human cytomegalovirus (HCMV).   *Virology*, *70*, 251-255

Hirai, K. & Watanabe, Y. (1976)   Induction of α-type DNA polymerases in human cytomegalovirus-infected WI-38 cells.   *Biochim. Biophys. Acta (Amst.)*, *447*, 328-339

Huang, E.-S. (1975a)   Human cytomegalovirus III. Virus-induced DNA polymerase.   *J. Virol.*, *16*, 298-310

Huang, E.-S. (1975b)   Human cytomegalovirus IV. Specific inhibition of virus-induced DNA polymerase activity and viral DNA replication by phosphonoacetic acid.   *J. Virol.*, *16*, 1560-1565

Plummer, G., Goodhert, C.R., Henson, D. & Bowling, C.P. (1969) A comparative study of the DNA density and behavior in tissue cultures of fourteen different herpesviruses.   *Virology*, *39*, 134-137

Smith, J.T. & De Harven, E. (1973)   Herpes simplex virus and human cytomegalovirus replication in WI-38 cells. I. Sequence of viral replication.   *J. Virol.*, *12*, 919-930

St. Jeor, S.C., Albrecht, T.B., Funk, F.D. & Rapp, F. (1974) Stimulation of cellular DNA synthesis by human cytomegalovirus. *J. Virol.*, *13*, 353-362

Tanaka, S., Furukawa, T. & Plotkin, S.A. (1975)   Human cytomegalovirus stimulates host RNA synthesis.   *J. Virol.*, *15*, 293-304

The, T.H., Klein, G. & Langenhuysen, M.M.M.C. (1974)   Antibody reactions to virus-specific early antigens (EA) in patients with cytomegalovirus (CMV) infection.   *Clin. exp. Immunol.*, *16*, 1-12

Weller, T.H. (1971)   The cytomegaloviruses: ubiquitous agents with protean clinical manifestations. *New Engl. J. Med.*, *285*, 203-214

CELL DNA INDUCTION BY HUMAN CYTOMEGALOVIRUS

S. ST. JEOR, L. HERNANDEZ & M. TOCCI

*Department of Microbiology and
Specialized Cancer Research Center,
The Milton S. Hershey Medical Center,
The Pennsylvania State University College of Medicine,
Hershey, Penn., USA*

Recently, this laboratory reported that cytomegalovirus (CMV) induces cell DNA synthesis following both productive and abortive infections and that induction was not dependent upon virus DNA synthesis (St. Jeor et al., 1974). These initial findings have been confirmed by a number of independent laboratories (DeMarchi & Kaplan, 1976; Furukawa et al., 1975a,b). Additional studies by St. Jeor & Hutt (1977) have indicated that a correlation exists between cell and virus DNA synthesis. Other studies have indicated that CMV replication is dependent upon host-cell function; however, whether or not CMV DNA synthesis can occur in the absence of cell DNA synthesis remains in question (DeMarchi & Kaplan, 1976; Furukawa et al., 1975b).

The studies to be reported in this manuscript deal with an analysis of cell DNA induction by human cytomegalovirus.

MATERIALS AND METHODS

Cell and virus culture

All studies to be reported were done in human embryonic lung cells (HEL) using the AD169 strain of human cytomegalovirus. The methods used for virus and cell culture, DNA labelling, and isolation and analysis in caesium chloride gradients and treatment of cells with 5-iodo-2'-deoxyuridine (IUDR) have been previously described (St. Jeor et al., 1974).

DNA-DNA reassociation

DNA-DNA hybridization was conducted as described by Huang & Pagano (1974).

RESULTS

Earlier studies had indicated that to detect the induction of cell DNA synthesis by cytomegalovirus it was necessary to arrest cell DNA synthesis by pretreatment of cells with 100 µgm/ml of IUDR.   After cell replication was arrested, cells in 25-cm^2 plastic tissue-culture flasks, were infected with human CMV at a multiplicity of infection (MOI) of 3 or mock-infected with growth medium.   Following infection the cells were pulsed with sequential 4-hour pulses of ^{3}H-thymidine. The DNA was then isolated, centrifuged to equilibrium in caesium chloride gradients and the total counts for ^{3}H-thymidine incorporated into cell and virus DNA determined.   The results of this study (Fig. 1) indicated a temporal relationship between cell and virus DNA synthesis.   In order to determine what fraction of the cell genome replicates following infection, a density shift study was initiated. This study was conducted in the following manner.   HEL cells were prelabelled with ^{14}C-thymidine, after which they were allowed to replicate in media containing 100 µgm/ml of IUDR.   The presence of IUDR completely inhibits cell DNA replication and cell DNA synthesis can be reinduced only by CMV infection.   The cells were then infected with human CMV and pulse-labelled with ^{3}H-thymidine for consecutive 24-hour periods.   Following the labelling period, the DNA was isolated and centrifuged to equilibrium in caesium chloride gradients.   The data from the 72-96-hour pulse are presented in Fig. 2, where panel B represents the uninfected control and panel A the infected culture. The open circles represent the ^{14}C-thymidine counts and the closed circles the ^{3}H-thymidine counts.   As can be seen in the control, there are two principal peaks containing ^{14}C-thymidine.   The material present in fractions 2-14 represents cell DNA containing IUDR in one strand and ^{14}C-thymidine in the other.   The increased density is due to the incorporation of IUDR into cell DNA.   If this material is placed in an alkaline gradient, the two strands separate and the ^{14}C-thymidine-labelled material bands with unsubstituted cell DNA.   If the entire cell genome were induced by the virus to replicate by semi-conservative DNA synthesis then the ^{14}C-thymidine-substituted strand would function as one parental strand and the IUDR-substituted material as the other parental strand.   Consequently, the ^{14}C-thymidine-substituted strand would separate from the IUDR-substituted strand and band at a density of 1.695 g/cm^3.   If only a portion of the genome was induced by the virus to replicate, then only that portion of the genome labelled with ^{14}C-thymidine and induced by the virus to replicate would shift from the dense to the light position.   New DNA replication is indicated by the presence of ^{3}H-thymidine.   As can be seen in

FIG. 1. RELATIONSHIP BETWEEN CMV AND CELL DNA REPLICATION

Human embryonic lung cells were pretreated with IUDR and infected with CMV. Following infection, cells were labelled with sequential 4-hour pulses of ^{3}H-thymidine. After the labelling period, the DNA was extracted and centrifuged to equilibrium in caesium chloride gradients. The total counts per minute of ^{3}H-thymidine incorporated into cell and virus DNA were determined from plots of the gradient profiles using a Hewlett Packard Calculator, tape reader and plotter. The closed circles (● - ●) represent cell DNA and the open boxes (□ - □) virus DNA.

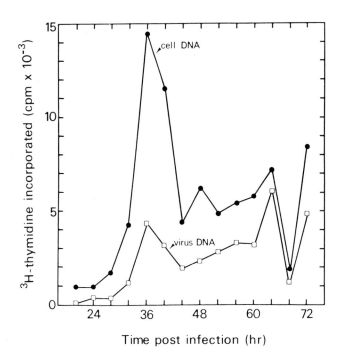

Figure 2, in the uninfected cells the principal area of the gradient where material containing ^{3}H-thymidine banded was in fractions 32-42 (density 1.695 g/cm^3). This represents DNA synthesis occurring only from a DNA template not substituted with IUDR. When the infected cultures are compared to the uninfected cells, it can be seen that cell

FIG. 2.   REPLICATION OF DNA IN IUDR-SUBSTITUTED, ^{14}C-THYMIDINE LABELLED HEL CELLS

Human embryonic lung (HEL) cells were prelabelled with ^{14}C-thymidine and grown in the presence of IUDR.   The cells were infected with the AD169 strain of human CMV and pulse-labelled with ^{3}H-thymidine for consecutive 24-hour periods.   The cultures were harvested, digested and centrifuged to equilibrium in neutral caesium chloride (40.3 rotor, 30 000 rpm, 20°C, 60 hours).   Panel A represents the infected cultures; panel B, the uninfected cultures from the 72-96-hour labelling period. The open circles represent ^{14}C-thymidine labelled material and the closed circles the ^{3}H-thymidine labelled material.

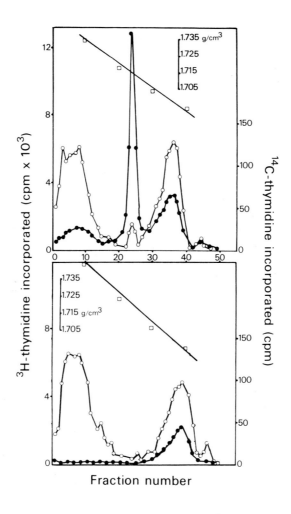

DNA synthesis in the infected cultures occurred at both the light and heavy positions. In addition, it appears that only a fraction of the cell genome was induced by the virus to replicate.

In order to determine the nature of the cell DNA induced by the virus to replicate, the induced cell DNA was examined by DNA-DNA reassociation. Uninfected-cell DNA labelled with ^{14}C-thymidine and infected-cell DNA labelled with ^{3}H-thymidine (purified in caesium chloride density gradients) were mixed. Approximately a 100-fold excess of unlabelled cold normal HEL-cell DNA was added to the reaction mixture. The material was denatured and the DNA-DNA reassociation carried out as described earlier (Huang & Pagano, 1974). The results (Fig. 3) indicated that the cell DNA induced by CMV to replicate contained primarily unique rather than repetitive DNA sequences. In contrast, 15% of the uninfected-cell DNA appeared to reassociate at a $C_{0}t$ of 10 with the majority of the DNA reassociating at a slower rate. The unique cell DNA sequences appear to be the primary species in the virus-induced system.

SUMMARY

The studies presented indicate that in cells pretreated with IUDR: (1) a temporal relationship exists between CMV and cell DNA synthesis; (2) in cells pretreated with IUDR only a fraction of the cell genome is induced by the virus to replicate; and (3) cell DNA induced by the virus to replicate represents unique rather than repetitive DNA sequences.

ACKNOWLEDGEMENTS

This work was supported in part by Contract N01 CP 53516 within the Virus Cancer Program of the National Cancer Institute and by Grant CA 18450 awarded by the National Cancer Institute. S. St. Jeor's work was aided by a Basil O'Connor Starter Research Grant from The National Foundation-March of Dimes.

FIG. 3. KINETICS OF REASSOCIATION OF CMV-INDUCED CELL DNA

Cells either pretreated with IUDR and infected with the AD169
strain of human CMV (^{3}H-thymidine-labelled) or untreated (^{14}C-
thymidine-labelled) were isolated and purified on caesium chloride
gradients (Fig. 1).   The cell DNA was further extracted with phenol,
precipitated with isopropanol and resuspended in 10 mM tris hydrochloride buffer.   A 100-fold excess of cell DNA was added to the
reaction.   The total DNA concentration was 1 mg/ml.   The DNA was
sheared by sonication, denatured by boiling and adjusted to 1.2 M
sodium chloride.   Hybridization was done at 66°C and the fraction
of DNA reassociated analysed by S_1 enzyme digestion.

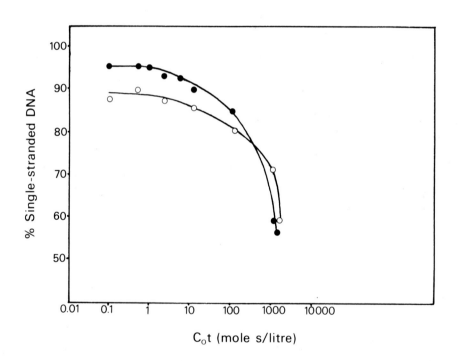

REFERENCES

DeMarchi, J.M. & Kaplan, A.S. (1976)   Replication of human cytomegalovirus DNA: Lack of dependence on cell DNA synthesis.   *J. Virol.*, *18*, 1063-1070

Furukawa, T., Tanaka, S. & Plotkin, S.A. (1975a)   Stimulation of macromolecular synthesis in guinea pig cells by human CMV. *Proc. Soc. exp. Biol. (N.Y.)*, *148*, 211-214

Furukawa, T., Tanaka, S. & Plotkin, S.A. (1975b)   Restricted growth of human cytomegalovirus in UV-irradiated WI-38 human fibroblasts. *Proc. Soc. exp. Biol. (N.Y.)*, *148*, 1248-1251

Huang, E.S. & Pagano, J.S. (1974)   Human cytomegalovirus.   II. Lack of relatedness to DNA of herpes simplex I and II, Epstein-Barr virus, and nonhuman strains of cytomegalovirus.   *J. Virol.*, *13*, 642-645

St. Jeor, S.C., Albrecht, T.B., Funk, F.D. & Rapp, F. (1974) Stimulation of cellular DNA synthesis by human cytomegalovirus. *J. Virol.*, *13*, 353-362

St. Jeor, S.C. & Hutt, R. (1977)   Cell DNA replication as a function in the synthesis of human cytomegalovirus.   *J. gen. Virol.*, *37*, 65-73

EFFECT OF CYCLIC NUCLEOTIDES ON THE RESPONSE OF CELLS TO INFECTION BY VARIOUS HERPESVIRUSES

A.A. NEWTON

Department of Biochemistry,
University of Cambridge,
Cambridge, UK

The same strain of herpesvirus may replicate in one type of cell and not in another; moreover the ability of any one type of cell to support replication of an herpesvirus may vary according to the growth state of the cell. It is therefore possible that factors affecting the growth regulation of cells may influence the replication of herpesviruses within the cell both *in vivo* and in tissue culture. Intracellular concentrations of cyclic nucleotides vary according to the state of growth and differentiation (Pastan et al., 1975) as well as in the response of cells to hormones and stress. We have therefore investigated the effects of alteration of intracellular cyclic nucleotide concentrations on the growth of herpes simplex virus type 1 (HSV-1) in mouse fibroblasts (strain L).

The results of treatment of these cells with agents known to alter the intracellular concentrations of 3'-5' cyclic adenosine monophosphate (cAMP) on the total yield of infectious HSV-1 at 24 hours post infection are shown in Table 1. All compounds tested that increased cAMP levels increased virus yields. However, significant increases were obtained only when cells were treated with compounds causing an increased cAMP level early in the infectious cycle. Of these compounds prostaglandin E_1 (PGE_1) is active at physiological concentrations. cGMP also gave increased virus yields. None of these compounds affected the number of plaques obtained in a standard plaque assay.

Synthesis of viral and cellular DNA in infected cells treated with these agents was studied by incubation of cells with ^{3}H-labelled thymidine; the DNA synthesized at various times after infection was analysed by separation using preparative caesium chloride density-gradient centrifugation. As shown in Figure 1, the early inhibition of host-cell DNA synthesis is enhanced in the presence of PGE_1, but synthesis of viral DNA occurs earlier and to a greater extent than in untreated controls. Infected cells treated with cGMP show no early inhibition of host DNA synthesis but synthesis of viral DNA is enhanced.

Table 1. Effect of cyclic nucleotides on yield of HSV-1 from mouse L cells[a]

Treatment	Yield, compared with control	Comment
0 (control)	1	
1 mM cAMP	1.8, 2.0, 2.9	Cells poorly permeable. Note high concentration.
1 mM cAMP (preincubate 1 hour)	5.2, 3.6, 3.8, 21.0	Cells poorly permeable. Note high concentration.
1 mM theophylline	1, 2.7, 2.0, 1.6	Inhibits phosphodiesterase. Transient elevation in cAMP.
10 μg/ml cholera toxin	1.4, 2.5	Activates adenyl cyclase after long lag.
1 μg/ml prostaglandin E_1	7.2, 8.0, 9.9	Physiological concentration. Rapid rise in cAMP.

[a] Monolayer cultures of L cells were infected with HSV-1 (strain FRA) at an input multiplicity of 1 PFU/cell After 1 hour cells were removed from culture using 0.1% trypsin, washed and resuspended in growth medium with additions as indicated at a density of 10^5/ml. After 24 hours at 37°C cells were collected and disrupted by sonication in 1 ml of distilled water. Cell lysates and growth medium were pooled and the infectivity determined by plaque assay using L-cell monolayers. Yield of virus in control cultures approximately 10 PFU/cell.

The effects of alterations in growth control on the behaviour of chick or duck embryo fibroblasts infected with various herpesviruses have been studied. We have shown previously (Newton & Ross, 1973) that infection of these cells with a tumour-producing strain of Marek's disease virus (MDV) (HPRS-16) results in a stimulation of host-cell DNA synthesis and cell division; cultivation of such infected cultures may be continued for many months (Newton, 1976), but only if cells are maintained under conditions where intracellular cAMP levels are low (sparse cultures, rich medium). Elevation of intracellular cAMP (low serum, theophylline) results in cessation of cell division and synthesis of viral DNA and viral antigens, as shown in Table 2. The attenuated, vaccine strain of MDV (att-HPRS-16) does not stimulate cell division; synthesis of viral DNA occurs under all growth conditions. Treatment with cGMP, however, allows both continued growth and concomitant synthesis of viral DNA, as shown in Figure 2.

These experiments suggest that synthesis of infectious virus and viral DNA may be affected by altering conditions that affect intra-cellular cyclic nucleotide levels in the cell. Furthermore, the effect of the virus on cell behaviour may be modified by altering these conditions. These effects are seen both with HSV-1 and MDV. The growth of herpes simplex virus type 2 (HSV-2) (Costa et al., 1974) and Epstein-Barr virus (EBV) (Zimmerman et al., 1973) is also enhanced

FIG. 1.   EFFECT OF cGMP AND PROSTAGLANDIN E_1 ON INCORPORATION
OF ^{3}H-THYMIDINE BY L CELLS INFECTED WITH HSV-1

Cells were infected at 5 PFU/cell; ^{3}H-thymidine (1 μCi/ml) and
either 1 mM cGMP or PGE_1 (1 μg/ml) were added at the time of
infection;   incorporation of radioactivity into acid-insoluble
material was determined.   ○——○ Control uninfected cells;
●——● Infected cells;   ⊗——⊗ Uninfected cells + mM cGMP;
—— Infected cells + 1 mM cGMP;   ◖——◖ Infected cells + 1 μg/
ml PGE_1

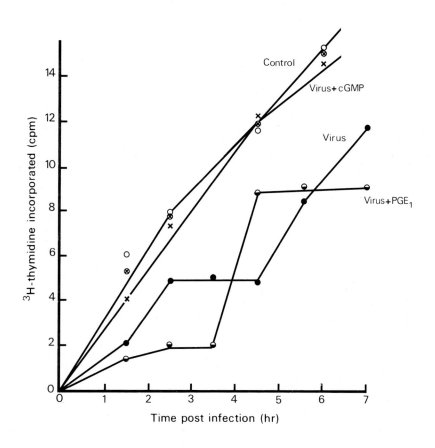

Table 2. Growth of chick cells infected with MDV or HVT[a]

Medium		Control	Virulent virus (HPRS-16)	Attenuated virus (Att-HPRS-16)	Herpesvirus of turkeys (HVT)
10% serum	CD	++	++++	0	0
	VDNA	0	0 continued growth	++	+++
1% serum	CD	0	0	0	0
	VDNA	0	++	++++	++++
10% serum + 1 mM theophylline	CD	0	0	0	ND
	VDNA	0	+++	+	ND
10% serum + 0.2 mM cGMP	CD	+++	ND	++	0
	VDNA	0	ND	+ continued growth	++++

[a] Experiments were initiated by mixing equal samples of control chick embryo fibroblasts with infected cells. Replicate cultures were established. Cell numbers were counted at daily intervals. Viral DNA synthesis was estimated by incubation of cells for 24-hour periods with ^{3}H-thymidine, followed by analysis of radioactive DNA by caesium chloride density-gradient centrifugation. CD: cell division; VDNA: viral DNA synthesis; ND: not done.

by treatments that may affect intracellular cAMP levels. It has also been suggested recently (Blyth et al., 1976) that prostaglandin E_2 may reactivate HSV-1 *in vivo*. It seems possible that the growth of several types of herpesvirus may be affected by cellular control mechanisms modulated by variation in cyclic nucleotide concentration.

FIG. 2.   GROWTH OF DUCK EMBRYO FIBROBLASTS
INFECTED WITH ATTENUATED (HPRS-16) MDV

Cultures were established at day 0 as described for Table 2.
Figures in parentheses denote viral DNA synthesized during the
24-hour period as a percentage of total DNA synthesis.

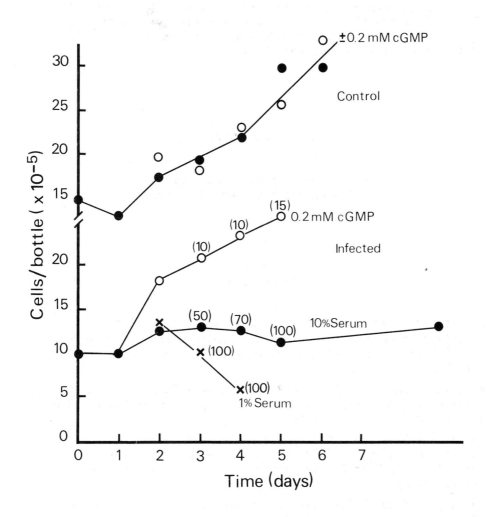

SUMMARY

The effect of varying the intracellular cyclic nucleotide concentration of mouse cells infected with HSV-1 or of duck embryo fibroblasts infected with Marek's disease virus has been studied.   It has
been shown in each case that agents that elevate the intracellular
cAMP levels increase the yield of infectious virus or viral DNA, but
inhibit cell division.   cGMP enhances synthesis of viral DNA but
allows continued synthesis of cell DNA.

ACKNOWLEDGEMENTS

This work was supported by a grant
from the Cancer Research Campaign.

REFERENCES

Blyth, W.A., Hill, T.J., Field, H.J. & Harbour, D.A. (1976)
    Reactivation of Herpes simplex infection by ultraviolet light and
    possible involvement of Prostaglandins.   *J. gen. Virol.*, *33*,
    547-550

Costa, J., Yee, C., Troost, T. & Rabson, A.S. (1974)   Effect of
    dexamethasone on Herpes simplex virus type 2 infection *in vitro*.
    Nature (Lond.), *252*, 745-746

Newton, A.A. (1976)   *Growth stimulation of duck fibroblasts infected
    with Marek's disease virus*.   In: *Abstracts, Third Meeting on
    Herpesviruses*, Cold Spring Harbor, N.Y., Cold Spring Harbor
    Laboratory, p. 59

Newton, A.A. & Ross, L.J.N. (1973)   Stimulation of cell division and
    DNA synthesis in duck cells infected with Marek's disease virus.
    J. gen. Microbiol., *77*, xiv

Pastan, I.H., Johnson, G.S. & Anderson, W.B. (1975)   Role of cyclic
    nucleotides in growth control.   *Ann. Rev. Biochem.*, *44*, 491–522

Zimmerman, J.E., Glaser, R. & Rapp, F. (1973)   Effect of dibutyryl
    cyclic AMP on the induction of Epstein-Barr virus in hybrid
    cells.   *J. Virol.*, *12*, 1442–1445

STUDIES ON EPSTEIN-BARR VIRUS DNA POLYMERASE ACTIVITIES IN VARIOUS HUMAN LYMPHOBLASTOID CELL LINES

T. OOKA & J. DAILLIE

*Département de Biologie Générale et Appliquée,
Université Claude Bernard (Lyon-I),
Villeurbanne, France*

O. COSTA & G. LENOIR

*International Agency for Research on Cancer,
Lyon, France*

INTRODUCTION

Following cell infection by herpes simplex virus (HSV) (Keir et al., 1966), human cytomegalovirus (CMV) (Huang, 1975), Marek's disease herpesvirus (MDV) (Boezi et al., 1974) and equine herpesvirus (Cohen et al., 1975; Kemp et al., 1974), all members of the herpes group, it is known that a new DNA polymerase, which differs with respect to activity and physical properties from the corresponding enzymes of uninfected cells (Allen et al., 1977; Weissbach et al., 1973), is induced.

Epstein-Barr virus (EBV), another herpesvirus, is known to convert normal human and New-World primate B-type lymphocytes into established lines with an unlimited capacity for continuous growth. However, little was known about EBV-induced DNA polymerase. Miller et al. (1977) have recently found an EBV-induced DNA polymerase in iododeoxy-uridine (IUDR)-treated cells which express early antigen (EA), but not in untreated cells. This EBV-induced DNA polymerase possesses the same properties in activity with regard to salt requirements and template-primer specificity as that of other herpesvirus-induced DNA polymerases.

In this paper, we have concentrated on the detection of EBV-directed DNA polymerase activity in three cell lines derived from Burkitt's lymphoma (BL): BJA-B (a negative EBV genome line), Raji (a non-producer line carrying the EBV genome), P3HR-1 (an EBV producer line) and EA-containing cells prepared from Raji cells superinfected with P3HR-1 virus and from P3HR-1 cells following chemical (IUDR) induction.

Our results showed that an EBV-induced DNA polymerase can be found in highly EA-positive cells only.

MATERIALS AND METHODS

Cells

Cells of BJA-B (Menezes et al., 1975), Raji (Pulvertaft, 1965), and the EBV producer P3HR-1 (Hinuma & Grace, 1967) were all grown in RPMI 1640 medium supplemented with 10% heat-inactivated fetal calf serum and antibiotics.

Preparation of cell extracts

All manipulations during the preparation were carried out at 0-4°C. The cells from suspension culture were centrifuged at 600 g for 6 minutes, washed with TKMD buffer (50 mM tris hydrochlo ide, pH 7.5, 10 mM potassium chloride, 1 mM magnesium chloride, 1mM dithiothreitol). After resuspension at 2-3 × 10^8 cells/ml in TKMD, the cells were sonicated with a MSE sonicator for 1 minute. The sonicated suspension was centrifuged at 105 000 g for 60 minutes. The supernatant after this centrifugation was used as a source of DNA polymerase.

DNA polymerase assays

DNA polymerase assays have been described previously (Ooka & Daillie, 1975). Briefly, the reaction mixture contained in a total volume of 125 µl was: 12.5 µmol tris hydrochloride buffer (pH 7.0 for α polymerase conditions and pH 8.5 for viral and β polymerase conditions); 0.5 µmol magnesium chloride; 12.5 µg of activated calf thymus DNA; 6.25 nmol each of dTTP, dGTP, dCTP and dATP containing 0.5 µCi of ^{3}H-dTTP (specific activity 24.5 Ci/mmol) and previously prepared enzyme. To detect viral DNA polymerase activity, 150 mM ammonium sulfate were added in a previous reaction mixture.

RESULTS AND DISCUSSION

Since herpesvirus-induced DNA polymerase activity can be stimulated at high salt concentration whereas cellular DNA polymerase α, β and γ are inhibited under the same conditions (Keir et al., 1966; Weissbach et al., 1973), we tried to use this fact to detect EBV-induced DNA polymerase activity. Potassium chloride, sodium chloride and ammonium sulfate were tested at concentrations of 250 mM for the former two and of 150 mM for the latter (Weissbach et al., 1973). With potassium chloride and sodium chloride, no differences were observed between the lymphoblastoid cell lines examined; about 95% of total activity was inhibited in all cases at both pH levels (data not shown). The results presented in Table 1, however, showed that superinfected Raji and IUDR-treated P3HR-1 cell extracts were partially resistant to 150 mM ammonium sulfate, representing up to 50% of the total DNA polymerase activity at pH 8.5 and 29% at pH 7 in the former and about 5% at any pH in the latter. These resistant activities at high salt concentration were sensitive to N-ethylmaleimide (NEM) (2 mM) and were thus

Table 1. DNA polymerase activities in human lymphoblastoid cell lines

Cell line	Antigen-positive cells (%)		DNA polymerase activity[a] (pmol dTTP incorporated in 30 minutes per mg of protein)			
	EBNA	EA	Total activity	Activity in the presence of 150 mM ammonium sulfate	% resistant	Activity in the presence of 2 mM NEM and 150 mM ammonium sulfate
BJA-B	0	0	pH 7 612	9	1.5	0
			pH 8.5 572	10	1.7	0
Raji	100	0	pH 7 1508	11	0.7	1
			pH 8.5 1143	9	0.8	0
Superinfected Raji[b]	100	60	pH 7 798	232	29.1	2
			pH 8.5 243	133	54.7	1
P3HR-1	100	8	pH 7 1038	11	1.0	1
			pH 8.5 607	6	0.9	0
IUDR-treated P3HR-1[c]	100	21	pH 7 1763	88	5.0	1
			pH 8.5 1149	60	5.2	2

[a] DNA polymerase was assayed as described in Materials and methods. Enzyme activities were tested at two different pH-values (7 and 8.5), using activated DNA as template. Activated DNA was prepared by limited digestion of calf thymus DNA with crystalline pancreatic DNase I following the procedure of Aposhian & Kornberg (1962).

[b] Superinfected with P3HR-1 virus in the presence of cytosine arabinoside (Ara-C) (20 μg/ml)

[c] Treated for 48 hours with IUDR (50 μg/ml)

not a residual activity of β polymerase, which is in general resistant
to NEM (2 mM).   This confirmed the results obtained by Allen et al.
(1977) demonstrating a specific inactivation of equine herpesvirus-
induced DNA polymerase activity by this inhibitor.

The above results show that, of the salts tested, ammonium sulfate
is a better means for the detection of virus-induced DNA polymerase.
It has been demonstrated that EBV-induced DNA polymerase has an optimal
activity at 50 mM ammonium sulfate (Miller et al., 1977) whereas herpesvirus-induced DNA polymerase was detected in 150 mM (Weissbach et al.,
1975).   In the course of our studies on the purification of EBV-induced
DNA polymerase[1] we have also observed a stimulation of EBV-induced DNA
polymerase activity at 50 mM ammonium sulfate in diethylaminoethyl
(DEAE)-cellulose fractions.   However, cellular DNA polymerases again
represent a significant residual activity at the same salt concentration (about 60% of the value observed for α polymerase).   With 150 mM
ammonium sulfate, cellular DNA polymerase activities are almost completely inhibited but virus-induced DNA polymerase is partly resistant.
This implies that the concentration used in our experiment provides the
right conditions specifically for detecting EBV-induced DNA polymerase
activity.

As shown in Table 1, no significant DNA polymerase activities were
detected in the BJA-B, Raji and P3HR-1 cell extracts in the presence of
150 mM ammonium sulfate, so that a correlation between the presence of
EBV-induced DNA polymerase activity and cultures exhibiting a high
level of EA could be expected.   It should be noted that Miller et al.
(1977) have also found EBV-induced polymerase in IUDR-treated D98/HR-1
cells which express about 20% of EA.

REFERENCES

Allen, G.P., O'Callaghan, D.J. & Randall, C.C. (1977)   Purification
    and characterization of equine herpesvirus-induced DNA polymerase.
    Virology, 76, 395-408

Aposhian, H.V. & Kornberg, A.J. (1962)   Enzymatic synthesis of DNA
    (IX) The polymerase found after T2 bacteriophage infection of
    E. Coli: A new enzyme. *J. biol. Chem., 237,* 519-525

Boezi, J.A., Lee, L.F., Blakesley, R.W., Koenig, M. & Towle, H.C. (1974)
    Marek's disease herpesvirus-induced DNA polymerase. *J. Virol.,*
    14, 1209-1219

---

[1] Unpublished data

Cohen, J.C., Perdue, M.L., Randall, C.C. & O'Callaghan, D.J. (1975) Replication of equine herpesvirus type 1: Resistance to hydroxyurea. *Virology, 67*, 56-67

Hinuma, Y. & Grace, J.I. (1967) Clonings of immunoglobulin-producing human leukemic and lymphoma cells in long-term cultures. *Proc. Soc. exp. Biol. (N.Y.), 124*, 107-111

Huang, E.S. (1975) Human cytomegalovirus III. Virus-induced DNA polymerase. *J. Virol., 16*, 298-310

Keir, H.M., Subak-Sharpe, H., Shedden, W.I.H., Watson, D.H. & Wildy, P. (1966) Immunological evidence for a specific DNA polymerase produced after infection by herpes simplex virus. *Virology, 30*, 154-157

Kemp, M.C., Perdue, M.L., Rogers, M.N., O'Callaghan, D.J. & Randall, C. C. (1974) Structural polypeptides of the hamster strain of equine herpesvirus type 1: Products associated with purification. *Virology, 61*, 361-375

Menezes, J., Leibold, W., Klein, G. & Clements, G. (1975) Establishment and characterization of an Epstein-Barr virus (EBV) negative lymphoblastoid B cell line (BJA-B) from an exceptional EBV-genome negative African Burkitt's lymphoma. *Biomedicine, 22*, 276-284

Miller, R.L., Glaser, R. & Rapp, F. (1977) Studies of an Epstein-Barr virus induced DNA polymerase. *Virology, 76*, 494-502

Ooka, T. & Daillie, J. (1975) Studies on changes in DNA polymerase activity during the cell cycle in synchronized KB cells. *Biochimie, 57*, 235-246

Pulvertaft, R.J.V. (1965) A study of malignant tumors in Nigeria by short term tissue culture. *J. clin. Pathol., 18*, 261-273

Weissbach, A., Hong, S.C.L., Aucker, J. & Muller, R. (1973) Characterization of Herpes Simplex Virus-induced deoxyribonucleic acid polymerase. *J. biol. Chem., 243*, 6270-6277

IDENTIFICATION AND PARTIAL PURIFICATION OF TWO EBV-ASSOCIATED DNA POLYMERASES

S.R. GOODMAN, C. PREZYNA & W. CLOUGH

*Sidney Farber Cancer Institute,
Boston, Mass., USA*

MATERIALS AND METHODS

A detailed description of all the experimental procedures will be published elsewhere.

RESULTS AND DISCUSSION

Diethylaminoethyl (DEAE)-cellulose chromatography was performed on crude extracts of log-phase cells in order to compare profiles of enzyme activity among various EBV-positive and EBV-negative lymphocyte lines. Figure 1 shows a new DNA polymerase activity eluting at 210-270 mM potassium metaphosphate, pH 7.5, in P3HR-1 virus producer cells [10% viral capsid antigen (VCA)], but absent in Raji (EBV-positive non-producer), Ramos, and CCRF-CEM (EBV-negative) cell lines. When P3HR-1 is grown under conditions in which the production of the viral capsid antigen (1% VCA) and viral production drops, this new EBV-associated polymerase activity drops correspondingly. This new activity has been found also in the B95-8 producer line (Liversidge[1]). A direct comparison has been made with DEAE-cellulose column profiles of enzymatically active sonicated viral preparations from B95-8 and P3HR-1 cells. Figure 2 shows that the virion-associated polymerase activity elutes from DEAE-cellulose at 45-60 mM potassium metaphosphate.

---

[1] Personal communication

FIG. 1. DEAE-CELLULOSE COLUMN CHROMATOGRAPHY
OF WHOLE-CELL EXTRACTS

Supernatants of crude whole-cell extracts of log-phase cells
(centrifuged at 10 000 rpm) were chromatographed according to the
method of Weissbach et al. (1971) as modified by Goodman & Benz
(unpublished data).

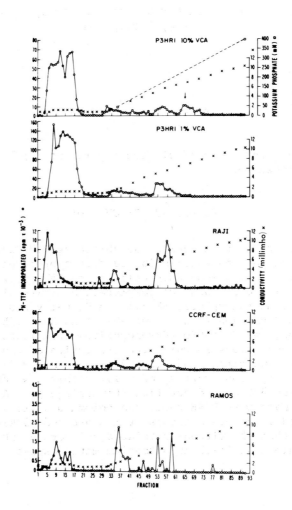

FIG. 2. DEAE-CELLULOSE COLUMN CHROMATOGRAPHY OF SONICATED VIRIONS

Virions from B95-8 or P3HR-1 were purified according to the method of
Dolyniuk et al. (1976).   A mock purification from Ramos cells was
performed using the identical procedure.   The chromatography was
performed as for Figure 1.

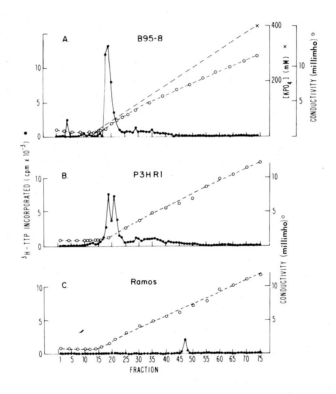

Both the virion-associated enzyme and the virus-induced intracellular enzyme were further characterized by chromatography on phosphocellulose columns.   The former enzyme eluted at 100 mM potassium
metaphosphate, pH 8.0, while the latter eluted at 200 mM potassium
metaphosphate pH 8.0 (data not shown).   The EBV-induced intracellular polymerase elutes from phosphocellulose at the same salt
concentration (200 mM) as the enzymes induced by herpes simplex virus
(Weissbach et al., 1973) and equine herpesvirus (Allen et al., 1977).
After phosphocellulose chromatography an 886-fold purification of the
EBV-induced intracellular polymerase has been achieved.

Sedimentation of both enzymes in 10-30% glycerol gradients in the
presence of 500 mM sodium chloride showed that the two EBV-associated
polymerases had larger S-values than the α, β or γ polymerases present
in lymphocytes (Lewis et al., 1974).   The virion-associated enzyme
formed a broad peak that centred at 9.5S (Fig. 3), and the intracellular EBV-induced polymerase sedimented at 8.3S (Fig. 4).   Both enzymes
are in the 8-10S size range of the intracellular enzyme activity reported by Twardzik et al. (1975) to be present in P3HR-1 producer cells but
not in Raji or Nunn non-producer lines.

FIG. 3. GLYCEROL GRADIENT SEDIMENTATION
OF VIRION-ASSOCIATED POLYMERASE

Concentrated material from the phosphocellulose column was sedimented
in 10-30% glycerol with 500 mM sodium chloride, as will be described
elsewhere.

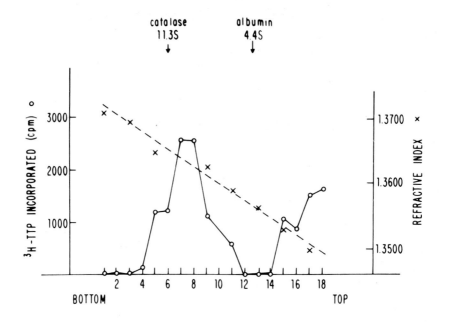

FIG. 4.   GLYCEROL GRADIENT SEDIMENTATION
OF INTRACELLULAR VIRUS-INDUCED POLYMERASE

For procedure, see Figure 3.

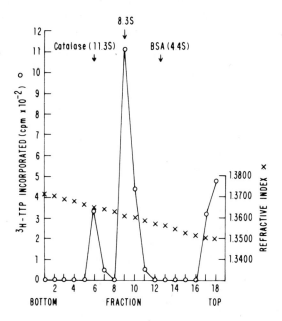

The preliminary biochemical characterization of the partially
purified EBV-induced, virion-associated, α and β polymerases purified
from lymphocytes will now be discussed (Figs 5 & 6 and Tables 1 & 2).
The EBV-induced polymerase can be clearly distinguished from α, β and
the virion-associated polymerase in: (1) being less sensitive to salt
inhibition (Fig. 5);   (2) having a more basic pH optimum in tris buffer
(pH 9.5) as compared with α (7.0), β (8.5) and virion-associated polymerase (8.0);   and (3) copying "activated DNA" far more efficiently
(Table 2).

The EBV virion-associated polymerase can be distinguished from the
other three polymerases because it cannot use artificial initiated
deoxy- and ribohomopolymers as template (Table 2).   The virion-
associated polymerase resembles the Marek's disease-induced polymerase

FIG. 5.   SALT INHIBITION OF DNA POLYMERASES

DNA polymerase assays in 100 μl final volume contained: 80 mM tris,
pH 8.0, 6 mM magnesium acetate, 1 mM dithiothreitol, 0.05% Triton X-100,
10 μM dGTP, 10 μM dATP, 10 μM dCTP, 5 μM ^{3}H-TTP (2000 cpm/pmol) and
15 μg of "activated DNA".   The incubation proceeded at 37°C for 60
minutes.   Detailed information on this assay will be published elsewhere.   Ammonium sulfate was added to the desired final concentration.
α and β polymerase were partially purified from P3HR-1 by the technique
of Weissbach et al. (1971).   100% DNA polymerase activity is the
activity obtained in the absence of ammonium sulfate.
■ EBV-induced DNA polymerase;   □ EBV virion-associated DNA polymerase;
○ α Polymerase;   △ β Polymerase.

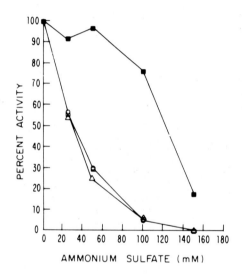

FIG. 6. PAA INHIBITION OF DNA POLYMERASES

DNA polymerase activity was measured using an activated DNA template as described in Figure 5. Disodium phosphonoacetate (Abbott Laboratories) was added to the desired final concentrations. Incubations were 60 minutes at 37°C. 100% Polymerase activity is the activity obtained in the absence of PAA. ■ EBV-induced DNA polymerase; □ EBV virion-associated DNA polymerase; ○ α Polymerase; △ β Polymerase.

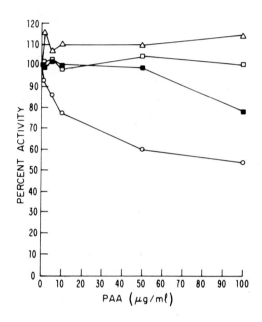

(Boezi et al., 1974) in template specificity (Table 2) and being highly sensitive to salt inhibition (Fig. 5). The virion-associated polymerase is partially inhibited (33%) by 1 mM N-ethyl maleimide, while the EBV-induced polymerase is resistant (3% inhibition) (Table 1).

Neither of the EBV-associated polymerases can copy the ribohomopolymers $dT_{10}poly(rA)$ or $dG_{12-18}poly(rC)$ efficiently as compared to "activated DNA", and therefore they can be distinguished from γ polymerase (Table 2).

GOODMAN ET AL.

Table 1. DNA polymerase reaction requirements[a]

System	EBV-induced polymerase	EBV virion-associated polymerase	α Polymerase	β Polymerase
Complete system	100	100	100	100
- Mg^{2+}	< 1	< 1	< 1	< 1
- Activated DNA	< 1	< 1	< 1	< 1
- dATP	14.2	29.4	27.5	22.2
- dATP, dGTP	10.1	19.9	16.3	13.8
- dATP, dGTP, dCTP	8.0	19.0	9.8	9.9
+ N-ethyl maleimide (1 mM)	97.1	67.1	27.2	88.1

[a] DNA polymerase assays were run using "activated DNA" as described in Figure 5, with the specified omissions and additions. Details of the DNA polymerase assay will be published elsewhere. Values are given as percentages of maximal activity.

Table 2. Template specificities[a]

Template	Final concentration of template (μg/ml)	EBV-induced polymerase	EBV virion-associated polymerase	α Polymerase	β Polymerase
Activated DNA	75	100	100	100	100
Activated DNA	15	76.3	23.7	30.0	25.7
Activated DNA	1	26.9	0.5	2.4	2.9
$dT_{10}poly(dA)$	75	< 1	< 1	3.6	< 1
$dT_{10}poly(rA)$	75	8.2	< 1	6.8	< 1
dT_{12-18}	75	< 1	< 1	< 1	< 1
$dG_{12-18}poly(dC)$	75	164.3	3.9	858.9	89.5
$dG_{12-18}poly(rC)$	75	< 1	< 1	< 1	< 1

[a] The total assay volume was 100 μl, and the final concentrations of components were as follows: 80 mM tris, pH 8.0, 0.5 mM manganese acetate, 1 mM dithiothreitol, 0.05% Triton X-100, 5 mM ^{3}H-GTP (2000 cpm/pmol) or ^{3}H-TTP (2000 cpm/pmol) and 7.5 μg of deoxy- or ribohomopolymer: the assay using activated DNA is described in Figure 5. More detailed information on the DNA polymerase assay will be published elsewhere. All incubations were at 37°C for 60 minutes. Values are percentages of maximal activity.

The EBV-induced, virion-associated, and β polymerases are unaffected by antibody prepared in rabbits against HeLa cell α polymerase, while α polymerase from P3HR-1 or Raji are substantially inhibited (40 and 44% inhibition) (Table 3).

Table 3.   Inhibition by α polymerase antibody[a]

Enzyme	Source	Antibody	^{3}H-TTP incorporated (cpm)	% Activity
α Polymerase	P3HR-1	-	97 312	100
-		+	58 746	60.4
α Polymerase	Raji	-	29 336	100
		+	16 520	56.3
β Polymerase	P3HR-1	-	83 435	100
		+	95 762	114.8
EBV-induced polymerase	P3HR-1	-	31 456	100
		+	33 313	105.9
EBV virion-associated polymerase	P3HR-1	-	6328	100
		+	6367	100.6
	B95-8	-	7011	100
		+	8652	123.4

[a] DNA polymerases were challenged with antibody prepared in rabbits against HeLa cell α polymerase.   10 μl of enzyme was preincubated with 5 μl of bovine serum albumin (10 mg/ml), 5 μl of 20 mM tris, pH 7.5, and 20 μl of antibody (8 mg/ml IgG protein). For control reactions, unimmunized rabbit IgG (8 mg/ml protein) was used in place of antibody.   Preincubation was for 10 minutes at 24°C; 160 μl of the activated DNA reaction mixture (see Fig. 5) was added, and the incubation was at 37°C for 60 minutes. The method of measuring the DNA polymerase activity will be described elsewhere.

Phosphonoacetic acid (PAA) inhibits several herpesvirus–induced DNA polymerases *in vitro* (Allen et al., 1977; Bolden et al., 1975; Huang, 1975b); host-cell α polymerase is also sensitive to PAA while β polymerase is highly resistant.   In the case of Epstein-Barr virus, PAA: (1) inhibits VCA production with no effect upon early antigen (EA); (2) inhibits the production of transforming virus; and (3) decreases the number of viral genome copies per cell in a producer line (Nyormoi et al., 1976; Summers & Klein, 1976).   As shown in Figure 6, the EBV-induced polymerase is inhibited by high levels of PAA (23% inhibition at 100 μg/ml PAA), but appears less sensitive than the host α polymerase (46% inhibition at 100 μg/ml).   Whether or not the EBV-induced DNA polymerase is the *in vivo* target site for PAA cannot yet be answered definitively.   It is, however, interesting that DNA synthesizing nuclei isolated from EBV-producer (P3HR-1 and B95-8), EBV-positive non-producer (Raji) and EBV-negative (CCRF-CEM) lines all show identical patterns of PAA inhibition (Benz[1]).

---

[1] Unpublished data

SUMMARY

   Virally induced DNA polymerases have been demonstrated in cells
infected with a variety of herpesviruses.   These include herpes
simplex virus (Weissbach et al., 1973), Marek's disease virus (Boezi
et al., 1974), equine herpesvirus (Allen et al., 1977), and cytomegalovirus (Huang, 1975a).   Recently a new iododeoxyuridine (IUDR)-induced
intracellular DNA polymerase in an Epstein-Barr virus (EBV)-producing
hybrid cell line has also been reported (Miller et al., 1977).   We
present evidence that there are two different DNA polymerase activities
associated with EBV, one intracellular and the other virion-associated.
Both of these enzymes have certain biochemical characteristics which
distinguish them from each other, and from the host-cell DNA polymerases found in lymphocytes.

ACKNOWLEDGEMENTS

This work was supported by the Sidney Farber Cancer Institute,
   National Institutes of Health grant No. 5T32CA09172, and the
   Medical Foundation Incorporated, Boston.   The authors wish
    to thank Arthur Weissbach for kindly sending antibody
       raised against HeLa cell α polymerase. We should
        also like to thank V. Celeste Carter for her help
                 in preparing the manuscript.

REFERENCES

Allen, G.P., O'Callaghan, D.J. & Randall, C.C. (1977)   Purification
    and characterization of equine herpesvirus-induced DNA polymerase.
    Virology, 76, 395-408

Boezi, J.A., Lee, L.F., Blakesley, R.W., Koenig, M. & Towle, H.C.
    (1974)   Marek's disease herpesvirus-induced DNA polymerase.
    J. Virol., 14, 1209-1219

Bolden, A., Aucker, J. & Weissbach, A. (1975)   Synthesis of herpes simplex virus, vaccinia virus, and adenovirus DNA in isolated HeLa cell nuclei. I. Effect of viral-specific antisera and phosphonoacetic acid. *J. Virol.*, *16*, 1584-1592

Dolyniuk, M., Pritchett, R. & Kieff, E. (1976)   Proteins of Epstein-Barr virus. I. Analysis of the polypeptides of purified enveloped Epstein-Barr virus. *J. Virol.*, *17*, 935-949

Huang, E.S. (1975a)   Human cytomegalovirus. III. Virus-induced DNA polymerase. *J. Virol.*, *16*, 298-310

Huang, E.S. (1975b)   Human cytomegalovirus. IV. Specific inhibition of virus-induced DNA polymerase activity and viral DNA replication by phosphonoacetic acid. *J. Virol.*, *16*, 1560-1565

Lewis, B.J., Abrell, J.W., Smith, R.G. & Gallo, R.C. (1974)   DNA polymerases in human lymphoblastoid cells infected with simian sarcoma virus. *Biochim. Biophys. Acta (Amst.)*, *349*, 148-160

Miller, R.L., Glaser, R. & Rapp, F. (1977)   Studies of an Epstein-Barr virus-induced DNA polymerase. *Virology*, *76*, 494-502

Nyormoi, O., Thorley-Lawson, D., Elkington, J. & Strominger, J.L. (1976)   Differential effect of phosphonoacetic acid on the expression of Epstein-Barr viral antigens and virus production. *Proc. nat. Acad. Sci. (Wash.)*, *73*, 1745-1748

Summers, W.C. & Klein, G. (1976)   Inhibition of Epstein-Barr virus DNA synthesis and late gene expression by phosphonoacetic acid. *J. Virol.*, *18*, 151-155

Twardzik, D.R., Aaslestad, H.G., Tureckova, M.I., Gravell, N., Ablashi, D.V. & Levine, P.H. (1975)   *Comparison of DNA polymerase activities from an American Burkitt's lymphoma cell line and EBV producer and nonproducer cells.* In: de-Thé, G., Epstein, M.A. & zur Hausen, H., eds, *Oncogenesis and Herpesviruses II, part 1*, Lyon, International Agency for Research on Cancer (*IARC Scientific Publications* No. 11), pp. 237-243

Weissbach, A., Schlabach, A., Fridlender, B. & Bolden, A. (1971)   DNA polymerases from human cells. *Nature new Biol.*, *231*, 167-170

Weissbach, A., Hong, S.L., Aucker, J. & Muller, R. (1973)   Characterization of herpes simplex virus-induced DNA polymerase. *J. biol. Chem.*, *248*, 6270-6277

HERPESVIRUS PRODUCTION BY ULTRAVIOLET-IRRADIATED HUMAN SKIN CELLS: A MARKER OF REPAIR

J. COPPEY & S. NOCENTINI

Fondation Curie-Institut du Radium,
Paris, France

G. MORENO

Institut de Pathologie Cellulaire,
Le Kremlin-Bicêtre, France

The impairment of herpes simplex virus (HSV) type 1 replication in cells irradiated with ultraviolet (UV) light just before infection is due to damage to host-cell DNA (Coppey, 1977; Coppey & Nocentini, 1976; Lytle & Benane, 1975; Lytle et al., 1976). When the time interval between UV exposure and infection is increased a recovery of HSV production capacity occurs in monkey cells (Bockstahler et al., 1976; Coppey & Nocentini, 1976) and in skin cells from normal subjects, but not in repair-deficient cells from xeroderma pigmentosum (XP) patients (Lytle et al., 1976).

We have measured here the HSV yield corresponding to the first cycle (18 hours) in human skin cells from different origins infected at various time intervals after UV-irradiation.

The following cultures were tested at passages 5-15 of subcultiva-- tion: CRL 1121 and CRL 1295 (normal donors), CRL 1200 (XP group D), from the American Type Culture Collection; Du..., mother of two XP patients, presumed heterozygous for XP, XP Du... (male, 2 years), and XP RU... (female, 8 years), three lines provided by Dr Schnitzler (France); and XP Di... (male, 15 years), provided by Professor Beurey (France).

Confluent cultures ($3\text{--}4 \times 10^4$ cells/cm^2) were UV-irradiated at indicated times before infection (= time 0) as described (Coppey & Nocentini, 1976).   All strains yielded $1\text{--}1.5 \times 10^3$ plaque-forming units per cell (for method, see Coppey, 1972).   The techniques used for autoradiography are described elsewhere (Nocentini, 1976).

RESULTS

Unscheduled DNA synthesis (UDS)

The initial UDS was comparable in the two normal, XP heterozygous and XP Di... lines, whereas it was low in XP lines Du..., CRL 1200 (10%) and Ru... (1%) (Table 1).

Table 1. Unscheduled DNA synthesis in cells in G_1 and G_2 phases after UV irradiation[a]

Cell line	Dose of UV (J/m^2)					
	0	2	5	10	24	48
CRL 1121 (normal)[b]	0.7 ± 0.1	8 ± 0.5	13.4 ± 1.2	15.6 ± 0.8	25.6 ± 1.2	18.8 ± 1.3
CRL 1295 (normal)[b]	0.3 ± 0.1	14.2 ± 1.2	23.4 ± 1.1	32.9 ± 1.2	50.2 ± 3.2	42.9 ± 3.3
Du... (XP heterozygote)[c]	0.7 ± 0.2	7.4 ± 0.4	16 ± 0.7	21 ± 1.5	23.6 ± 1.6	24 ± 1.2
Du... (XP)[c]	0.6 ± 0.1	1.6 ± 0.1	1.5 ± 0.2	2.1 ± 0.2	2 ± 0.1	3.8 ± 0.3
Ru... (XP)[c]	0.5 ± 0.1	0.7 ± 0.2	0.4 ± 0.1	0.3 ± 0.1	0.3 ± 0.1	0.4 ± 0.1
1200 (XP group D)[b]	0.2 ± 0.1	1.5 ± 0.1	1 ± 0.2	2.5 ± 0.2	-	3 ± 0.3
Di... (XP)[d]	0.4 ± 0.1	-	16.6 ± 1.2	26.2 ± 1.6	35.6 ± 2.2	41.4 ± 3.5

[a] Average number of grains per nucleus ± the standard error of the mean.   Only nuclei with 60 or less grains were included.

[b] From the American Type Culture Collection

[c] From Angers, France

[d] Fram Nancy, France

UDS decreased faster 24 and 48 hours after irradiation in XP heterozygous than in normal and XP Di... cultures (Table 2).

HSV production

At time 0, HSV production capacity was more resistant to UV-irradiation in XP heterozygous than in normal cultures.   This capacity was progressively recovered after irradiation (Fig. 1). The extent of recovery decreased with increasing UV doses and was

Table 2. Unscheduled DNA synthesis at different time intervals after UV irradiation (24 J/m^2)^a

Cell line	Time interval after UV exposure (hr)			
	0 - 3	12 - 15	24 - 27	48 - 51
CRL 1121 (normal)	100 (6.9^b)	24.6 ± 3.1	15.9 ± 2.8	5.8 ± 1.4
CRL 1295 (normal)	100 (7.6^b)	15.8 ± 2.5	7.9 ± 2	11 ± 2.2
Du... (mother of XP patient)	100 (6.3^b)	17.5 ± 2.8	1.4 ± 0.8	2.4 ± 0.6
Di... (XP patient)	100 (9.9^b)	16.2 ± 2	9.3 ± 3.1	5 ± 1.3

^{a} Values are expressed as percentages of the initial amounts of UDS (0-3 hours) ± the standard error.

^{b} Actual average number of grains per nucleus

FIG. 1.   EFFECT OF UV-IRRADIATION BEFORE HSV INFECTION
ON VIRUS YIELD

Virus yields per petri dish from different cultures exposed to a single UV dose of 24 J/m^2 at the indicated times before infection with HSV (time 0).   (●) CRL 1295 (normal);   (■) Du... mother (XP heterozygote)

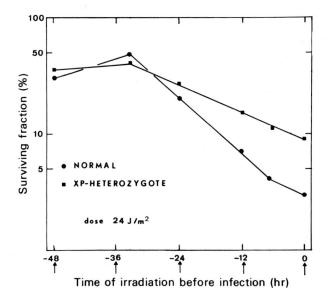

lower in XP heterozygous than in normal cells (Table 3).   In contrast,
in UDS-deficient strains, this capacity decreased with increasing time
intervals between UV-exposure and infection (Fig. 2A).   A linear

Table 3. Recovery of herpesvirus synthetic capacity in UV-irradiated
human skin cells[a]

Cell line	Donor	UV dose (j/m^2)			
		24	36	48	60
CRL 1121	Normal	16	8.5	2.2	2.1
CRL 1295	Normal	19	5.7	3	2
Du...	Mother of XP patient	5.2	4.5	1.3	1.4

[a] Recovery ratio of HSV production capacity =

$$\frac{\text{Virus yield in cells UV-irradiated 36 hr before infection}}{\text{Virus yield in cells UV-irradiated at time 0}}$$

(mean values of two separate experiments)

relation was obtained when the 24-hour rate of decrease (graphically
calculated) was plotted against the UV dose for the three XP lines
tested (Fig. 3).

    In UDS-competent XP Di... cells, HSV production capacity, which
was highly resistant to UV at time 0, recovered after an initial
fall over a period of six hours.   The final extent of recovery was
very low, as compared with that of the normal lines (Fig. 2B).

                              DISCUSSION

    The HSV yield corresponding to the first cycle (18 hours) is
related to the extent of the lesions remaining in the DNA of UV-
irradiated CV-1 cells during the time of viral DNA synthesis (Coppey
& Nocentini, 1976).   We have measured this production as a probe for
analysing the repair process in UV-irradiated human cells.   We have
observed a lower extent of recovery in a XP heterozygous line (which
has a normal UDS) than in those of two normal donors.   It has been
shown that the repair synthesis of such XP heterozygous lines was
slightly reduced (Cleaver, 1970; Kleijer et al., 1973), whereas
their capacity to repair UV-irradiated adenovirus was not impaired

FIG. 2. EFFECT OF UV-IRRADIATION BEFORE HSV INFECTION
ON VIRUS YIELD (VARIOUS UV DOSES)

Virus yields per petri dish from different cultures exposed to a
single UV dose of the amounts shown at the indicated times before
infection with HSV.
(A) Du... XP;   (B) Di... XP

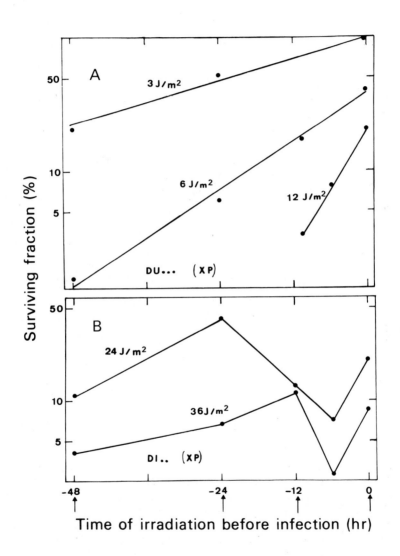

FIG. 3.   RATE OF DECREASE OF VIRUS YIELDS PER PETRI DISH PER DAY AS
A FUNCTION OF UV DOSE IN THE THREE EXCISION REPAIR-DEFICIENT XP LINES
(■) Du...;   (●) CRL 1200 group D;   (▲) Ru...

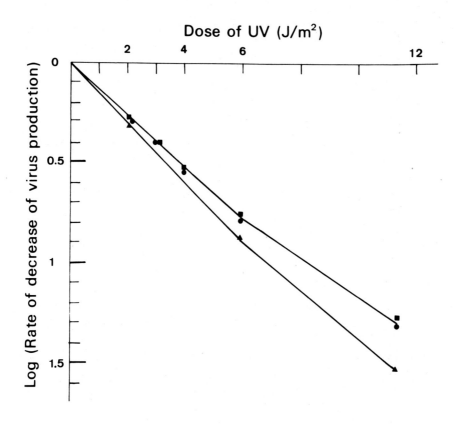

(Day, 1974).   Moreover, in a UDS-competent XP line, i.e., probably a
variant (Cleaver, 1972; Robbins et al., 1974), recovery of HSV production capacity was impaired by 80-90%.   Survival of other variants
was only 20-30% more sensitive to UV (Lehman et al., 1977) and their
capacity to repair UV-irradiated adenovirus was decreased by 30-40%
(Day, 1975).   Finally, in UDS-deficient XP lines, a "negative"
recovery of HSV production capacity was observed.

Thus, the measurement of this cellular capacity appears to be a very sensitive probe for detecting differences in the ability of UV-irradiated human skin cell lines to repair damaged DNA.

ACKNOWLEDGEMENTS

This work was supported by grants ATP-76-60 and
CRL 74.5.006.01 from INSERM. Thanks are due
to C. Baroche and F. Vinzens for
technical assistance.

REFERENCES

Bockstahler, L.E., Lytle, C.D., Stafford, J.E. & Haynes, K.F. (1976) Ultraviolet enhanced reactivation of a human virus: effect of delayed infection. *Mutation Res., 35,* 189-198

Cleaver, J.E. (1970) DNA repair and radiation sensitivity in human (xeroderma pigmentosum) cells. *Int. J. radiat. Biol., 18,* 557-565

Cleaver, J.E. (1972) Xeroderma Pigmentosum: variants with normal DNA repair and normal sensitivity to ultraviolet light. *J. invest. Dermat., 58,* 124-128

Coppey, J. (1972) Growth of Newcastle disease and herpes virus and interferon production in a monkey-mouse hybrid line. *J. gen. Virol., 14,* 9-14

Coppey, J. (1977) Common precursor pathways of Herpes DNA and of repair synthesis in ultraviolet irradiated cells. *Nature (Lond.), 265,* 260-262

Coppey, J. & Nocentini, S. (1976) Herpes virus and viral DNA synthesis in ultraviolet light irradiated cells. *J. gen. Virol., 32,* 1-15

Day, R.S. (1974) Studies on repair of adenovirus 2 by human fibroblasts using normal, xeroderma pigmentosum, and xeroderma pigmentosum heterozygous strains. *Cancer Res., 34,* 1965-1970

Day, R.S. (1975)   Xeroderma pigmentosum variants have decreased
    repair of ultraviolet-damaged NDA.   *Nature (Lond.), 253,* 748-749

Kleijer, W.J., de Weerd-Kastelein, E.A., Sluyter, M.L., Keijzer, W.,
    de Wit, J. & Bootsma, D. (1973)   UV-induced DNA repair synthesis
    in cells of patients with different forms of xeroderma pigmentosum
    and of heterozygotes.   *Mutation Res., 20,* 417-428

Lehman, A.R., Kirk-Bell, S., Arlett, C.F., Harcourt, S.A., de Weerd-
    Kastelein, E.A., Keijzer, W. & Hall-Smith, P. (1977)   Repair of
    ultraviolet light damage in a variety of fibroblast cell strains.
    Cancer Res., 37, 904-910

Lytle, C.D. & Benane, S.G. (1975)   Effect of photoreactivating light
    on virus infection of UV-exposed potoroo cells.   *Int. J. radiat.
    Biol., 26,* 487-491

Lytle, C.D., Day, R.S., Hellman, K.B. & Bockstahler, L.E. (1976)
    Infection of UV-irradiated xeroderma pigmentosum fibroblasts by
    herpes simplex virus: study of capacity and Weigle reactivation.
    Mutation Res., 36, 257-264

Nocentini, S. (1976)   Inhibition and recovery of ribosomal RNA
    synthesis in ultraviolet irradiated mammalian cells.   *Biochim.
    Biophys. Acta (Amst.), 454,* 114-128

Robbins, J.H., Kraemer, K.H., Lutzner, M.A., Festoff, B.W. & Coon, H.
    G. (1974)   Xeroderma pigmentosum.   An inherited disease with sun
    sensitivity, multiple cutaneous neoplasms and abnormal DNA repair.
    Ann. intern. Med., 80, 221-248

REPAIR OF SINGLE-STRANDED BREAKS IN HOST DNA WHEN RABBIT KIDNEY CELLS ARE INFECTED WITH HERPES SIMPLEX VIRUS TYPE 2

A.D. KELMAN, C.M. GUNDBERG & F. MAROTT SINEX

Boston University School of Medicine,
Boston, Mass., USA

We have recently described a preformed herpes simplex virus type 2 (HSV-2) virion-associated factor, probably an endonuclease, which scissions host chromosomes in rabbit kidney (RK) cells infected by HSV-2 (Gundberg et al., 1977). We now report on the ability of RK cells to repair this HSV-2 induced damage. Demonstration of un- scheduled DNA synthesis was first recognized as follows. Confluent plates of RK cells were pulsed for two hours with 15 μc/ml ^{3}H-thymidine at timed intervals after infection. The cells were immediately lysed and tritium-labelled DNA was then examined analytically by the use of rate zonal alkaline sucrose gradient centrifugation under optimal conditions for sedimentation of mammalian cell DNA. At 0-2 hours post infection, there was an 18($\pm$ 2)% increase of ^{3}H-thymidine incorporation into high molecular-weight DNA as compared to mock-infected cells; 2-4 hours post infection the increase was 25($\pm$ 2)%; 4-6 hours post infection the increase was 45($\pm$ 3)%; while 6-8 hours post infection there was only a 5($\pm$ 1)% increase of incorporated radioactivity as compared with mock-infected cells.

To distinguish between semi-conservative replication or repair of DNA, a modification of the methods of Painter & Cleaver (1967) and Roberts et al. (1971) was used. Incorporation of bromodeoxyuridine (BUDR) plus ^{3}H-thymidine produces no increase in density of the DNA for repair synthesis, yet significantly increases the density of DNA during semi-conservative replication. "Light" DNA can be distinguished from "heavy" DNA by equilibrium density-gradient centrifugation. To exclude "fork" artefacts of labelling of DNA, cells were grown in the presence of BUDR for one hour prior to and one hour following the addition of the ^{3}H-thymidine plus BUDR pulse.

When rabbit kidney cells were infected with HSV-2 for a total of six hours and pulsed with BUDR and ^{3}H-thymidine, as described above, the amount of DNA yielded was 47 ± 5 µg (specific activity = 0.76 µCi/µmol). Mock-infected cells yielded 53.2 ± 4.0 µg of DNA (specific activity = 0.42 µCi/µmol). HSV-2 infected ^{3}H-RK DNA (7.0 µg) or the same amount of mock-infected ^{3}H-RK DNA was combined with 0.3 µg of marker ^{14}C-RK DNA and banded on an alkaline caesium chloride gradient. Mock-infected ^{3}H-RK DNA banded at a density of 1.834 g/cm[3] whereas the marker ^{14}C-RK DNA banded at a density of 1.720 g/cm[3]. This indicates that any incorporation of label into mock-infected RK DNA was a consequence of semiconservative replication. In the HSV-2 infected ^{3}H-RK DNA 45(± 3)% of the DNA banded at a density of 1.832 g/cm[3] whereas 51(± 3)% of the DNA banded at a lower density (see Fig. 1). This means that, in HSV-2 infected cells, the entire amount of increase of ^{3}H-thymidine incorporation as compared with mock-infected cells was due to a stimulation of repair synthesis. This is in good agreement with the higher specific activity of the DNA of HSV-2 infected cells (0.76 µCi/µmol versus 0.42 µCi/µmol in infected versus mock-infected cells).

The DNA peaks from these caesium chloride gradients were pooled, and recentrifuged on another alkaline caesium chloride gradient as before. Figures 1C and 1D show the results of this experiment. All the DNA from HSV-2 infected RK cells which originally banded in the region of light DNA remained in that region upon rebanding. Similar results were achieved when ^{3}H-deoxycytidine was substituted for ^{3}H-thymidine in the pulse label with BUDR. Therefore, we conclude that ^{3}H-deoxynucleoside incorporation into RK DNA after HSV-2 infection was indeed a consequence of repair replication.

Some bacteriophages have the capability of adding nucleotides to the terminal ends of the DNA of their host (Kornberg, 1974). The possibility exists that herpesvirus also has this ability. If this is the case, then the activity observed in the "light" fraction of the caesium chloride gradients may have been due to short fragments of terminally added nucleotides in RK DNA. To test this possibility the prepared RK DNA was subjected to a 3' or 5' limited digestion with spleen and venom phosphodiesterase. Uniformly ^{3}H-labelled RK DNA was used as a standard for comparison with mock-infected or virally infected RK DNA. ^{3}H-RK DNA (1.6 µg) was used as substrate for these enzymes. Table 1 shows the results of these experiments.

Digestion of RK DNA with spleen or venom phosphodiesterase is linear up to one minute. At 0.5 minutes, 0.6% of the radioactivity from both mock-infected or HSV-infected RK DNA was solubilized by either enzyme. This is inconsistent with the hypothesis that HSV-2 causes the terminal addition of free nucleotides to the host DNA. There was a 45% increase in incorporated radioactivity into host DNA after viral infection, which was attributed to repair synthesis. If the radioactive nucleotides were in fact added to the 3' and 5' ends, digestion of the terminal portions of the HSV-2 RK DNA would have produced a large increase in solution radioactivity.

FIG. 1.   DEMONSTRATION OF REPAIR OF RK CHROMOSOMES
AFTER HSV-2 INFECTION

RC cells were infected with HSV-2 (multiplicity of infection = 1) for
a total of six hours.   During this period they were treated with BUDR
(one hour) then BUDR + ^{3}H-thymidine (four hours) then BUDR alone (one
hour) and then total DNA was prepared.   Alkaline caesium chloride
density gradients of DNA labelled with ^{3}H-thymidine contained 0.3 μg
of ^{14}C-RK DNA (16 000 dpm) as a marker (open circles) and 7.0 μg of
mock-infected ^{3}H-RK DNA (21 000 dpm) or 7.0 μg of HSV-2 infected
^{3}H-RK DNA (35 000 dpm) closed circles.   A. Mock-infected cells;
B. HSV-2 infected cells; C. Reband of A (light band); D. Reband of
B (light band).

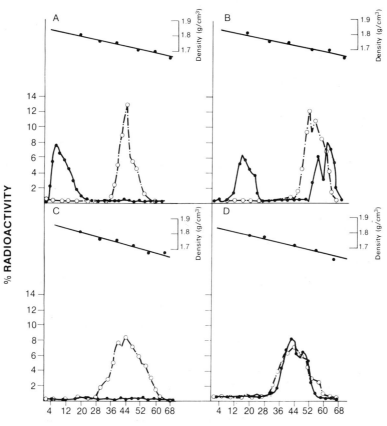

Table 1. Attempts to preferentially remove incorporated ^{3}H-thymidine "repair" label from DNA by exonuclease attack

A. Spleen phosphodiesterase digestion[a]

Incubation time (min)	% Radioactivity released from uniformly labelled DNA (100% = 90 000 dpm)	% Radioactivity released from MI-RK DNA (100% = 5 000 dpm)	% Radioactivity released from HSV-RK DNA (100% = 8 000 dpm)
0	0	0	0
0.5	6.2 ± 0.4	0.6 ± 0.1	0.6 ± 0.1
1.0	17.1 ± 0.4	9.2 ± 0.3	6.1 ± 0.3
2.0	21.8 ± 0.6	11.7 ± 0.3	7.5 ± 0.3
5.0	26.8 ± 0.8	15.0 ± 0.4	10.2 ± 0.3
10.0	27.4 ± 0.8	16.6 ± 0.4	10.8 ± 0.3

B. Venom phosphodiesterase digestion[b]

0	0	0	0
0.5	5.0 ± 0.3	0.6 ± 0.1	0.6 ± 0.1
1.0	10.5 ± 0.3	9.7 ± 0.3	6.6 ± 0.2
2.0	21.0 ± 0.6	16.5 ± 0.4	10.8 ± 0.3
5.0	27.3 ± 0.8	20.4 ± 0.6	13.6 ± 0.3
10.0	29.3 ± 0.8	22.9 ± 0.6	14.3 ± 0.3

[a] 1.6 µg of ^{3}H-labelled RK DNA incubated at 37°C with 7×10^{-4} µg enzyme. The reaction was stopped at intervals shown.

[b] 1.6 µg of ^{3}H-labelled RK DNA incubated at 37°C with 1.1×10^{-5} units enzyme. The reaction was stopped at intervals showns.

MI = Mock-infected

Molar concentrations of 10^{-5}, 10^{-6}, and 10^{-7}, 17 β-oestradiol were added to mock-infected and HSV-2 infected cells during the entire six-hour BUDR incubation period. In mock-infected cells, the amount of radioactivity incorporated into DNA was not affected by oestrogen. This radioactivity represents semi-conservative replication as seen in Figure 2A, C and E. In HSV-2 infected RK cells, 10^{-5} M oestradiol completely inhibited repair replication (Fig. 2B) while 10^{-6} M oestradiol decreased it by approximately 11% (Fig. 2D), and 10^{-7} M oestradiol had no effect upon DNA repair in this system (Fig. 2F).

FIG. 2. HORMONAL SUPPRESSION OF REPAIR OF HOST DNA
IN HSV-2 INFECTED CELLS

Effect of oestradiol on repair synthesis in HSV-2 infected RK cells.
Gradients contained 0.3 μg of ^{14}C-RK DNA (16 000 dpm) as a marker
(open circles), 7.0 μg of HSV-2 infected ^{3}H-RK DNA (25 000-35 000 dpm)
(closed circles), and 7.0 μc of mock-infected ^{3}H-RK DNA (21 000 dpm)
(triangles). A. Mock-infected RK cells, 10^{-5} M oestradiol;
B. HSV-2 infected RK cells, 10^{-5} M oestradiol; C. mock-infected RK
cells, 10^{-6} M oestradiol; D. HSV-2 infected RK cells, 10^{-6} M
oestradiol; E. Mock-infected RK cells, 10^{-7} M oestradiol; F. HSV-2
infected RK cells, 10^{-7} M oestradiol.

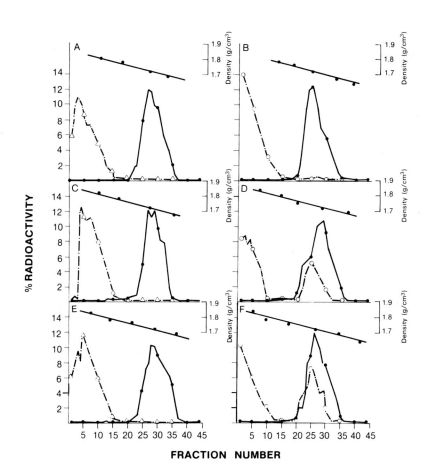

Although repair synthesis was diminished at these levels of oestrogen, the amount of semi-conservative replication was increased by 6% with 10^{-6} M oestradiol and 20% with 10^{-5} M oestradiol. These concentrations of oestradiol have no effect, however, on the plaquing efficiency of HSV-2 in RK cells.

CONCLUSIONS

^{3}H-thymidine is incorporated into the DNA of HSV-2 infected RK cells to a greater extent than into the DNA of mock-infected cells. This occurs maximally up to six hours post infection. At 6-8 hours post infection there is onset of viral DNA synthesis[1]. At this time, unscheduled host DNA synthesis is still detectable but is diminished. Furthermore, density-shift studies demonstrate that increase in nucleotide incorporation after HSV-2 infection is a result of repair synthesis. This interpretation is also suggested by the pattern of nucleotide release after digestion of the RK DNA with 3' or 5' specific phosphodiesterases (Table 1).

Repair synthesis in RK cells during productive infection may be related to the initiation of latency and transformation by herpesviruses. Two mechanisms, insertion and mutation, exist which are consistent with the necessity for repair activity. During the initial infection, some host DNA damage is caused by the virus. This damage may induce cellular repair enzymes. The presence of open-stranded regions and an active repair system could possibly facilitate viral DNA integration into host DNA. The host cell is able to survive, carrying the viral information for a later manifestation of the virus.

We have also demonstrated that oestradiol in the culture medium, at concentrations of 10^{-6} M, will decrease repair synthesis by 11%. At levels of 10^{-5} M, repair synthesis was completely inhibited. Furthermore, at 10^{-6} M oestradiol, semi-conservative replication was stimulated by 6% while at 10^{-5} M oestradiol semi-conservative replication was stimulated by 20%. Therefore, in this system, 10^{-5} M oestradiol has the capability not only of inhibiting normal repair but also of stimulating semi-conservative replication, and hence facilitating "error-prone" post-replication repair. In women, infection with HSV-2 may produce damage to DNA of the cervix. Hormonal action (as yet uncharacterized) may inhibit the cellular repair processes and stimulate DNA synthesis with error-prone post-replicative repair. The resulting mutations might promote HSV-2 transformation and accelerate the progression: normal ⇄ dysplasia → cancer *in situ* →

---

[1] Unpublished data

invasive cancer.   This hypothesis is consistent with the reported
progression of chromosome aberrations in human cervical carcinoma
in situ in women taking birth control pills for seven years (Stern
et al., 1977) and the findings that tumour promoters have been demonstrated to inhibit repair synthesis and stimulate semi-conservative
replication (Trosko & Chang, 1975).

REFERENCES

Cellier, K.M., Kirkland, J.A. & Stanley, M.A. (1970)   Statistical
    analysis of cytogenetic data in cervical neoplasia.   *J. nat.
    Cancer Inst.*, *44*, 1221-1230

Gundberg, C.M., Sinex, F.M. & Kelman, A.D. (1977)   *A UV resistant
    HSV-2 virion associated factor which damages host chromosomes.*
    In: *Abstr., Annual Mtg Amer. Soc. Microbiol.* (Abstract S-374)

Kornberg, A. (1974)   *DNA synthesis*, San Francisco, Freeman

Painter, R.B. & Cleaver, J.E. (1967)   Repair replication in HeLa
    cells after large doses of X-irradiation.   *Nature (Lond.), 216*,
    369-370

Roberts, J.J., Pascoe, J.M., Smith, B.A. & Cathorn, A.R. (1971)
    Quantitative aspects of the repair of alkylated DNA in cultured
    mammalian cells.   *Chem biol. Interactions, 3*, 49-68

Stern, E., Forsythe, A.B., Youkeles, L. & Coffelt, C.F. (1977)
    Steroid contraceptive use and cervical dysplasia: increased
    risk of progression.   *Science, 196*, 1460-1462

Trosko, J.E. & Chang, C.C. (1975)   *Role of DNA repair in mutation
    and cancer production.*   In: Smith, K., ed., *Aging, Carcinogenesis
    and Radiation Biology*, New York, Plenum Press, pp. 346-382

DISCUSSION SUMMARY

Y. BECKER

Laboratory for Molecular Virology,
Hebrew University,
Hadassah Medical School,
Jerusalem, Israel

The studies presented provided information on some
of the molecular events occurring during the replication
of three herpesviruses (herpes simplex virus, cytomegalovirus, and Epstein-Barr virus) in permissive and semi-
permissive cells. These studies increased our understanding both of the mode of replication of these
viruses leading to lytic cycles and of the behaviour
of herpesviruses in lymphoid cells capable of preventing them from developing such a cycle except when a change
of cellular control is evident [e.g., the case of the
expression of Epstein-Barr virus (EBV) in lymphoid cells].
The abundant information on the lytic cycle of herpes
simplex virus (HSV) in permissive cells has made it
possible to define the molecular processes involving
virus replication to the point where the information
still needed for an understanding of the molecular
biology of this virus can clearly be seen. Our understanding of the molecular processes involved in the
replication of cytomegalovirus (CMV) is still in
process of development, but it is clear that there
are both similarities to, and differences from those
seen with HSV. The biology and molecular biology of
the expression of EBV in lymphoid cells and the mechanisms
which prevent the virus from replicating in such cells
remain a mystery, perhaps because experiments to determine
the properties of human lymphoid cells and especially of
lymphoid cell lines that do not carry EBV have yet to be
performed. Although our picture of the molecular biology
of EBV is still in part somewhat blurred, studies in this
field are continuously adding to our understanding of the

unique relationship between this virus and its host, the lymphoid cell.

From the data presented, four points of major importance emerge; these will be discussed, not only in terms of their scientific interest, but also with a view to defining the areas where further work is needed in order to increase our understanding of the viruses concerned.

Analysis of the virion: the viral DNA

Our understanding of the viral genome, which is present in the virion, has increased markedly over the last two years. The genetic map of HSV has been constructed and 24 viral polypeptides, out of a total of 44, have been mapped to date. In addition to refined genetic procedures, to which many of the participants in the Symposium have contributed, this achievement was also the result of refinements in molecular techniques. It is becoming clear at this stage that a large part of the viral genetic information is involved in the regulation of the structural polypeptides. This involves processes taking place both before and after the synthesis of the polypeptide chains. Further studies are needed to increase our understanding of these genes and to determine their positions in the HSV genetic map. It is also clear that studies on CMV will have to follow a path similar to that taken in the case of HSV; studies on EBV DNA and the isolation of mutants are hampered by the absence of a cell permitting EBV replication in a lytic cycle.

Molecular events in lytically infected cells

The molecular processes in the infected cells were reviewed and new information on some of the processes reported.

Four subjects were considered:

1. *Transcription of viral mRNA*.   After entry of the viral DNA into the nucleus of the infected cell, transcription of the DNA is initiated.   Recent studies have demonstrated that the cellular RNA polymerase II of the host cell is responsible for transcription of the viral DNA, a process that results in the synthesis of symmetrical copies, since both strands of the viral DNA are transcribed. This is a puzzling process, since the HSV genome is 100×10^6 daltons in size and has an abundance of viral

genes.   Our understanding of this phenomenon still
awaits further studies.

The early and late viral RNA transcripts present
in lytically infected cells have been mapped and
information obtained on the map locations of the viral
genes that provided the stable portions of the viral
mRNA species.   Essentially, it was demonstrated that
the entire viral genome is involved in transcription,
both early and late, but the primary viral transcripts
are processed.   By the use of the R-loop technique
(electron microscopy of viral RNA transcripts hybridized to viral DNA), it was also possible to detect the
viral genes transcribed to stable mRNA species.
Evidence is available from other studies to show that
the viral mRNA is processed after transcription, polyadenylated at the 3' end of the molecule and capped by
7mG at the 5' end.   Recent studies on adenovirus and
SV40 mRNAs have revealed a new mechanism of splicing
a capped leader sequence to the viral mRNA.   Since
degradation of the primary transcripts of HSV mRNA has
been observed, it will be of interest to determine
whether splicing of leader sequences to the viral mRNA
is a control mechanism in herpesviruses.

2. *Translation of viral mRNA*.   The analysis of the
viral peptides in cells infected with wild-type virus
and temperature-sensitive (*ts*) mutants reported during
the last few years has provided information on some of
their properties.   A study of such polypeptides has been
carried out using 13 *ts* mutants belonging to different
complementation groups.   The mechanisms that control the
synthesis and possibly the post-translational modifications
of polypeptides are not yet known.   Thus the mechanisms
which lead to the shut-off of cellular protein synthesis
and to the establishement of viral polyribosomes are not
fully understood.   The use of *in vitro* subcellular systems
to study protein synthesis and possibly the factors
involved in it might be of use.

The mechanisms involved in the transport of the viral
peptides from the site of synthesis in the cytoplasm to
the site of action in the nucleus are still not known and
await further studies.   The regulation of the synthesis
of viral proteins in three distinct groups was studied
and evidence found to suggest that the synthesis of
different peptides provides a mechanism of regulation of
transcription of different genes.   There are other ways
in which regulation of protein synthesis can be explained,
and further experiments in this area are needed to determine

how the virus cycle is controlled. Studies on CMV
proteins have provided information on CMV comparable
with that on the HSV lytic cycle.

    3. *Control of viral DNA replication.*   The synthesis
of viral DNA in the infected nucleus triggers off the
synthesis of late viral functions involved in the production of viral progeny.   Recent studies have provided
information on the mode of HSV DNA replication.   The
control of HSV DNA replication by viral and cellular
processes was indicated in some studies.   Attention was
drawn to the role of cyclic nucleotides present in the
infected cells in the control of viral DNA synthesis.
It was also reported that treatment of HSV-infected
lymphoid cells by the polypeptide hormone insulin, which
produces a decrease in cAMP and an increase in cGMP in
lymphoid cells, suppressed cellular and viral DNA
synthesis.   These studies clearly suggest the involvement of cyclic nucleotides and cellular enzymatic systems
involved in their synthesis and degradation, in the
process of DNA replication.

    The polypeptides, enzymes and non-enzymatic proteins
involved in DNA replication constitute a class of DNA-
binding proteins.   These proteins have been further
characterized, and a HSV nuclease has been isolated and
characterized.   The various enzymes (DNA polymerase,
DNase, ligase, etc.) as well as the unwinding proteins
of HSV still remain to be studied.

    4. *Recombination of HSV DNA.*   Recombinants of HSV
with specific genetic markers and characterized genomes
are available for the analysis of viral functions.   The
mechanisms and enzymes involved in the process of DNA-DNA
recombination are not yet known; the elucidation of this
process will lead to an understanding of the mechanisms
of intermolecular recombination and possibly to the integration of viral DNA fragments into host-cell DNA, when
interaction of the herpesvirus with the cell leads to cell
transformation.

Semi-permissive interactions of herpesviruses with cells

    The replication of a herpesvirus in a cell that
supports the synthesis of viral progeny requires cellular
processes, some of which have already been discussed.   It
seems possible that certain cells may have the ability to
regulate the viral genetic information in a way that
prevents the virus from expressing its full genetic information.   This might result from a modification of the

viral genome (e.g., fragmentation of the viral DNA
into small pieces, circularization of the complete
viral genome in such a way as to prevent transcription or replication).   The phenomena involved in
the restricted behaviour of EBV in the lymphoid
host cell were described.   In the absence of any
understanding of the molecular processes in the
lymphoid cell, we are in the process of identifying
virus-coded proteins (e.g., EBNA, DNA polymerase,
and other antigens) with a view to determining to
what extent the expression of the viral genetic
information is restricted.   Information was presented
on the presence of a virus-coded DNA polymerase in
EBV DNA-carrying human lymphoid cells.   These and
other studies on the biochemistry of EBV in lymphoid
cells clearly show that the virus is closely controlled
by the host cell; the mechanisms involved, however,
are not yet fully understood.

CELL-VIRUS INTERACTIONS: INTEGRATION AND EXPRESSION OF THE VIRAL GENOME

TRANSFORMATION OF NON-LYMPHOID CELLS BY HERPESVIRUSES: A REVIEW

F. RAPP & E.J. SHILLITOE

Department of Microbiology and Specialised Cancer Research Center,
The Milton S. Hershey Medical Center,
The Pennsylvania State University College of Medicine,
Hershey, Penn., USA

Herpesviruses have been suspected for several years of inducing tumours in man, on the basis of clinical and sero-epidemiological evidence. Direct inoculation of laboratory animals with human herpesviruses has been consistently uninformative as to their possible oncogenicity, but indirect approaches have yielded a large amount of information. Susceptible cell cultures have been transformed *in vitro* by a number of herpesviruses, using a variety of techniques, and the transformed cells have often behaved in a malignant fashion after reinoculation into the host species. No satisfactory single definition of transformation has yet been devised, and the transformed cells are generally recognized by acquisition of a variety of features (Rapp & Westmoreland, 1976).

The present review will describe a number of cell types which have become transformed following herpesvirus infection, and their relationship to malignant disease will be considered.

CELL TRANSFORMATION BY HERPES SIMPLEX VIRUS

Infection of permissive cells by herpes simplex virus (HSV) leads to replication of the virus and death of the cell. Few mammalian cells are resistant to such infection and attempts to transform cells have usually been carried out with virus which has been partially inactivated (Table 1). This was originally achieved by irradiation of the virus with ultraviolet light (Duff & Rapp, 1971), or by exposure to heterotricyclic dyes, and then to white light (Rapp et al., 1973).

Table 1. Summary of studies showing cell transformation by HSV and
properties of the transformed cells

Virus	Treatment of virus to prevent cell lysis	Cell species	Marker of HSV in transformed cells	Oncogenicity of transformed cells	References
HSV-2	UV[a]	Hamster	Antigens, DNA	+	Duff & Rapp, 1971 Frenkel et al., 1976
HSV-1	UV[a]	Hamster	Antigens, poly-peptides	+	Duff & Rapp, 1973 Gupta & Rapp, 1977
HSV-1	UV[a]	Mouse	Thymidine kinase	NT[b]	Munyon et al., 1971
HSV-1 & HSV-2	Neutral red + white light	Hamster	Antigens	+	Rapp et al., 1973 Li et al., 1975
HSV-2	Incubation at 42°C	Human	Antigens	NT[b]	Darai & Munk, 1973
HSV-2	Incubation at 40°C	Chicken	Antigens	NT[b]	Geder et al., 1973
HSV-2 ts mutant[c]	None	Hamster and human	Antigens	+	Takahashi & Yamanishi, 1974
HSV-1 & -2 ts mutant[c]	None	Rat	Antigens	+	Macnab, 1975
HSV-2	UV[a]	Mouse	Antigens	+	Boyd et al., 1975
HSV-1 & HSV-2	Incubation at 42°C	Rat	Antigens	+	Darai & Munk, 1976
HSV-1 & HSV-2	Incubation at 20°C	Rat	Antigens	+	Darai et al., 1977

[a] UV: Ultraviolet light irradiation
[b] NT: Not tested
[c] ts: Temperature-sensitive

Following these procedures (Fig. 1) the virus loses the ability to lyse
cells; however, infected hamster embryo fibroblasts develop foci of
transformed cells with oncogenic properties (Duff & Rapp, 1971, 1973;
Li et al., 1975).

        After permissive cells have been infected with infectious HSV, it
may still be possible to inhibit virus production and allow transformation by incubating at non-optimal temperatures.   Darai & Munk (1973)
established four lines of transformed human cells by infecting embryo
lung fibroblasts with HSV-2 and incubating the cultures at 42°C for
eight days.   The temperature of the surviving cells was then reduced
to 37°C and lines of transformed cells could be established.   Geder
et al. (1973) transformed chicken embryo fibroblasts after incubating
HSV-2 infected cells at 40°C for 25 days.   Similarly, incubation of
infected rat embryo fibroblasts at the reduced temperature of 20°C
resulted in malignant transformation of the cells (Darai et al., 1977).

        Temperature-sensitive (ts) mutants of HSV have been described and
can transform cells without prior inactivation.   Macnab (1975)
established lines of rat cells and Takahashi & Yamanishi (1974) transformed hamster and human cells by infection and culture at the non-
permissive temperature.

FIG. 1. DIAGRAMMATIC REPRESENTATION OF SYSTEMS USED
TO DEMONSTRATE MORPHOLOGICAL TRANSFORMATION OF
MAMMALIAN CELLS BY HERPES SIMPLEX VIRUS

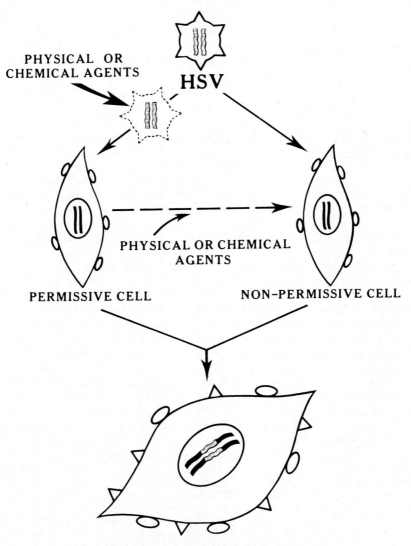

TRANSFORMED CELL

PROPERTIES OF CELLS TRANSFORMED BY HERPES SIMPLEX VIRUS

Morphology

Cells transformed by HSV may show either fibroblastoid or epithelioid morphology. Hamster embryo fibroblasts transformed by HSV-2
retained their basic morphology, but when transformed by HSV-1 they
became epithelioid (Duff & Rapp, 1973). However, later observations
have shown that cells transformed by either HSV-1 or HSV-2 can yield
fibroblastoid or epithelioid lines (Darai et al., 1977; Rapp & Li,
1974).

Oncogenicity

Unlike normal cells, HSV-2 transformed cells grow in soft agar or
methylcellulose (Boyd et al., 1975; Darai et al., 1977; Kucera &
Gusdon, 1976); this is a property associated in other cell types with
malignancy (Risser et al., 1974). Inoculation of HSV-transformed
cells into the homologous host has produced tumours in hamsters
(Duff & Rapp, 1971), mice (Boyd et al., 1975) and rats (Darai et al.,
1977; Macnab, 1975) (Table 1). Not all transformed lines are oncogenic, but oncogenicity frequently increases during culture *in vitro*
or *in vivo*. When hamster cells transformed by the same strain of
HSV-2 were inoculated into newborn hamsters, the percentage developing
tumours varied from 36% to 100% with different lines (Duff & Rapp,
1973; Rapp & Duff, 1973). The oncogenicity changed during growth
in vivo; cells isolated from tumours induced by the less oncogenic
line were more oncogenic, in terms of dose and latent period, than
cells from tumours induced by more oncogenic lines (Rapp & Duff, 1973).
Macnab (1974) observed changes in oncogenicity of HSV-2 transformed
cells during culture *in vitro*. The cells were non-oncogenic in newborn hamsters until passage 34 when two of 10 animals developed tumours
after a 13-week latent period following inoculation with 10^5 or 10^6
transformed cells. An *in vivo* increase in oncogenicity then occurred
since cells from the primary tumours produced tumours in all newborn
and weanling hamsters, and the latent period became reduced to one
week. HSV-1 and HSV-2 transformed cell-induced tumours frequently
metastasize to distant sites in the host animal; hamster tumours
not only invaded surrounding bone and muscle, but frequently produced
metastases in lungs, kidneys and liver (Duff et al., 1974).

The histological appearance of tumours induced by HSV-transformed
cells seems to vary according to the morphology of the cells *in vitro*.
Fibroblastoid lines induced tumours resembling fibrosarcomas with interlacing bundles of pleomorphic fibroblasts. Most tumours were predominantly anaplastic although some were well differentiated in certain
areas (Duff et al., 1974). Epithelioid cells transformed by HSV-1
gave rise to tumours resembling adenocarcinomas. The epithelioid cells
also gave rise to metastases which appeared in lungs, kidneys and lymph-

nodes and showed a similar histological appearance to the primary tumour.

Presence of HSV genes in transformed cells

Infectious HSV cannot be isolated from cells transformed by the virus, and electron microscopic examination has revealed the presence of only very occasional HSV particles (Glaser et al., 1972; Rapp & Duff, 1972). This is undoubtedly due to the transformed cells containing less than the complete virus genome. Frenkel et al. (1976) studied the kinetics of hybridization of radio-labelled HSV-2 DNA with HSV-transformed cell DNA and concluded that, although all the lines tested contained virus DNA sequences, only 8-32% of the genome was present. Cells derived from tumours had a lower sequence complexity than the original transformed cell line. Repeated passage *in vitro* can also lead to loss of HSV DNA. At passage 48, about 40% of the HSV-2 genome was found in 333-8-9 cells but by passage 78 this had decreased to less than 10% (Minson et al., 1976). Studies of cells transformed by SV40 or adenovirus have shown that the genetic information required to maintain the transformed state can be contained in less than 2×10^6 daltons of DNA. This corresponds to about 2% of the HSV genome and is below the limits of detection of current techniques (Frenkel et al., 1976). Therefore, it is unknown at present whether HSV-transformed cells eventually lose all HSV genes or whether they retain a minimal set of sequences which are necessary to maintain transformation. This question may be resolved in the future by the use of restriction endonuclease fragments as probes. An alternative approach is to examine HSV RNA, since transcription involves amplification of virus-specific nucleic acid sequences. Collard et al. (1973) found HSV-specific RNA in HSV-transformed hamster cells, and the RNA was detected even in clones which lost all detectable HSV DNA (Copple & McDougall, 1976).

In one experimental system the presence of a specific virus gene is the required transformation marker. Munyon et al. (1971) demonstrated that, when mouse L-cells which lacked thymidine kinase (TK) were infected with ultraviolet (UV)-inactivated HSV, the enzyme was permanently induced in the cells. The enzyme was of virus, and not cellular type (Davidson et al., 1973; Davis et al., 1974; Munyon et al., 1972) and HSV DNA was found in the cells by measurement of DNA reassociation kinetics (Kraiselburd & Weissbach, 1975). However, since latently infected ganglia cells also contain this enzyme without undergoing morphological transformation (Yamamoto et al., 1977) it is unclear how closely this biochemical transformation is related to malignancy.

Antigens of HSV-transformed cells

Although cells transformed by HSV do not release virus particles, they nevertheless synthesize virus proteins that can be detected by immunofluorescence (IF) tests and with HSV neutralizing sera. Rapp

& Duff (1972) detected HSV antigens by this method in the cytoplasm of up to 5% of HSV-transformed hamster cells.   Similarly, 5-10% of transformed chicken fibroblasts (Geder et al., 1973) or human embryo fibroblasts (Kucera & Gusdon, 1976) were stained by HSV neutralizing serum.   Macnab (1975), however, reported that 50% of transformed rat cells stained with an anti-HSV-2 serum.   The surface of HSV-1 transformed cells was stained by an antiserum to a purified virion-associated antigen of HSV-1 (CP-1) by Reed et al. (1975).   About 50% of cells were stained, but cells transformed by HSV-2 did not react at all with the serum.

More recent studies have attempted to characterize in greater detail the HSV-related antigens associated with transformed cells. Flannery et al. (1977) stained 10-15% of HSV-2 transformed hamster cells with a hyperimmune rabbit serum raised against a single polypeptide (VP143).   When the transformed cells were synchronized in mitosis and stained later at various times, the expression of the antigen was shown to be cell-cycle dependent; maximum intensity of staining was seen before and again after the time of maximum DNA synthesis when up to 90% of cells were stained.   Gupta & Rapp (1977) detected ten polypeptides on the surface of the virion of HSV-1 by polyacrylamide gel electrophoresis of surface-labelled envelope proteins.   Hamster cells transformed by HSV-1 contained three of these ten polypeptides.

Evidence for the presence of HSV-associated antigens on the surface of HSV-transformed cells is further provided by studies of the immune responses of animals bearing tumours induced by the cells. Animals with HSV-2 transformed cell-induced tumours develop serum antibody capable of neutralizing infectious HSV-2 particles (Boyd et al., 1975; Kimura et al., 1975; Rapp & Duff, 1972), provided that the virus was inactivated by UV light, and not photodynamically (Li et al., 1975).   The titre was directly proportional to the length of time the tumour had been present (Rapp & Duff, 1972).   Spleen cells from the tumour-bearing hamsters were cytotoxic to the transformed cells, although this response was lost as the tumour increased in size. Spleen cells from animals bearing isografts of HSV-2 transformed cells also killed HSV-1 transformed cells, as did spleen cells from animals immunized with HSV-1 infected rabbit kidney cells (Lausch et al., 1975).   Sera from the tumour-bearing or virus-immunized host blocked the cytotoxic response of the spleen cells.

Despite the evidence for the presence of HSV-associated antigens on and within HSV-transformed cells, immunization of hamsters with the cells has not protected them from such tumour isografts.   Indeed, in immunized animals tumours appear earlier (Lausch et al., 1976), grow more rapidly (Thiry et al., 1975), and metastasize to the lungs more frequently (Duff et al., 1973).   Serum blocking factors may be the cause of such enhancement (Duff et al., 1973) although evidence for this is still lacking.

CELL TRANSFORMATION BY CYTOMEGALOVIRUS

The human cytomegalovirus (CMV), like HSV, is widespread through-out the population. Infection with CMV *in utero* can result in congenital brain defects, but can presumably occur without fetal damage since about 1% of "normal" newborns excrete CMV in the urine (Weller, 1971). In adults CMV infections cause less well-defined diseases than HSV, although latent infections are probably common since in immunosuppressed patients the virus frequently appears in the urine or sputum (Weller, 1971).

Infection of cells in culture by CMV can lead to stimulation of DNA and RNA synthesis (St. Jeor et al., 1974) and this is a character-istic of oncogenic viruses such as SV40, polyoma, and of adenoviruses and Epstein-Barr virus (EBV). Cell transformation by CMV was first demonstrated by Albrecht & Rapp (1973). Hamster embryo fibroblasts were infected by CMV which had been previously irradiated to prevent cytolysis. After 20 days incubation, foci of morphologically altered cells were seen which were not contact-inhibited. One focus could be subcultured repeatedly, and was designated Cx-90-3B. These cells were oncogenic in syngeneic weanling hamsters and could be recovered from the tumours. Morphologically, the transformed cells were fibroblastoid and the tumours they produced were poorly differentiated, metastasizing fibrosarcomas. The tumour cells were frequently multi-nucleated, with prominent nuclei, and very frequent mitotic figures. No virus particles were either recoverable, or visible in the trans-formed cells by electron microscopy (Albrecht & Rapp, 1973).

IF studies utilizing sera from human patients convalescing from CMV infections revealed the presence of CMV antigens on the membrane of 47% of cells, and in the cytoplasm of 0.5% of cells (Albrecht & Rapp, 1973). CMV antigen was also detected on the cell membrane by haemag-glutination and ^{125}I-antiglobulin studies (Lausch et al., 1974). After passage through hamsters, the cytoplasmic antigen could no longer be detected and the membrane antigen was found on only 17% of cells, as compared to the 47% originally observed (Albrecht & Rapp, 1973).

Syngeneic hamsters carrying Cx-90-3B derived tumours develop an immune response to the cells, as shown by their acquisition of serum antibody which reacts with the transformed cells, the tumour cells, or CMV-infected cells in IF assays (Albrecht & Rapp, 1973). Spleen cells from the hamsters are specifically cytotoxic for the transformed cells (Murasko & Lausch, 1974). Curiously, the tumour-bearing hamsters do not develop antibody which can neutralize infectious CMV particles (Albrecht & Rapp, 1973) and so the nature of the tumour-cell antigen detected in the various immunological tests is uncertain.

A suggestion that CMV could transform human cells came from obser-vations by Rapp et al. (1975) on cultured prostate cells from a three-

year-old boy.   The cells initially released infectious CMV, but at
higher passage numbers underwent morphological transformation and
ceased to release virus.   CMV antigens and DNA were, however,
retained by the transformed cells.   The CMV isolated from the cells
was used to infect human embryo lung (HEL) cells at a very low multiplicity of infection (Geder et al., 1976).   The infection persisted
during frequent passaging of the cells but eventually, foci of transformed cells emerged which showed no cytopathic effect and from which
infectious virus could not be rescued.   The transformed cells were a
mixture of fibroblastoid and epithelioid cells and were oncogenic in
athymic mice (Geder et al., 1977).   The tumours consisted of small
polygonal cells with large nuclei set in a collagenous matrix.
Invasion of surrounding tissues was observed, but only rarely.   The
tumour cells were possibly epithelioid, but were not well differentiated.

        IF staining of the transformed cells and of cells recovered from
the tumours showed CMV antigens in the cytoplasm and on the membrane.
The transformed cells were specifically killed by spleen lymphocytes
from hamsters bearing Cx-90-3B induced tumours (Geder et al., 1976).
In addition, the transformed HEL cells were shown by the highly
sensitive anticomplement immunofluorescence technique to bear a nuclear
antigen, when stained with appropriate human sera (Geder & Rapp, 1977).
Each serum which stained the nuclear antigen also reacted with an early
antigen present shortly after infection of cells by CMV (Geder & Rapp,
1977).   The transformed cells therefore carry an antigen which may be
analogous to EBNA, an early antigen present in EBV-infected cells,
EBV-transformed cells and Burkitt's lymphoma cells.

                CELL TRANSFORMATION BY GUINEAPIG HERPES-LIKE VIRUS

        Guineapig herpes-like virus (GPHLV) was originally isolated from
leukaemia-susceptible guineapigs by Hsiung et al. (1971) and from the
leukaemic cells by Nayak (1971).   The virus persists in guineapig
leukocytes *in vitro* and induces morphological transformation (Fong et
al., 1973).   Non-lymphoid cells can also be transformed.   Fong &
Hsiung (1973) infected hamster embryo cells with GPHLV and maintained
the cultures for three weeks.   At the end of this time, 10-50% of
cultures contained foci of transformed cells, which were mainly
epithelioid but occasionally fibroblastoid.   Antiserum to GPHLV
stained the cytoplasm of 7-20% of the cells in IF tests.   Initially
the transformed cells were non-oncogenic in hamsters, but after 37
passages *in vitro* induced tumours in 42% of animals (Michalski et al.,
1976).   The tumours occasionally invaded adjacent muscle and skin, and
metastasized to the lungs in 6/28 animals examined.   Histologically,
these were fibrosarcomas showing marked pleomorphism: epithelioid,
spindle-shaped and transitional cells were present.   Cells isolated
from the hamster tumours were cultured, and resembled the parent cell

line in that up to 10% could be stained on the surface by anti-GPHLV
serum.

Rhim (1977) transformed rat embryo cells with GPHLV and induced
tumours in newborn rats by inoculation of the transformed cells.
He observed some antigenic cross-reactivity between HSV and GPHLV,
and the rat tumour cells expressed a complement-fixing HSV-related
antigen.   The rat tumour cells resembled the hamster tumour cells
(Michalski et al., 1976) in that co-cultivation experiments did not
isolate infectious virus.

CELL TRANSFORMATION BY EPSTEIN-BARR VIRUS

The range of host cells which can be infected by EBV is extremely
narrow.   The virus has been found only in human lymphoblastoid cells
with B-cell markers, and can infect only B-lymphocytes of man (Jondal
& Klein, 1973) or certain other primates (Falk et al., 1974; Miller
et al., 1972).   However, the nucleic acid hybridization studies of
Wolf et al. (1973) detected the presence of EBV DNA in epithelial cells
derived from nasopharyngeal carcinomas, and treatment of the epithelial
cells with iododeoxyuridine (IUDR) can induce the expression of EBV
early antigens (Glaser et al., 1976).   It is possible therefore that
non-lymphoid cells can be transformed by EBV under certain conditions.

Glaser and his colleagues fused lymphoid cells carrying the EBV
genome with either human or mouse cells to form human-human or human-
mouse hybrid cells (Glaser & Nonoyama, 1973; Glaser & O'Neill, 1972;
Glaser & Rapp, 1972).   The hybrid cells grew continuously as monolayers, unlike the lymphoid parent cells, and the human-mouse hybrids
grew in the absence of aminopterin, unlike the mouse parent cells.
Similar hybrids were formed by Klein et al. (1974) between an EBV
DNA-containing line, and mouse fibroblast L-cells.   None of the
several hybrid lines which were produced expressed the EBV membrane
antigen, the early antigen, or the viral capsid antigen, and they
further resembled the mouse parent cells in lacking EBV receptors and
surface immunoglobulin.   Klein et al. (1974) did find the EBV nuclear
antigen in some cells, and the proportion of cells with that antigen
was related to the number of copies of the EBV genome present in the
cells.   Klein et al. (1974) were unable to induce virus antigens in
the cells by treatment with IUDR, although this could be done in the
human parent cells.   Glaser & Rapp (1972), on the other hand, found
that IUDR induced the virus to replicate and to synthesize complete
particles, and also depending on the parent lymphoid line used, induced
several EBV antigens (Glaser, 1975).

Al-Moslih et al. (1976) infected monolayers of primary human amnion
cells, and rat embryo cells with a Burkitt's lymphoma cell line which
had been disrupted by ultrasonication.   Transformed foci were obtained
but only if the monolayer had been pretreated with diethylaminoethyl

(DEAE)-dextran, using a technique known to enhance transfection by
poliovirus RNA.   The cells of the transformed foci grew as enlarging
mounds of rapidly dividing cells and could be subcultured as continuous lines.   The transformed human cells showed a modal chromosome
number of 65 instead of the normal 46, and 30-50% of the cells were
stained in indirect IF tests by human sera containing EBV antibody.
The staining was located in both the nuclei and cytoplasm of the
transformed cells, but exactly which of the EBV antigens were present
is unknown.   The nature of the transforming agent is also unknown, but
since transformation was prevented by DNAse or trypsin and not by anti-
EBV serum, the agent was probably EBV DNA with some necessary protein.

The experiments with hybrid cells have shown that the EBV genome
can be maintained and expressed in transformed cells with non-lymphoid
morphology, and fibroblasts and amnion cells have been transformed by
an EBV DNA-containing preparation.   It is therefore possible that
transformation of non-lymphoid cells *in vivo* could occur if the EBV
genome were transferred from infected B-cells to non-lymphoid cells:
this was postulated to occur in nasopharyngeal carcinomas by Henle &
Henle (1973).

TRANSFORMATION BY FROG RENAL TUMOUR VIRUSES

Adenocarcinomas of the kidney occur naturally in North American
leopard frogs and were suggested by Lucké in 1938 to be caused by a
virus.   Fawcett (1956) later described virus-like particles in the
tumours, and a unique association between warm weather and tumour
growth;   an association between cold weather and lytic infection by the
virus is now recognized (McKinnell & Ellis, 1972).   Herpesviruses have
been recognized in the Lucké tumours, and cell-free tumour extracts
which contain such viruses will induce new tumours in susceptible frogs.
Tweedell et al. (1972) demonstrated that infection of frog embryo cells
in vitro, with extracts of frog tumours, led to formation of localized
areas of proliferation within the monolayer.   The proliferating cells
grew continuously following inoculation of the eye chamber of adult
frogs, while control implants of uninfected cells failed to survive.
Nevertheless, other viruses were present in the tumour extracts, and
direct proof that it is the Lucké herpesvirus that causes cell transformation and tumours is still lacking.

CONCLUSIONS

Examination of the above data reveals a number of similarities
between cell transformation systems employing different herpesviruses
(Tables 1 and 2).   Exposure of the virus to UV light or other agents
is not essential for the expression of transforming ability: cells
can be transformed by *ts* mutants of HSV (Macnab, 1975;   Takahashi &

Table 2. Summary of studies showing transformation of non-lymphoid cells by herpesviruses other than HSV, and properties of the transformed cells

Virus	Treatment of virus to prevent cell lysis	Cell species	Marker of HSV in transformed cells	Oncogenicity of transformed cells	References
LHV[a]	None	Frog	NT[b]	+	Tweedell et al., 1972
EBV	Fusion of transformed lymphoid cells with fibroblast lines	Mouse and human	Virus induced by IUDR[c] Antigens induced by IUDR[c]	NT[b]	Glaser & O'Neil, 1972; Glaser & Rapp, 1972; Klein et al., 1974
CMV	UV[d]	Hamster	Antigens	+	Albrecht & Rapp, 1973; Lausch et al., 1974
	None	Human	Antigens	NT[b]	Geder et al., 1976; Geder & Rapp, 1976
GPHLV	None	Hamster	Antigens	+	Fong & Hsiung, 1973; Michalski et al., 1976

[a] LHV: Lucké herpesvirus
[b] NT: Not tested
[c] IUDR: Iododeoxyuridine
[d] UV : Ultraviolet light irradiation

& Yamanishi, 1974), by the Mj strain of CMV (Geder et al., 1976), by GPHLV (Fong & Hsiung, 1973) and by EBV, and in all of these cases unmodified virus was used.   After transformation has occurred the cells may shed infectious virus particles for a number of passages, but then cease to do so.   This has been observed in experiments with HSV (Kutinová et al., 1973), CMV (Geder et al., 1976), and following animal passage of cells transformed by GPHLV (Michalski et al., 1976).
Animal passage of cells transformed by HSV can result in a reduction of gene sequence complexity (Frenkel et al., 1976) and in the case of cells transformed by CMV, can result in loss of cytoplasmic virus antigens and a reduction in membrane antigen (Albrecht & Rapp, 1973).   In parallel with the loss of viruses, virus genes, or antigens, the oncogenicity of the transformed cells can increase with continued growth.   HSV-transformed cells became more oncogenic following animal passage (Macnab, 1974; Rapp & Duff, 1973) and GPHLV-transformed cells acquired oncogenic properties after passage *in vitro*.   Whether the increase in oncogenicity is a consequence of the loss of antigens, or due to some other selective process is presently unknown.

Since herpesviruses are suspected of playing a role in the etiology of certain human cancers, any similarities between herpesvirus-transformed cells and human cancer cells could be of the greatest significance.   Very little research into such similarities appears to have

been carried out, however, and in fact, might be unproductive due to
the apparent loss of virus genes and antigens seen in certain experimental systems.   Human tumours are clearly a large number of cell
divisions away from the original transformed cell from which they
originate, and spontaneous loss of virus-associated features could
have occurred.   Indeed, although one cervical tumour was reported
to contain a portion of the HSV genome (Frenkel et al., 1972), this
finding still awaits confirmation.   Since the fraction of the virus
genome remaining in tumour cells may be at or below the present limits
of detection, future studies of nucleic acid hybridization will have
to place particular emphasis on maximizing the sensitivity of the
technique (zur Hausen et al., 1974).   An alternative approach might
consist of an examination of the immune status of the patient, since
a response generated against a virus-specified tumour-associated antigen
should persist even after loss of such an antigen from the tumour.
Using this approach, Notter & Docherty (1976) detected complement-fixing
antibody against HSV-transformed cell antigens in sera of 94% of patients
with squamous-cell carcinoma, compared to about 45% of sera from patients
with other tumours and 16% of controls.   Preliminary efforts to detect
responses of patients with prostate carcinomas against CMV-transformed
cells have been made, but have so far failed to demonstrate specificity
of the response (Sanford et al., 1977).   The nature of the virus
antigen carried by transformed cells and which might also be expressed
at some stage of growth of human cancers is uncertain.   However,
Burkitt's lymphoma is characterized by the presence of antibody to
early antigens of EBV (Henle et al., 1971) and cervical carcinoma may
have an associated antibody to an early antigen of HSV (Aurelian et
al., 1975).   Early antigens of CMV also exist, and are immunogenic in
man (The et al., 1974).   Therefore it seems important that the attention
of future research programmes be turned toward the study of early virus
antigens in herpesvirus-transformed cells (Fig. 2), and toward study
of the immune response of cancer patients against such antigens.

ACKNOWLEDGEMENTS

This investigation was supported by Contract NO1 CP 53516
within the Virus Cancer Program of the National Cancer
Institute, Grant CA 18450 awarded by the National
Cancer Institute, and by Grant CA 16365 awarded
by the National Cancer Institute.
E.J. Shillitoe is a Leukemia
Society of America Fellow.

FIG. 2. RATIONALE FOR STUDYING ANTIGENS IN TRANSFORMED CELLS AND THE IMMUNE RESPONSES

Note amplification of the integrated virus DNA by subsequent transcription and translation.

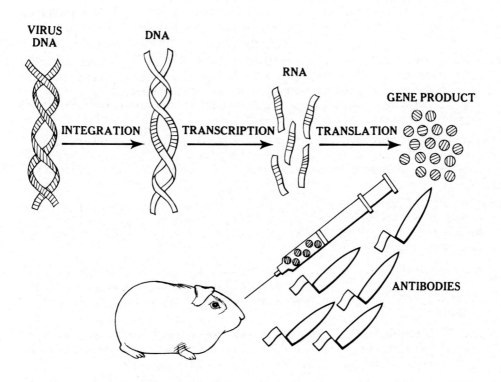

REFERENCES

Albrecht, T. & Rapp, F. (1973)   Malignant transformation of hamster embryo fibroblasts following exposure to ultraviolet-irradiated human cytomegalovirus. *Virology, 55,* 53-61

Al-Moslih, M.I., White, R.J. & Dubes, G.R. (1976)   Use of a trans-
    fection method to demonstrate a monolayer cell transforming agent
    from the EB3 line of Burkitt's lymphoma cells.   *J. gen. Virol., 31,*
    331-345

Aurelian, L., Cornish, J.D. & Smith, M.F. (1975)   *Herpesvirus type*
    2-induced tumour-specific antigen (AG-4) and specific antibody in
    patients with cervical cancer and controls.   In: de-Thé, G.,
    Epstein, M.A. & zur Hausen, H., eds, *Oncogenesis and Herpesviruses*
    II, part 2, Lyon, International Agency for Research on Cancer
    (*IARC Scientific Publications* No. 11), pp. 79-87

Boyd, A., Orme, T. & Boone, C. (1975)   *Transformation of mouse cells*
    with herpes simplex virus type 2.   In: de-Thé, G., Epstein, M.A.,
    & zur Hausen, H., eds, *Oncogenesis and Herpesviruses II, part 1,*
    Lyon, International Agency for Research on Cancer (*IARC Scientific*
    Publications No. 11), pp. 429-435

Collard, W., Thornton, H. & Green, M. (1973)   Cells transformed by
    human herpesvirus type 2 transcribe virus specific RNA sequences
    shared by herpesvirus types 1 and 2.   *Nature (Lond.), 243,* 264-
    266

Copple, C.D. & McDougall, J.K. (1976)   Clonal derivatives of a herpes
    type 2 transformed hamster cell line (333-8-9):   cytogenetic
    analysis, tumorigenicity and virus sequence detection.   *Int. J.*
    Cancer, 17, 501-510

Darai, G., Braun, R., Flügel, R.M. & Munk, K. (1977)   Malignant
    transformation of rat embryo fibroblasts by herpes simplex virus
    types 1 and 2 at suboptimal temperature.   *Nature (Lond.), 265,*
    744-746

Darai, G. & Munk, K. (1973)   Human embryonic lung cells abortively
    infected with herpes virus hominis type 2 show some properties of
    cell transformation.   *Nature (Lond.), 241,* 268-269

Davidson, R.L., Adelstein, S.J. & Oxman, M.N. (1973)   Herpes simplex
    virus as a source of thymidine kinase for thymidine kinase-
    deficient mouse cells: suppression and reactivation of the viral
    enzyme.   *Proc. nat. Acad. Sci. (Wash.), 70,* 1912-1916

Davis, D.B., Munyon, W., Buchsbaum, R. & Chawda, R. (1974)   Virus
    type-specific thymidine kinase in cells biochemically transformed
    by herpes simplex virus types 1 and 2.   *J. Virol., 13,* 140-145

Duff, R., Doller, E. & Rapp, F. (1973)   Immunologic manipulation of
    metastases due to herpesvirus transformed cells.   *Science, 180,*
    79-81

Duff, R., Kreider, J.W., Levy, B.M., Katz, M. & Rapp, F. (1974)
    Comparative pathology of cells transformed by herpes simplex
    virus type 1 or type 2.   *J. nat. Cancer Inst., 53,* 1159-1164

Duff, R.G. & Rapp, F. (1971) Oncogenic transformation of hamster cells after exposure to herpes simplex virus type 2. *Nature (Lond.), 233,* 48-50

Duff, R. & Rapp, F. (1973) Oncogenic transformation of hamster embryo cells after exposure to inactivated herpes simplex virus type 1. *J. Virol., 12,* 209-217

Falk, L., Wolfe, L., Deinhardt, F., Paciga, J., Dombos, L., Klein, G., Henle, W. & Henle, G. (1974) Epstein-Barr virus: transformation of nonhuman primate lymphocytes *in vitro. Int. J. Cancer, 13,* 363-376

Fawcett, D.W. (1956) Electron microscope observations on intracellular virus like particles associated with the cells of the Lucké renal adenocarcinoma. *J. biophys. biochem. Cytol., 2,* 725-742

Flannery, V.L., Courtney, R.J. & Schaffer, P.A. (1977) Expression of an early, nonstructural antigen of herpes simplex virus in cells transformed *in vitro* by herpes simplex virus. *J. Virol., 21,* 284-291

Fong, C.K.Y. & Hsiung, G.D. (1973) *In vitro* transformation of hamster embryo cells by a guinea pig herpes-like virus. *Proc. Soc. exp. Biol. (N.Y.), 144,* 974-978

Fong, C.K.Y., Tenser, R.B., Hsiung, G.D. & Gross, P.A. (1973) Ultrastructural studies of the envelopment and release of guinea pig herpes-like virus in cultured cells. *Virology, 52,* 468-477

Frenkel, N., Locker, H., Cox, B., Roizman, B. & Rapp, F. (1976) Herpes simplex virus DNA in transformed cells: sequence complexity in two hamster cell lines and one derived hamster tumor. *J. Virol., 18,* 885-893

Frenkel, N., Roizman, B., Cassai, E. & Nahmias, A. (1972) A DNA fragment of herpes simplex 2 and its transcription in human cervical cancer tissue. *Proc. nat. Acad. Sci. (Wash.), 69,* 3784-3789

Geder, L., Kreider, J. & Rapp, F. (1977) Human cells transformed *in vitro* by human cytomegalovirus: tumorigenicity in athymic nude mice. *J. nat. Cancer Inst., 58,* 1003-1009

Geder, L., Lausch, R., O'Neill, F. & Rapp, F. (1976) Oncogenic transformation of human embryo lung cells by human cytomegalovirus. *Science, 192,* 1134-1347

Geder, L. & Rapp, F. (1977) Evidence for nuclear antigens in cytomegalovirus-transformed human cells. *Nature (Lond.), 265,* 184-186

Geder, L., Vaczi, L. & Boldogh, I. (1973) Development of cell lines after exposure of chicken embryonic fibroblasts to herpes simplex virus type 2 at supraoptimal temperature. *Acta Microbiol. Acad. Sci. Hung., 20,* 119-125

Glaser, R. (1975)   *Expression and regulation of the Epstein-Barr-virus early antigen component(s) in Burkitt-epithelial hybrid cells*.   In: Ablashi, D.V., Aaslestad, H.G. & de-Thé, G., eds, *Epstein-Barr Virus Production, Concentration and Purification*, Lyon, International Agency for Research on Cancer (*IARC Internal Technical Report* No. 75 003), pp. 225-234

Glaser, R., de-Thé, G., Lenoir, G. & Ho, J.H.C. (1976)   Superinfection of epithelial nasopharyngeal carcinoma cells with Epstein-Barr virus.   *Proc. nat. Acad. Sci. (Wash.), 73*, 960-963

Glaser, R., Duff, R.G. & Rapp, F. (1972) Ultrastructural characterization of hamster cells transformed following exposure to ultra-violet-irradiated herpes simplex virus type 2.   *Cancer Res., 32*, 2803-2806

Glaser, R. & Nonoyama, M. (1973)   Epstein-Barr virus: detection of genome in somatic cell hybrids of Burkitt lymphoblastoid cells.   *Science, 179*, 492-493

Glaser, R. & O'Neill, F.J. (1972)   Hybridization of Burkitt lymphoblastoid cells.   *Science, 176*, 1245-1247

Glaser, R. & Rapp, F. (1972)   Rescue of Epstein-Barr virus from somatic cell hybrids of Burkitt lymphoblastoid cells.   *J. Virol., 10*, 288-296

Gupta, P. & Rapp, F. (1977)   Identification of virion polypeptides in hamster cells transformed by herpes simplex virus type 1.   *Proc. nat. Acad. Sci. (Wash.), 74*, 372-374

Henle, W. & Henle, G. (1973)   Evidence for an oncogenic potential of the Epstein-Barr virus.   *Cancer Res., 33*, 1419-1423

Henle, G., Henle, W., Klein, G., Gunven, P., Clifford, P., Morrow, R.H. & Ziegler, J.L. (1971)   Antibodies to early Epstein-Barr virus-induced antigens in Burkitt's lymphoma.   *J. nat. Cancer Inst., 46*, 861-871

Hsiung, G.D., Kaplow, L.S. & Booss, J. (1971)   Herpes virus infection of guinea pigs. I. Isolation, characterization and pathogenicity.   *Amer. J. Epidem., 93*, 298-307

Jondal, M. & Klein, G. (1973)   Surface markers on human B- and T-lymphocytes.   II. Presence of Epstein-Barr virus receptors on B lymphocytes.   *J. exp. Med., 138*, 1365-1378

Kimura, S., Flannery, V.L., Levy, B. & Schaffer, P.A. (1975)   Oncogenic transformation of primary hamster cells by herpes simplex virus type 2 (HSV-2) and an HSV-2 temperature-sensitive mutant.   *Int. J. Cancer, 15*, 786-798

Klein, G., Wiener, F., Zech, L., zur Hausen, H. & Reedman, B. (1974)   Segregation of the EBV-determined nuclear antigen (EBNA) in somatic cell hybrids derived from the fusion of a mouse fibroblast and a human Burkitt lymphoma line.   *Int. J. Cancer, 14*, 54-64

Kraiselburd, E. & Weissbach, A. (1975) *Presence of a herpes simplex virus type 1 genome fragment in HSV-transformed cells.* In: de-Thé, G., Epstein, M.A. & zur Hausen, H., eds, *Oncogenesis and Herpesviruses II, part 1*, Lyon, International Agency for Research on Cancer, (*IARC Scientific Publications* No. 11), pp. 415-419

Kucera, L.S. & Gusdon, J.P. (1976) Transformation of human embryonic fibroblasts by photodynamically inactivated herpes simplex virus type 2 at supraoptimal temperature. *J. gen. Virol., 30*, 257-261

Kutinová, L., Vonka, V. & Broucek, J. (1973) Increased oncogenicity and synthesis of herpesvirus antigens in hamster cells exposed to herpes simplex virus type-2. *J. nat. Cancer Inst., 50*, 759-765

Lausch, R.N., Murasko, D.M., Albrecht, T. & Rapp, F. (1974) Detection of specific surface antigens on cells transformed by cytomegalovirus with the techniques of mixed hemagglutination and ^{125}I-labelled antiglobulin. *J. Immun., 112*, 1680-1684

Lausch, R.N., Jones, C., Christie, D., Hay, K.A. & Rapp, F. (1975) Spleen cell-mediated cytotoxicity of hamster cells transformed by herpes simplex virus: evidence for virus specific membrane antigen. *J. Immun., 114*, 459-465

Lausch, R.N., Murasko, D.M. & Hay, K.A. (1976) *Host response to hamster cells transformed by cytomegalovirus and herpes simplex virus type 2.* In: Weiss, L., ed., *Fundamental Aspects of Metastases*, New York, Roswell Park Institute, pp. 327-340

Li, J.L.H., Jerkofsky, M.A. & Rapp, F. (1975) Demonstration of oncogenic potential of mammalian cells transformed by DNA-containing viruses following photodynamic inactivation. *Int. J. Cancer, 15*, 190-202

Lucké, B. (1938) Carcinoma in the leopard frog: its probable causation by a virus. *J. exp. Med., 68*, 457-468

Macnab, J.C.M. (1974) Transformation of rat embryo cells by temperature-sensitive mutants of herpes simplex virus. *J. gen. Virol., 24*, 143-153

Macnab, J.C.M. (1975) *Transformed cell lines produced by temperature-sensitive mutants of herpes simplex types 1 and 2.* In: de-Thé, G., Epstein, M.A. & zur Hausen, H., eds, *Oncogenesis and Herpesviruses II, part 1*, Lyon, International Agency for Research on Cancer (*IARC Scientific Publications* No. 11), pp. 227-236

McKinnell, R.G. & Ellis, V.L. (1972) *Epidemiology of the frog renal tumour and the significance of tumour nuclear transplantation studies to a viral aetiology of the tumour - a review.* In: Biggs, P.M., de-Thé, G. & Payne, L.N., eds, *Oncogenesis and Herpesviruses*, Lyon, International Agency for Research on Cancer (*IARC Scientific Publications* No. 2), pp. 183-197

Michalski, F.J., Fong, C.K.Y., Hsiung, G.D. & Schneider, R.D. (1976)   Induction of tumors by a guinea pig herpesvirus-transformed hamster cell line.   *J. nat. Cancer Inst.*, *56*, 1165-1170

Miller, G., Shope, T., Lisco, H., Stitt, D. & Lipman, M. (1972) Epstein-Barr virus: transformation, cytopathic changes and viral antigens in squirrel monkey and marmoset leukocytes.   *Proc. nat. Acad. Sci. (Wash.)*, *69*, 383-387

Minson, A.C., Thouless, M.E., Eglin, R.P. & Darby, G. (1976)   The detection of virus DNA sequences in a herpes type 2 transformed hamster cell line (333-8-9).   *Int. J. Cancer*, *17*, 493-500

Munyon, W., Kraiselburd, E., Davis, D. & Mann, J. (1971)   Transfer of thymidine kinase to thymidine kinaseless L cells by infection with ultraviolet-irradiated herpes simplex virus.   *J. Virol.*, *7*, 813-820

Munyon, W., Buchsbaum, R., Paoletti, E., Mann, J., Kraiselburd, E. & Davis, D. (1972)   Electrophoresis of thymidine kinase activity synthesized by cells transformed by herpes simplex virus.   *Virology*, *49*, 683-689

Murasko, D. & Lausch, R.N. (1974)   Cellular immune response to virus specific antigen in hamsters bearing isografts of cytomegalovirus-transformed cells.   *Int. J. Cancer*, *14*, 451-460

Nayak, D.P. (1971)   Isolation and characterization of a herpesvirus from leukemic guinea pigs.   *J. Virol.*, *8*, 579-588

Notter, M.F.D. & Docherty, J.C. (1976)   Antigens isolated from herpes simplex virus transformed cells react with sera of squamous cell carcinoma patients.   *Cancer Res.*, *36*, 4394-4401

Rapp, F. & Duff, R. (1972)   *In vitro* cell transformation by herpesviruses.   *Fed. Proc.*, *31*, 1660-1668

Rapp, F. & Duff, R. (1973)   Transformation of hamster embryo fibroblasts by herpes simplex viruses type 1 and type 2.   *Cancer Res.*, *33*, 1527-1534

Rapp, F., Li, J.L.H. & Jerkofsky, M. (1973)   Transformation of mammalian cells by DNA-containing viruses following photodynamic inactivation.   *Virology*, *55*, 339-346

Rapp, F. & Li, J.L.H. (1974)   Demonstration of the oncogenic potential of herpes simplex viruses and human cytomegalovirus.   *Cold Spring Harb. Symp. quant. Biol.*, *39*, 747-763

Rapp, F., Geder, L., Murasko, D., Lausch, R., Ladda, R., Huang, E. & Webber, M. (1975)   Long term persistence of cytomegalovirus genome in cultured human cells of prostatic origin.   *J. Virol.*, *16*, 982-990

Rapp, F. & Westmoreland, D. (1976)   Cell transformation by DNA-containing viruses. *Biochim. Biophys. Acta (Amst.)*, *458*, 167-211

Reed, C.L., Cohen, G.H. & Rapp, F. (1975)   Detection of a virus-specific antigen on the surface of herpes simplex virus-transformed cells. *J. Virol.*, *15*, 668-670

Rhim, J.S. (1977)   Malignant transformation of rat embryo cells by a herpesvirus isolated from L_2C guinea pig leukemia. *Virology*, *82*, 100-110

Risser, R., Rifkin, D. & Pollack, R. (1974)   The stable classes of transformed cells induced by SV40 infection of established 3T3 cells and primary rat embryonic cells. *Cold Spring Harb. Symp. quant. Biol.*, *39*, 317-324

Sanford, E.J., Dagen, J.E., Geder, L., Rohner, T.J. & Rapp, F. (1977)   Lymphocyte reactivity against virally transformed cells in patients with urologic cancer. *J. Urol.*, *118*, 809-810

St. Jeor, S.C., Albrecht, T.B., Funk, F.D. & Rapp, F. (1974)   Stimulation of cellular DNA synthesis by human cytomegalovirus. *J. Virol.*, *13*, 353-362

Takahashi, M. & Yamanishi, K. (1974)   Transformation of hamster embryo and human embryo cells by temperature sensitive mutants of herpes simplex virus type 2. *Virology*, *61*, 306-311

The, T.H., Klein, G. & Langenhuysen, M.M.A.C. (1974)   Antibody reactions to virus-specific early antigens (EA) in patients with cytomegalovirus (CMV) infection. *Clin. exp. Immunol.*, *16*, 1-12

Thiry, L., Sprecher-Goldberger, S., Tack, L., Jacques, M. & Stienon, J. (1975)   Comparison of the immunogenicity of hamster cells transformed by adenovirus and herpes simplex virus. *Cancer Res.*, *35*, 1022-1029

Tweedell, K.S., Michalski, F.J. & Morek, D.M. (1972)   *Bioassay of frog renal tumour viruses.*   In: Biggs, P.M., de-Thé, G. & Payne, C.N., eds, *Oncogenesis and Herpesviruses*, Lyon, International Agency for Research on Cancer (*IARC Scientific Publications* No. 2), pp. 198-205

Weller, T.H. (1971)   The cytomegaloviruses: ubiquitous agents with protean clinical manifestations. I. *New Engl. J. Med.*, *285*, 203-214

Wolf, H., zur Hausen, H. & Becker, B.V. (1973)   EB viral genomes in epithelial nasopharyngeal carcinoma cells. *Nature new Biol.*, *244*, 245-247

Yamamoto, H., Walz, M.A. & Notkins, A.L. (1977)   Viral specific thymidine kinase in sensory ganglia of mice infected with herpes simplex virus. *Virology*, *76*, 866-869 zur Hausen, H., Schulte-Holthausen, H., Wolf, H., Dörries, K. & Egger, H. (1974)   Attempts to detect virus-specific DNA in human tumors.   II. Nucleic acid hybridizations with complement-ary RNA of human herpes group viruses.   *Int. J. Cancer, 13,* 657–664

TRANSFORMATION OF LYMPHOID CELLS BY HERPESVIRUSES: A REVIEW WITH SPECIAL REFERENCE TO THE PHENOTYPIC PROPERTIES OF TRANSFORMED CELLS

K. NILSSON

Department of Tumor Biology,
The Wallenberg Laboratory,
University of Uppsala,
Uppsala, Sweden

INTRODUCTION

The possibility that Epstein-Barr virus (EBV), originally detected in Burkitt's lymphoma (BL) cells *in vitro* (Epstein et al., 1964), is a tumour virus has stimulated extensive studies which have shown that EBV:

(*a*) is the cause of heterophil antibody-positive infectious mononucleosis (IM) in man (Henle et al., 1968; Niederman et al., 1968);

(*b*) is present in all tumour biopsy cells of BL *in vivo* and *in vitro* and in nasopharyngeal carcinoma cells *in vivo* (Lindahl et al., 1974; Nonoyama et al., 1973; zur Hausen et al., 1970, 1972);

(*c*) can cause permanent growth transformation ("immortalization") of human and non-human primate lymphocytes *in vitro* (for a review, see Miller, 1974); and

(*d*) induces a fatal lymphoproliferation when injected into several species of New-World primates (Epstein et al., 1973; Falk et al., 1976b; Miller, 1974; Shope et al., 1973; Werner et al., 1975). A causative role of EBV in BL is suggested by the above features of the virus but remains, however, to be proved.

In animal systems a few other types of lymphotropic herpesviruses have been proved to be oncogenic. Marek's disease virus (MDV) causes a fatal lymphoproliferation in chicken)for a recent review see

Nazerian et al., 1976a).   Herpesvirus saimiri (HVS) (Meléndez et al.,
1968) and herpesvirus ateles (HVA) (Deinhardt et al., 1973; Falk et
al., 1974a; Meléndez et al., 1972) are not oncogenic in the natural
host but cause leukaemia and lymphoma in other non-human primates
(for reviews, see Ablashi et al., 1976; Deinhardt et al., 1974).
These systems have provided interesting models for the study of the
possible oncogenic role of herpesviruses, and especially EBV, in
humans.

Recently herpesvirus strains have also been isolated from Old-
World monkeys (baboon and chimpanzee) (Falk et al., 1976a; Gerber et
al., 1976; Lapin et al., 1976; Rabin et al., 1976).   These viruses
[herpesvirus papio (HVP) and "chimpanzee agent"] have a DNA which is
approximately 40% homologous to HR-1 EBV DNA.   Like EBV they can
immortalize lymphocytes *in vitro*.   Chimpanzee and baboon lymphocyte
cell lines, carrying the respective types of herpesviruses, have
biological properties which are closely similar to those of the EBV-
carrying human B-lymphoblastoid lines.   The Old-World monkey viruses
may therefore prove to be even more important as models than MDV, HVS
and HVA in the study of EBV's putative oncogenic role in man.

This review will deal with the transformation of lymphocytes by
herpesviruses *in vitro* with particular reference to the properties of
the established EBV-carrying B-lymphoid cell lines.   The emphasis on
EBV-induced lymphoproliferation simply reflects the fact that present
knowledge of EBV and its interaction with lymphoid cells is far more
advanced than that of the animal lymphotropic herpesviruses.

TRANSFORMATION *IN VITRO*

EBV is a lymphotropic virus *in vitro*.   So far no other cell type
has been found susceptible to EBV infection.   However, the most
relevant non-lymphoid cell type, the epithelial cell of the nasopha-
rynx, has not been tested extensively since it grows poorly *in vitro*.
The principal target cell seems to be an EBV and complement receptor-
expressing B-lymphocyte (Greaves et al., 1975; Jondal & Klein, 1973;
Pattengale et al., 1973).   Other types of lymphocytes lack the EBV
receptor (Greaves et al., 1975) and infection is consequently impossible.   In line with these experimental observations is the fact
that no continuous haematopoietic lines other than lymphoid lines
expressing B-cell markers have been found to carry EBV genomes.

EBV can also convert lymphocytes from some non-human primate
species (gibbon, marmoset, squirrel and woolly monkey) into indefinitely proliferating cell lines (zur Hausen, 1975).   Lymphocytes
from other species are resistant to EBV infection.

EBV-carrying cell lines can be established *in vitro* from human
blood and reticulolymphoid tissue either "spontaneously" or by
infection with "immortalizing" strains of EBV (for a review, see

Miller, 1974).   Spontaneous establishment is observed only with
biopsy material from anti-EBV seropositive donors (Chang et al., 1971;
Gerber et al., 1970; Nilsson et al., 1971; Pope et al., 1968).

It has been suggested that the spontaneous establishment of an
EBV-carrying cell line is the result of a direct outgrowth of the few
EBV-carrying lymphoblastoid cells present in the original explant
(Klein, 1973).   However, recent studies by Epstein's group (Epstein,
1975; Rickinson et al., 1974, 1975, 1977) have shown that, at least
in the case of blood from normal donors and patients with infectious
mononucleosis (IM), the outgrowth of a polyclonal lymphoblastoid cell
line (LCL) is mainly the result of a two-step *in vitro* event.
Epstein and his co-workers suggest that lymphocytes, latently infected
by EBV but not expressing EBV-related antigens *in vivo*, will liberate
immortalizing EBV during a lytic cycle when explanted *in vitro*.   The
released virus will then infect normal B-lymphocytes which eventually
undergo EBV-induced immortalization *in vitro*.   Although these studies
certainly demonstrate that the vast majority of the established cells
in a LCL are derived from cells infected *in vitro*, unequivocal evidence
that *in vivo* infected cells never grow out *in vitro* seems to be lacking
(Dalens et al., 1975).   This, together with the demonstration that
some lymphoid cells in the blood of IM patients and in tonsils express
EBV-determined nuclear antigen (EBNA) (Klein et al., 1976; Veltri et
al., 1976), suggest that the important question whether a different
type of cell-virus interaction may exist in Burkitt's lymphoma (BL)
cells than in EBV-carrying lymphocytes in normal EBV seroreactive
individuals, as suggested by Epstein & Achong (1973), therefore seems
to await its final answer.

The molecular events leading to immortalization of lymphocytes
after EBV infection have not been worked out in detail.   However, it
is clear that the interaction between the virus and host-cell genomes
must be such that virus replication is prevented.   Viral protein
synthesis always leads to irreversible cell damage and eventual cell
death.   Studies with phosphonoacetic acid indirectly suggest that EBV
has a DNA polymerase (Summers & Klein, 1976; Thorley-Lawson & Strominger, 1976) which may be required during the early events of the
immortalization (Thorley-Lawson & Strominger, 1976).

LCL and BL lines typically contain multiple copies (10-100) of the
EBV genome (Pagano, 1974; zur Hausen, 1975).   The EBV genomes
replicate synchronously with the host cells (Hampar et al., 1974), and
the number of genomes is kept remarkably constant during continuous
cultivation *in vitro* (zur Hausen, 1975).   Intracellular EBV DNA is
present both as integrated and free, circular virus DNA (Adams &
Lindahl, 1975; Kaschka-Dierich et al., 1976; Lindahl et al., 1976).
No difference in the physical state of the intracellular EBV DNA was
demonstrated in BL lines and lines established spontaneously from
donors without lymphoproliferative disease (Kaschka-Dierich et al.,
1977).   However, differences in integration sites and/or in integrated
fragments could not be excluded for technical reasons.

Several antigenic changes have been detected in lymphocytes immortalized by EBV (for a review, see Klein, 1975).   (1) EBV-determined nuclear antigen (EBNA) can be demonstrated in all EBV DNA-containing lymphoid cell lines.   EBNA appears to be associated with chromosomes *in vivo*.   Recently Ohno et al. (1977) characterized EBNA as a protein which binds to fixed metaphase chromosomes *in vitro*.   It was suggested that EBNA may be a non-histone protein which interacts with the EBV genomes in the host cell.   If so, the EBNA protein may play a role in the EBV-induced immortalization and in maintaining the transformed state.   (2) The complement-fixing soluble (S) antigen is identical to EBNA (Ohno et al., 1977).   (3) The membrane antigen (MA) has several antigenically distinct components and is found only in EBV producer lines.   (4) Early antigens (EA), detectable in a small fraction of producer cells, have two components [restricted (R) and diffuse (D)].   The chemical nature and function of MA and EA have not been clarified.   (5) The viral capsid antigen (VCA) can be demonstrated in a small minority of cells within producer lines. (6) The lymphocyte-detected antigen (LYDMA) (Jondal, 1976) is present in all EBV genome-carrying cell lines and appears to be an antigen recognized by cytotoxic T-cells.   LYDMA has not been chemically defined.

Little is known about the mechanisms that restrict the production of virus but allow the expression of EBNA and LYDMA in EBV genome-containing cells.   In non-producer lines, virus production is at a non-detectable level.   Even in producer lines, with the exception of the P3HR-1 and marmoset lines (Hinuma & Grace, 1967; Miller & Lipman, 1973), the fraction of cells replicating virus is very low.   EBV-determined antigen(s) can be induced in some non-producer lines by:

(*a*) superinfection by P3HR-1 virus (Henle et al., 1971);

(*b*) the use of halogenated nucleotide analoges (iododeoxyuridine, bromodeoxyuridine) (IUDR, BUDR) (Gerber, 1972; Hampar et al., 1972; Sugawara et al., 1972); or

(*c*) by fusion with other types of cells (Glaser & O'Neill, 1972; Klein et al., 1974).   The general picture that has emerged from these studies so far is that virus antigen expression is controlled mainly by cellular repressive mechanisms operating at different parts of the viral cycle.

PROPERTIES OF HUMAN EBV-CARRYING CELL LINES

Comparative studies on morphology, cell-surface characteristics, chromosomes, tumorigenicity and functional properties of EBV-carrying lines established from African BL and reticulolymphoid tissue of EBV sero-positive donors demonstrate that two main types of lines can be distinguished (Fagraeus et al., 1975; Nilsson & Pontén, 1975;

Nilsson et al., 1977a; Zech et al., 1976).   One type, the BL line, can be obtained only from BL biopsies while the other type, here termed lymphoblastoid cell line (LCL), can be derived from normal as well as from neoplastic lymphoid tissue including, in rare cases, BL biopsies. The cell lines established by EBV infection *in vitro* (e.g., from the QIMR-WIL, QIMR-GOR and B95-8 lines) have biological properties indistinguishable from those of LCL derived "spontaneously" from blood and lymphoid tissue (Nilsson, 1976; Pope, 1975).   Cells of BL lines are progeny of the neoplastic cells *in vivo* and are monoclonal at the initiation of the culture (Bechét et al., 1974; Fialkow et al., 1970). The LCL, in contrast, are polyclonal shortly after establishment (Bechét et al., 1974).   At "spontaneous" establishment they seem to be derived from B-lymphocytes that have been converted into established cells by EBV *in vitro* (Epstein & Achong, 1973) and perhaps also from *in vivo* immortalized EBV-carrying lymphoblastoid cells displaying their capacity for infinite growth when explanted *in vitro* (Klein, 1973).

Both types of lines will undergo secondary chromosomal alterations during prolonged culture *in vitro* (Nilsson & Pontén, 1975; Steel[1]; Zech[1]).   These alterations are sometimes followed by phenotypic change(s) and classification of any cell line should therefore be performed shortly after its establishment.   The properties listed in Tables 1 and 2 are those found in fresh lines (less than six months in culture).

Generally the LCL form a very homogeneous group of lines with regard to the various phenotypic properties.   This contrasts to the marked morphological heterogeneity within each LCL.   The difference sometimes noted between individual lines in the frequency of cells expressing a certain surface marker, or in the functional properties, generally reflects a difference in growth conditions rather than a stable phenotypic difference.   The BL lines, on the other hand, are more heterogeneous with regard to the different characteristics listed in Tables 1 and 2 when considered as a group.   This is probably due to aneuploidy which, in addition to the common 14q+ marker, is unique for each lymphoma line.

LCL cells are highly motile cells with great morphological flexibility.   They grow in large clumps in stationary suspension cultures or attach strongly and move about on feeder cells when such are present. BL lines generally contain uniformly round cells growing in loose small clumps or as single cells.   They attach poorly to feeder cells and are comparatively immotile, with the motility confined to short, thin, surface villi.

---

[1] Personal communication

Table 1. Properties of human EBV-carrying lymphoid cell lines

Characteristics	LCL	BL Lines	Reference
Morphology			
Cell type (diameter)	Lymphoblastoid (12-13 µ)	Lymphoblastoid (10-11 µ)	Nilsson & Pontén, 1975
Morphological diversity: between lines within lines	None Marked	Present Slight	
Ultrastructure (TEM)[a]	Moderate development of endoplasmic reticulum	Sparsely developed Golgi apparatus and endoplasmic reticulum	
Surface morphology (SEM)[b]	Long villi often with asymmetric location	Thin, short villi covering the entire surface	
Time-lapse cinematography	Highly motile. Translocation	Low motility. No translocation	
Growth characteristics			
Efficiency of establishment	High	High	Nilsson & Pontén, 1975
Attachment to feeder cells	Strong and rapid, most cells	Loose and slow, only some cells	
Growth in suspension	Large, dense clumps	Single cells or small, loose clumps	
Population doubling time (hr)	24-48	18-30	
Colony formation in agarose	All lines; low cloning efficiency	Some lines; often high cloning efficiency	
Surface characteristics			
Lymphocyte markers (% positive cells)			Huber et al., 1976
SRBC[c]	0	0	
C3 (EAC)	60-100	0-100	
Fc (EA)	0-5	0-60	
Fc (Aggr. Ig)	2+	2-3+	
Ig	70-90	70-100	
Surface glycoprotein (GP) pattern	B-blast-like, GP 160 and GP 115 prominent	B-cell-like, GP 210 prominent. B-lymphoma pattern, GP 87/85, GP 71/69	Gahmberg et al., 1977 Nilsson et al., 1977b
Functional markers			
Ig surface ($ng/10^6$ cells)	0.7	0-20	Nilsson, 1977
Ig secretion ($µg/10^6$ cells in 24 hr)	1-3	0	
Lysozyme secretion ($µg/10^6$ cells in 24 hr)	0	0	
β_2-microglobulin secretion	300-400	0-150, highly variable	
Interferon production	Yes	Yes	

[a] TEM: Transmission electron microscope

[b] SEM: Scanning electron microscope

[c] Sheep red blood cells

Table 2. Distinguishing characteristics of newly established LCL and BL lines

Characteristic	LCL	BL Lines	Reference
Clonality	Polyclonal	Monoclonal	Bechét et al., 1974
Karyotype	Normal diploid	Aneuploid, chromosome 14 marker	Jarvis et al., 1974 Zech et al., 1976
Tumorigenicity	-	+ or -	Nilsson et al., 1977a
Surface glycoprotein pattern	GP 160, GP 115	GP 210, GP 87/85, GP 71/69	Gahmberg et al., 1978[a] Nilsson et al., 1977b

[a] See p. 649

Both types of lines are composed of B-lymphocytes which, however, seem to have been frozen at different stages of B-lymphoid differentiation, as judged from the immunological surface-marker characteristics (Huber et al., 1976), the type of immunoglobulin (Ig) production (Nilsson, 1977), the surface glycoprotein pattern (Nilsson et al., 1977b), and the ultrastructural features (Nilsson, 1977). The LCL type of cell characteristically expresses complement (C) receptor and only a small amount of Fc receptor and surface Ig, and always secretes Ig into the medium. The BL cells often express both C and Fc receptor and generally have a larger amount of surface Ig, commonly of IgM type. The BL lines typically do not secrete Ig and some do not synthesize Ig at all (Bechét et al., 1974). Ultrastructural studies reveal that LCL cells have some endoplasmic reticulum and a fairly well-developed Golgi apparatus while BL cells have polyribosomes unattached to membranes. The recent studies of the surface glycoprotein pattern by galactose oxidase catalysed-tritiated borohydride labelling (Gahmberg et al.[1]; Nilsson et al., 1977a) also suggest a greater similarity of BL cells to B-lymphocytes than to mitogen-stimulated B-blasts while the reverse was true for the LCL cells. On the whole, the BL cell resembles a resting B-lymphocyte, although of course having many abnormal features, while the LCL cell has many similarities to mitogen-stimulated B-lymphoblasts.

[1] See p. 649

An important difference between the two types of lines is the karyotype.   LCL are normal diploid while the BL lines always are aneuploid on establishment (Jarvis et al., 1974; Zech et al., 1976). Manolov & Manolova (1972) described a chromosome 14 marker in most BL lines.   The characteristic abnormality was later identified as a 8q–; 14q+ translocation by Zech et al. (1976); up to the present, this marker has been identified in 27/30 BL biopsies and derived lines (Jarvis et al., 1974; Manolov & Manolova, 1972; Zech et al., 1976). It should be noted, however, that the chromosome 14 marker is not BL-specific, since it was also detected in other human lymphomas of B-cell origin (Zech et al., 1976).

Analysis of the surface glycoprotein pattern by galactose oxidase catalysed-tritiated borohydride labelling (Gahmberg, 1976) has proved to be a method sensitive enough to detect differences between various types of haematopoietic cell lines (Andersson et al., 1977; Nilsson et al., 1977a) and as reported separately the LCL and BL types of lines have characteristically different patterns (Gahmberg et al.[1]).

The LCL, when still polyclonal and normal diploid, are not tumori-genic when transplanted subcutaneously into nude mice while BL lines will usually grow (Nilsson et al., 1977b).   This is in contrast to some previous findings that lymphoid lines immortalized by EBV may be tumorigenic when transplanted into an immunosuppressed or newborn heterologous host (e.g., Adams et al., 1971; Christofinis, 1969; Deal et al., 1971; Southam et al., 1969).   This difference is probably best explained by the fact that old LCL with secondary chromo-somal alterations, which may be tumorigenic (Nilsson et al., 1977b), have been used in these experiments but it is also possible that the nude mouse differs from other animals in accepting grafted cells.

The most important characteristics for use in distinguishing between the two types of human EBV-carrying cell lines are listed in Table 2.

Cell lines immortalized *in vitro* by other isolates of EBV than the B95-8 virus have not been characterized by the same parameters which have formed the basis for the subdivision of EBV-carrying cell lines into two main groups (LCL and BL lines) described above.   It is therefore possible that lines obtained by immortalization with other EBV isolates may give rise to lines with phenotypic properties different from the prototype LCL (Hinuma & Katsuki, 1975).

In a series of experiments with two EBV-genome negative BL lines and their EBV-converted sublines attempts were made to determine which phenotypic properties could be related to the presence of EBV (Steinitz & Klein, 1975, 1976, 1977; Yefenof & Klein, 1976; Yefenof et al.,

---

[1]   See p. 649

1977). So far, the comparative studies of growth properties have demonstrated that the EBV-converted sublines differed from the parental lines in being less serum-dependent and less sensitive to saturation conditions. The presence of the EBV genome may also impair the lateral diffusion of glycoproteins in the plasma membrane as shown by the reduced ability to form caps in the EBV-converted sublines after staining with anti-IgM and concanavalin A (con A). An effect of the EBV genome on the plasma membrane dynamics was also suggested by an increased con A agglutinability in the sublines.

TRANSFORMATION BY PRIMATE HERPESVIRUSES AND PROPERTIES OF ESTABLISHED LINES

Herpesvirus saimiri (HVS) and herpesvirus ateles (HVA)

These horizontally transmitted viruses cause no known disease in the natural host (Table 3). They can be propagated in vitro in various types of primate cells (for reviews, see Ablashi et al., 1976; Deinhardt et al., 1974). Cytopathic effect (CPE) assays on monkey kidney cells are available for both viruses.

Table 3. Comparison of EBV, HVS and HLA-induced lymphoproliferation in vivo and in vitro

Characteristic	EBV	HVS	HVA
Transmission	Horizontal	Horizontal	Horizontal
Disease in natural host	Subclinical seroconversion or infectious mononucleosis; wide-spread infection	Not known; wide-spread infection	Not known; wide-spread infection
Suggested oncogenicity in natural host	Burkitt's lymphoma; nasopharyngeal carcinoma	Not known	Not known
Experimental oncogenicity	Lymphoma induction in non-human primates	Causes T-cell lymphomas in subhuman primates and rabbits	Causes T-cell lymphomas in subhuman primates and rabbits
In vitro transformation	B-lymphocytes (polyclonal)	Not found	Human and marmoset T-lymphocytes, polyclonal
Viral antigen expression in cell line	VCA, MA, EA, EBNA, CF	EA, LA, MA	EA, LA, MA
Viral production	Producers and non-producers	Producers (a small fraction of cells)	Producers (a small fraction of cells)
Viral genomes	Present in tumours and established lines	Present in tumours and established lines	Present in tumours and established lines

Like EBV, the simian viruses are lymphotropic and cause a sometimes fatal lymphoproliferation when inoculated into primates other than the natural host (Ablashi et al., 1971; Deinhardt et al., 1974; Meléndez et al., 1972) and also into New Zealand white rabbits (Rangan et al., 1976). The induced malignancies have clinical and

histopathological similarities to leukaemia and lymphoma but since
they are polyclonal (Chu & Rabson, 1972; Marczynska et al., 1973)
they may well represent a fatal form of a disease equivalent to IM
in man.

In contrast to EBV, HVS and HVA transform T-cells (Deinhardt et
al., 1974; Falk et al., 1974a,b; Wallen et al., 1973). Explanted
tissue from HVS and HVA-induced tumours gives rise to cell lines with
a lymphoblastoid morphology and T-cell surface markers (Falk et al.,
1974a; Oie et al., 1973; Rabson et al., 1971). As in established
EBV-carrying cell lines, the cells contain multiple copies of viral
genomes which seem to be associated with the cell genome both as
integrated sequences and as episomal DNA (Fleckenstein et al., 1976;
Werner et al., 1977). Viral antigens are expressed in a small
percentage of cells (Ablashi et al., 1976; Deinhardt et al., 1974).
HVS-infected cells express early antigen (EA), late antigen (LA) and
membrane antigen (MA) while EA and LA have been found in HVA-carrying
cells. In neither case has a nuclear antigen similar to EBNA been
demonstrated. Most lines become non-producers after prolonged cultivation *in vitro*, a development often encountered also in human EBV-
carrying lymphoid cell lines.

The HVS lines established from experimentally induced tumours
share some important features with the LCL type of human EBV-carrying
cell lines (e.g., IM-derived lines):

(*a*) they are polyclonal on establishment but may become monoclonal
during long-term cultivation; and

(*b*) no specific chromosome aberrations have been found
(Marczynska et al., 1973).

Similar information is not available for tumour-derived HVA-
containing lines.

Immortalization *in vitro* has been accomplished only with HVA (Falk
et al., 1974b). Lines from blood and splenic marmoset lymphocytes and
human lymphocytes were established by co-cultivation with lethally X-
irradiated HVA-producing lymphoblastoid cells. The established
splenic lines seem to have properties similar to those of HVS-containing,
tumour-derived lines. They were polyclonal, and cells expressed T-
lymphocyte surface characteristics.

Herpesvirus papio (HVP) and chimpanzee agent

The Old-World non-human primates seem to carry EBV-likeviruses.
HVP, as judged from serological studies, is widespread among several
baboon species (Deinhardt & Ablashi, 1977). The natural host of the
chimpanzee agent is the chimpanzee. The incidence of natural infection with chimpanzee agent is unknown. The mode of transmission for
HVP and chimpanzee agent is probably horizontal, as for EBV.
Nothing is known about the pathogenicity and possible oncogenicity in
the natural host for the chimpanzee agent and knowledge is still
fragmentary for HVP. However, as with EBV, HVS and HVA, lymphomas

can be induced by experimental inoculation of HVP into marmosets (Deinhardt & Ablashi, 1977).

Gerber et al. (1976) failed to establish human and marmoset lymphocytes by supernatant from chimpanzee agent-containing cell lines. Transformation *in vitro* has, however, been successfully achieved with HVP (Falk et al., 1977). The host range for HVP was similar to that of EBV.

Cell lines carrying HVP and chimpanzee agent have been spontaneously established *in vitro* from baboon and chimpanzee lymphocytes, respectively (Falk et al., 1976b; Gerber et al., 1976; Landon et al., 1968). The properties of these cell lines (Table 4) are closely similar to those of lines established spontaneously from normal donors or by infection of human lymphocytes *in vitro* by B95-8 virus. Information on the clonality and tumorigenicity of the baboon and chimpanzee lines is still lacking but existing data suggest that such lines resemble the LCL type of human EBV-carrying cell lines more than BL lines.

Table 4. Comparison of lymphoblastoid cell lines (LCL) established from lymphocytes

Characteristic	Human LCL	Chimpanzee LCL[a]	Baboon LCL[b]
Establishment	Lag phase ⟶ rapid growth	Lag phase ⟶ rapid growth	Lag phase ⟶ rapid growth
Growth pattern	Clumps, in suspension	Clumps, in suspension	Clumps, in suspension
Doubling time (hr)	24-48	24-36	24-72
Virus particles[c]	+	+	+
Viral genome	EBV	34-45% homology with HR-1 EBV DNA	40% homology with HR-1 EBV DNA
Viral antigens	MA, VCA, EA, EBNA, soluble antigen	VCA-like and/or EA-like C-NA (nuclear antigen)	VCA-, MA-, EA-like
Surface markers (% positive cells)			
SRBC[d]	-	-	-
Ig	70-90	20-30	20
C3	60-100	85-95	45-55
Fc	0-5 (EA)	Not tested	90 (Aggr. Ig)
Karyotype	Diploid	Diploid	Diploid

[a] Spontaneously established from blood (Gerber et al., 1976; Landon et al., 1968)

[b] Established from splenic lymphocytes by a co-cultivation method (Falk et al., 1976a, 1977)

[c] By electron microscopy

[d] Sheep red blood cells

TRANSFORMATION BY MAREK'S DISEASE VIRUS (MDV)
AND PROPERTIES OF CELL LINES ESTABLISHED

Marek's disease virus (MDV), first isolated from MD tumour cells
(Churchill & Biggs, 1967), is a herpesvirus which like EBV infects
both lymphoid and epithelial cells *in vivo* (for a recent review, see
Nazerian et al., 1976a).   The virus is horizontally transmitted and
causes MD in chickens.   MDV, like HVS and HVA, also replicates in
kidney cells and fibroblasts *in vitro* and plaque assays exist.   MDV
has not been found to immortalize lymphoid cells *in vitro*.   The properties of MDV-infected lymphoid cells can therefore be studied only
in a limited number of cell lines spontaneously established from MD
tumours (Akiyama et al., 1973; Akiyama & Kato, 1974; Nazerian et
al., 1976b; Nazerian & Witter, 1975; Powell et al., 1974).

MDV-transformed lymphoid cells contain multiple copies of the
virus genome (Nazerian & Lee, 1974) and, like cells in lines established
by other lymphotropic herpesviruses, production of virus-determined
antigens and viral particles can be detected in a small minority of the
cells.   In all cells in the lymphoblastoid lines a surface antigen
[Marek's-associated tumour-specific antigen (MATSA)] can be demonstrated (Witter et al., 1975).   In addition "early" antigens can be
induced by treatment with IUDR or BUDR (Nazerian, 1976b).   Removal
of these nucleotide analogues leads to expression of "late" antigens.
The physical state of MDV in genome-containing lymphoblastoid cells is
unknown, but like EBV the association with the host-cell genome seems
to be stable generation after generation *in vitro* (Nazerian et al.,
1976a).   The target cell for MDV in the development of MD seems to
be a lymphoid cell with T-cell surface characteristics (Nazerian &
Sharma, 1975; Powell et al., 1974).

Cell lines have been established with a low success rate after a
varying latent period (Powell et al., 1975).   A characteristic
difference between the avian and primate lymphoid lines is the short
population doubling time at 40-41°C of the former (Nazerian & Witter,
1975; Powell et al., 1975).   The MDV lines, like the primate lymphoid
lines, grow in suspension and have a similar maximum cell density.
Morphological studies, including electron microscopy, have shown that
the cells closely resemble BL cells (Frazier & Powell, 1975).
Nazerian et al. (1976b) have described the successful transplantation
of one cell line into MD-susceptible chickens.   Information on
clonality and chromosomes is lacking and no further conclusions can
be drawn, therefore, as to the possibility that MD lymphoid cell lines
may be more similar to the BL than to the LCL type of human EBV-carrying cell lines, as perhaps suggested by the morphological and transplantation studies.

SUMMARY AND CONCLUSIONS

B-lymphocytes, when exposed to EBV *in vitro*, become established
as permanent cell lines. The molecular events leading to this
immortalization remain to be clarified. In addition, information
on virus/cell interaction and the mechanisms controlling the expression of viral gene functions is still fragmentary.

The *in vitro* infection of B-lymphocytes, at least with the EBV
isolates used so far, leads to the establishment of the LCL and not
the BL type of line. This shows that *in vitro* "transformation" by
EBV is not equivalent to full malignant transformation of BL precursor cells *in vivo*.

The experiments by Epstein's group suggest that the development
of an LCL may be an exclusively *in vitro* event. However, it remains
to be proved that this means that the nature of the virus/cell interaction is different in BL cells and EBV-carrying lymphocytes in
normal donors and in those with IM.

HVP and the chimpanzee agent are recently described herpesviruses
which seem to be closely related to EBV. The lymphoid cell lines
carrying these viruses have biological properties closely similar to
those of the human EBV-carrying lines, especially the LCL type.
These viruses therefore promise to become even better models than HVS,
HVA, and MDV for the study of EBV-associated diseases in man.

ACKNOWLEDGEMENTS

I thank Dr G. Klein for helpful discussions.

REFERENCES

Ablashi, D.V., Easton, J.M. & Guegan, J.H. (1976)   Herpesviruses and
    cancer in man and subhuman primates. *Biomedicine, 24*, 268-305

Ablashi, D.V., Loeb, W.F., Valerio, M.G., Adamson, R.H., Armstrong, G.
    R., Bennett, D.G. & Herne, U. (1971)   Malignant lymphoma with
    lymphocytic leukemia induced in owl monkey by Herpes virus saimiri.
    J. nat. Cancer Inst., 47, 837-856

Adams, A. & Lindahl, T. (1975)   Epstein-Barr virus genomes with
    properties of circular DNA molecules in carrier cells.   *Proc.*
    nat. Acad. Sci. (Wash.), 72, 1477-1481

Adams, R.A., Hellerstein, E.E., Pothier, L., Foley, G.E., Lazarus, H.
    & Stuart, A.B. (1971)   Malignant potential of a cell line isolated
    from the peripheral blood in infectious mononucleosis.   *Cancer,*
    27, 651-657

Akiyama, Y., Kato, S. & Iwa, N. (1973)   Preliminary report.
    Continuous cell culture from lymphoma of Marek's disease.
    Biken J., 16, 177-179

Akiyama, Y. & Kato, S. (1974)   Two cell lines from lymphomas of
    Marek's disease.   *Biken J., 17*, 105-116

Andersson, L.C., Gahmberg, C.G., Nilsson, K. & Wigzell, H. (1977)
    Surface glycoprotein patterns of normal and malignant human
    lymphoid cells. I. T cells, T blasts and leukemic T cell lines.
    Int. J. Cancer, 20, 702-707

Bechét, J.M., Fialkow, P., Nilsson, K. & Klein, G. (1974)   Immuno-
    globulin synthesis and glucose-6-phosphate dehydrogenase as cell
    markers in human lymphoblastoid cell lines.   *Exp. Cell Res., 89*,
    275-282

Chang, R.S., Hsiek, M.W. & Blankenship, W.J. (1971)   Cell line
    initiation from cord blood leukocytes treated with viruses,
    chemicals and radiation.   *J. nat. Cancer Inst., 47*, 479-483

Christofinis, G.J. (1969)   Chromosome and transplantation results
    of a human leukocyte cell line derived from a healthy individual.
    Cancer, 24, 649-651

Chu, E.W. & Rabson, A.S. (1972)   Chimerism in lymphoid cell culture
    line derived from lymph node of marmoset infected with Herpes-
    virus saimiri.   *J. nat. Cancer Inst., 48*, 771-775

Churchill, A.E. & Biggs, P.M. (1967)   Agent of Marek's disease in
    tissue culture.   *Nature (Lond.), 215*, 528-530

Dalens, M., Zech, L. & Klein, G. (1975)   Origin of lymphoid lines
    established from mixed cultures of cord-blood lymphocytes and
    explants from infectious mononucleosis, Burkitt lymphoma and
    healthy donors.   *Int. J. Cancer, 16*, 1008-1014

Deal, D.R., Gerber, P. & Chisari, F.V. (1971)   Heterotransplantation
    of two human lymphoid cell lines transformed *in vitro* by Epstein-
    Barr virus.   *J. nat. Cancer Inst., 47*, 771-780

Deinhardt, F. & Ablashi, D.V. (1977)   Epstein-Barr like viruses of
    primates.   *IARC Newsletter No. 5*

Deinhardt, F., Falk, L. & Wolfe, L. (1973)   Simian Herpesviruses.
    Cancer Res., 33, 1424-1426

Deinhardt, W.F., Falk, A.L. & Wolfe, G.L. (1974)   Simian herpesviruses and neoplasia.   *Advanc. Cancer Res.*, *19*, 167-205

Epstein, M.A. (1975)   *Transformation* in vivo - *a review*.   In: de-Thé, G., Epstein, M.A. & zur Hausen, H., eds, *Oncogenesis and Herpesviruses II*, *part 2*, Lyon, International Agency for Research on Cancer (*IARC Scientific Publications* No. 11), pp. 141-152

Epstein, M.A. & Achong, B.G. (1973)   Various forms of Epstein-Barr virus infection in man: established facts and a general concept. *Lancet*, *ii*, 836-839

Epstein, M.A., Achong, B.G. & Barr, Y.M. (1964)   Virus particles in cultured lymphoblasts from Burkitt's lymphoma.   *Lancet*, *i*, 702-703

Epstein, M.A., Hunt, R.D. & Rabin, H. (1973)   Pilot experiments with EB virus in owl monkeys (*Aotus trivigartus*). I. Reticuloproliferative disease in an inoculated animal.   *Int. J. Cancer*, *12*, 309-318

Fagraeus, A., Nilsson, K., Lidman, K. & Norberg, R. (1975)   Reactivity of smooth muscle antibodies, surface ultrastructure, and mobility in cells of human hematopoietic cell lines.   *J. nat. Cancer Inst.*, *55*, 783-789

Falk, L., Deinhardt, F., Nonoyama, M., Wolfe, L.G., Bergholz, C., Lapin, B., Yakovleva, L., Agrba, V., Henle, G. & Henle, W. (1976a) Properties of a Baboon lymphotropic Herpesvirus related to Epstein-Barr virus.   *Int. J. Cancer*, *18*, 798-807

Falk, L., Deinhardt, F., Wolfe, L., Johnson, D., Hilgers, J. & de-Thé, G. (1976b)   Epstein-Barr virus: experimental infection of *Callithrix jacchus* marmosets.   *Int. J. Cancer*, *17*, 785-788

Falk, L.A., Henle, G., Henle, W., Deinhardt, F. & Schindel, A. (1977) Transformation of lymphocytes by Herpesvirus Papio.   *Int. J. Cancer*, *20*, 219-226

Falk, A.L., Nigida, M.S., Deinhardt, F., Wolfe, G.L., Cooper, W.R. & Hernandez-Camacho, I.J. (1974a)   Herpesvirus Ateles: Properties of an oncogenic herpesvirus isolated from circulating lymphocytes of spider monkeys (*Ateles* sp.).   *Int. J. Cancer*, *14*, 473-482

Falk, L., Wright, J., Wolfe, L. & Deinhardt, F. (1974b)   Herpesvirus ateles: Transformation *in vitro* of marmoset splenic lymphocytes. *Int. J. Cancer*, *14*, 244-251

Fialkow, P.J., Klein, G., Gartler, S.M. & Clifford, P. (1970) Clonal origin for individual Burkitt tumours.   *Lancet*, *i*, 384-386

Fleckenstein, B., Bornkamm, G.W. & Werner, F.J. (1976)   *The role of Herpesvirus saimiri genomes in oncogenic transformation of primate cells.*   In: Clemmesen, J. & Yohn, D., eds, *Comparative Leukemia Research*, Basel, Karger (*Bibliotheca Haematologica*, Vol. 43), pp. 308-312

Frazier, J.A. & Powell, P.C. (1975)   The ultrastructure of lymphoblastoid cell lines from Marek's disease lymphomata.   *Brit. J. Cancer, 31*, 7-14

Gahmberg, C.G. (1976)   External labeling of erythrocyte glycoproteins. Studies with galactose oxidase and fluorography.   *J. biol. Chem., 251*, 510-515

Gerber, P. (1972)   Activation of Epstein-Barr virus by 5-Bromodeoxyuridine in "virus-free" human cells.   *Proc. nat. Acad. Sci. (Wash.), 69*, 83-85

Gerber, P., Pritchett, R.F. & Kieff, E.D. (1976)   Antigens and DNA of a Chimpanzee agent related to Epstein-Barr virus.   *J. Virol., 19*, 1090-1099

Gerber, P., Whang-Peng, J. & Monroe, J.H. (1970)   Lymphoproliferative effect of Epstein-Barr virus on normal human lymphocytes in culture.   *Bibl. Haemat., 36*, 739-750

Glaser, R. & O'Neill, F.J. (1972)   Hybridization of Burkitt lymphoblastoid cells.   *Science, 176*, 1245-1247

Greaves, M.F., Brown, G. & Rickinson, A.B. (1975)   Epstein-Barr virus binding sites on lymphocyte subpopulations and the origin of lymphoblasts in cultured lymphoid cell lines and in the blood of patients with infectious mononucleosis.   *Clin. Immunol. Immunopathol., 3*, 514-524

Hampar, B., Derge, J.G., Martos, L.M. & Walker, J. (1972)   Synthesis of Epstein-Barr virus after activation of the viral genome in a viral genome in a virus negative human lymphoblastoid cell (Raji) made resistant to 5-bromodeoxyuridine.   *Proc. nat. Acad. Sci. (Wash.), 69*, 78-82

Hampar, B., Tanaka, A., Nonoyama, M. & Derge, J.G. (1974)   Replication of the resistent repressed Epstein-Barr virus genome during the early S phase (S-1 period) of nonproducer Raji cells.   *Proc. nat. Acad. Sci. (Wash.), 71*, 631-633

Henle, G., Henle, W. & Diehl, V. (1968)   Relation of Burkitt's tumor-associated herpes type virus to infectious mononucleosis.   *Proc. nat. Acad. Sci. (Wash.), 59*, 94-101

Henle, G., Henle, W., Klein, G., Gunvén, P., Clifford, P., Morrow, R.H. & Ziegler, J. (1971)   Antibodies to early Epstein-Barr virus induced antigens in Burkitt's lymphoma.   *J. nat. Cancer Inst., 46*, 861-871

Hinuma, Y. & Grace, J.T. (1967) Cloning of immunoglobulin-producing human leukemic and lymphoma cells in long term cultures. *Proc. Soc. exp. Biol. (N.Y.), 124,* 107-111

Hinuma, Y. & Katsuki, T. (1975) Characteristics of cell lines derived from human leukocytes transformed by different strains of Epstein-Barr virus. *Int. J. Cancer, 15,* 203-210

Huber, C., Sundström, C.C., Nilsson, K. & Wigzell, H. (1976) Surface receptors on human haematopoietic cell lines. *Clin. exp. Immunol., 25,* 367-378

Jarvis, J.E., Ball, G., Rickinson, A.B. & Epstein, M.A. (1974) Gytogenetic studies on human lymphoblastoid cell lines from Burkitt's lymphomas and other sources. *Int. J. Cancer, 14,* 716-721

Jondal, M. (1976) Antibody-dependent cellular cytotoxicity (ADCC) against Epstein-Barr virus-determined membrane antigens. I. Reactivity in sera from normal persons and from patients with acute infectious mononucleosis. *Clin. exp. Immunol., 25,* 1-5

Jondal, M. & Klein, G. (1973) Surface markers on human B and T lymphocytes. II. Presence of Epstein-Barr virus receptors on B lymphocytes. *J. exp. Med., 138,* 1365-1378

Kaschka-Dierich, C., Adams, A., Lindahl, T., Bornkamm, G.W., Bjursell, G., Klein, G., Giovanella, B.C. & Singh, S. (1976) Intracellular forms of Epstein-Barr virus DNA in human tumour cells *in vivo. Nature (Lond.), 260,* 302-306

Kaschka-Dierich, C., Falk, L., Bjursell, G., Adams, A. & Lindahl, T. (1977) Human lymphoblastoid cell lines derived from individuals without lymphoproliferative disease contain the same latent forms of Epstein-Barr virus DNA as those found in tumor cells. *Int. J. Cancer, 20,* 173-180

Klein, G. (1973) Tumor immunology. *Transplant. Proc., 5,* 31-41

Klein, G. (1975) *Virus-induced antigens - a review.* In: de-Thé, G., Epstein, M.A. & zur Hausen, H., eds, *Oncogenesis and Herpesviruses II, part 1,* Lyon, International Agency for Research on Cancer (*IARC Scientific Publications* No. 11), pp. 293-308

Klein, G., Svedmyr, E., Jondal, M. & Persson, P.O. (1976) EBV-determined nuclear antigen (EBNA)-positive cells in the peripheral blood of infectious mononucleosis patients. *Int. J. Cancer, 17,* 21-26

Klein, G., Wiener, F., Zech, L., zur Hausen, H. & Reedman, B. (1974) Segregation of the EBV-determined nuclear antigen (EBNA) in somatic cell hybrids derived from the fusion of a mouse fibroblast and a human Burkitt lymphoma line. *Int. J. Cancer, 14,* 54-64

Landon, J.C., Ellis, L.B., Zeve, V.H. & Fabrizio, D.P.A. (1968)
Herpes-type virus in cultured leukocytes from Chimpanzees.
J. nat. Cancer Inst., 40, 181-192

Lapin, B.A., Kokosha, L.V., Agrba, V.Z., Yakovleva, L.A., Arshba, N.N.,
Markova, T.P. & Timanovskaya, V.V. (1976) Immunological study
of suspension cultures prepared from cells of hemopoietic organs
of baboons with lymphomas. *Vop. Virus, 2*, 141-145

Lindahl, T., Adams, A., Bjursell, G., Bornkamm, G.W., Kaschka-Dierich,
C. & Jehn, U. (1976) Covalently closed circular duplex DNA of
Epstein-Barr virus in a human lymphoid cell line. *J. molec. Biol.,
102*, 511-530

Lindahl, T., Klein, G., Reedman, B.M., Johansson, B. & Surjit, S. (1974)
Relationships between Epstein-Barr virus (EBV) DNA and the EBV-
determined nuclear antigen EBNA in Burkitt lymphoma biopsies and
other lymphoproliferative malignancies. *Int. J. Cancer, 13*, 764-
772

Manolov, G. & Manolova, Y. (1972) Marker band in one chromosome 14
from Burkitt lymphomas. *Nature (Lond.), 237*, 33-34

Marczynska, B., Falk, L., Wolfe, L. & Deinhardt, F. (1973) Transplantation and cytogenetic studies of herpesvirus saimiri.
Induced disease in marmoset monkeys. *J. nat. Cancer Inst., 50*,
331-337

Meléndez, L.V., Daniel, M.D., Hunt, R.D. & Garcia, F.G. (1968)
An apparently new herpesvirus from primary kidney cultures of the
squirrel monkey (*Saimiri sciureus*). *Lab. Anim. Care, 18*, 374-
381

Meléndez, L.V., Hunt, R.D., King, N.W., Barakova, N.H., Daniel, M.D.,
Fraser, C.E.O. & Garcia, F.G. (1972) Herpesvirus ateles. A new
lymphoma virus of monkeys. *Nature new Biol., 235*, 182-184

Miller, G. (1974) The oncogenicity of Epstein-Barr virus. *J. infect.
Dis., 130*, 187-205

Miller, G. & Lipman, M. (1973) Release of infectious Epstein-Barr
virus by transformed marmoset leukocytes. *Proc. nat. Acad. Sci.
(Wash.), 70*, 190-194

Nazerian, K. & Lee, L.F. (1974) Deoxyribonucleic acid of Marek's
disease virus in a lymphoblastoid cell line from Marek's disease
tumors. *J. gen. Virol., 25*, 317-321

Nazerian, K. & Sharma, I.M. (1975) Detection of T-cell surface
antigens in a Marek's disease lymphoblastoid cell line. *J. nat.
Cancer Inst., 54*, 277-286

Nazerian, K. & Witter, R.L. (1975) Properties of a chicken lymphoblastoid cell line from Marek's disease tumor. *J. nat. Cancer
Inst., 54*, 453-458

Nazerian, K., Lee, F.L. & Sharma, M.J. (1976a)   The role of herpes-
    viruses in Marek's disease lymphoma of chickens.   *Progr. med.*
    Virol., 22, 123-151

Nazerian, K., Stephens, E.A., Sharma, I.M., Lee, F.L., Gailitis, M.
    & Witter, R.L. (1976b)   A nonproducer T-lymphoblastoid cell line
    from Marek's disease transplantable tumor (IMV).   *Avian Dis., 21*,
    69-76

Niederman, J.C., McCollum, R.V., Henle, G. & Henle, W. (1968)
    Infectious mononucleosis: Clinical manifestations in relation
    to EB virus antibodies.   *J. Amer. med. Ass., 205*, 205-209

Nilsson, K. (1976)   *Establishment of permanent human lymphoblastoid*
    cell lines in vitro.   In: David, J. & Bloom, B.R., eds, In vitro
    Methods in Cell Mediated and Tumor Immunity, New York, Academic
    Press, Vol. II, pp. 713-721

Nilsson, K. (1977)   *Established cell lines as tools in the study of*
    human, lymphoma and myeloma cell characteristics.   In:
    Thierfelder, S., Rodt, H. & Thiel, E., eds, *Immunological Diagnosis*
    Diagnosis of Leukemias and Lymphomas, Berlin, Springer-Verlag,
    Vol. 20, pp. 253-264

Nilsson, K., Andersson, L.C., Gahmberg, C.G. & Wigzell, H. (1977a)
    Surface glycoprotein patterns of normal and malignant human lymphoid
    cells.   II. B cells, B blasts and Epstein-Barr virus (EBV) positive
    and negative B-lymphoid cell lines.   *Int. J. Cancer, 20*, 703-716

Nilsson, K., Giovanella, B.C., Stehlin, J.S. & Klein, G. (1977b)
    Tumorigenicity of human hematopoietic cell lines in athymic nude
    mice.   *Int. J. Cancer, 19*, 337-344

Nilsson, K., Klein, G., Henle, G. & Henle, W. (1971)   The establishment
    of lymphoblastoid cell lines and its dependence on EBV.   *Int. J.*
    Cancer, 8, 443-450

Nilsson, K. & Pontén, J. (1975)   Classification and biological nature
    of established human hematopoietic cell lines.   *Int. J. Cancer, 15*,
    321-341

Nonoyama, M., Huang, C.H., Pagano, J.S., Klein, G. & Singh, S. (1973)
    DNA of Epstein-Barr virus detected in tissue.   *Proc. nat. Acad.*
    Sci. (Wash.), 70, 3265-3268

Ohno, S., Luka, J., Lindahl, T. & Klein, G. (1977)   Identification of
    a purified complement-fixing antigen as the Epstein-Barr-virus-
    determined nuclear antigen (EBNA) by its binding to metaphase
    chromosomes.   *Proc. nat. Acad. Sci. (Wash.), 74*, 1605-1609

Oie, H.K., Ablashi, D.V., Armstrong, G.R., Pearson, G.R., Orr, T. &
    Heine, U. (1973)   A continuous "*in vitro*" source of herpes virus
    saimiri.   *J. nat. Cancer Inst., 51*, 1077-1080

Pagano, J.S. (1974)   *The Epstein-Barr viral genome and its interactions with human lymphoblastoid cells and chromosomes.*   In: Kurstak, E. & Maramorosch, K., eds, *Viruses, Evolution and Cancer*, New York, Academic Press, pp. 79-116

Pattengale, P.K., Smith, R.W. & Gerber, P. (1973)   Selective transformation of B lymphocytes by E.B. virus.   *Lancet, ii*, 93-94

Pope, J.H. (1975)   *Transformation* in vitro *by herpesviruses - A review* In: de-Thé, G., Epstein, M.A. & zur Hausen, H., eds, *Oncogenesis and Herpesviruses II, part 1*, Lyon, International Agency for Research on Cancer (*IARC Scientific Publications* No. 11), pp. 367-378

Pope, J.H., Horne, M.K. & Scott, W. (1968)   Transformation of foetal human leucocytes *in vitro* by filtrates of a human leukemic cell line containing herpes-like virus.   *Int. J. Cancer, 3*, 857-866

Powell, P.C., Payne, L.N., Frazier, I.A. & Rennie, M. (1974) T-lymphoblastoid cell lines from Marek's disease lymphomas. *Nature (Lond.), 251*, 79-80

Powell, P.C., Payne, L.N., Frazier, I.A. & Rennie, M. (1975) *T-lymphoblastoid cell lines from Marek's disease lymphomas.*   In: de-Thé, G., Epstein, M.A. & zur Hausen, H., eds, *Oncogenesis and Herpesviruses II, part 2*, Lyon, International Agency for Research on Cancer (*IARC Scientific Publications* No. 11), pp. 89-99

Rabin, H., Neubauer, R.H., Hopkins, R.F., Dzhikidze, E.K., Shevtsova, Z. V. & Lapin, B.A. (1977)   Transforming activity of an Epstein-Barr like virus from lymphoblastoid cell lines of baboons with lymphoid disease.   *Intervirology*

Rabson, A.S., O'Conor, G.T., Lorenz, D.E., Kirschstein, R.L., Legallais, F.Y. & Tralka, T.S. (1971)   Lymphoid cell culture line derived from lymph node of marmoset infected with herpesvirus saimiri.   A preliminary report.   *J. nat. Cancer Inst., 46*, 1099-1109

Rangan, S.R.S., Martin, L.N., Enright, F.M. & Allen, W.P. (1976) Herpesvirus saimiri-induced malignant lymphoma in rabbits. *J. nat. Cancer Inst., 57*, 151-156

Rickinson, A.B., Epstein, M.A. & Crawford, D.H. (1975)   Absence of infectious Epstein-Barr virus in blood in acute infectious mononucleosis.   *Nature (Lond.), 258*, 236-238

Rickinson, A.B., Finerty, S. & Epstein, M.A. (1977)   Comparative studies on adult donor lymphocytes infected by EB virus *in vivo* or *in vitro*: origin of transformed cells arising in cocultures with foetal lymphocytes.   *Int. J. Cancer, 19*, 775-782

Rickinson, A.B., Jarvis, J.E., Crawford, D.H. & Epstein, M.A. (1974) Observations on the type of infection by Epstein-Barr virus in peripheral lymphoid cells of patients with infectious mononucleosis. *Int. J. Cancer, 14*, 704-715

Shope, T., Dechairo, D. & Miller, G. (1973)   Malignant lymphoma in cotton-top marmosets after inoculation with Epstein-Barr virus. *Proc. nat. Acad. Sci. (Wash.), 70,* 2487-2491

Southam, C.M., Burchenal, J.H., Clarkson, B., Tanzi, A., Mackey, R. & McComb, V. (1969)   Heterotransplantation of human cell lines from Burkitt's tumors and acute leukemia into newborn rats. *Cancer, 23,* 281-299

Steinitz, M. & Klein, G. (1975)   Comparison between growth characteristics of an Epstein-Barr virus (EBV)-genome-negative lymphoma line and its EBV-converted subline *in vitro.   Proc. nat. Acad. Sci. (Wash.), 72,* 3518-3520

Steinitz, M. & Klein, G. (1976)   Epstein-Barr virus (EBV)-induced change in the saturation sensitivity and serum dependence of established EBV-negative lymphoma lines *in vitro.   Virology, 70,* 570-573

Steinitz, M. & Klein, G. (1977)   Further studies on the differences in serum dependence in EBV negative lymphoma lines and their *in vitro* EBV converted, virus-genome carrying sublines. *Eur. J. Cancer, 13,* 1269-1275

Sugawara, K., Mizuno, F. & Osato, T. (1972)   Demonstration of Epstein-Barr virus-associated antigens in all the clones from non-producing human lymphoblastoid cell lines by 5-bromodeoxyuridine and 5-iododeoxyuridine. *Nature new Biol., 239,* 242-243

Summers, W.C. & Klein, G. (1976)   Inhibition of EBV DNA synthesis and late gene expression by phosphonoacetic acid. *J. Virol., 18,* 151-155

Thorley-Lawson, D. & Strominger, J.L. (1976)   Transformation of human lymphocytes by Epstein-Barr virus is inhibited by phosphonoacetic acid. *Nature (Lond.), 263,* 332-334

Veltri, R.W., McClung, I.E. & Sprinkle, P.M. (1976)   Epstein-Barr nuclear antigen (EBNA) carrying lymphocyte in human palatine tonsils. *J. gen. Virol., 32,* 455-460

Wallen, W.C., Neubauer, R.H., Rabin, H. & Ciemanec, J.L. (1973)   Non-immune rosette formation by lymphoma and leukemia cells from herpesvirus saimiri-infected owl monkeys. *J. nat. Cancer Inst., 51,* 967-975

Werner, F.J., Bornkamm, G.W. & Fleckenstein, B. (1977)   Episomal viral DNA in a herpesvirus saimiri-transformed lymphoid cell line. *J. Virol., 22,* 794-803

Werner, J., Wolf, H., Apodaca, J. & zur Hausen, H. (1975)   Lymphoproliferative disease in a cotton-top marmoset after inoculation with infectious mononucleosis-derived Epstein-Barr virus. *Int. J. Cancer, 15,* 1000-1008

Witter, R.L., Stephens, E.A., Sharma, J.M. & Nazerian, K. (1975)
    Demonstration of a tumor associated surface antigen in Marek's
    disease. *J. Immun., 115*, 177-183

Yefenof, E. & Klein, G. (1976)   Difference in antibody induced
    redistribution of membrane IgM in EBV-genome free and EBV-positive
    human lymphoid cells. *Exp. Cell Res., 99*, 175-178

Yefenof, E.S., Klein, G., Ben Bassat, H.S. & Lundin, L. (1977)
    Difference in the Con A induced redistribution and agglutination
    patterns of EBV genome free and EBV carrying human lymphoma lines.
    Exp. Cell Res., 108, 185-190

Zech, L., Haglund, U., Nilsson, K. & Klein, G. (1976)   Characteristic
    chromosomal abnormalities in biopsies and lymphoid-cell lines from
    patients with Burkitt and non-Burkitt lymphomas. *Int. J. Cancer,
    17*, 47-56

zur Hausen, H. (1975)   Oncogenic herpes viruses. *Biochim. Biophys.
    Acta (Amst.), 417*, 25-53

zur Hausen, H., Diehl, V., Wolf, H., Schulte-Holthausen, H. & Schneider,
    U. (1972)   Occurrence of Epstein-Barr virus genomes in human
    lymphoblastoid cell lines. *Nature new Biol., 237*, 189-190

zur Hausen, H., Schulte-Holthausen, H., Klein, G., Henle, W., Henle,
    G., Clifford, P. & Santesson, L. (1970)   EBV DNA in biopsies
    of Burkitt tumours and anaplastic carcinomas of the nasopharynx.
    Nature (Lond.), 228, 1056-1058

MAPPING OF THE HERPES SIMPLEX VIRUS DNA SEQUENCES IN THREE HERPES SIMPLEX VIRUS THYMIDINE KINASE-TRANSFORMED CELL LINES

J.M. LEIDEN, N. FRENKEL & D. POLACEK

Committee on Virology,
The University of Chicago,
Chicago, Ill., USA

F. RAPP

Department of Microbiology and Specialized Cancer Research Center,
Pennsylvania State University College of Medicine,
Hershey, Penn., USA

INTRODUCTION

Transformation of cells in culture by herpes simplex viruses has been reported for cells from a variety of hosts including hamster, mouse, rat, and human. Such herpes simplex virus (HSV)-transformed cells have been selected in two ways. First, HSV-transformed cells exhibiting altered growth properties have been selected by their ability to form foci in culture (Duff & Rapp, 1971; Darai & Munk, 1973; Kutinova et al., 1973; MacNab, 1974; Takahashi & Yamanishi, 1974; Boyd & Orme, 1975; Kimura et al., 1975; Kucera & Gudson, 1976). It has been reported that cell lines selected in this way exhibit variable degrees of tumorigenicity (Rapp & Duff, 1973).

The second type of selection system which has been used to generate HSV-transformed cell lines has been referred to as biochemical transformation and involves the transfer of the HSV-encoded thymidine kinase (TK) gene using either UV-irradiated HSV (Munyon et al., 1971; Davidson et al., 1973), sheared HSV DNA (Bacchetti & Graham, 1977; Minson et al., 1978) or restriction enzyme fragments of HSV DNA (Maitland & McDougall, 1977; Wigler et al., 1977), to cells previously lacking this enzyme.

Such HSV-TK[+] transformants continue to express the virus-specific TK when selected and maintained in HAT medium[1].

The studies described in this paper deal with the identification and mapping of the HSV DNA sequences present in HSV-TK[+] transformants. Previous studies have addressed this question by using reassociation kinetics hybridization tests employing whole HSV DNA probes. All HSV-TK[+] transformants thus far examined with this technique have been shown to contain HSV DNA sequences corresponding to between 9% and 23% of the viral genome present in a small number of copies per cell (less than six) (Davis & Kingsbury, 1976; Kraiselburd et al., 1975). Although only a limited portion of the HSV genome has been shown to be present in these cell lines, these viral DNA sequences have not yet been mapped. In the studies described below we have mapped the HSV-1 and HSV-2 DNA sequences present in three different HSV-TK[+] transformed cell lines, one transformed with UV-irradiated HSV-2, and two others transformed with sheared HSV-1 DNA. In mapping the HSV DNA sequences present in these cell lines, we have made use of a novel filter hybridization approach in which transformed cell DNA labelled *in vitro* with ^{32}P is first preselected and enriched for viral DNA sequences; it is then hybridized to nitrocellulose strips containing various restriction enzyme fragments of unlabelled HSV DNA which have been blotted on to the nitrocellulose strips by the method of Southern (1974). After autoradiography, the bands are identified by comparing the pattern of hybridization of blots hybridized to preselected transformed cell DNA to the pattern of hybridization of replicate control blots which have been hybridized to purified *in vitro* labelled HSV DNA.

RESULTS

Specificity and sensitivity of the hybridization approach

In order to determine the specificity of the hybridization approach described above, DNA extracted from Vero, HEp-2, or mouse CL1D LTK[-] cells, as well as commercially available calf thymus DNA, was hybridized to nitrocellulose blots containing the *Kpn*I or *Eco*RI/*Hpa*I restriction enzyme fragments of HSV-2 DNA or the *Bgl*II or *Bgl*II/*Hin*dIII restriction enzyme fragments of HSV-1 DNA. No bands were seen in any of these hybridizations (data not shown).

In order to determine the sensitivity of this hybridization approach the following reconstruction experiment was performed. HSV-2 (G) DNA was mixed with either a 10^5 or 10^4-fold excess of Vero cell DNA. Assuming a molecular weight of 10^{13} for cell DNA and 10^8 for HSV-2 DNA, these ratios represent one copy and 10 copies per cell respectively. DNA from each of these mixtures was then labelled *in vitro* with ^{32}P and hybridized, as described above, to *Kpn*I and *Eco*RI/*Hpa*I blots of

---

[1] Medium containing hypoxanthine, aminopterin and thymidine

HSV-2 (G) DNA.   The results are shown in Figures 1 and 2.   Several points are noteworthy.

(1) As seen in Figure 1 the hybridization approach has the necessary sensitivity to detect a 2×10^6 dalton sequence of HSV DNA present once per cell.

FIG. 1. RECONSTRUCTION EXPERIMENT

Vero cell DNA was mixed with HSV-2 DNA in ratios of either 10^5 or 10^4 representing one copy and 10 copies per cell of the viral genome respectively. Purified *in vitro* ^{32}P-labelled HSV DNA or *in vitro* labelled DNA from the reconstruction mixtures, which was preselected to enrich for viral DNA sequences, was hybridized to nitrocellulose strips containing the *Kpn*I or *Eco*RI/*Hpa*I restriction enzyme fragments of HSV-2 (G) DNA (Southern, 1974).   C=control, purified *in vitro* labelled HSV-2 DNA; 10= *in vitro* labelled DNA from the 10 copies per cell reconstruction mixture; 1= *in vitro* labelled DNA from the one copy per cell reconstruction mixture; 1d= one day of autoradiographic exposure; 5d= five days of autoradiographic exposure.

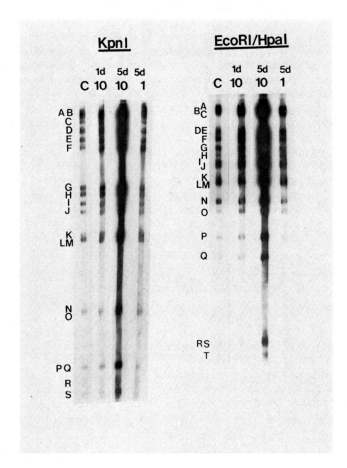

(ii) In Figure 2 we have compared the relative molarities of the
virus-specific hybridization bands seen in the one copy and 10 copies
per cell reconstruction experiments (as determined by densitometry
scanning) to those of their counterparts from autoradiograms of
replicate control nitrocellulose strips which were hybridized to
purified *in vitro* labelled HSV-2 (G) DNA.   As seen in Figure 2 there
is no significant difference between the molarities of the control and
reconstruction bands, indicating that the preselection and hybridization
steps do not result in the loss of specific subsets of viral DNA sequences.   It is interesting to note that in two cases the relative molarities of the control bands themselves do not correspond to the expected
value of 1.   First, the small fragments (molecular weights less than
4×10^6) seem to be under-represented, i.e., they are usually present
in molarities of less than 1.   This is probably due to the selective
loss of smaller fragments from the nitrocellulose strips during the
high-temperature hybridization (Southern, 1974).   The second group of
control bands which display relative molarities which differ significantly from 1 are the 0.5 and 0.25 molar fragments which form the
boundaries of the S and L components (Hayward et al., 1975;   Skare &
Summers, 1977;   Wilkie, 1976).   The bands corresponding to these
fragments are consistently present in molarities of greater than 1.
The reason for this observation is not entirely clear.   However, our
previous experience has shown that our blot hybridizations are sensitive to both the amount of unlabelled viral DNA on the nitrocellulose
strips and the amount of labelled viral probe DNA in the hybridization
solution.   Thus, in calculating the relative molarities of the 0.5 and
0.25 molar bands, we have divided the autoradiographic intensities of
these bands by two and four respectively in order to normalize for
their lower relative abundances on the filters.   The observation that
the relative molarities obtained after such normalization are consistently greater than 1 most likely reflects the fact that the *ab* and
ac repeated sequences are present in greater than unit molarity in the
labelled probe DNA and, therefore, confirms the hypothesis that the
hybridization is sensitive to the amounts of labelled probe DNA in the
hybridization solution.   It should again be emphasized that, although
the molarities of some control bands differ from 1, there is no
significant difference between the calculated molarities of a given
control band and that of the same band in the one copy and 10 copies
per cell reconstruction experiments.

(iii) it was of interest to determine whether the hybridization
approach described above would not only allow us to identify the viral
DNA sequences present in a given transformed cell line but could also
yield information concerning the number of copies per cell of these
viral DNA sequences.   Towards this end it was necessary to compare
the absolute intensities (as determined from densitometric scans) of
corresponding bands in the one copy and 10 copies per cell reconstruction experiments.   If the intensity of a given band was determined
solely by the amount of homologous labelled sequences in the hybridization solution, we would have expected the ratio of the intensity of a

FIG. 2. RELATIVE ABUNDANCES OF HYBRIDIZED BANDS IN CONTROL AND RECONSTRUCTION HYBRIDIZATIONS

Upper panels: Densitometric scans of the autoradiograms shown in Figure 1. Scanning was done using a Transidyne 2955 scanning densitometer equipped with an automatic integrator. Bottom panels: The relative molarities of the various bands were calculated by dividing the percentage area under each peak of the densitometric scan by the expected percentage area as determined from the fractional weight and known molarities of the fragments contained in each peak, i.e.: % area × 10^6/molecular weight for a 1.0 molar fragment; (% area × 10^6/ molecular weight) × 0.5 for a 0.5 molar fragment; (% area × 10^6/ molecular weight) × 0.25 for a 0.25 molar fragment.
Each triplet of bars contains, from left to right, the relative molarities of the bands from the 10 copies per cell reconstruction, the control (purified HSV DNA), and the one copy per cell reconstruction experiments.   An asterisk indicates a group of fragments containing either a 0.5 or a 0.25 molar fragment.

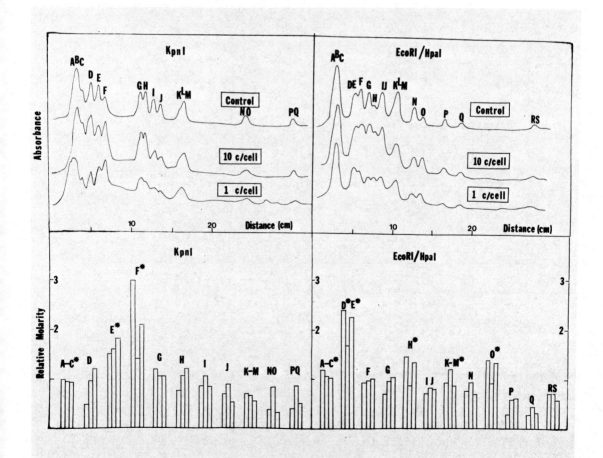

LEIDEN ET AL.

a band in the 10 copies per cell reconstruction to that of the corresponding band in the one copy per cell reconstruction to be 10.   Table
1 shows that these ratios ranged between 7.9 and 21.9 (with an average
of 10.95).   Thus the technique is quantitative with an error of less
than two-fold.

Table 1. Comparison of the absolute intensities of the bands from
the one copy and 10 copies per cell reconstruction experiments

Restriction endonuclease	Fragment	Ratio intensity$_{10}$: intensity$_1$[a]	Restriction endonuclease	Fragment	Ratio intensity$_{10}$: intensity$_1$[a]
KpnI	A B C	8.3	EcoRI/HpaI	A B C	7.99
	D	16.44		D E	9.03
	E	10.08		F	9.94
	F	8.43		G	13.91
	G H	12.3		H	8.54
	I	8.27		I J	10.55
	J	8.86			
	K L M	8.03		K L M	9.27
	N O	7.89		N	8.84
	P	12.2		O	9.45
				P	20.74
				Q	21.96
				R S	10.0

[a] Ratios of the intensities of the corresponding bands (as determined by
densitometric scanning; see legend to Figure 2) of the 10 copies and
one copy per cell reconstruction experiments shown in Figure 1.   The
five-day autoradiographic exposures were used for the densitometric
scanning

*Mapping of the HSV-2 DNA sequences present in the HSV-TK[+] transformed
cell line 33A+*

Cell line 33A+ was produced by infection of TK[−] 3T3 cells with
UV-irradiated HSV-2 (333) and subsequent selection and propagation in
HAT medium.   Three separate preparations of DNA were made from this

cell line after 50-70 passages and hybridized, as described above, to
*Kpn*I and *Eco*RI/*Hpa*I blots of HSV-2 (G) DNA.   The results of these
hybridizations are shown in Figures 3 and 4 and can be summarized as
follows.

FIG. 3.   MAPPING OF THE HSV-2 DNA SEQUENCES PRESENT
IN CELL LINE 33A+

Top panels: Control (purified *in vitro* labelled HSV-2 (G) DNA) (C) or
in vitro labelled 33A+ DNA (33A+), which was preselected to enrich for
viral DNA sequences, was hybridized to nitrocellulose strips containing
either the *Kpn*I or *Eco*RI/*Hpa*I restriction enzyme fragments of HSV-2 (G)
DNA. A, B, and C show the autoradiograms from three separate hybridization experiments, each done with a separate preparation of 33A+ DNA
(passages 50, 60, and 70 of the cell line) and a separate set of nitrocellulose blots.   In experiment C, a one copy per cell reconstruction
mixture (see legend to Figure 1) was hybridized to a replicate nitrocellulose strip (R).   In experiment A, autoradiography was performed for
either five days (panels 2 and 10) or three weeks (panels 3 and 11)
using Dupont high-speed intensifying screens.   Bottom panel:
Schematic representation of the regions of homology between 33A+ DNA and
the *Kpn*I or *Eco*RI/*Hpa*I restriction enzyme fragments of HSV-2 (G) DNA.
The restriction enzyme maps were taken from G.S. Hayward, T.G. Buchman
& B. Roizman (unpublished data). Dotted lines represent an uncertain
region of homology.

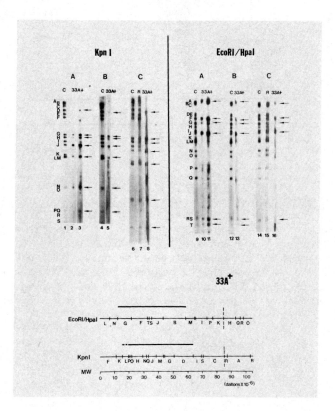

480   LEIDEN ET AL.

FIG. 4.   RELATIVE ABUNDANCES OF THE HSV-2 DNA SEQUENCES
PRESENT IN CELL LINE 33A+

Schematic representation of the relative molarities of the transformed
cell DNA sequences which are homologous to the various HSV-2 (G) *KpnI*
and *EcoRI/HpaI* restriction enzyme fragments.   The autoradiograms shown
in Figure 3 were scanned as described in the legend to Figure 2.
Relative molarities were calculated as the percentage area under each
peak divided by the fractional weight of the fragments known to be
contained in that peak, i.e., % area × 10^6/molecular weight.   The
letters correspond to the restriction enzyme maps shown in Figure 3.

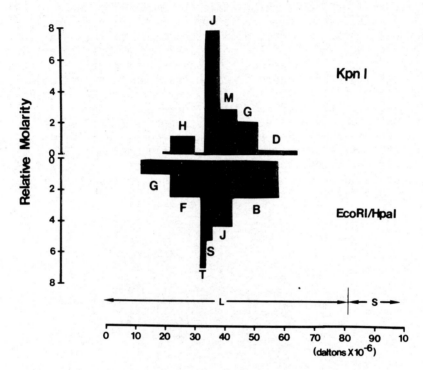

(i) HSV-2 DNA sequences corresponding to approximately 40% of the
viral genome were detected in the DNA of this cell line.   The maps
generated from the two different restriction enzyme digests used in
these experiments were in complete agreement and indicated that this
cell line contains DNA sequences corresponding to the entire set of
HSV-2 (G) DNA sequences located between map units 0.15 and 0.57.
However, it should be noted that we cannot rule out the existence of
small deletions of viral DNA sequences within this region – deletions
which are too small to be detected with the particular restriction
enzymes used in these experiments.

(ii) As shown in Figure 3 identical band patterns have been obtained using three different preparations of 33A+ transformed cell DNA and three different sets of nitrocellulose blots.

(iii) If all of the viral DNA sequences in the 33A+ cell line were present in an equal number of copies per cell, and if the transformed cell DNA sequences corresponding to each restriction enzyme fragment were present in their entirety, we would expect the calculated molarities of all bands from a given blot to be identical. However, an analysis of the densitometric scans of the autoradiograms shown in Figure 3 revealed significant differences in the relative molarities of the transformed cell DNA sequences corresponding to the various bands seen in these autoradiograms. Both restriction enzyme maps agreed and allowed us to construct the relative abundance maps seen in Figure 4. There are two, not mutually exclusive, explanations for these observed differences in relative abundance. First, this cell line may contain sequences which are only homologous to a portion of a given restriction enzyme fragment, resulting in bands of apparently low molarity. This was clearly exemplified in the case of both the KpnI fragment D and the EcoRI/HpaI fragment G, in that a comparison of the KpnI and EcoRI/HpaI maps of the HSV-2 (G) DNA sequences present in cell line 33A+ revealed that only a portion of each of these fragments is present in this cell line. The second possible explanation for the observed differences in relative abundance is that certain transformed cell DNA sequences were indeed present in a larger number of copies per cell than others. This explanation is more likely to explain the higher relative molarities of the transformed cell DNA sequences which were homologous to the KpnI fragment J and EcoRI/HpaI fragments S and T, all of which seemed to be present in their entirety in this cell line.

(iv) As seen in Figure 3, a comparison of the intensities of the bands produced by 33A+ DNA with those produced by the one copy and 10 copies per cell reconstruction mixtures which were hybridized to replicate nitrocellulose blots, revealed that this transformed cell line contains 1-5 copies per cell of these HSV-2 DNA sequences.

Mapping of the HSV-1 DNA sequences present in two HSV-1 TK[+] transformed cell lines

Cell lines 5A and 8N are HSV-TK[+] transformed cell lines produced by transfection of TK[-] mouse CL1D cells with sheared HSV-1 (1023) DNA and selection and propagation in HAT medium. DNA from passage 15 of these cell lines was extracted and hybridized, as described above, to nitrocellulose blots containing the BglII restriction enzyme fragments of HSV-1 (Justin) DNA and the HindIII/BglII restriction enzyme fragments of HSV-1 (F) DNA. The results of these hybridizations shown in Figure 5, revealed the following.

(i) Cell line 5A contained sequences mapping between 0.26 and 0.41 on the wild-type HSV-1 genome. These sequences are known to

FIG. 5. MAPPING OF THE HSV-1 DNA SEQUENCES PRESENT
IN CELL LINES 5A AND 8N

Left-hand panels: Control [purified *in vitro* labelled HSV-1 (F) DNA]
or *in vitro* labelled 8N or 5A DNA, which was preselected to enrich for
viral DNA sequences, was hybridized to replicate nitrocellulose strips
containing either the *Bgl*II restriction enzyme fragments of HSV-1
(Justin) DNA or the *Bgl*II/*Hind*III restriction enzyme fragments of
HSV-1 (F) DNA. After hybridization, autoradiography was performed for
5-10 days using Dupont high-speed intensifying screens and medical
X-ray film.   Right-hand panels: Schematic representation of the
regions of homology between 8N or 5A DNA and the *Bgl*II or *Bgl*II/*Hind*III
restriction enzyme fragments of HSV-1 DNA.   The restriction enzyme maps
were taken from G.S. Hayward, T.G. Buchman & B. Roizman (unpublished
data).

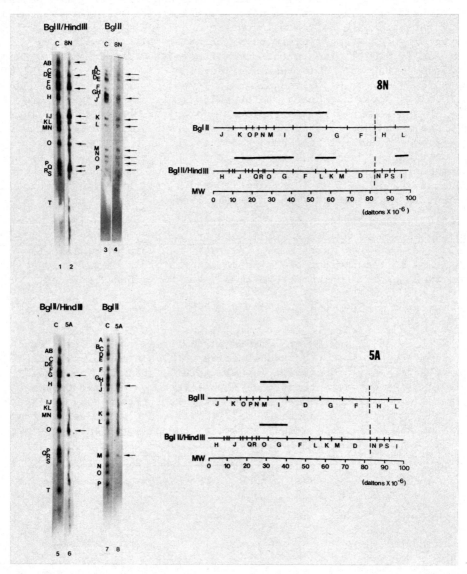

contain the viral TK gene, which has been mapped on the basis of HSV-1 × HSV-2 recombinants between 0.25 and 0.35 map units of the HSV-1 genome (Morse et al., 1978). It should be noted that these 14.2×10^6 daltons of viral DNA sequences represent a maximum estimate of the viral DNA sequences present in this cell line. Further hybridization studies utilizing different restriction enzyme fragments will be needed to more precisely map the HSV-1 DNA sequences present in this cell line.

In contrast to cell line 5A, cell line 8N appears to contain two sets of non-contiguous L-region viral DNA sequences mapping between coordinates 0.09 and 0.41, and 0.53 and 0.58, as well as sequences which are homologous to the 0.5 molar *Bgl* II fragment L from the right-hand side of the S region of HSV-1 (F) DNA (spanning coordinates 0.94 - 1.0). In the light of the fact that the DNA from cell line 8N shows little, if any, hybridization to the 0.5 molar fragment from the left-hand side of S or to the 0.25 molar fragments containing sequences from the left-hand side of S, we conclude that the hybridization of 8N DNA to the 0.5 molar fragment from the right-hand side of S (fragment L) is due to the presence of predominantly *Us* rather than *ac* DNA sequences in this cell line.

DISCUSSION

In the studies described in this report, we have employed a novel filter hybridization approach to identify and map the HSV DNA sequences present in three different HSV-TK[+] transformants.

Because HSV is such a highly lytic virus, it was of interest to find such a large proportion (40%) of the HSV-2 genome present in the 33A+ cell line. One could envision at least two possible explanations for this finding. First, it is possible that there are viral control genes located at some distance from the viral TK gene. The presence of such control genes could promote the expression of higher levels of the viral thymidine kinase enzyme. Thus, cells containing such positive control elements might have a selective advantage during propagation in HAT medium. This possibility is especially attractive in the light of the findings of Lin & Munyon (1974) and Leiden et al. (1976) that the viral TK gene in one HSV-TK[+] transformed cell line remains responsive to viral control genes. Alternatively, it is possible that the incorporation of viral DNA sequences during HSV-mediated biochemical transformation is a random event which can result in the incorporation of a wide variety of different viral sequences (in addition to the necessary viral TK gene sequences).

In the light of the fact that the viral TK gene has been mapped between 0.25 and 0.35 on the HSV-1 genome, it was extremely interesting to find this portion of the genome (0.31-0.37) represented in higher relative abundance than the other viral DNA sequences present in cell

line 33A+.   The finding of different viral DNA sequences present in
different relative abundances within a single transformed cell line is
similar to the finding that specific regions of the SV40 genome are
represented in different relative abundances within cloned SV40-
transformed cell lines (Botchan et al., 1974).   One could envision
several possible mechanisms each of which could result in the abundance
pattern which was observed for this cell line.   First, the transformed
cells could all contain identical sets of viral DNA sequences, some of
which could be present in a greater number of copies per cell than
others.   Alternatively, the observed abundance pattern could be due to
the presence of several subpopulations of cells, all containing TK gene
sequences, but each containing a different set of non-TK-gene viral DNA
sequences.   We currently favour the latter possibility, because several
investigators have reported that the amount of viral DNA sequences in
several HSV morphologically transformed cell lines varies with
passaging both in animals and in tissue culture (Frenkel et al., 1976;
Minson et al., 1976).   Several possible mechanisms could account for
the presence of different subpopulations of 33A+ cells, each containing
a different set of viral DNA sequences.   First, this cell line could
have arisen from several independently transformed cells.   This possibility must be considered, given that this cell line has not been
extensively cloned.   Second, it is possible that a single transformation
event (involving a single cell) was followed by a transient period of
loss and rearrangement of viral DNA sequences in the progeny of the
original transformed cell.   This initial period of sorting out of viral
DNA sequences could have been followed by stabilization of the viral DNA
in the cells, resulting in the propagation of subpopulations of cells
containing different amounts of viral DNA sequences.   Finally, it is
possible that HSV DNA sequences are continuously lost from the transformed cells, resulting in continuous changes in the transformed cell
population even following prolonged propagation in culture.

     In contrast to cell line 33A+, cell line 8N appears to contain
several non-contiguous stretches of viral DNA sequences.   This is
not unexpected in that cell line 8N was biochemically transformed
using sheared HSV-1 DNA, as opposed to cell line 33A+, which was
transformed using UV-irradiated virus.   The finding of these non-
contiguous viral DNA sequences in cell line 8N implies that several
groups of HSV DNA sequences can be stably incorporated and propagated
in the biochemically transformed cells.   In this light, it will be of
interest to follow the fate of the non-TK viral DNA sequences upon
further passaging of this cell line.   As discussed above, the non-TK
viral DNA sequences present in cell line 8N may represent unexpressed
viral genes which can be lost with no selective disadvantage, or alternatively may represent advantageous positive control elements.

     Finally, the finding of only 14.2×10^6 daltons of HSV DNA sequences
in cell line 5A establishes an upper limit to the amount of the viral
DNA sequences which are necessary for the stable HSV-mediated TK transformation of cultured cells, as well as providing further confirmation of
the map location of the HSV-1 TK gene.

SUMMARY

We have made use of a novel filter hybridization approach in order
to map the herpes simplex virus (HSV) DNA sequences which are present in
three HSV thymidine kinase (TK)-transformed cell lines.   The cell line
33A+ which was produced by infection of 3T3 TK⁻ cells with UV-irradiated
HSV-2 (333) was found to contain one contiguous stretch of viral DNA
sequences which maps between 0.15 and 0.57 on the HSV-2 genome.   The
sequences mapping from 0.31 to 0.37 were present in 3-4-fold higher
abundance than the rest of the viral DNA sequences in this cell line.
Cell lines 5A and 8N were produced by transfection of mouse CL1D cells
with sheared HSV-1 (1023) DNA.   The cell line 5A was found to contain
a contiguous set of viral DNA sequences mapping between 0.26 and 0.41
on the HSV-1 genome.   The cell line 8N was found to contain three
non-contiguous sets of viral DNA sequences, mapping between 0.09 and
0.41, 0.53 and 0.58, and 0.94 and 1.0 on the HSV-1 genome.   These
results seem to indicate that many different sets of viral DNA sequences can be incorporated into the cell during HSV-mediated biochemical
transformation.

ACKNOWLEDGEMENTS

These studies were aided by grants from the National
Cancer Institute (University of Chicago Cancer
Research Center) CA-19264,   project 404, and
from the American Cancer Society (VC-204)
and by Contract No. CP 53516 within the
Virus Cancer Program of the National
Cancer Institute.   J.M. Leiden is
a pre-doctoral trainee supported
by USPHS 5-T32 HD-07009-03.

REFERENCES

Bacchetti, S. & Graham, F.L. (1977)   Transfer of the gene for thymidine kinase to thymidine kinase-deficient human cells by purified herpes simplex viral DNA.   *Proc. nat. Acad. Sci. (Wash.), 74*, 1590-1594

Botchan, M., Ozanne, B., Sugden, B., Sharp, P. & Sambrook, J. (1974) Viral DNA in transformed cells.   III. The amounts of differing regions of the SV40 genome present in a line of transformed mouse cells.   *Proc. nat. Acad. Sci. (Wash.), 71*, 4183-4187

Boyd, A.L. & Orme, T.W. (1975)   Transformation of mouse cells after infection with ultraviolet irradiation-inactivated herpes simplex virus type 2.   *Int. J. Cancer, 16*, 526-538

Darai, G. & Munk, K. (1973)   Human embryonic lung cells abortively infected with herpes virus hominis type 2 show some properties of cell transformation.   *Nature new Biol., 241*, 268-269

Davidson, R.L., Adelstein, S.J. & Oxman, M.M. (1973)   Herpes simplex virus as a source of thymidine kinase for thymidine kinase-deficient mouse cells: suppression and reactivation of the viral enzyme. *Proc. nat. Acad. Sci. (Wash.), 70*, 1912-1916

Davis, D.B. & Kingsbury, D.T. (1976)   Quantitation of the viral DNA present in cells transformed by ultra-violet irradiated herpes simplex virus.   *J. Virol., 17*, 788-793

Duff, R. & Rapp, F. (1971)   Properties of hamster embryo fibroblasts transformed *in vitro* after exposure to ultraviolet-irradiated herpes simplex virus type 2.   *J. Virol., 8*, 469-477

Frenkel, N., Locker, H., Cox, B., Roizman, B. & Rapp, F. (1976) Herpes simplex virus DNA in transformed cells: sequence complexity in five hamster cell lines and one derived hamster tumor. *J. Virol., 18*, 885-893

Hayward, G.S., Jacob, R.J., Wadsworth, S.C. & Roizman, B. (1975) Anatomy of herpes simplex virus DNA: Evidence for four populations of molecules that differ in the relative orientation of their long and short components.   *Proc. nat. Acad. Sci. (Wash.), 72*, 4243-4247

Kimura, S., Flannery, V., Levy, B. & Schaffer, P. (1975)   Oncogenic transformation of primary hamster cells by herpes simplex virus type 2 (HSV-2) and an HSV-2 temperature-sensitive mutant.   *Int. J. Cancer, 15*, 786-798

Kraiselburd, E., Gage, L.P. & Weissbach, A. (1975)   Presence of a
    herpes simplex virus DNA fragment in an L cell clone obtained
    after infection with irradiated herpes simplex virus type 1.
    J. molec. Biol., *97*, 533-542

Kucera, L.S. & Gudson, J.P. (1976)   Transformation of human embryonic
    fibroblasts by photodynamically inactivated herpes simplex virus
    type 2 at supraoptimal temperature.   *J. gen. Virol.*, *30*, 257-261

Kutinova, L., Vonka, V. & Broucek, J. (1973)   Increased oncogenicity
    and synthesis of herpesvirus antigens in hamster cells exposed to
    herpes simplex type 2 virus.   *J. nat. Cancer Inst.*, *50*, 759-766

Leiden, J.M., Buttyan, R. & Spear, P.G. (1976)   Herpes simplex virus
    gene expression in transformed cells.   I. Regulation of the viral
    thymidine kinase gene in transformed L cells by products of super-
    infecting virus.   *J. Virol.*, *20*, 413-424

Lin, S.-S. & Munyon, W. (1974)   Expression of the viral thymidine
    kinase gene in herpes simplex virus-transformed L cells.   *J. Virol.*,
    14, 1199-1208

MacNab, J.C.M. (1974)   Transformation of rat embryo cells by
    temperature-sensitive mutants of herpes simplex virus.   *J. gen.*
    Virol., *24*, 143-153

Maitland, N.J. & McDougall, J.K. (1977)   Biochemical transformation
    of mouse cells by fragments of herpes simplex virus DNA.   *Cell*, *11*,
    233-241

Minson, A.C., Thouless, M.E., Eglin, R.P. & Darby, G. (1976)   The
    detection of virus DNA sequences in a herpes type 2 transformed
    hamster cell line (333-8-9).   *Cancer*, *17*, 493-500

Minson, A.C., Wildy, P., Buchan, A. & Darby, G. (1978)   Introduction
    of the herpes simplex virus thymidine kinase gene into mouse cells
    using virus DNA or transformed cell DNA.   *Cell*, *13*, 581-587

Morse, L.S., Pereira, L., Roizman, B. & Schaffer, P.A. (1978)
    Anatomy of HSV DNA.   X. Mapping of viral genes by analysis of
    polypeptides and functions specified by HSV-1 × HSV-2 recombinants.
    J. Virol., *26*, 389-410

Munyon, W., Kraiselburd, E., Davis, D. & Mann, J. (1971)   Transfer of
    thymidine kinase to thymidine kinaseless L cells by infection
    with ultraviolet-irradiated herpes simplex virus.   *J. Virol.*, *7*,
    813-820

Rapp, F. & Duff, R. (1973)   Transformation of hamster embryo fibro-
    blasts by herpes simplex viruses type 1 and 2.   *Cancer Res.*, *33*,
    1527-1534

Skare, J. & Summers, W.C. (1977)   Structure and function of herpesvirus
    genomes.   II. EcoRI, XbaI and HindIII endonuclease cleavage sites on
    herpes simplex virus type 1 DNA.   *Virology*, *76*, 581-596

Southern, E.M. (1974)   Detection of specific sequences among DNA
    fragments separated by gel electrophoresis.   *J. molec. Biol.,*
    98, 503-517

Takahashi, M. & Yamanishi, K. (1974)   Transformation of hamster embryo
    and human embryo cells by temperature-sensitive mutants of herpes
    simplex virus type 2.   *Virology, 61,* 306-311

Wigler, M., Silverstein, S., Lee, L., Pellicer, A., Cheng, Y. &
    Axel, R. (1977)   Transfer of purified herpes virus thymidine
    kinase gene to cultured mouse cells.   *Cell, 11,* 223-232

Wilkie, N.M. (1976)   Physical maps for herpes simplex virus type 1
    DNA for restriction endonucleases HindIII, HpaI, and Xba I.
    J. Virol., 20, 222-233

INCORPORATION OF THE HERPES SIMPLEX VIRUS THYMIDINE-KINASE GENE INTO A MAMMALIAN CELL LINE USING FRAGMENTS OF THE VIRUS GENOME

G. DARBY, A.C. MINSON & P. WILDY

*Department of Pathology,
University of Cambridge,
Cambridge, UK*

The demonstration by Munyon and his colleagues (1971) that the thymidine-kinase gene of herpes simplex virus could be introduced into a mammalian cell which lacked that gene provides an ideal system for studying the interaction of a fragment of virus DNA with the eukaryotic chromosome. Rather than using UV-irradiated virus as in these early studies we have preferred the use of virus DNA fragments to achieve the transformation (Bacchetti & Graham, 1977; Maitland & McDougall, 1977; Wigler et al., 1977).

LTK$^-$ cells were transformed with herpes simplex virus type 2 DNA sheared to approximately 20×10^6 molecular weight. The calcium phosphate technique developed by Graham et al. (1973) to demonstrate the infectivity of herpesvirus DNA was used. The transformation was dose-dependent below about 0.2 µg/dish (5×10^5 cells) yielding about 10 transformants per µg. At higher concentrations a maximum of 1 cell in 10^5 was transformed.

A number of clonally unrelated lines were established in selective medium (Munyon et al., 1971) and all were shown by serological neutralization to possess herpesvirus-specific thymidine kinase. A number of lines were examined to determine the stability of the gene, and several interesting features emerged. Shortly after the lines were established they contained a significant proportion of thymidine kinase-negative cells as judged by their ability to plate in 50 µg/ml bromodeoxyuridine (BUDR). This appeared to be a relatively stable character, since passage in selective or non-selective medium for 50 generations did not significantly alter the proportion of kinase-negative cells in the population. (For example, in the case of line

$D2_1$, 13% were kinase-negative after passage in selective, and 18% after passage in non-selective medium). As TK^- cells cannot survive in selective medium these results imply that they are generated from TK^+ cells at each division. Furthermore, as the proportion remains fairly stable, even in non-selective medium, we have to conclude that possession of the TK gene imparts a selective advantage to the cells. This stability of the TK gene in the cell population was further confirmed by direct measurement of enzyme activity as it was shown that in the case of the three lines tested ($D2_1$, $D2_5$ and $D2_6$) continuous passage in either selective or non-selective medium did not significantly affect the levels of thymidine kinase.

In an attempt to determine whether the lines carry herpesvirus genetic information in addition to the TK gene their ability to support the growth of several temperature-sensitive (*ts*) mutants of type 1 virus at the restrictive temperature ($38.5^{\circ}C$) was tested. The line $D2_1$ produced almost wild-type yields of the mutants N102 and N103 (DNA-negative mutants isolated by Dr A. Buchan). No other mutants were complemented by this cell line and neither mutant grew at the restrictive temperature in any other lines (11 were tested in all). Similar results have been obtained independently by Dr Buchan.

We isolated DNA from $D2_1$ cells and used it to transform further LTK^- cells. Table 1 shows the results obtained. Five clonally unrelated lines were established from the colonies obtained in dishes

Table 1. Transformation of LTK^- cells by DNA from $D2_1$ cells[a]

Treatment	Colonies/10 dishes	Proportion of dishes containing colonies
0.5 µg/dish HSV-2 DNA 9.5 µg/dish salmon sperm DNA	9	6/10
10 µg/dish $D2_1$ DNA	28	9/10
10 µg/dish salmon sperm DNA	0	0/10

[a] Monolayers of 5×10^5 LTK^- cells were inoculated with DNA and after 48 hours in non-selective medium (ETC: Eagle's medium supplemented with 10% calf serum and 10% tryptose phosphate broth) the cells were subsequently incubated in selective medium (Munyon et al., 1971). Colonies were counted at three weeks.

treated with $D2_1$ DNA and it was confirmed by serological neutralization that all possessed herpesvirus-specific thymidine kinase. One remarkable feature of this experiment was the high efficiency with which $D2_1$ DNA transformed. Virus DNA was only 10-fold more efficient than

Table 2. Growth of mutants in various cell lines[a]

Cell line	Virus yield (PFU × 10^{-4})		Mutant yield
	Wild type	Mutant	(% wild type)
LTK⁻	300	0.1	0.03
D2$_1$	390	190	50
D2$_1$T1[b]	760	0.05	
D2$_1$T2[b]	820	0.08	< 0.1
D2$_1$T3[b]	750	0.33	
D2$_1$T4[b]	420	0.08	
D2$_1$T5[b]	510	0.30	
D2$_1$R1[c]	200	0.15	
D2$_1$R2[c]	450	0.08	< 0.1
D2$_1$R3[c]	440	0.18	

[a] 2×10^5 cells were infected with 5×10^6 PFU of mutant at 38.5°C and harvested at 20 hours post infection. The yield was assayed at 33°C in BHK cells. The virus recovered from D2$_1$ infected with N103 was temperature-sensitive.

[b] Line obtained by transformation with DNA from D2$_1$

[c] TK⁻ revertant of D2$_1$ selected in BUDR

the cell DNA on a weight basis.   To explain this result simply on the basis of multiple copies of the TK gene, $D2_1$ must carry several thousand copies.   This explanation seems unlikely as $D2_1$ does not produce abnormally high levels of thymidine kinase when compared to other lines; in addition, where the herpesvirus DNA content of trans- formed lines has been measured directly only a few copies per cell have been detected (Davis & Kingsbury, 1976; Kraiselburd et al., 1975).

Two alternative explanations for the high frequency of transforma- tion with $D2_1$ DNA are either that the transforming DNA is a fragment of virus DNA flanked by host sequences, or that the virus DNA is carried in a circular form in transformed cells and that this is a far more efficient transforming element than the original linear DNA fragments.   Both explanations predict that cells transformed with $D2_1$ DNA would carry the N103 gene in addition to the TK gene.   In fact the data in Table 2 show that none of the lines transformed with $D2_1$ DNA would support the growth of N103.   There still remained the possibility that the two genes were carried independently in $D2_1$.   A number of revertant lines were selected in BUDR for loss of the TK gene.   These revertant lines had also lost the ability to complement N103, thus providing good evidence for the linkage of the two genes in $D2_1$.

We therefore have to consider other explanations for the high transformation efficiency of $D2_1$ DNA.   The only other reasonable hypothesis appears to be that the virus DNA carried in $D2_1$ is modified by the cell so that it receives a more favourable reception than normal virus DNA fragments when it enters an LTK^- cell.

ACKNOWLEDGEMENTS

This research was supported by the Cancer Research Campaign.

REFERENCES

Bacchetti, S. & Graham, F.L. (1977) Transfer of the gene for thymidine kinase to thymidine kinase-deficient human cells by purified herpes simplex viral DNA. *Proc. nat. Acad. Sci. (Wash.), 74*, 1590-1594

Davis, D.B. & Kingsbury, D.T. (1976) Quantitation of the viral DNA present in cells transformed by u.v.-irradiated herpes simplex virus. *J. Virol., 17*, 788-793

Graham, F.L., Veldhuisen, G. & Wilkie, N.M. (1973) Infectious herpes virus DNA. *Nature new Biol., 245*, 265-266

Kraiselburd, E., Gage, L.P. & Weissbach, A. (1975) Presence of a herpes simplex virus DNA fragment in an L-cell clone obtained after infection with irradiated herpes simplex virus 1. *J. molec. Biol., 97*, 533-542

Maitland, N.J. & McDougall, J.K. (1977) Biochemical transformation of mouse cells by fragments of herpes simplex virus DNA. *Cell, 11*, 233-241

Munyon, W., Kraiselburd, E., Davis, S. & Mann, J. (1971) Transfer of thymidine kinase to thymidine kinaseless L cells by infection with ultraviolet-irradiated herpes simplex virus. *J. Virol., 7*, 813-820

Wigler, M., Silverstein, S., Lee, L-S., Pellicer, A., Cheng, Y. & Axel, R. (1977) Transfer of a purified herpes thymidine kinase gene to cultured mouse cells. *Cell, 11*, 223-232

DNA-MEDIATED TRANSFER OF HERPES SIMPLEX VIRUS TK GENE TO HUMAN TK⁻ CELLS: PROPERTIES OF THE TRANSFORMED LINES

S. BACCHETTI & F.L. GRAHAM

*Departments of Pathology and Biology,
McMaster University,
Hamilton, Ontario, Canada*

Human cells carrying the herpes simplex virus type 2 (HSV-2) TK gene have been generated by infection of 143-BU TK⁻ cells with sheared viral DNA, followed by selection of TK⁺ transformants in medium containing hypoxanthine, aminopterin and thymidine (HAT medium; Littlefield, 1964) (Bacchetti & Graham, 1977). All of the transformed lines thus isolated are able to grow continuously in this selective medium and express a TK activity of viral origin. The specific activity of the viral enzyme in the transformed lines is in most cases lower than the activity of the human enzyme expressed in the grandparental TK⁺ line (Table 1). When the transformed lines were

Table 1. Specific activity of TK in control and transformed lines[a]

Cell line	Origin of TK	TK activity
R970-5	Human	0.68
AC1	HSV-2	0.52
AC2	HSV-2	0.31
AC3	HSV-2	0.83
AC4	HSV-2	0.39
AC5	HSV-2	0.35

[a] TK activity in crude cell extracts was assayed according to Munyon et al. (1972). The enzymatic activity is expressed in picomoles of thymidine phosphorylated in 45 minutes at 37°C per μg of protein.

tested at early times after transformation for their ability to survive in medium containing bromodeoxyuridine (BUDR) (selecting for TK⁻
cells) significant differences among them were observed in the fraction
of TK⁻ cells (Table 2).

Table 2. Relative proportion of TK^+ and TK^- cells in transformed
lines[a]

Cell line	No. of passages in HAT medium	% TK^+ cells	% TK^- cells
AC1	5	76	24
AC2	10	88	12
AC3	10	99	1
AC4	10	99.94	0.06
AC5	5	99.8	0.2
DC1	5	92.7	8.3
DC2	4	77	23
DC3	5	94.6	5.4
DC4	6	94.1	5.9
DC5	5	66	44

[a] Transformed lines grown in HAT medium were plated in either HAT
or BUDR medium and the relative plating efficiencies were taken as
a measure of the fraction of TK^+ and TK^- cells in the population.

Moreover successive subcloning of the transformed lines has shown
that the degree of stability of TK expression is an inherited property.

     In order to understand whether the ability to survive in BUDR
reflects a stable phenotypic change, eight TK⁻ clones, derived from
different transformed lines by cloning either in BUDR medium or in
non-selective medium (Eagle's minimum essential medium: MEM), were
plated in HAT medium and their reversion rate to the TK^+ phenotype
was measured.   In no instances were survivors observed among
5-40 x 10⁶ cells plated, suggesting that the expression of the viral
TK gene was permanently suppressed or that the gene was lost.   This
latter hypothesis is somewhat supported by the observation that reinfection of TK⁻ clones with viral DNA gives rise to TK^+ transformants
with efficiencies similar to those obtained in the original transformation[1].

---

[1] Unpublished data

Three of the original transformed lines were analysed in detail for their stability of TK expression when grown continuously under selective (HAT) or non-selective (MEM) conditions (Fig. 1).   For both the AC1 and AC5 lines, which originally contained 20 and 0.2% of TK$^+$ cells respectively, prolonged growth in HAT results in a steady decrease in the fraction of cells expressing the TK$^-$ phenotype.

FIG. 1.   VARIATION IN THE FRACTION OF TK$^-$ CELLS
UNDER SELECTIVE AND NON-SELECTIVE CONDITIONS

The fraction of TK$^-$ cells in transformed lines grown in HAT or MEM was calculated from the ratio of the plating efficiency in BUDR medium to the sum of the plating efficiencies in BUDR and HAT medium. (A) AC1 line;   (B) AC5 line

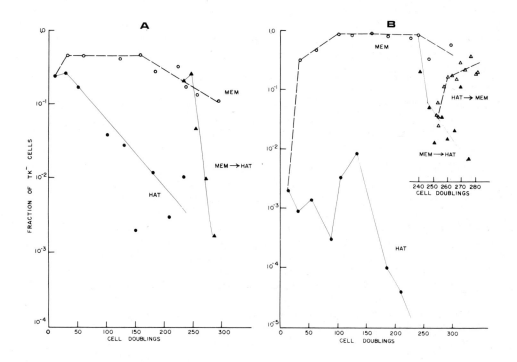

Growth in MEM on the other hand increases significantly the fraction of TK$^-$ cells, to 45% in the AC1 line and to 80% in the AC5 line. These patterns are again repeated when cells are switched from MEM to HAT and back to MEM.   For both lines grown in MEM the percentage of TK$^-$ cells, after the initial increase, remains constant at 45% and 80% respectively for more than 100 cell doublings and then declines again.

Measurement of the relative doubling time of the two cell types in
the AC1 line grown in MEM has indicated that the TK^+ cells grow at a
rate about 20% faster than the TK^- cells (possibly because the medium
is supplemented with undialysed fetal calf serum containing thymidine).
Thus the plateau in the fraction of TK^- cells is probably due to an
equilibrium between the two cell types resulting from a balance
between differential growth rates and TK^+ to TK^- conversion.   As a
result of their faster growth rate TK^+ cells are slowly selected for,
even in "non-selective" conditions, as indicated by the eventual
decline in the fraction of TK^- cells in lines grown in MEM.

A third line, AC4, similarly analysed, behaves in a quite different
manner in that in either HAT or MEM it contains never more than 1-2%
TK^- cells and thus is the most stable line so far isolated.

Several hypotheses can be put forward to explain the variability
of expression of the viral TK gene in the transformed lines:

(1) The viral gene exists as an episome which is randomly lost
at each cell division.   This contention, however, is not fully
supported by the fact that transformed lines growing in HAT can be
easily established and that no crisis or reduction in growth rate has
been observed in any of them.

(2) The viral TK gene is retained by the TK^- cells in an integrated but stably suppressed form.   Although no evidence for or
against this hypothesis is as yet available, the fact that TK^- to TK^+
reversion has not been observed and that TK^- cells can be supertrans-
formed with efficiencies similar to those obtained in the original
transformation is not in direct support of this hypothesis.

(3) The viral TK gene is integrated in transformed cells into one
chromosome (possibly a different chromosome in different lines)
present in several copies per cell (but only one copy containing the
TK gene).   Reversion from TK^+ to TK^- would result from loss of the
chromosome bearing the TK gene and occur with different frequency
according to the ploidy of the cells for such a chromosome.   We
favour this hypothesis since a number of our observations are
consistent with this model: firstly, all transformed lines can be
cultured indefinitely in TK^+ selective medium implying that the viral
TK gene is inherited by a majority of the progeny at each cell division;
secondly, loss of TK activity appears to be irreversible; and thirdly,
the degree of stability of transformants varies from one line to another
but seems to be an inherent trait of each line.

SUMMARY

Human TK⁻ cells carrying the HSV-2 TK gene express a TK activity
of viral origin and maintain the TK⁺ phenotype when grown in HAT
medium.   Under non-selective or counterselective conditions, however, reversion to a TK⁻ phenotype occurs with a significant frequency
characteristic of each transformed line.   The TK⁻ phenotype appears
to be stable since no instances of TK⁻ to TK⁺ reversion have been
observed.

ACKNOWLEDGEMENTS

This work was supported by the National Cancer Institute
of Canada.   The authors are Research Scholars of
the National Cancer Institute of Canada.

REFERENCES

Bacchetti, S. & Graham, F.L. (1977)   Transfer of the gene for
    thymidine kinase to thymidine kinase-deficient human cells
    by purified Herpes simplex viral DNA.   *Proc. nat. Acad. Sci.
    (Wash.), 74*, 1590-1594

Littlefield, J.W. (1964)   Selection of hybrids from matings of
    fibroblasts *in vitro* and their presumed recombinants.   *Science,
    145*, 709-710

Munyon, W., Buchsbaum, R., Paoletti, E., Mann, J., Kraiselburd, E.
    & Davis, D. (1972)   Electrophoresis of thymidine kinase activity
    synthesized by cells transformed by Herpes simplex virus.
    Virology, 49, 683-689

IDENTIFICATION OF SEQUENCES CODING FOR THYMIDINE KINASE IN HERPES SIMPLEX VIRUS AND TRANSFORMED CELL DNA

S. SILVERSTEIN, M. WIGLER, A. PELLICER & R. AXEL

*Departments of Microbiology and Pathology,
and The Institute for Cancer Research,
Columbia University,
Health Sciences Center,
New York, N.Y., USA*

Infection of mouse LTK⁻ cells deficient in cytoplasmic thymidine kinase (Kit et al., 1963) with ultraviolet-irradiated herpes simplex virus (HSV) results in the introduction and stable expression of viral thymidine kinase activity (Munyon et al., 1971). Davidson et al. (1973) demonstrated that it was possible to suppress phenotypic expression of the TK gene by growing LTK⁺ transformants in medium containing bromodeoxyuridine (BUDR). Phenotypically LTK⁻ cells were shown to contain the TK gene in a form that could be reactivated by subsequent recloning in medium containing hypoxanthine, aminopterin and thymidine (HAT) (Littlefield, 1963). Recently, Leiden et al. (1976) and Kit & Dubbs (1977) demonstrated that expression of the resident viral TK in biochemical transformants could be regulated by superinfecting these cells with TK⁻ HSV. We are interested in investigating the mechanisms that control the expression of HSV genes in transformed cells. In particular, we are concentrating on the expression of HSV TK in biochemical transformants. Towards this end, we have isolated a 3.4 kilobase (Kb) fragment generated by *Bam*H1 restriction endonuclease that contains the gene coding for TK (Wigler et al., 1977). The specific fragment containing the TK gene was identified by transfecting LTK⁻ cells with restriction endonuclease-derived fragments and selecting for the TK⁺ phenotype by growth in HAT.

Isolation of the specific fragment containing the TK gene required the identification of a restriction endonuclease that digests HSV DNA without cleaving the structural gene. Initially, limit digests of viral DNA were prepared using *Bam*H1 and *Eco*R1. When DNA digested

with these enzymes was examined in transfection assays for the
ability to convert LTK⁻ cells to the TK⁺ phenotype only cultures
treated with *Bam*-digested DNA displayed surviving colonies in HAT
(Table 1).   DNA digested with both enzymes was inactive in transfection assays indicating that the *Eco*R1 enzyme cleaves within the *Bam*
fragment containing the TK gene.

Table 1. Transfection of LTK⁻ cells with unfractionated restriction-
endonuclease digests of HSV-1 DNA*a*

Restriction-endonuclease digest	HSV-1 DNA per dish (μg)	Colonies per 10^6 cells
*Eco*R1-digested HSV-1 DNA	4.00	0
	2.00	0
	1.00	0
	0.50	0
	0.25	0
*Bam*H1-digested HSV-1 DNA	4.00	3.5
	2.00	3.0
	1.00	1.0
	0.50	0
	0.25	0.75
*Bam*H1-, *Eco*R1- digested HSV-1 DNA	2.00	0
*Hpa*1-digested HSV-1 DNA	5.00	3.0

a All dishes received 10 μg of DNA in 0.5 ml, salmon sperm DNA being
used as carrier

To demonstrate that the TK⁺ transformants had acquired and were
stably expressing the viral TK gene, cells were cloned in HAT, grown
into mass culture and tested for virus-specific TK by neutralization
of the TK activity with specific antisera and by examining the electrophoretic mobility of the TK activity (Wigler et al., 1977).   In all

cases the enzyme activity proved to be indistinguishable from HSV-1 TK.

To isolate the *Bam* fragment that contained the TK gene from the total *Bam* digest we fractionated the digest into size classes on the basis of electrophoretic mobility in agarose gels.   Each size class was examined for the ability to convert LTK$^-$ cells to the TK$^+$ phenotype by employing the calcium phosphate transfection technique described by Graham & van der Eb (1973).   These experiments demonstrated that the activity resided within five well separable bands.   The components of this size class were isolated and tested for the ability to transform LTK$^-$ cells to the TK$^+$ phenotype.   The activity was found to reside within a 3.4 Kb fragment (Wigler et al., 1977).   Of interest was the observation that the specific activity (i.e., number of transformants per μg equivalent of total digested DNA) of the isolated *Bam* 3.4 Kb fragment was some 40-fold higher than that of DNA derived either from a total *Bam* digest or from *Bam*-digested DNA containing the five components in the size class from which the fragment was originally isolated (Table 2).   Subsequently, we demonstrated that this 3.4 Kb fragment is a doublet composed of one band that contains the TK gene and can be cleaved by *Eco*R1 and *Hind*II, and another band which is derived from a terminal fragment (N. Wilkie [1]) and persists after digestion with *Eco*R1.

Table 2. Transfection with fractionated restriction-endonuclease cleaved HSV-1 DNA

Fragment	μg equivalents per dish[a]	Colonies per 10^6 cells
Bam 3.4 Kb	1.5	24.00
	0.5	19.00
	0.15	6.00
	0.05	3.34
Hpa 8.8 Kb	5.0	3.50
Hpa, *Bam* 3.4 Kb	5.0	1.00
Kpn 5.2 Kb	5.0	TMTC

[a] A μg equivalent represents the amount of DNA present in a specific fragment multiplied by the reciprocal of the amount of the total genome that any particular fragment represents.

---

[1] Personal communication

To purify the fragment containing the TK gene to homogeneity we identified other enzymes that, after cleavage, left the TK activity intact.   Cleavage with either *Hpa*1 or *Kpn* yields such a product. The *Hpa* fragment that contains the TK gene is 8.3 Kb while the *Kpn* fragment is 5.2 Kb.   Each of these fragments when digested with *Bam* yields a unique 3.4 Kb fragment that contains the gene coding for TK.   To understand why DNA digested with *Eco*R1 is inactive in trans- fection assays we cleaved the unique 3.4 Kb fragment with *Eco*R1 and demonstrated that this enzyme cleaved at two points within the frag- ment resulting in bands that were 2.27, 0.53 and 0.68 Kb respectively. The 2.27 Kb fragment is internal and can be isolated as a unique frag- ment from total *Eco*R1 digests of HSV-1 DNA.

To analyse the stability of the TK gene within biochemical trans- formants two types of experiments were performed.   In the first we examined the capacity of individual TK^+ clones derived by transfection to grow in either HAT or BUDR.   Unlike the parental LTK^- cell line, the transformants cloned with equal efficiency in HAT or non-selective medium (Table 3).   A low but reproducible number of cells lost the ability to express TK as indicated by their ability to grow in BUDR. Unlike cells transformed by UV-inactivated virus (Davidson et al., 1973) these BUDR-resistant cells do not possess the capacity to reexpress the TK gene, i.e., they cannot be recloned in HAT.

Table 3. Cloning efficiency of various cell lines in selective and non-selective media[a]

Cell line	BUDR[b]	DME[c]	HAT[d]
TK^-	7.3×10^{-1}	7.5×10^{-1}	$10 - 8$
LH7	3.3×10^{-2}	5.8×10^{-1}	5.4×10^{-1}
$LH5C_2$	6.0×10^{-3}	6.9×10^{-1}	5.4×10^{-1}
LH2-1	1.4×10^{-2}	6.2×10^{-1}	5.9×10^{-1}
LH2b	2.0×10^{-4}	4.5×10^{-1}	4.5×10^{-1}

[a] Cells were plated in replicate, and colonies stained with Giemsa and counted after incubation for 12 days.

[b] TK- selective medium (DME, 10% calf serum, 30 µg/ml BUDR)

[c] Non-selective medium (DME, 10% calf serum)

[d] TK+ selective medium (DME, 10% calf serum, 15 µg/ml hypoxanthine, 1 µg/ml aminopterin, 5 µg/ml thymidine)

In the second series of experiments we analysed the transformed cells for the number of copies of viral DNA that codes for TK.   In these experiments the unique *Eco*R1 2.27 Kb fragment was isolated from a total *Eco*R1 digest and labelled *in vitro* with ^{32}P-deoxyribonucleotide triphosphates employing the procedure described by Maniatis et al. (1975). The DNA probe was then annealed to DNA extracted from LTK$^-$ or transformed cell DNA and the rate of reassociation was monitored using S$_1$ nuclease. As a control ^{3}H-globin cDNA was annealed in the same reaction. As there are three globin genes expressed in the adult mouse we were able to compare the kinetics of annealing of the globin probe with the TK probe and demonstrate that in a cell line (LH1b) transformed using the isolated *Bam* 3.4 Kb doublet there was only one copy of the TK gene per diploid quantity of transformed cell DNA (Fig. 1). The data for hybridization of the probe to the DNA from three other cell lines and LH1b are shown in Figure 2. In this

FIG. 1. HYBRIDIZATION OF *Eco*R1 2.27 Kb FRAGMENT
WITH TRANSFORMED CELL DNA

^{3}H-labelled globin cDNA (10^4 cpm) and the ^{32}P-labelled *Eco*R1 2.27 Kb fragment of HSV-1 DNA were reassociated in the presence of transformed cell (LH1b) or LTK$^-$ DNA. The labelled probes in 1 mM tris, pH 7.9, 0.2 mM EDTA, mixed with sonicated cell DNAs were boiled for 10 minutes, 5 M sodium chloride was added to a final concentration of 0.4 M and the reactions were overlaid with mineral oil and permitted to reassociate at 68°C. At various intervals aliquots were removed and assayed using S$_1$ nuclease. O——O Hybridization of ^{3}H-labelled globin cDNA to DNA extracted from LH1b. △——△ Hybridization of ^{32}P-labelled *Eco*R1 fragment to DNA extracted from LH1b (3.9 mg of DNA in 150 μl). ●——● Hybridization of ^{32}P-labelled *Eco*R1 fragment to DNA extracted from LTK$^-$ cells (4.2 mg of DNA in 170 μl).

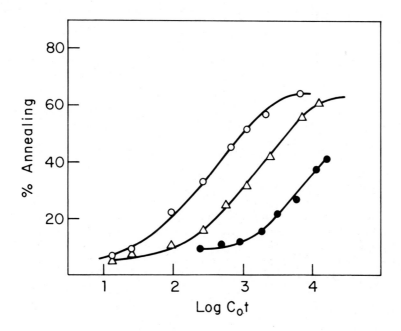

FIG. 2.   HYBRIDIZATION OF *Eco*R1 2.27 Kb FRAGMENT
WITH THE DNA EXTRACTED FROM FOUR CELL LINES DERIVED
BY TRANSFECTION WITH THE *Bam* 3.4 Kb DOUBLET

The hybridizations were performed as described in the legend to Figure
1.   The data are plotted as $1/f$ (where f is the fraction of ^{32}P-
labelled probe remaining single-stranded) against $t/t_{\frac{1}{2}P}$ where $t_{\frac{1}{2}P}$ is
the time required for 50% of the ^{32}P-labelled probe to reanneal in the
presence of untransformed cell DNA.   The closed circles represent
hybridization in the presence of DNA extracted from LTK$^-$ cells;   the
open circles represent the reannealing that occurred in the presence of
transformed cell DNA.   (A) DNA from LH1b (3.9 mg in 150 μl);
(B) DNA from LH2b (3.7 mg in 170 μl);   (C) DNA from LH3b (3.9 mg in
150 μl);   and (D) DNA from LH7 (4.8 mg in 150 μl).

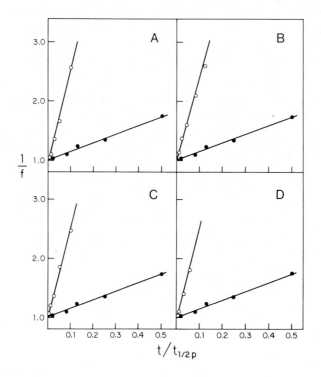

instance, the renaturation kinetics were analysed using the equations
derived by Sharp et al. (1974).   As shown in Figure 2 each of the
transformed cells contains base sequences homologous to the 2.27
*Eco*R1 fragment;   each of them appears to contain approximately one
copy of this fragment per diploid quantity of cell DNA.

Previously (Wigler et al., 1977) we demonstrated that mouse LTK⁻ cells could be stably transformed to the TK⁺ phenotype using a restriction endonuclease fragment derived by cleavage of HSV-1 DNA with *Bam*H1. The TK⁺ transformants isolated by growth in a selective medium expressed the viral TK enzyme as judged by neutralization with specific antisera and by the electrophoretic mobility of the enzyme activity. In this paper we have extended our results by demonstrating that a unique fragment derived by double digestion with *Hpa*1 and *Bam*H1 contains the TK gene. The viral TK gene is present in a stable form in these transformed cells at the level of one copy per cell. Currently we are analysing the BUDR-resistant revertants to determine whether the inability subsequently to clone in HAT represents loss of the sequences coding for TK or a reorientation of these viral sequences within the cellular genome.

ACKNOWLEDGEMENTS

We gratefully acknowledge the assistance of Ms Mary Chen for maintaining the cell lines used in these studies. This work was supported by grants from the National Institutes of Health to S. Silverstein (No. CA17477) and R. Axel (No. CA16346).

REFERENCES

Davidson, R.L., Adelstein, S.J. & Oxman, M.N. (1973)   Herpes simplex virus as a source of thymidine kinase for thymidine kinase-deficient mouse cells: Suppression and reactivation of the viral enzyme. *Proc. nat. Acad. Sci. (Wash.)*, *70*, 1912-1916

Graham, F.L. & van der Eb, A.J. (1973)   A new technique for the assay of infectivity of human adenovirus 5DNA. *Virology*, *52*, 456-467

Kit, S., Dubbs, D., Piekarski, L. & Hsu, T. (1963)   Deletion of thymidine kinase activity from L cells resistant to bromodeoxy-uridine. *Exp. Cell Res.*, *31*, 297-312

Kit, S. & Dubbs, D. (1977)   Regulation of herpesvirus thymidine kinase activity in LM(TK⁻) cells transformed by ultraviolet light-irradiated herpes simplex virus. *Virology*, *76*, 331-340

Leiden, J.M., Buttyan, R. & Spear, P.G. (1976) Herpes simplex virus gene expression in transformed cells. I. Regulation of the viral thymidine kinase gene in transformed L cells by products of super-infecting virus. *J. Virol., 20,* 413-424

Littlefield, J. (1963) The inosinic acid pyrophosphorylase activity of mouse fibroblasts partially resistant to β-azaguanine. *Proc. nat. Acad. Sci. (Wash.), 50,* 568-573

Maniatis, T., Jeffrey, A. & Kleid, D.G. (1975) Nucleotide sequence of the rightward operator of phage λ. *Proc. nat. Acad. Sci. (Wash.), 72,* 1184-1188

Munyon, W., Kraiselburd, E., Davies, D. & Mann, J. (1971) Transfer of thymidine kinase to thymidine kinaseless L cells by infection with ultraviolet-irradiated herpes simplex virus. *J. Virol., 7,* 813-820

Sharp, P.A., Pettersson, U. & Sambrook, J. (1974) Viral DNA in trans-formed cells. I. A study of the sequences of adenovirus 2 DNA in a line of transformed rat cells using specific fragments of the viral genome. *J. molec. Biol., 86,* 709-726

Wigler, M., Silverstein, S., Lee, L.-S., Pellicer, A., Cheng, Y.-C. & Axel, R. (1977) Transfer of purified herpes virus thymidine kinase gene to cultured mono cells. *Cell, 11,* 223-232

ONCOGENIC TRANSFORMATION OF NON-PERMISSIVE MURINE CELLS BY VIABLE EQUINE HERPESVIRUS TYPE 1 (EHV-1) AND EHV-1 DNA

G. ALLEN, D. O'CALLAGHAN & C. RANDALL

*University of Mississippi Medical Center,
Jackson, Miss., USA*

INTRODUCTION

Because many herpesviruses have a wide *in vitro* host range and replicate in cells derived from most mammalian species, the use of non-permissive cells has not become a popular model for the study of herpesvirus transformation. However, it would be advantageous to have a cell system which could be transformed by viable herpesvirus or intact viral DNA without resort to prior inactivation of the virus's lytic functions. In this report, we describe such a system by demonstrating that viable equine herpesvirus type 1 (EHV-1) as well as intact EHV-1 DNA have the capacity to oncogenically transform cells (primary BALB/c mouse embryo fibroblasts; MEF) that are non-permissive for virus replication.

TRANSFORMATION OF BALB/c MEF BY EHV-1 AND EHV-1 DNA

That infection of BALB/c MEF with EHV-1 was both non-productive and non-cytopathic was demonstrated by adding 1, 10, or 100 PFU of virus per cell to subconfluent monolayers of cells. No cytopathology was observed, no virus replication could be demonstrated either by infectivity assays or by electron microscopy, and the cells could be serially subcultured with continued growth. After four such sub-cultures, EHV-1 could no longer be detected in the cells by assay of culture medium or cell sonicates in permissive horse cells. Furthermore, cells infected in the presence of 100 µCi/ml of ^{3}H-uridine did not synthesize ^{3}H-RNA that would hybridize to EHV-1 DNA.

EHV-1 DNA was introduced into secondary cultures of BALB/c MEF cells by the calcium phosphate precipitation technique of Graham & Van der Eb

(1972).   That the viral DNA was intact and infectious was demonstrated by its transfectivity for permissive horse cells (Fig. 1A).

FIG. 1. ADDITION OF EHV-1 DNA TO PERMISSIVE AND NON-PERMISSIVE CELLS

Viral plaques (A) or foci of transformed cells (B) resulting from the addition of EHV-1 DNA to permissive horse (A) or non-permissive BALB/c MEF cells (B).

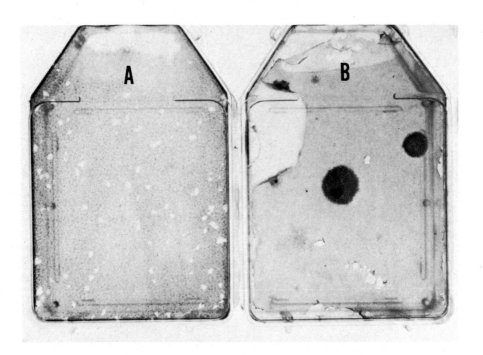

No high-density viral DNA characteristic of that found in defective interfering herpesvirions (Campbell et al., 1976) could be detected in the preparation of EHV-1 DNA by analytical ultracentrifugation in caesium chloride.

Approximately 3-6 weeks after addition of EHV-1 virions (100 PFU per cell) or DNA (1-2 µg) to BALB/c monolayers, foci of densely packed, piled-up cells were visible in 10-20% of the cultures (Fig. 1B). Although most flasks contained only 1-2 foci, some contained as many as 10.   Foci were never observed in uninoculated control MEF.

Seven independently transformed cell lines were established from single foci and were maintained for further study.   The transformed cells propagated rapidly in culture (doubling time 12–30 hours) to high saturation densities (3–6 x 10^5 cells/cm^2) and formed multilayered sheets of fibroblast-like cells with occasional multinucleate giant cells (Fig. 2).   Cells of all lines had lost the property of contact inhibition of growth and exhibited the irregular arrangement and crisscrossing observed for most types of transformed cells.   All the transformed cultures have been passaged more than 70 times (> 500 cell doublings), thus demonstrating their potential for unlimited culture *in vitro*.   Although the cells from all transformed lines had the capacity to grow in 1.2% methylcellulose medium (Shin et al., 1975), the fraction of total cells forming colonies (plating efficiency) varied from one line to another (< 1% to > 10%).   Normal MEF cells were unable to grow in methylcellulose medium.   Cytogenetic analysis of the cell lines transformed by EHV-1 DNA demonstrated that all lines displayed aneuploid and subtetraploid karyotypes with modal chromosome numbers ranging from 72 to 79.   In contrast, cultures of MEF at low passage levels had predominantly diploid karyotypes (40 ± 5 chromosomes).

FIG. 2.   MONOLAYER CULTURES OF TRANSFORMED AND TUMOUR-DERIVED CELLS

(A) Monolayer cultures of control MEF cells;   (B) EHV-1 transformed MEF cells;   (C) tumour-derived cells.   (Giemsa's stain) (x 75)

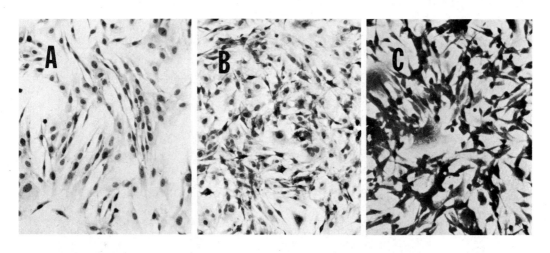

Electron microscopic examination of cells from the transformed lines revealed no evidence of herpesvirus or C-type virus particles. Moreover, viable EHV-1 could not be recovered from sonicates of the transformed cells by *in vitro* culture or by inoculation into susceptible animals (weanling hamsters), nor could the virus be rescued from the cells by induction with iododeoxyuridine (IUDR) or by co-cultivation with permissive horse cells.   Attempts to detect EHV-1 specific bio-chemical markers (thymidine kinase, DNA polymerase, or ribonucleotide reductase) in the transformed cells were also not successful.

ONCOGENICITY OF TRANSFORMED CELLS

The ability of the seven lines of EHV-1 transformed cells to produce tumours in animals was tested by the subcutaneous (s.c.) injection of cells into newborn BALB/c mice.   Six to ten mice were used for each line of cells, and the challenge dose was 10^6 cells in 0.05 ml of phosphate-buffered saline (PBS).   Palpable subcutaneous tumours at the site of inoculation were discernible in some mice as early as 30 days post implantation, and most animals had developed tumours by 60 days post implantation (Fig. 3A).   The tumours grew rapidly, were serially transplantable into adult mice, and were inva-riably fatal to their hosts.   They were well circumscribed and only

FIG. 3.   TUMOUR PRODUCTION BY EHV-1 TRANSFORMED CELLS

(A) Induced tumour 50 days after s.c. inoculation of newborn mouse with 10^6 EHV-1 transformed cells;   (B) histological section of tumour.

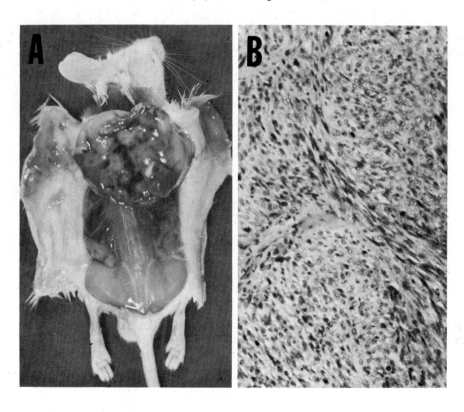

loosely adherent to the adjacent muscle and skin; small tumours were generally solid with firm gray-white tissue whereas large tumours became cystic with haemorrhagic necrosis at the centre.   The largest tumour measured 5 cm in diameter and weighed 25 g.   Although metastasis into the lungs was noted in only three of more than 50 tumour-bearing animals examined, tumour invasion of the musculature of the shoulders and front legs was frequently observed.

The histological appearance of all the tumours induced by EHV-1 transformed cells was that of highly undifferentiated fibrosarcomas consisting of interlacing bundles of closely spaced pleiomorphic spindle cells (Fig. 3B).

In general, cell lines established from the primary tumours grew more rapidly, were more pleiomorphic, and exhibited higher plating efficiencies in methylcellulose than did the original transformed cell lines.   Such tumour-derived cells were also more oncogenic, both by dose and by latent period, than were cells from the parent transformed lines.

No tumours developed over a period of eight months in newborn mice inoculated with 10^6 normal MEF or with an established line of BALB/c 3T3 cells.

VIRUS-SPECIFIC ANTIGENS IN TRANSFORMED, TUMOUR, AND CONTROL CELL LINES

Cells were examined for the presence of EHV-1 antigens by the indirect viable cell-membrane immunofluorescence assay utilizing antiserum elicited in mice against sonicates of EHV-1 infected mouse L-M cells.   The EHV-1 specific antiserum reacted with the surfaces of 10-40% of cells in all transformed and tumour-derived lines but not with control MEF cells (Fig. 4).   Internal viral antigens could not be detected in fixed cell preparations from any of the transformed or tumour lines utilizing the same antiserum.

VIRUS DNA IN TRANSFORMED LINES AND TUMOURS

Three of the EHV-1 transformed cell lines and their corresponding tumours were examined for the presence of the EHV-1 genome utilizing the technique of DNA-DNA reassociation kinetics (Frenkel et al., 1976). The strategy of this kinetic hybridization test was to allow a small amount of denatured, highly radioactive EHV-1 probe DNA (2×10^8 cpm/µg), prepared by enzymatic repair of DNAse-nicked EHV-1 DNA with _E. coli_ DNA polymerase and ^{125}I-dCTP (Shaw et al., 1975), to reassociate in the presence of transformed or tumour-cell DNA (test hybridization) or in the presence of identical concentrations of unrelated DNAs (control hybridization).   As shown in Figure 5, transformed or tumour cell DNA accelerated the initial rate of probe reassociation, indicating the

FIG. 4.   IMMUNOFLUORESCENT MEMBRANE STAINING OF TRANSFORMED CELLS

Immunofluorescent membrane staining of non-fixed EHV-1 transformed
BALB/c MEF cells with mouse anti-EHV-1 serum and fluorescein-conjugated
rabbit anti-mouse IgG serum.   (A) Fluorescent cell;   (B) non-fluorescent
cell.

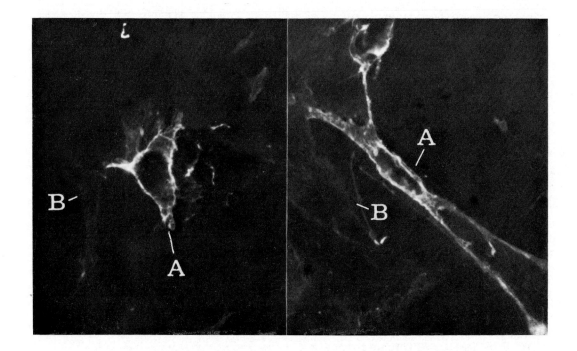

presence of EHV-1 DNA sequences within the transformed (and tumour)
cells.   Analysis of the hybridization data for each of the examined
cell lines by the method of Fujinaga et al.(1974) revealed that
multiple copies (1-4) of a fragment of EHV-1 DNA representing 8-15%
of the total genome were present in each transformed and tumour cell.

In summary, these results indicate that cells non-permissive for
replication of EHV-1 remain susceptible to neoplastic transformation
by both the virus and the viral genome, and that such transformed cells
retain a small portion of the viral genome whose continuous expression
can be detected as antigenic modification of the transformed cell
surface.

FIG. 5.   DNA-DNA REASSOCIATION OF DENATURED LABELLED EHV-1 DNA
IN THE PRESENCE OF TRANSFORMED OR TUMOUR-CELL DNA

Reassociation of 1 ng/ml of denatured EHV-1 ^{125}I-DNA fragments
(2×10^8 cpm/µg) in the presence of 5 mg/ml of DNA from MEF cells
(passage 1-7), transformed cells (passage 18-23), or tumour cells
(derived from mice inoculated with passage-15 transformed cells).
Hybridizations were performed at 63°C in 0.1 M tris hydrochloride
(pH 8.1), 0.025 M EDTA, 1.0 M sodium chloride, and 20% (v/v) formamide.
The fraction of DNA remaining single-stranded (f_{ss}) after various times
of annealing was determined by hydroxyapatite chromatography.

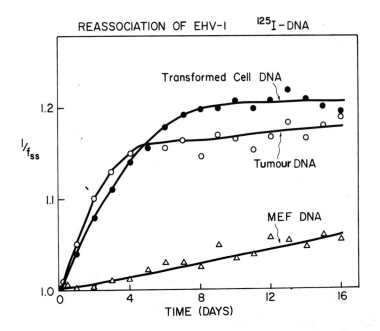

SUMMARY

    Primary cultures of BALB/c mouse embryo fibroblasts infected with as
much as 100 PFU per cell of EHV-1 do not exhibit cytopathology or
synthesize detectable amounts of EHV-1 specific RNA, DNA, or infectious
virus.   Addition of 1-2 µg of non-fragmented EHV-1 DNA as a co-precipi-
tate with calcium phosphate to monolayers of such non-permissive mouse

cells resulted in the appearance, after 4-6 weeks, of foci of piled-up,
morphologically altered cells.   Cell lines established from such transformed foci exhibited a greatly increased growth rate, unlimited growth
potential, aneuploid karyotype, and grew with colony formation in soft
agar.   Inoculation of 10^6 transformed cells into newborn syngeneic
mice resulted in the formation of serially transplantable tumours
(undifferentiated fibrosarcomas) with a 100% incidence within eight
weeks.   Infectious virus could not be rescued from the EHV-1 transformed
or tumour-derived cell lines by growth in the presence of IUDR, by co-
cultivation with permissive horse cells, or by attempts to transfect
permissive cells with transformed or tumour cell DNA.   However, EHV-1
specific membrane antigens were detected in the transformed cells by
immunofluorescence with hyperimmune anti-EHV-1 mouse serum, and the
presence of a fragment of the EHV-1 genome was demonstrated in both the
transformed and tumour cells.   These results indicate that cells non-
permissive for replication of EHV-1 remain susceptible to neoplastic
transformation by the EHV-1 genome.

REFERENCES

Campbell, D.E., Kemp, M.C., Perdue, M.L., Randall, C.C. & Gentry, G.A.
    (1976)   Equine herpes virus *in vivo*: cyclic production of a DNA
    density variant with repetitive sequences.   *Virology, 69*, 737-750

Frenkel, N., Locker, H., Cox, B., Roizman, B. & Rapp, F. (1976)
    Herpes simplex virus DNA in transformed cells: sequence complexity
    in five hamster cell lines and one derived hamster tumor.   *J.
    Virol., 18*, 885-893

Fujinaga, K., Sekikawa, K., Yamazaki, H. & Green, M. (1974)   Analysis
    of multiple viral genome fragments in adenovirus 7-transformed
    hamster cells.   *Cold Spring Harb. Symp. quant. Biol., 39*, 633-636

Graham, F.L. & Van der Eb, A.J. (1972)   A new technique for the assay
    of infectivity of human adenovirus 5 DNA.   *Virology, 52*, 456-467

Shaw, J.E., Huang, E.S. & Pagano, J.S. (1975)   Iodination of herpes-
    virus nucleic acids.   *J. Virol., 16*, 132-140

Shin, S.I., Freedman, V.H., Risser, R. & Pollack, R. (1975)   Tumor-
    igenicity of virus-transformed cells in nude mice is correlated
    specifically with anchorage independent growth *in vitro*.
    Proc. nat. Acad. Sci. (Wash.), 72, 4435-4439

REGULATION OF THE HERPES SIMPLEX VIRUS GENE FOR THYMIDINE KINASE IN CLONAL DERIVATIVES OF TRANSFORMED MOUSE L-CELLS

R. BUTTYAN & P.G. SPEAR

*Department of Microbiology and the Committee on Virology,
The University of Chicago,
Chicago, Ill., USA*

The herpes simplex virus (HSV) gene for thymidine kinase (TK) may be either expressed or suppressed in clonal derivatives of HSV-transformed mouse L-cell lines (Davidson et al., 1973) whose selection and isolation from TK-deficient L-cells depended originally on the incorporation and expression of the HSV TK gene supplied by UV-irradiated virus (Munyon et al., 1971). Identification of the factors that regulate viral TK synthesis in clonal derivatives of HSV-transformed L-cells is one focus of our investigation into the regulation of viral gene expression in transformed cells.

We have isolated from an HSV-1 transformed cell line, according to the protocol shown in Figure 1, several phenotypically TK⁻ clones and also TK⁺ clones that express different levels of HSV TK. In this report, we present evidence that the HSV TK gene is retained by both the phenotypically TK⁻ and TK⁺ clones and that expression of the viral TK gene may depend on the concomitant expression of other products, possibly viral in genetic origin, that enhance HSV replication.

The ability of the clonal derivatives identified in Figure 1 to form colonies in selective media was consistent with the levels of TK activity detectable in cell extracts. Specifically, the relative cloning efficiencies in HAT media[1] compared with non-selective media were essentially 1.00 for LVTK/F4, 0.16 for LVTK/F10 and 1×10^{-4} for LVTK/F10/B. Conversely, the relative cloning efficiencies in

---

[1] Hypoxanthine, aminopterin and thymidine

FIG. 1. PROTOCOL FOR THE ISOLATION OF CLONAL VARIANTS FROM
THE LVTK PARENTAL LINE

Obtained from R. Davidson, Harvard Medical School, Boston, Mass.

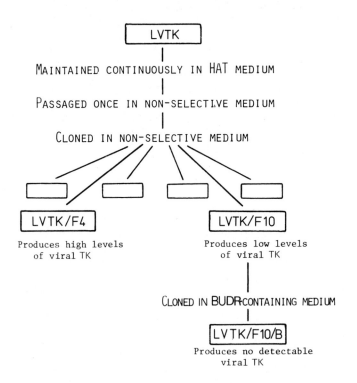

bromodeoxyuridine (BUDR)-containing medium were 0.01 for LVTK/F4,
0.65 for LVTK/F10 and 0.94 for LVTK/F10/B.   Although clone LVTK/F10/B
was phenotypically TK⁻ based on two criteria (low and high cloning
efficiencies in HAT medium and BUDR-containing medium respectively,
and absence of detectable viral TK activity in cell extracts), we
found that viral TK could be synthesized by these cells under certain
conditions.   Superinfection of LVTK/F10/B with HSV-1 (TK⁻), a procedure which has previously been shown to enhance expression of the
resident viral TK gene of LVTK cells (Kit & Dubbs, 1977;   Leiden et
al., 1976;   Lin & Munyon, 1974), resulted in the induction of TK
synthesis (Fig. 2).   Antibody neutralization tests revealed that
the enzyme made was viral in genetic origin;   it was presumably
specified by the resident HSV-TK gene because the superinfecting
virus was TK⁻.   These results demonstrate not only the retention of

FIG. 2.   INDUCTION OF TK ACTIVITY IN PHENOTYPICALLY TK$^+$
(LVTK/F4) OR TK$^-$ (LVTK/F10/B) CLONES DERIVED
FROM HSV-1 TRANSFORMED MOUSE CELLS

The TK assays were done according to Leiden et al. (1976) on extracts
prepared from cells infected with HSV-1 (TK$^-$) at 2 PFU per cell (●),
or from mock-infected cells (○).   The TK$^-$ virus used (*B2006*) was
obtained from S. Kit, Baylor University, Houston, Texas.

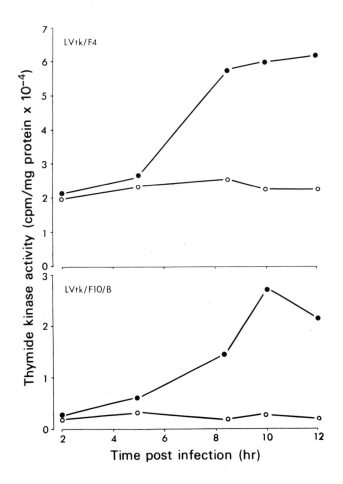

the viral TK gene in the phenotypically TK$^-$ clone but also the
apparently unaltered susceptibility of this viral gene to regulation
by products of the superinfecting virus.

The clonal variants differed from one another, not only in the levels of viral TK synthesized (in the absence of superinfection), but also in their ability to support HSV replication.   We found that, during a productive infection of the TK$^+$ LVTK/F4 cells with HSV-1 (TK$^+$), progeny virus could be detected earlier and significantly higher yields of virus were produced than during equivalent infections of LVTK/F10/B cells or untransformed LTK$^-$ cells (data not shown). That this effect was due to greater yields of HSV per LVTK/F4 cell rather than differential adsorption or penetration of input virus was demonstrated by the results shown in Figure 3.   HSV-1 ultimately formed approximately the same number of plaques on monolayers of LVTK/F4, LVTK/F10/B or LTK$^-$ cells; however, visible plaques are detectable much earlier and grow larger on monolayers of LVTK/F4 cells.

FIG. 3.   PLAQUE FORMATION AFTER EXPOSURE TO HSV-1 (TK$^+$)

Detection of plaques at various times after exposure of LVTK/F4 cells (●), LVTK/F10/B cells (■) or LTK$^-$ cells (○) to identical aliquots of HSV-1 (TK$^+$).   Neutral red was added to the agarose-containing media on these cultures 24 hr prior to the enumeration of plaques.

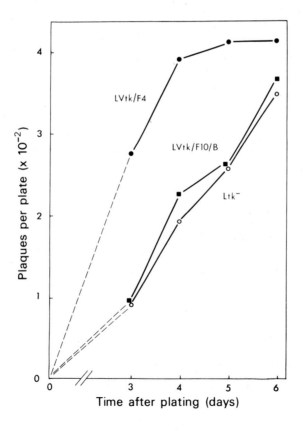

The correlation between high levels of HSV TK synthesis by the LVTK/F4 cells and enhanced expression of an input viral genome suggests that the same factor or factors may be responsible for both phenomena. This consideration, in addition to our finding that the HSV TK gene in both the LVTK/F4 and LVTK/F10/B cells can be regulated by products of superinfecting virus, supports our hypothesis that viral gene products may play a role in regulating HSV TK synthesis in the transformed cells even in the absence of superinfection (Leiden et al., 1976). If this hypothesis is correct, it remains to be determined why the relevant HSV regulatory products are expressed in LVTK/F4 cells but not in LVTK/F10/B cells.

ACKNOWLEDGEMENTS

This work was supported by a grant from the United States
Public Health Service (1 P01 CA 19264-01).   R. Buttyan
is a predoctoral fellow supported by Virology Training
Grant 5 T01 AI 00238-13 and P.G. Spear is the recipient
of USPHS Research Career Development
Award 5 K04 CA 00035-02.

REFERENCES

Davidson, R., Adelstein, S. & Oxman, M. (1973)   Herpes simplex virus
    as a source of thymidine kinase for thymidine kinase deficient
    mouse cells: suppression and reactivation of the viral enzyme.
    Proc. nat. Acad. Sci. (Wash.), *70*, 1912-1916

Kit, S. & Dubbs, D.R. (1977)   Regulation of herpesvirus thymidine
    kinase activity in LM (tk) cells transformed by ultraviolet
    light-irradiated herpes simplex virus.   *Virology*, *76*, 331-340

Leiden, J.M., Buttyan, R. & Spear, P.G. (1976)   Herpes simplex virus
    gene expression in transformed cells.   I. Regulation of the viral
    thymidine kinase gene in transformed L cells by products of super-
    infecting virus.   *J. Virol.*, *20*, 413-424

Lin, S.-S. & Munyon, W. (1974)   Expression of the viral thymidine
    kinase gene in herpes simplex virus-transformed L cells.   *J.
    Virol.*, *14*, 1199-1208

Munyon, W., Kraiselburd, E., Davis, D. & Mann, J. (1971)   Transfer of
    thymidine kinase to thymidine kinaseless L cells after infection
    with ultraviolet-irradiated herpes simplex virus.   *J. Virol.*, *7*,
    813-820

ENHANCED EFFICIENCY OF TRANSFECTION OF HSV DNA IN HSV-1 DNA-TRANSFORMED HAMSTER CELLS

F. COLBERE-GARAPIN & F. HORODNICEANU

Virology Department,
Institut Pasteur,
Paris, France

Herpes simplex virus type 1 (HSV-1) and type 2 (HSV-2) replication has been shown to be delayed in UV-inactivated HSV-transformed cells, virus titres in HSV-transformed cells infected by HSV being lower than those obtained in control cells (Doller, 1977). Our previous experiments showed that HSV-1, HSV-2 and herpesvirus eidolon (HVE) grew more slowly in HSV DNA-transformed hamster cells (EH/A44) than in spontaneously transformed hamster cells (EHT), although the same maximum titres were obtained with both cell lines (Colbère-Garapin et al., 1978). In order to determine whether this delay involved an early step in HSV infection, transfection experiments with purified herpesvirus DNA were performed.

The efficiency of transfection, i.e., the number of plaques per µg of DNA, was compared for EH/A44, UV-inactivated HSV-1 transformed (14.012.8.1) and EHT cells (Fig. 1). The efficiency of transfection obtained with HSV-1 DNA was 5.3 times higher in EH/A44 cells [3000 plaque-forming units (PFU)/µg of DNA] than in EHT cells (560 PFU/µg). In 14.012.8.1 cells this efficiency was 360 PFU/µg. Plaques were always smaller in HSV-transformed cells than in control cells. The results were similar when a different transfection technique was used: the diethylaminoethyl (DEAE)-dextran technique (Sheldrick et al., 1973). Progeny of plaques induced in EH/A44 cells by HSV-1 DNA were infectious in EHT cells, and thus non-defective.

In order to determine whether the high efficiency of transfection of HSV-1 DNA was specific to HSV-1 DNA and HSV-transformed cells, the efficiency of transfection of HSV-1, HSV-2 and HVE DNAs was studied in various cell systems and compared with that of intact viruses (Table 1). HSV-1 and HSV-2 DNAs had similar high transfection efficiencies in EH/A44 clones. In contrast, HVE DNA had approximately the same

FIG. 1. DOSE-RESPONSE CURVE OF HSV-1-A44 DNA ON HSV-1 DNA-TRANSFORMED
HAMSTER CELLS (EH/A44), UV-INACTIVATED HSV-1 TRANSFORMED HAMSTER CELLS
   (14.012.8.1), AND SPONTANEOUSLY TRANSFORMED HAMSTER CELLS (EHT)

Cell and virus culture, virus DNA extraction, establishment and
properties of EH/A44 and EHT cell lines are described elsewhere
(Colbère-Garapin et al., 1978).   The transfection technique used
was described by Graham et al. (1973).   Plaques were scored after
four days at 37°C.   Range is indicated by vertical bars.

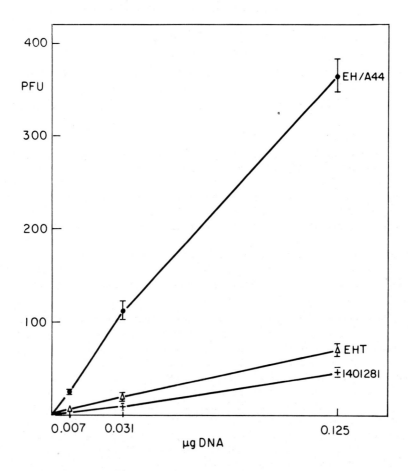

transfection efficiency in EH/A44 and EHT cells.   The efficiency of
transfection of HSV-1 DNA was not higher in 14.012.8.1 cells than in
EHT cells.   However, the ratio of infectivity of HSV-1 DNA in 14.012.
8.1 cells to the infectivity of the same DNA in EHT cells was seven
times higher than the ratio of infectivity of intact HSV-1 in 14.012.
8.1 cells to the infectivity of the same virus in EHT cells.

Table 1. Ratio of DNA infectivity and virus infectivity in various cell types to infectivity in spontaneously transformed EHT cells[a]

| Cell types | Ratio of infectivity in various cell types to infectivity in EHT cells | | | | | |
| | Ratio obtained with viral DNA | | | Ratio obtained with virus | | |
	HSV-1 A44 DNA	HSV-2 DNA	HVE DNA	HSV-1 A44	HSV-2	HVE
EHT	1	1	1	1	1	1
EHT C10[b]	1	1	-	1	1	-
RSF[c]	0.80	-	-	0.80	-	-
BHK/Py[d]	1	-	-	0.25	-	-
CX903B (CMV)[e]	0.10	-	-	0.25	-	-
14.012.8.1 (HSV-1)	0.70	-	-	0.10	-	-
EH/A44 (HSV-1)	5	-	0.9	0.15	0.24	0.06
EH/A44 C1[f]	4	5	-	0.15	-	-
EH/A44 C2[f]	7.5	6	-	0.15	0.20	-
EH/A44 AG1[f]	7.5	3.5	-	0.15	0.12	-
EH/A44 AG4[f]	2	1	-	0.20	0.27	-
EH/A44 AG5[f]	7.5	-	-	0.17	0.36	-
TUM EH/A44[g]	5	-	-	0.15	-	-

[a] Ratio = $\dfrac{\text{PFU in cell types}}{\text{PFU in EHT cells}}$

[b] Clone of EHT cells

[c] Rabbit skin fibroblasts

[d] BHK21 cells transformed by polyoma virus

[e] Hamster cells transformed by cytomegalovirus

[f] Clone of EH/A44 cells

[g] Cells derived from a tumour induced in a hamster after injection of EH/A44 cells

In conclusion, the transfection efficiency of HSV-1 DNA was 2-8 times higher in our HSV DNA-transformed clones than in controls, while the same EH/A44 clones were partially resistant to superinfection by intact herpesviruses. This indicates that infection of HSV-transformed cells by intact herpesviruses was partially blocked at an early step.

The mechanism by which infection of EH/A44 cells is enhanced by transfection with HSV DNA is being studied further.

SUMMARY

The efficiency of transfection, i.e., the number of plaques per µg of DNA, was compared for herpes simplex virus (HSV) type 1 and type 2, and herpesvirus eidolon (antigenically unrelated to HSV) DNAs in HSV DNA-transformed cells (EH/A44) and control hamster cells (EHT). The efficiency of transfection of HSV-1 and HSV-2 DNAs was significantly higher in EH/A44 cells than in EHT cells, showing that an early step in HSV infection was involved in the partial resistance of HSV DNA-transformed cells to superinfection by various intact herpesviruses.

ACKNOWLEDGEMENTS

The 14.012.8.1 and CX903B cell lines were kindly provided
by Dr F. Rapp and the BHK/Py cells by Dr C. Cremisi.
We wish to thank Dr A. Garapin and Dr S. Michelson
for helpful discussions. This investigation was
supported by INSERM grant 009 ATP
Virus et Cancer.

REFERENCES

Colbère-Garapin, F., Horodniceanu, F. & Tardy-Panit, M. (1978)
Comparison of HSV-1-DNA-induced and spontaneous transformation of
hamster cells. *Ann. Microbiol.*, *129A* (in press)

Doller, E. (1977) Evidence for an inhibitor of herpes simplex virus in
transformed hamster cells. *Proc. Soc. exp. Biol. (N.Y.)*, *154*,
168-170

Graham, F.L., Veldhuisen, G. & Wilkie, N.M. (1973) Infectious herpesvirus DNA. *Nature new Biol.*, *245*, 265-266

Sheldrick, P., Laithier, M., Lando, D. & Ryhiner, M.L. (1973)
Infectious DNA from herpes simplex virus: infectivity of double-
stranded and single-stranded molecules. *Proc. nat. Acad. Sci.
(Wash.)*, *70*, 3621-3625

MAPPING OF PUTATIVE TRANSFORMING SEQUENCES OF EBV DNA

E. KIEFF, N. RAAB-TRAUB, D. GIVEN, W. KING,
A.T. POWELL, R. PRITCHETT & T. DAMBAUGH

*The Section of Infectious Disease of the Department of Medicine,
and the Committee on Virology,
University of Chicago,
Chicago, Ill., USA*

INTRODUCTION

Preparations of Epstein-Barr virus (EBV) from most EBV-producing continuous lymphoblastoid cell lines (Gerber et al., 1969; Pope et al., 1968) and from the throat washings of infected humans (Gerber, 1973) have in common the ability to "transform" uninfected lymphocytes with limited growth potential *in vitro* into lymphoblasts which can be grown indefinitely as continuous lymphoblastoid cell lines. The data contained in this report represent the current status of two ongoing programmes aimed at defining the EBV DNA sequences needed to initiate and maintain lymphocytes in the lymphoblastoid state. The objectives are: (1) to determine whether there are specific viral DNA sequences essential to the ability of EBV to transform; and (2) to determine which viral DNA sequences are expressed in (restringently infected) "transformed cells". The rationale for these two approaches is as follows.

Comparison of the DNA of transforming and non-transforming strains of EBV

Two EBV-infected continuous lymphoblastoid cell lines, HR-1 and B95-8, in which an unusually high percentage of cells are permissive of virus replication, have been utilized for biological and chemical studies of EBV (Dolyniuk et al., 1976; Hayward & Kieff, 1977; Hayward et al., 1976; Menezes et al., 1975; Miller et al., 1974; Pritchett et al., 1975). The HR-1 cell line is a subculture of the Jijoye line which was established from a Burkitt tumour biopsy (Hinuma et al., 1967). The B95-8 cell line was obtained by incubation

of marmoset lymphocytes with EBV from a lymphoblastoid culture
established from a patient with transfusion-acquired infectious mononucleosis (Miller et al., 1972).   Recently, another partially permissive continuous lymphoblastoid cell line (W91) was established by
infecting marmoset leukocytes with EBV obtained from Burkitt lymphoma
cells grown in culture (Miller et al., 1976).   Virus from the HR-1
line, EBV (HR-1), can be used to superinfect Raji cells, thereby
inducing the synthesis of early antigen (Henle et al., 1970), but this
virus cannot transform normal lymphocytes into cells possessing
capacity for long-term growth *in vitro* (Menezes et al., 1975;
Miller et al., 1974).   In contrast, virus from the B95-8 line,
EBV (B95-8) (Miller & Lipman, 1973), and from other recently
established EBV-infected marmoset lymphoblastoid cultures, including
the W91 cell line, EBV (W91) (Miller et al., 1976), cannot induce
early antigen in Raji cells but can transform normal lymphocytes into
cells capable of long-term replication in culture.   Although the
HR-1 strain could have latent transforming capability, attempts to
uncover the putative transforming potential of EBV (HR-1) by irradiation have not been successful suggesting that this strain lacks DNA
needed to initiate transformation (Henderson & Miller[1]).

    In initial studies no differences have been found between the
antigens (Miller et al., 1972, 1976) and polypeptides (Dolyniuk et
al., 1976) of the B95-8 and HR-1 strains of EBV.   Comparisons of
their DNAs have indicated the following: (*a*) EBV (B95-8) and (HR-1)
DNAs are linear, double-stranded molecules with the length and sedimentation properties indicative of a size of 100×10^6 daltons
(Pritchett et al., 1975).   (*b*) Kinetic and absorptive hybridization
analyses with *in vitro* labelled purified viral DNAs indicated that
EBV (B95-8) DNA lacks approximately 15% of the DNA sequences of EBV
(HR-1) DNA (Pritchett et al., 1975; Sugden et al., 1976) and that EBV
(HR-1) DNA contains more than 95% of the DNA sequences of EBV (B95-8)
DNA (Pritchett et al., 1975).   In one study, kinetic hybridization
data suggested that EBV (B95-8) DNA might contain sequences which EBV
(HR-1) DNA lacked (Sugden et al., 1976).   No attempt was made in this
study, however, to demonstrate that the residual labelled EBV (B95-8)
DNA which did not hybridize to EBV (HR-1) DNA could hybridize to EBV
(B95-8) DNA.   (*c*) EBV (B95-8) DNA is relatively enriched for DNA
sequences with a buoyant density in neutral caesium chloride of
1.720-1.721 g/cm^3 (Pritchett et al., 1975).   (*d*) The molecular weights
of some restriction enzyme-produced fragments of EBV (B95-8) and (HR-1)
DNA are similar but others differ between the strains (Hayward & Kieff,
1977; Hayward et al., 1976).

    The distinctive biological properties of the B95-8 and HR-1 strains
of EBV could arise from the presence or absence of specific DNA
sequences or as a consequence of differences in the arrangement of

---

[1] Unpublished data

DNA sequences.   A long-range objective of this series of experiments is to discriminate between these alternative possibilities by identifying which fragments of EBV (HR-1) DNA contain DNA which is known to be missing from the B95-8 strain and which, if any, fragments of EBV (B95-8) DNA contain DNA missing from the HR-1 strain.

Mapping of EBV DNA sequences encoding polyribosomal and poly-adenylated RNA of restringently infected cells

Most EBV-infected cell lines contain more than 90% of the EBV genome (Kawai et al., 1973; Kieff & Levine, 1974; Nonoyama & Pagano, 1973; Pritchett et al., 1976) and an EBV-determined intra-nuclear antigen, EBNA (Lindahl et al., 1974; Reedman & Klein, 1973), at least one component of which is a DNA-binding protein of approximately 1.75×10^5 daltons (Ohno et al., 1977).   Most EBV-infected cell lines do not contain progeny virus or antigens associated with productive infection.   Expression of EBV DNA in these cells must therefore be under tight control which permits the expression of a few viral functions, i.e., EBNA and cellular growth enhancement, while prohibiting the expression of many others.   This state of EBV infection is referred to as restringent.   Restringently infected Namalwa and Raji cultures contain RNA encoded by 16 and 30% of EBV DNA, respectively (Hayward & Kieff, 1976; Orellana & Kieff, 1977).   The polyadenylated (Orellana & Kieff, 1977) and polyribosomal (Hayward & Kieff, 1976) RNA fractions of Raji and Namalwa cells are enriched for a class of RNA encoded by approximately 5% of EBV DNA.   Summation hybridizations indicated that the same EBV DNA sequences encode the polyadenylated and polyribosomal RNA of both Raji and Namalwa cells (Orellana & Kieff, 1977).   These findings favour the hypothesis that the viral RNA which is selectively processed in restringently infected cells specifies functions related to maintenance of the transformed state.   The second objective of the studies reported here is to map the DNA encoding these polyribosomal and polyadenylated RNA species of restringently infected cells.

RESULTS

Identification of EBV DNA fragment which contains DNA sequences deleted in EBV (B95-8) DNA

In order to identify those DNA sequences deleted in EBV (B95-8) DNA, a specific probe for these sequences was prepared.   EBV (HR-1) DNA was labelled *in vitro* (Rigby et al., 1977), denatured, and hybridized in the presence of a 50- to 100-fold excess of (B95-8) DNA to at least 4 $C_0 t_{50}$ of the unlabelled EBV DNA.   Under these conditions the residual single-stranded DNA should be enriched for sequences deleted in (B95-8) DNA.   Following hybridization, 10% of the labelled EBV (HR-1) DNA eluted as single-stranded DNA from hydroxyapatite. Further incubation of the single-stranded DNA with additional (B95-8)

DNA failed to increase the rate of hybridization of the labelled single-
stranded EBV (HR-1) DNA indicating that all of the sequences homologous
to (B95-8) DNA had been removed.   Hybridization of this labelled
single-stranded DNA to filters (Southern, 1975) containing restriction
enzyme fragments of EBV (HR-1) DNA (Hayward & Kieff, 1977) indicated
that the DNA sequences not present in (B95-8) DNA are located in EBV
(HR-1) DNA *Eco*RI C and D fragments (Fig. 1) and *Hsu*I E and N fragments
(Fig. 2) and in a minor heterogeneous *Hsu*I fragment smaller than fragment C.   Exposure of the autoradiograms for longer intervals did not
indicate hybridization to other fragments of EBV (HR-1) DNA.

Previous hybridization studies using EBV (HR-1) DNA have consistently demonstrated that this DNA possesses more than 90% homology to the
DNA of cells infected with most strains of EBV and no homology to uninfected cell DNA (Kawai et al., 1973; Kieff & Levine, 1974; Nonoyama
& Pagano, 1973; Pritchett et al., 1976).   Nevertheless, it is important to determine whether the sequences present in EBV (HR-1) DNA and
missing in EBV (B95) DNA are present in the DNA of other strains of
EBV.   Analysis of the complexity of EBV DNA in the W91 cell line by
hybridization of W91 cellular DNA with labelled denatured EBV (HR-1)
DNA suggested that this DNA contains more than 90% (94 ± 6%, mean ± S.D.
of five separate experiments) of the sequences of EBV (HR-1) DNA
(Fig. 3).   Electrophoresis of the fragments produced by cleavage of the
DNA of the W91 strain of EBV with *Eco*RI and *Hsu*I restriction endonucleases yields a pattern distinct from that of B95-8 or HR-1 DNA (Figs 4
& 5).   All fragments produced by cleavage of EBV (W91) DNA with *Hsu*I
and *Eco*RI nucleases are present in equimolar amounts.   The molecular
weight of the fragments, estimated by electrophoresis with intact and
digested DNA, agrees well,fragment by fragment,with previous estimates
of the molecular weight of *Hsu*I and *Eco*RI fragments of EBV (B95-8) DNA
(Given & Kieff[1]).   The major difference observed was that the molecular
weight of the W91 *Eco*RI fragment C is approximately 8×10^6 larger than
B95-8 *Eco*RI fragment C and W91 has two *Hsu*I fragments, D and E, whose
aggregate molecular weight exceeds that of the single corresponding
B95-8 *Hsu*I fragment D by approximately 8×10^6 daltons.   Experiments
in which the denatured labelled EBV (HR-1) DNA, from which sequences
homologous to EBV (B95-8) DNA had been removed, was hybridized to
blots of EBV (W91) DNA,as in the preceding experiment, indicate that
EBV DNA sequences deleted from B95-8 DNA are located primarily in EBV
(W91) DNA *Eco*RI fragment C (Fig. 4) and *Hsu*I fragments D and E (Fig. 5).
Some hybridization was seen to *Eco*RI fragment A or B (Fig. 4).   However,
since fragments A and B are most efficient in hybridizing with unabsorbed
labelled EBV (HR-1) DNA it is possible that the hybridizations observed
to A and B are an artefact of incomplete removal of EBV (B95-8) homologous sequences.   The data indicate that most of the DNA sequences
deleted from EBV (B95-8) DNA are present not only in the HR-1 but also
in the W91 strain of EBV.

---

[1] Unpublished data

FIG. 1.   IDENTIFICATION OF *Eco*RI FRAGMENT(S) OF EBV (HR-1)
DNA WHICH CONTAIN DNA SEQUENCES NOT PRESENT IN DNA OF THE
B95-8 STRAIN

EBV (HR-1) DNA was incubated with *Eco*RI restriction enzyme, subjected
to electrophoresis in 0.4% agarose gels, stained with ethidium bromide
and photographed under ultraviolet light (Hayward & Kieff, 1977)
(above, left of lettering).   The DNA fragments were transferred on
to nitrocellulose filters (Southern, 1975) which were then cut in
half lengthwise.   One-half of the filter was incubated with 80 000
cpm ^{32}P-EBV (HR-1) DNA (above, far right of lettering).   The other
half of the filter was incubated with 35 000 cpm of the residual
single-stranded ^{32}P-EBV (HR-1) DNA from which sequences homologous to
EBV (B95-8) DNA had been removed (above, near right of lettering).
The filters were washed and exposed to X-ray film for four days.

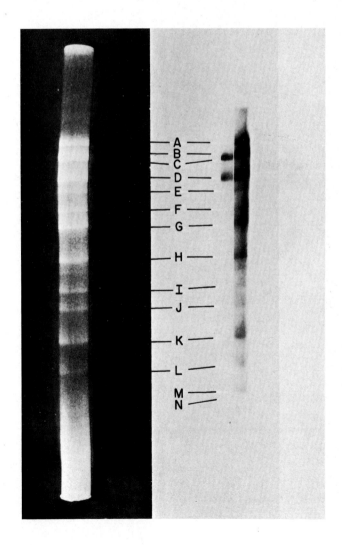

FIG. 2.   IDENTIFICATION OF *Hsu*I FRAGMENT(S) OF EBV (HR-1)
DNA WHICH CONTAIN DNA SEQUENCES NOT PRESENT IN THE DNA OF
THE B95-8 STRAIN

EBV (HR-1) DNA *Hsu*I fragments (above, left of lettering) were transferred on to nitrocellulose filters which were then cut in half lengthwise.   One-half of the filter was incubated with 80 000 cpm ^{32}P-EBV
(HR-1) DNA (above, far right of lettering).   The other half of the
filter was incubated with 45 000 cpm of the residual single-stranded
^{32}P-EBV (HR-1) DNA from which sequences homologous to EBV (B95-8) DNA
had been removed (above, near right of lettering).   The filters were
washed and exposed to X-ray film for four days.

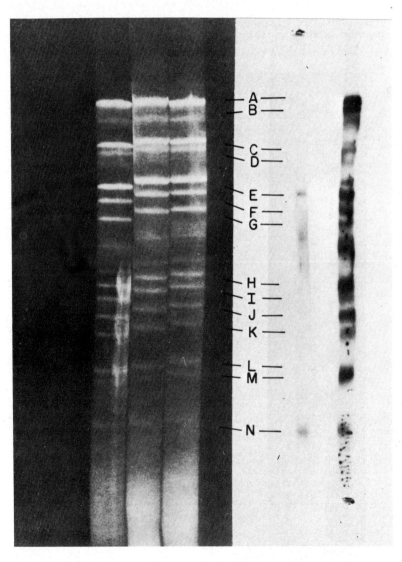

FIG. 3. KINETICS OF HYBRIDIZATION OF ^{32}P-LABELLED EBV
(HR-1) DNA WITH EBV HOMOLOGOUS DNA IN HR-1 OR W91 CELLS

Approximately 0.005 µg ^{32}P-labelled EBV (HR-1) DNA, specific activity,
2×10^7 cpm/µg, was mixed with 0.2 mg of HR-1, W91, or calf thymus DNA
and denatured in 0.2 M sodium hydroxyde.   The denatured DNA was
neutralized and incubated at 68°C in 100 µl of a solution consisting
of 0.005 M EDTA, 1.5 M sodium chloride and 0.025 M tris hydrochloride,
pH 7.4.   At the indicated time intervals the pipettes were removed
and frozen at -30°C until analysed.   Single-stranded DNA was differentiated from double-stranded DNA by digestion with S_1 nuclease as
previously described (Pritchett et al., 1976).   HR-1: ●——●;
W91:△——△.

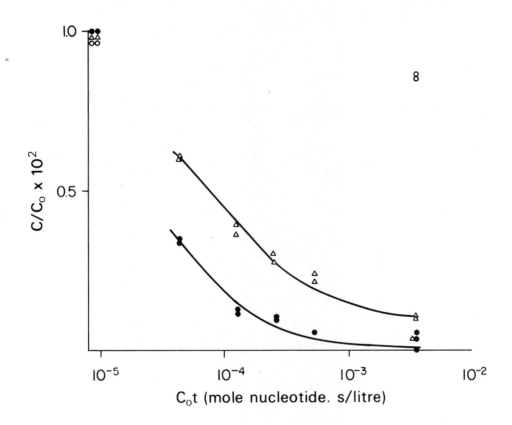

FIG. 4.   IDENTIFICATION OF *Eco*RI FRAGMENTS OF EBV (W91)
DNA WHICH CONTAIN DNA SEQUENCES HOMOLOGOUS TO EBV (HR-1)
DNA SEQUENCES NOT PRESENT IN THE DNA OF THE B95-8 STRAIN

EBV (W91) DNA *Eco*RI fragments (above, left of lettering) were transferred on to nitrocellulose filters which were than cut in half lengthwise.   One-half of the filter was incubated with 30 000 cpm ^{32}P-EBV
(HR-1) DNA (above, near right of lettering).   The other half of the
filter was incubated with 45 000 cpm of the residual single-stranded
^{32}P-EBV (HR-1) DNA from which sequences homologous to EBV (B95-8) DNA
had been removed (above, far right of lettering).   The filters were
exposed to X-ray film for ten days.

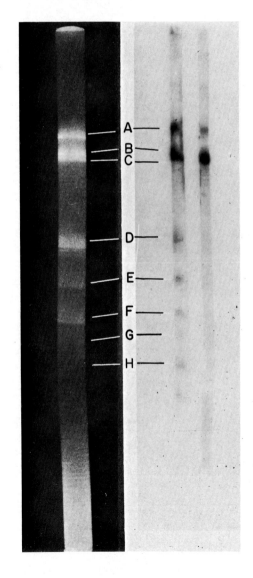

FIG. 5.   IDENTIFICATION OF *Hsu*I FRAGMENTS OF EBV (W91) DNA
WHICH CONTAIN DNA SEQUENCES HOMOLOGOUS TO THE EBV (HR-1)
DNA SEQUENCES NOT PRESENT IN THE DNA OF THE B95-8 STRAIN

EBV (W91) DNA *Hsu*I fragments (above, left of lettering) were transferred
on to nitrocellulose filters which were then cut in half lengthwise.
One-half of the filter was incubated with 30 000 cpm ^{32}P-EBV (HR-1) DNA
(above, near right of lettering).   The other half of the filter was
incubated with 45 000 cpm of the residual single-stranded ^{32}P-EBV (HR-1)
DNA from which sequences homologous to EBV (95-8) DNA had been removed
(above, far right of lettering).   The filters were washed and exposed
to X-ray film for ten days.

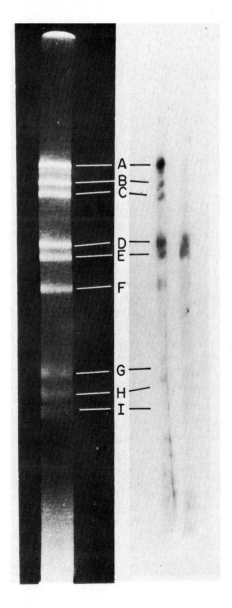

Identification of the EBV DNA sequences deleted from the DNA of the HR-1 strain of EBV

To determine whether EBV (B95-8) DNA contains sequences not present in the DNA of the HR-1 strain and to identify the fragments of EBV (B95-8) DNA which contain these sequences, EBV (B95-8) DNA was labelled *in vitro* (Rigby et al., 1977), denatured, incubated with a 50-fold excess of denatured DNA from HR-1 cells for at least 6 C_ot_{50} of the unlabelled EBV DNA and the residual single-stranded DNA which would be enriched for sequences not present in HR-1 DNA was separated by chromatography on hydroxyapatite. Of the labelled EBV (B95-8) DNA, 2% eluted as single-stranded DNA from hydroxyapatite. Incubation of the labelled single-stranded DNA with additional HR-1 DNA failed to increase the rate of hybridization of the single-stranded EBV (B95-8) DNA, indicating that all of the sequences homologous to (HR-1) DNA had been removed. Autoradiograms prepared from blots of *Eco*RI fragments of EBV (B95-8) DNA which had been hybridized to the residual labelled single-stranded DNA revealed hybridization to an *Eco*RI fragment between J and K and to fragment A (Fig. 6); blots of *Hsu*I fragments revealed hybridization to fragment B and to a lesser extent to fragment A (Fig. 7). Since the A fragments of both the EBV (B95-8) DNA *Eco*RI and *Hsu*I digests are the fragments detected most efficiently by the unabsorbed probe (Figs 6 & 7), we cannot be certain from these data that the hybridization seen to band A with the absorbed probe specifically identifies a component of band A missing from EBV (HR-1) DNA or reflects an incomplete absorption of the sequences homologous to EBV (HR-1) DNA. With regard to *Hsu*I fragment A we favour the latter possibility since the small amount of hybridization to fragment A evident in some experiments was not seen in all experiments.

In order to demonstrate that the DNA sequences missing from the HR-1 strain but present in the B95 strain of EBV were viral sequences, the labelled EBV (B95-8) DNA from which sequences homologous to EBV (HR-1) DNA had been absorbed out was incubated with blots of EBV (W91) DNA. Autoradiograms prepared from the hybridized blots revealed hybridization to *Eco*RI fragment A and to a lesser extent to *Eco*RI fragments B and D hetero (Fig. 8) and to *Hsu*I fragment B.

Identification of the fragment of EBV (B95-8) DNA encoding polyribosomal and polyadenylated RNA of restringently infected cells

Attempts to identify the DNA fragment encoding polyribosomal and polyadenylated RNA from restringently infected cells using blots of agarose gels containing separated restriction enzyme fragments of EBV (B95-8) DNA and polyadenylated polyribosomal RNA labelled with ^{32}P-orthophosphate *in vivo* or cDNA to polyadenylated polyribosomal RNA have not yielded definitive results. Autoradiograms prepared by hybridizing labelled DNA homologous to polyadenylated RNA from restringently infected cells to blots of fragments of viral DNA indicate hybridization to *Hsu*I fragment A (Fig. 9). Much less

FIG. 6.   IDENTIFICATION OF *Eco*RI FRAGMENTS OF EBV (B95-8)
DNA WHICH CONTAIN DNA SEQUENCES NOT PRESENT IN DNA
OF THE HR-1 STRAIN

EBV (B95-8) DNA was incubated with *Eco*RI restriction enzyme, subjected
to electrophoresis in 0.4% agarose gels, stained with ethidium bromide
and photographed under ultraviolet light (above, right of lettering).
The DNA fragments were transferred on to nitrocellulose filters which
were then cut in half lengthwise.   One-half of the filter was incubated
with 20 000 cpm ^{32}P-EBV (B95-8) DNA (above, far left of lettering).
The other half of the filter was incubated with 25 000 cpm of the
residual single-stranded ^{32}P-EBV (B95-8) DNA from which those sequences
homologous to EBV (HR-1) DNA had been removed (above, near left of
lettering).   The filters were exposed to X-ray film for eight days.

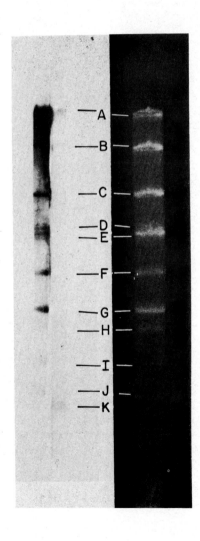

FIG. 7.   IDENTIFICATION OF *Hsu*I FRAGMENTS OF EBV (B95-8)
DNA WHICH CONTAIN DNA SEQUENCES NOT PRESENT IN DNA
OF THE HR-1 STRAIN

EBV (B95-8) DNA *Hsu*I fragments (above, left of lettering) were transferred on to nitrocellulose filters which were then cut in half lengthwise.   One-half of the filter was incubated with 20 000 cpm ^{32}P-EBV
(B95-8) DNA (above, far right of lettering).   The other half of the
filter was incubated with 20 000 cpm of the residual single-stranded
^{32}P-EBV (B95-8) DNA from which those sequences homologous to EBV (HR-1)
DNA had been removed (above, near right of lettering).   The filters
were exposed to X-ray film for ten days.

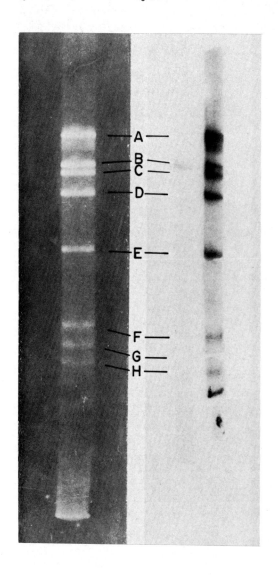

FIG. 8.   IDENTIFICATION OF *Eco*RI FRAGMENT(S) OF EBV (W91)
DNA WHICH CONTAIN DNA SEQUENCES HOMOLOGOUS TO EBV (B95-8)
DNA NOT PRESENT IN THE DNA OF THE HR-1 STRAIN

EBV (W91) DNA was incubated with *Eco*RI restriction enzyme, subjected
to electrophoresis in 0.4% agarose gels, stained with ethidium bromide
and photographed under ultraviolet light (above, left of lettering).
The DNA fragments were transferred on to nitrocellulose filters which
were then cut in half lengthwise.   One-half of the filter was incubated
with 140 000 cpm ^{32}P-EBV (B95-8) DNA (above, far right of lettering).
This filter was exposed to X-ray film with a Cronex screen for four
hours.   The other half was incubated with 190 000 cpm of the residual
single-stranded ^{32}P-EBV (B95-8) DNA from which those sequences homologous to EBV (HR-1) DNA had been removed (above, near right of
lettering).   This filter was exposed to X-ray film with a Cronex
screen for two days.

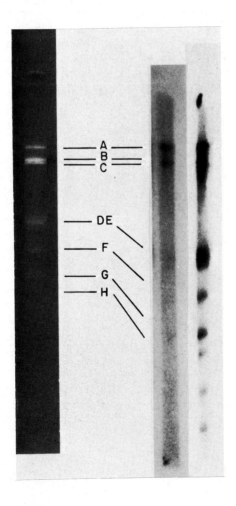

FIG. 9.   IDENTIFICATION OF THE B95 *Hsu*I FRAGMENTS ENCODING
POLYSOMAL POLYADENYLATED RNA FROM RESTRINGENTLY
INFECTED RAJI CELLS

Labelled ^{32}P-EBV (B95-8) DNA, 1.36 × 10^6 cpm, specific activity,
10^8 cmp/μg, was hybridized to Raji polysomal polyadenylated RNA at a
concentration of 1.0 mg/ml in 165 μl under conditions previously
described (Orellana & Kieff, 1977).   The hybridization mixture was
diluted into 0.05 M phosphate buffer (PB) and passed directly over a
hydroxyapatite (HAP) column.   Unhybridized RNA and DNA were washed
from the column with 0.12 M PB.   All duplexed DNA-DNA and RNA-DNA were
eluted with 0.5 M PB.   The pooled peak fractions of about 35 000 cpm
were diluted to 0.05 M PB and treated with RNase A at a final concentration of 10 μg/ml for 20 hours at 37°C.   This mixture was passed
over hydroxyapatite in 0.04 M PB.   Labelled DNA which eluted from HAP
with 0.04 M PB (1.5 × 10^4 cpm) was incubated with half of a *Hsu*I blot
of EBV (B95-8) DNA.   The blot was then exposed to X-ray film (Kodak
SB54) with a Cronex screen at -70°C for four days (right side of
figure).   The other half of the blot was incubated with 8 × 10^4 cpm
of ^{32}P-labelled EBV (B95-8) DNA and exposed to X-ray film without a
screen for one day (left side of figure).

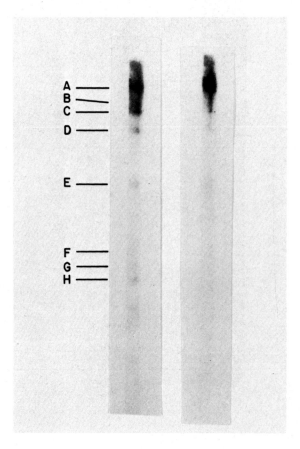

hybridization is seen to *Hsu*I fragments B and C. It is not possible to determine whether the residual hybridization of fragments B and C is due to incomplete separation of labelled DNA which had hybridized to RNA from that which had hybridized to complementary labelled DNA. A second approach using separated *Hsu*I fragments of EBV (B95-8) DNA which are eluted from agarose (Wigler et al., 1977) labelled *in vitro* with polymerase I of *E. coli* (Rigby et al., 1977), and hybridized in solution to excess polyadenylated polyribosomal RNA (Orellana & Kieff, 1977) has confirmed these results. These data indicate that the *Hsu*I A, and to a lesser extent, B, fragments of EBV (B95-8) DNA (Fig. 10) contain DNA encoding polyadenylated polyribosomal RNA of restringently infected cells.

Linkage of restriction enzyme fragments of EBV (B95-8) DNA

The order of restriction enzyme fragments of EBV (B95-8) DNA was determined using *Hsu*I, *Eco*RI, or *Sal*I fragments which had been separated on agarose gels (Hayward & Kieff, 1977) and labelled *in vitro* using DNA polymerase I of *E. coli*. The specificity of each separated and labelled fragment was first demonstrated by hybridization to a blot of an agarose gel containing all of the fragments produced by incubating EBV (B95) DNA with the same restriction enzyme (Fig. 11). The labelled fragments were then individually hybridized to blots of agarose gels containing separated *Eco*RI, *Sal*I, *Hsu*I, or *Kpn*I fragments (Fig. 12). The data for the hybridization of separated and labelled *Hsu*I fragments to *Eco*RI digests are shown in Figure 13. The linkage data for (B95-8) DNA are summarized in Table 1. The map (Fig. 14) was constructed using the linkage data from Table 1 and a previous determination of fragment size (Hayward & Kieff, 1977). The *Sal*I A and D and *Hsu*I A fragments of EBV (B95-8) DNA had been determined to be near termini by their sensitivity to λ exonuclease (Hayward & Kieff, 1977). These and other end fragments frequently appeared as multiple discrete bands in the agarose gels indicating that there is variation in the length of the terminal DNA fragments.

DISCUSSION

A prerequisite to identifying functions of parts of the EBV genome is the ability to separate specific fragments of a viral DNA and knowledge of the order of these fragments in the intact molecule. The problem is complicated by the limited quantities of EBV DNA available and by the presence of single-stranded nicks in the DNA of virus which has accumulated in the extracellular media in the several-day interval needed to obtain a significant harvest. The strategy that we have employed has been to determine the linkage of restriction enzyme-cleaved fragments of EBV (B95-8) DNA by their hybridization with separated, labelled, restriction enzyme fragments. The resulting linkage data have permitted the ordering of the *Hsu*I, *Sal*I, and *Eco*RI

FIG. 10.   HYBRIDIZATION OF POLYADENYLATED POLYRIBOSOMAL RNA
FROM RESTRINGENTLY INFECTED CELLS TO SEPARATED HsuI FRAGMENTS
A TO E OF EBV (B95-8) DNA

Purified viral DNA was digested with HsuI restriction enzyme, electrophoresed on 0.4% agarose gels (Hayward & Kieff, 1977), eluted from the
gels with 5 M perchlorate (Wigler et al., 1977) and labelled in $vitro$
(Rigby et al., 1977).   The preparation of polyribosomes (Hayward &
Kieff, 1976), separation of polyadenylated RNA (Orellana & Kieff, 1977),
and the conditions for hybridization of RNA in excess to labelled DNA
and the procedures employed to differentiate between single- and double-
stranded nucleic acid were those described previously (Orellana & Kieff,
1977). D_0 is the concentration of single-stranded DNA at time zero
and D_t the concentration of single-stranded DNA at each time.

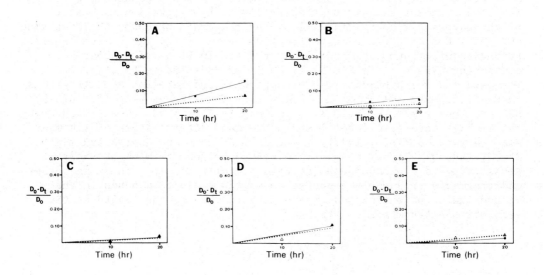

FIG. 11. SPECIFICITY OF SEPARATED ^{32}P-LABELLED *Hsu*I FRAGMENTS

Autoradiograms of DNA blots of 0.4% agarose gels containing *Hsu*I digests of EBV (B95-8) DNA.   The blots had been hybridized with separated *Hsu*I fragments A to E (left to right) which had been cut out of 0.4% agarose gel (far right), eluted from the gel with perchlorate (Wigler et al., 1977) and labelled *in vitro* with DNA polymerase I of *E. coli* (Rigby et al., 1977).

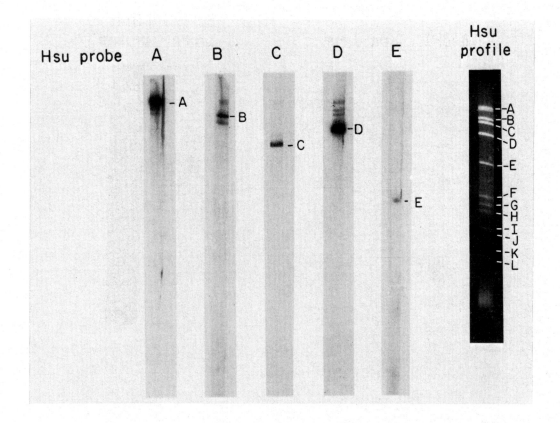

fragments of EBV (B95-8) DNA in a unique linear array.   The data indicate that the relative position of *Sal*I, *Hsu*I, and *Eco*RI endonuclease sites is constant in EBV (B95-8) DNA.

Direct approaches which have been useful in defining the viral DNA sequences needed to transform cells by adeno- and papovaviruses, such as isolation and characterization of viral mutants defective in transformation and transformation with specific fragments of viral DNA, are difficult to pursue in this system.   Two sets of experiments are described in this communication which may provide an indirect

FIG. 12.   LINKAGE DATA DERIVED BY HYBRIDIZATION OF ^{32}P-LABELLED
*Sal*I E FRAGMENT TO BLOTS OF *Eco*RI, *Hsu*I, *Sal*I or *Kpn*I FRAGMENTS

The autoradiograms were obtained by hybridization of labelled
separated *Sal*I E fragment of EBV (B95-8) DNA to blots of agarose gels
containing *Eco*RI, *Kpn*I, *Hsu*I and *Sal*I (left to right) fragments of
EBV (B95-8) DNA.

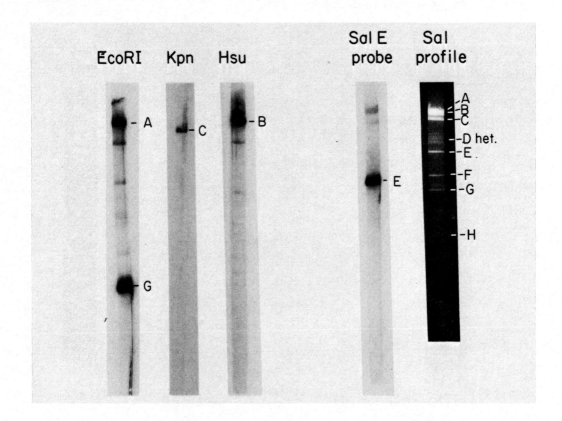

approach to identify DNA sequences important for transformation of
Epstein-Barr virus.   The objective of the first series of experiments
is to determine whether there were differences in the DNA sequences of
the transformation-positive (B95-8 and W91) and transformation-
negative (HR-1) strains of Epstein-Barr virus.   The results indicate
that the transformation-positive strains (both B95-8 and W91) contain
within the *Hsu*I B and *Eco*RI A fragments several million daltons of
DNA missing from the transformation-negative HR-1 strain.   The *Hsu*I
B and *Eco*RI A fragments overlap over a 15×10^6 dalton stretch from
27 to 42×10^6 daltons from the *Hsu*I A end of the map, as plotted in

FIG. 13. LINKAGE DATA DERIVED BY HYBRIDIZATION OF ^{32}P-LABELLED
SEPARATED *Hsu*I FRAGMENTS TO BLOTS OF *Eco*RI FRAGMENTS

The autoradiograms were obtained by hybridization of labelled separated *Hsu*I A to E (left to right) fragments of EBV (B95-8) DNA to blots of agarose gels containing *Eco*RI fragments of EBV (B95-8) DNA.

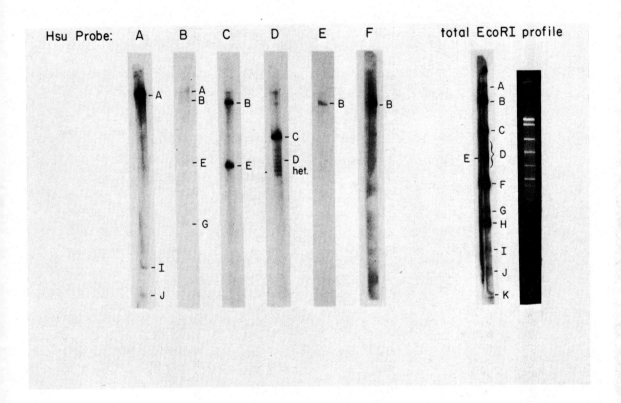

Figure 14.   While this result is unambiguous, there are several aspects of the data and the approach which require discussion.   First, hybridization was also seen to a small, previously undetected fragment of about 1×10^6 daltons located between *Eco*RI fragments J and K in agarose gels, the map position of which is as yet undetermined.   We also cannot be certain that the small amount of hybridization seen to *Hsu*I fragment A was due to incomplete removal of all of the sequences common to the transforming and non-transforming strains.   Second, the B95-8, W91, and HR-1 strains are each independent isolates. Although the failure of radiation to uncover putative latent transforming ability in HR-1 virus suggests that its unusual phenotype is

Table 1. Linkage data for *Eco*RI, *Sal*I, *Hsu*I, and *Kpn*I restriction enzyme fragments of EBV (B95-8) DNA

Probe	Fragments on blot			
	Sal	*Eco* I	*Kpn*	*Hsu*
Hsu A	A,D,het	A,I,J,D,het	A,B,H?	A,het
B	E,G,A,C	A,G,	A,C,H,(F)	A,B
C	B,F,H	E,B	C,E,F	C
D	B,D	C,D	(DE) hetero, G,L,O	D
E	C	B,K	C,D,K,N	E
F	C	B	K,N,(CD)	-
G	-	F	D,F,(CKMN)	-
H	-	C,(H)	F?,M	-
Sal A	A	A,I,J	A,B,H	A
B	B	C,E,B.H	E,F,L,M	C,D,F
C	C	B,F	D,J,K,(C)	E,G,H,I,J
D	D,het	C,D,het	-	D,het
E	E	A,G	C	B
F	F	-	-	C,I
G	G	-	-	-
H	H,D,het	B,het,D	-	C,het
Eco A	A,E,G	A	A,B,D,H,I	A,B
B	B,C,F,H	B	C,E,K,N	C,E,I
C	B,D	-	-	D,F
D,E	B,D,het	-	-	C,D, het
F	C	F	D	G,H
G	C,E	G	C,D,F,J	B,J,G
H	B	H	F	F,K,L
I	A,het	I	het(IJ)	A
J	A	J	(H)	A
K	C	K	D	E

due to the lack of DNA necessary for transformation, it is possible that there is more than a single phenotypic difference between the HR-1 strain and the B95-8 and W91 strains. Previous kinetic and absorptive hybridization experiments indicated that the B95 strain was itself lacking DNA which was present in the transformation-negative HR-1 strain. Presumably, this DNA is not necessary for transformation of cells *in vitro* although it could, in small part, conceivably

FIG. 14. MAP OF *SaL*I, *Hsu*I, AND *Eco*RI FRAGMENTS
OF EBV (B95-8) DNA

The molecular weight of fragments was established by electrophoresis
of fragments in agarose gels containing fragments of T5bl and HSV
(MP) DNA of known size (Hayward & Kieff, 1977).   The length of each
fragment was drawn relative to its molecular weight.   The order of
the fragments was determined from the linkage data (Table 1) obtained
by hybridizing blots of agarose gels containing *SaL*I, *Hsu*I, or *Eco*RI
fragments of EBV (B95-8) DNA with individual *SaL*I, *Hsu*I, or *Eco*RI
fragments of EBV (B95-8) DNA which had been labelled *in vitro* with
DNA polymerase I of *E. coli*.

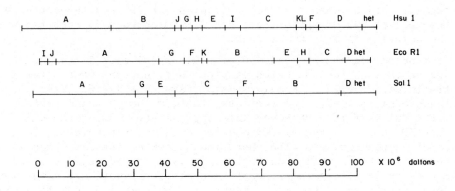

be related to possible differences between strains of virus from
Burkitt tumour tissue (HR-1 and W91) and those derived from non-
malignant cells (B95-8).   Previous data using probes with an
approximate complexity of 10^8 daltons (Kawai et al., 1973; Kieff &
Levine, 1974; Nonoyama & Pagano, 1973) have shown that there is more
than 90% homology between the HR-1 strain and viral DNA in EBV-infected
cells from a variety of non-malignant EBV-infected cells.   However,
this possibility needs to be reassessed as more sophisticated techniques
become available.   DNA missing from the B95-8 strain is located in
the HR-1 *Eco*RI C and D and *Hsu*I E and N fragments.   The W91 strain of
EBV has at least 90% of the sequences of the HR-1 strain.   It is of
interest that at least some of the "extra" DNA which the HR-1 strain
contains is also contained in the *Eco*RI C and *Hsu*I D and E fragments

of the W91 strain.   In cross-hybridization experiments with fragments
of EBV (B95-8) DNA (Given & Kieff[1]), it has been possible to show that
*Eco*RI fragments A to K of the B95-8 strain specifically hybridized to
only a single corresponding *Eco*RI fragment of the W91 strain.   The
only difference observed was that the C fragment of the W91 strain
was approximately 8×10^6 daltons larger than that of the B95 strain.
Furthermore, the only difference observed between the *Hsu*I digests of
B95 and W91 was that W91 contained two fragments, D and E, whose total
molecular weight was approximately 8×10^6 daltons larger than that
of the single corresponding fragment D of the B95 strain.   The *Eco*RI
C fragment overlaps *Hsu*I fragment D in the B95-8 map (Fig. 14).   Taken
together, these data lead us to conclude that the B95-8 strain has at
least one major deletion in the *Hsu*I D, *Eco*RI C overlap.   The simplest
explanation for the difference in size between the *Eco*RI B95-8 and W91
C fragments and between the *Hsu*I D fragment of B95 and the corresponding
DE fragment of W91 of approximately 8×10^6 daltons is that the size
of the deletion is 8×10^6 daltons.

The objective of the second series of experiments is to map the
DNA which encodes the RNA which is processed in transformed, restringently infected cells.   Previous data (Hayward & Kieff, 1977;
Orellana & Kieff, 1977) had indicated that, although transcription
of viral DNA is more extensive, only approximately 5% of the DNA
encodes RNA which is adenylated and found on polyribosomes.   Two
types of experiments described here indicate that the RNA which is
processed in the transformed, restringently infected cell is encoded
primarily by *Hsu*I fragment A.   Additional experiments are under way
to determine whether the small amount of hybridization seen to *Hsu*I
fragment B and to other more distant fragments is reproducible.   It
is, however, of interest that most of the RNA which is processed in
restringently infected cells is encoded by DNA contained in the
fragment lying adjacent to that which contains the DNA which we
infer from the first series of experiments may be important in
initiation of transformation.

SUMMARY

The linkage of restriction enzyme fragments of DNA of the B95-8
strain of Epstein-Barr virus has been determined.   Two approaches
are being employed to define which EBV DNA sequences are needed to
initiate and maintain the transformation of lymphocytes to lymphoblasts
capable of long-term growth in culture.   The first approach is to

---

[1] Unpublished data

determine the differences between the DNA of strains of EBV which possess transforming capacity and the DNA of the HR-1 strain which cannot transform. The data indicate that EBV (HR-1) DNA lacks approximately 2-3 × 10^6 daltons of DNA contained largely in the HsuI B and EcoRI (J-K) and A fragments of EBV (B95-8) DNA and in the EcoRI A and HsuI B fragment of the W91 strain. The DNA common to HsuI B and EcoRI A fragments lies between 27 and 42 × 10^6 daltons from the HsuI A end of the molecule. This finding is compatible with the hypothesis that the inability of the HR-1 strain to transform is due to the absence of DNA needed for transformation. The second approach is to identify and map the DNA encoding polyadenylated viral RNA in cultures of restringently infected cells which contain the EBNA antigen and show no evidence of abortive or productive infection. Previous data indicated that viral RNA species encoded by 5% of the viral DNA are adenylated and identified in the polyribosomes of restringently infected cells. The data indicate that these RNAs are encoded primarily by the HsuI A (and to a lesser extent, B) fragment of EBV (B95-8) DNA. This would place the DNA encoding the viral RNA processed in restringently infected cells adjacent to and possibly overlapping the small DNA segment deleted from the DNA of the non-transforming HR-1 strain.

ACKNOWLEDGEMENTS

We wish to thank George Miller for the gift of the W91 cell line and R. Foy, D. Morse, M. Hawke, and J. Woodruff for their excellent assistance. This work is supported by Grant No. VC-113C from the American Cancer Society and Grants Nos CA-17281-03 and CA-19264-02 from the US Public Health Service. Ann Powell is a Research Postdoctoral Awardee of the US Public Health Service, Grant No. CA-05891-01. W. King, D. Given, and N. Raab-Traub are predoctoral trainees supported by the US Public Health Service. W. King is supported by Grant No. AI-00238-14; N. Raab-Traub by GM-07183-02; and D. Given by HD-07009-03.

REFERENCES

Dolyniuk, M., Pritchett, R. & Kieff, E. (1976)   Proteins of Epstein-Barr virus.   I. Analysis of the polypeptides of purified enveloped Epstein-Barr virus.   *J. Virol., 17*, 935-949

Gerber, P. (1973)   Oral excretion of Epstein-Barr virus.   *Lancet, i*, 1001

Gerber, P., Whang-Peng, J. & Monroe, J.H. (1969)   Transformation and chromosome changes induced by Epstein-Barr virus in normal human leukocyte cultures.   *Proc. nat. Acad. Sci. (Wash.), 63*, 740-747

Hayward, S.D. & Kieff, E. (1976)   Epstein-Barr virus-specific RNA. I. Analysis of viral RNA in cellular extracts and in the poly-ribosomal fraction of permissive and nonpermissive lymphoblastoid cell lines.   *J. Virol., 18*, 518-525

Hayward, S.D. & Kieff, E. (1977)   DNA of Epstein-Barr virus.   II. Comparison of the molecular weights of restriction endonuclease fragments of the DNA of Epstein-Barr virus strains and identifi-cation of end fragments of the B95-8 strain.   *J. Virol., 23*, 421-429

Hayward, D., Pritchett, R., Orellana, T., King, W. & Kieff, E. (1976) *The DNA of Epstein-Barr virus fragments produced by restriction enzymes: Homologous DNA and RNA in lymphoblastoid cells.*   In: Baltimore, D., Huang, A. & Fox, C.F., eds, *Animal Viruses*, New York, Academic Press (ICN-UCLA Symposia on Molecular and Cellular Biology, Vol. 4), pp. 619-640

Henle, W., Henle, G., Zajac, B., Pearson, G., Waubke, R. & Scriba, M. (1970)   Differential reactivity of human serums with early antigens induced by Epstein-Barr virus.   *Science, 169*, 188-190

Hinuma, Y., Konn, M., Yamaguchi, J., Wudarski, D., Blakeslee, J. & Grace, J. (1967)   Immunofluorescence and herpes type virus particles in the [3]P HR-1 Burkitt lymphoma clone.   *J. Virol., 1*, 1045-1051

Kawai, Y., Nonoyama, M. & Pagano, J. (1973)   Reassociation kinetics for Epstein-Barr virus DNA: Nonhomology to mammalian DNA and homology of viral DNA in various diseases.   *J. Virol., 12*, 1006-1012

Kieff, E. & Levine, J. (1974)   Homology between Burkitt herpes viral DNA and DNA in continuous lymphoblastoid cells from patients with infectious mononucleosis.   *Proc. nat. Acad. Sci. (Wash.), 71*, 355-358

Lindahl, T., Klein, G., Reedman, B.M., Johansson, B. & Singh, S. (1974) Relationship between Epstein-Barr virus (EBV) DNA and the EBV determined nuclear antigen (EBNA) in Burkitt's lymphoma biopsies and other lymphoproliferative malignancies. *Int. J. Cancer*, *13*, 764-772

Menezes, J., Leibold, W. & Klein, G. (1975) Biological differences between different Epstein-Barr virus (EBV) strains with regard to lymphocyte transforming ability. *Exp. Cell Res.*, *92*, 478-484

Miller, G. & Lipman, M. (1973) Comparison of the yield of infectious virus from clones of human and simian lymphoblastoid lines transformed by EBV. *J. exp. Med.*, *138*, 1398-1412

Miller, G., Coope, D., Niederman, J. & Pagano, J. (1976) Biological properties and viral surface antigens of Burkitt lymphoma and mononucleosis-derived strains of Epstein-Barr virus released from transformed marmoset cells. *J. Virol.*, *18*, 1071-1080

Miller, G., Shope, T., Lisco, H., Still, D. & Lipman, M. (1972) Epstein-Barr virus: Transformation, cytopathic changes, and viral antigens in squirrel monkey and marmoset leukocytes. *Proc. nat. Acad. Sci. (Wash.)*, *69*, 383-387

Miller, G., Robinson, J., Heston, L. & Lipman, M. (1974) Differences between laboratory strains of Epstein-Barr virus based on immortalization, abortive infection and interference. *Proc. nat. Acad. Sci. (Wash.)*, *71*, 4006-4010

Nonoyama, M. & Pagano, J.S. (1973) Homology between Epstein-Barr virus DNA and viral DNA from Burkitt's lymphoma and nasopharyngeal carcinoma determined by DNA-DNA reassociation kinetics. *Nature (Lond.)*, *242*, 44-47

Ohno, S., Luka, J., Lindahl, T. & Klein, G. (1977) Identification of a purified complement fixing antigen as the EBV determined nuclear antigen (EBNA) by its binding to metaphase chromosomes. *Proc. nat. Acad. Sci. (Wash.)*, *74*, 1605-1609

Orellana, T. & Kieff, E. (1977) Epstein-Barr virus specific RNA. II. Analysis of polyadenylated viral RNA in restringent, abortive and productive infection. *J. Virol.*, *22*, 321-330

Pope, J.H., Horne, M.K. & Scott, W. (1968) Transformation of foetal human leukocytes *in vitro* by filtrates of a human leukaemic cell line containing herpes-like virus. *Int. J. Cancer*, *3*, 857-866

Pritchett, R.F., Hayward, S.D. & Kieff, E.D. (1975) DNA of Epstein-Barr virus. I. Comparison of DNA of virus purified from HR-1 and B95-8 cells. *J. Virol.*, *15*, 556-569

Pritchett, R., Pedersen, M. & Kieff, E. (1976) Complexity of EBV homologous DNA in continuous lymphoblastoid cell lines. *Virology*, *74*, 227-231

Reedman, B.M. & Klein, G. (1973)   Cellular localization of an
    Epstein-Barr virus (EBV)-associated complement-fixing antigen
    in producer and non-producer lymphoblastoid cell lines.   *Int.
    J. Cancer, 11*, 499-520

Rigby, P., Dieckmann, M., Rhodes, C. & Berg, P. (1977)   Labeling DNA
    to high specific activity *in vitro* by nick translation with DNA
    polymerase I.   *J. molec. Biol., 113*, 237-252

Southern, E.M. (1975)   Detection of specific sequences among DNA
    fragments separated by gel electrophoresis.   *J. molec. Biol.,
    98*, 503-517

Sugden, B., Summers, W.C. & Klein, G. (1976)   Nucleic acid renatura-
    tion and restriction endonuclease cleavage analyses show that the
    DNAs of a transforming and a non-transforming strain of Epstein-
    Barr virus share approximately 90% of their nucleotide sequences.
    J. Virol., 18, 765-775

Wigler, M., Silverstein, S., Lee, S.-S., Pellicer, A., Cheng, Y.-C.
    & Axel, R. (1977)   Transfer of purified herpes virus thymidine
    kinase gene to cultured mouse cells.   *Cell, 11*, 223-232

IN VITRO LYMPHOCYTE TRANSFORMATION BY EPSTEIN-BARR VIRUS (EBV)-LIKE VIRUSES ISOLATED FROM OLD-WORLD NON-HUMAN PRIMATES

H. RABIN, R.H. NEUBAUER & R.F. HOPKINS III

Viral Oncology Program,
NCI Frederick Cancer Research Center,
Frederick, Md, USA

S. RASHEED

Department of Pathology,
School of Medicine,
University of Southern California,
Los Angeles, Calif., USA

Lymphoid cell lines have been established and EBV-like viruses isolated from three species of Old-World non-human primates: chimpanzees (*Pan troglodytes*), baboons (*Papio hamadryas*), and an orangutan (*Pongo pygmaeus*). In this paper we shall describe properties of the baboon and orangutan cell lines and present information on *in vitro* lymphocyte transformation and *in vivo* infectivity.

Several lymphoid cell lines have been established from baboons from the colony at the Institute of Experimental Pathology and Therapy, Sukhumi, USSR (Agrba et al., 1975; Falk et al., 1976; Rabin et al., 1977), where over 30 cases of leukaemia have been observed since 1967. Cell lines have also been initiated from normal baboons. Cells of the baboon lines have been shown to have properties of B-lymphocytes. Chimpanzee lines established from normal animals also have characteristics of B-lymphocytes (Gerber et al., 1976). The orangutan cell line, designated CP-81, was initiated from a peripheral blood sample taken six months prior to death from a 13-year-old female ape with a diagnosis of myelomonocytic leukaemia (Rasheed et al., 1977). The cells are positive for surface kappa light-chain and Fc receptors but lack receptors for sheep cells and activated complement. They are positive for N-alkaline phosphatase activity, a lymphoid cell marker (Neumann et al., 1976), but are negative for lysozyme activity, a human monocyte-granulocyte-associated enzyme (Ralph et al., 1976). The CP-81 cells have shown the capacity to transplant successfully to nude mice by both the subcutaneous and intracranial routes.   The resulting tumours histologically resembled lymphomas and showed the same karyological characteristics as the parent line.   CP-81 cells have shown a limited capacity to grow in semi-solid medium giving cloning efficiencies of 3.6 colonies per 1000 single cells plated in 0.35% agar and 9.8 colonies per 1000 cells plated in 0.35% agarose. Cells of baboon line 594S have not plated in semi-solid medium.

Cell lines of all three simian species show evidence, by antigenic analysis and DNA hybridization, of the presence of EBV-related viruses. Cross-reacting antigens include virus capsid (VCA), early, membrane, neutralizing, and, with the exception of baboon cells, nuclear antigens. Nuclear antigen in CP-81 cells was demonstrated with human, orangutan, and chimpanzee sera by use of anticomplement immunofluorescence. Similar results were obtained by Gerber et al. (1976) on chimpanzee cells.   Molecular hybridization using EBV DNA from P3HR-1 cells or virus showed 40-50% homology with DNA prepared from the various simian cell lines.

Using concentrated cell culture fluids, attempts were made to demonstrate *in vitro* lymphocyte transforming activity, defined as increased cell clumping, increased metabolic activity, and sustained cell growth, of virus associated with baboon and orangutan cell lines. EBV from B95-8 cells was included in these assays as a representative of a high titred transforming human virus.   Baboon virus transformed peripheral blood lymphocytes (PBL) from all simian species tested, namely baboons (*P. hamadryas* and *P. cynocephalus*), rhesus monkeys (*Macaca mulatta*), stump-tailed macaques (*M. arctoides*), and gibbons (*Hylobates lar*), as well as human cord lymphocytes.   In fewer trials, virus from CP-81 cells induced transformation only in gibbon PBL. B95-8 virus consistently transformed gibbon PBL and human cord lymphocytes.   Transformed cells had characteristics of B-lymphocytes. Continuous cell lines have been developed from PBL of individual gibbon donors transformed with each of these viruses.   These cell lines are positive for virus-associated cytoplasmic antigens at levels similar to or slightly below each of the parent lines.   In a preliminary report, Gerber et al. (1977) have shown transforming activity for chimpanzee virus and confirmed such activity for baboon virus.

In animal inoculation studies, cell-free baboon virus induced sustained antibody (anti-VCA) production in both baboons (*P. cynocephalus*) and rhesus monkeys.   Inoculated white-lipped marmosets (*Saguinus fuscicollis*) failed to develop an antibody response.   Inoculation of baboons with cells of baboon line KMPG-1 induced an antibody response to VCA as did the inoculation of autologous *in vitro* transformed cells in one out of two rhesus monkeys.   Inoculation with allogeneic *in vitro* transformed lymphocytes failed to induce an antibody response in two other rhesus monkeys.   No virus-related disease has been observed in these monkeys in over one year.   Similar results were reported by Gerber et al. (1977) with chimpanzee and baboon virus.   Deinhardt et al. (1978) reported that inoculation of high levels of baboon lymphoid cells in cotton-top marmosets (*Saguinus oedipus*) induced an acute lymphoproliferative disease of apparent recipient origin in some animals.   It has also been reported that inoculated baboon lymphoid cells induced splenomegaly and lymphadenopathy in stump-tailed macaques (Djatchenko et al., 1976).   The orangutan virus has not yet undergone infectivity trials in primates.

The isolation of these simian EBV-like viruses indicates that EBV is a member of a family of primate lymphotropic herpesviruses which are related to each other antigenically and by DNA homology and which share biological activity including the ability to transform cells *in vitro*.   The continued study of these viruses is of importance, especially in the light of the association of EBV with several types of human disease.

SUMMARY

EBV-like viruses and lymphoid cell lines have been isolated from baboons and an orangutan.   The cell lines have properties of B- or undifferentiated lymphocytes and have antigens and DNA related to those of EBV.   The baboon virus has a broad *in vitro* transformation host range among lymphocytes of Old-World simian species whereas the orangutan isolate has a narrower host range.   Baboon and orangutan viruses as well as EBV have shown transforming activity for gibbon lymphocytes.   Baboon virus is infectious for rhesus monkeys and baboons but has not induced neoplastic disease in these species.

ACKNOWLEDGEMENTS

We should like to thank Dr Peter Ralph of the Sloan Kettering
Institute for Cancer Research for collaboration in enzyme
assays, Dr Murray Gardner of the University of Southern
California for assistance in histopathology, Dr Walter
A. Nelson-Rees of the University of California at
Berkeley for aid in cytogenetic analysis, and
Dr Meihan Nonoyama of Life Sciences, Inc., for
collaboration in molecular hybridization. This
work was supported in part by Contracts
NO1-CO-25423 and NO1-CP53500 with the
National Cancer Institute.

REFERENCES

Agrba, V.A., Yakovleva, L.A., Lapin, B.A., Sangulija, I.A.,
    Timanovskaya, V.V., Markaryan, D.S., Chuvirov, G.N. & Salmanova,
    E.A. (1975)   The establishment of continuous lymphoblastoid
    suspension cell cultures from hematopoietic organs of baboon
    (*Papio hamadryas*) with malignant lymphoma.   *Exp. Path., 10,*
    318-332

Deinhardt, R., Falk, L., Wolfe, L.G., Nonoyama, M., Schudel, A.,
    Lapin, B. & Yakovleva, L. (1978)   Susceptibility of marmosets
    to the EBV-like baboon herpesvirus.   *Prim. Med., 10,* 163-170

Djatchenko, A.G., Kakubava, V.V., Lapin, B.A., Agrba, V.Z.,
    Yakovleva, L.A. & Samilchuk, E.I. (1976)   Continuous lympho-
    blastoid suspension cultures from cells of hematopoietic organs
    of baboons with malignant lymphoma — Biological characterization
    and biological properties of the herpesvirus associated with
    culture cells. *Exp. Path., 12,* 163-168

Falk, L., Deinhardt, F., Nonoyama, M., Wolfe, L.G., Bergholz, C.,
    Lapin, B., Yakovleva, L., Agrba, V., Henle, G. & Henle, W. (1976)
    Properties of a baboon lymphotropic herpesvirus related to Epstein-
    Barr virus. *Int. J. Cancer, 18,* 798-807

Gerber, P., Pritchett, R.F. & Kieff, E.D. (1976)   Antigens and DNA of a chimpanzee agent related to Epstein-Barr virus.   *J. Virol.*, *19*, 1090-1099

Gerber, P., Kalter, S.S., Schidlovsky, G., Peterson, W.D., Jr & Daniel, M.D. (1977)   Biologic and antigenic characteristics of Epstein-Barr virus-related herpesviruses of chimpanzees and baboons.   *Int. J. Cancer*, *20*, 448-459

Neumann, H., Klein, E., Hauck-Granoth, R., Yachnin, S. & Ben-Bassat, H. (1976)   Comparative study of alkaline phosphatase activity in acute myeloid leukemia, and chronic lymphatic leukemia cells. *Proc. nat. Acad. Sci. (Wash.)*, *73*, 1432-1436

Rabin, H., Neubauer, R.H., Hopkins, R.F., III, Dzhikidze, E.K., Shevtosova, Z.V. & Lapin, B.A. (1977)   Transforming activity and antigenicity of an Epstein-Barr-like virus from lymphoblastoid cell lines of baboons with lymphoid disease.   *Intervirology*, *8*, 240-249

Ralph, P., Moore, M.A.S. & Nilsson, K. (1976)   Lysozyme synthesis by established human murine histiocytic lymphoma cell lines.   *J. exp. Med.*, *143*, 1528-1533

Rasheed, S., Rongey, R.W., Nelson-Rees, W.A., Rabin, H., Neubauer, R.H., Bruszweski, J., Esra, G. & Gardner, M.B. (1977)   Establishment of a cell line with associated Epstein-Barr-like virus from a leukemic orangutan.   *Science*, *198*, 407-409

TRANSCRIPTION OF EPSTEIN-BARR VIRUS GENOMES IN HUMAN LYMPHOBLASTOID CELLS AND IN SOMATIC-CELL HYBRIDS OF BURKITT'S LYMPHOMA

M. NONOYAMA, A. TANAKA & S. SILVER

*Life Sciences Biomedical Research Institute and Life Sciences, Inc.,
St. Petersburg, Fla, USA*

R. GLASER

*Department of Microbiology and Special Cancer Research Center,
The Milton S. Hershey Medical Center,
Pennsylvania State University,
Hershey, Penn., USA*

Epstein-Barr virus (EBV) is suspected to induce nasopharyngeal carcinoma (NPC) as well as Burkitt's lymphoma. A number of human lymphoblastoid cell lines have been established for the study of latent virus genomes but, so far, it has been impossible to establish an epithelial cell line from an NPC tumour. However, human somatic hybrid cells, which have been established by fusing EBV-carrying lymphoblastoid cells and monolayer cells, are available as a model for the study of the relationship of carcinoma cells to EBV (Glaser & O'Neill, 1972). D98/HR-1 and D98/Raji cells, hybrid cells of human D98 monolayer cells and HR-1 or Raji lymphoblastoid cells, are mono-layer cultures and contain seven and 17 EBV genomes per cell respect-ively. They are virus non-productive cells but virus antigens and virus DNA replication can be induced by iododeoxyuridine (IUDR) (Table 1). Raji cells, on the other hand, can produce only early antigen (EA) by the same treatment. Virus DNA replication and virus capsid antigen (VCA) formation were not observed. This indicates that different cellular control mechanisms over EBV genomes exist in D98/Raji and Raji cells (Glaser & Nonoyama, 1974). HR-1 clone No. 9, derived from virus-productive HR-1 cells by treatment with cyclo-hexamide, contains one EBV genome per cell and is not inducible by IUDR for the virus antigen (Tanaka et al., 1976).

NONOYAMA ET AL.

Table 1. EA and VCA formation, virus DNA replication and virus genome transcription

Cell line	Control				IUDR (three days on)[a]				IUDR (three days on and off)[b]			
	EA	VCA	Virus DNA replication	% Virus genome transcribed	EA	VCA	Virus DNA replication	% Virus genome transcribed	EA	VCA	Virus DNA replication	% Virus genome transcribed
Raji	-	-	-	25	+	-	-	30	+	-	-	50
D98/Raji	-	-	-	23	+	-	-	30	+	+	+	50
D98/HR-1	-	-	-	25	+	-	-	30	+	+	NT[c]	50
HR-1 clone No. 9	-	-	-	> 16	-	-	-	NT[c]	-	-	-	> 16

[a] Cells were treated with IUDR (50 μg/ml) for three days.

[b] Cells were treated with IUDR (50 μg/ml) for three days and further incubated without IUDR for three more days.

[c] NT: Not tested

This series of cell lines has been examined for the level of virus genome transcription by DNA-RNA reassociation kinetics (Frenkel & Roizman, 1972). As shown in Table 1, Raji, D98/Raji and D98/HR-1 cells contain virus-specific RNA transcribed from 20-25% of virus DNA. HR-1 clone No. 9 shows only 16% genome transcription. The reaction, however, may reach 20-25% at a higher R_0t value. After induction with IUDR, Raji, D98/Raji and D98/HR-1 cells produced virus mRNA transcribed from 50% of virus DNA, which may be a reflection of complete genome transcription, whereas HR-1 clone No. 9 did not show any sign of enhancement of virus genome transcription. DNA-RNA hybridization kinetics of Raji and D98/Raji cell RNA mixed together showed that hybridization did not exceed 50%, indicating that the virus-specific RNAs in Raji and D98/Raji cells after IUDR induction are of the same species. Thus, the studies of antigen induction and virus genome transcription after IUDR treatment show that the status of the latent virus genome varies in at least three ways: (1) latent virus DNA readily inducible by IUDR (D98/HR-1 and D98/Raji); (2) latent virus DNA inducible at the level of transcription but not at the level of translation (Raji); and (3) latent-virus non-inducible at the level of transcription (HR-1 clone No. 9).

It has been questioned whether all of the multiple copies of the EBV genomes present in transformed cells are transcribed or if only some of them are active. Since DNA-RNA hybridization kinetics gives the information concerning the amount of virus-specific RNA present in cells, a correlation was made between the amount of virus mRNA and the number of virus genomes in each cell line (Table 2). The amounts of virus-specific RNA in D98/Raji, D98/HR-1 and HR-1 clone No. 9 are 28, 14 and 1.8% respectively of virus-specific RNA in Raji cells, whereas the numbers of virus genomes are 24, 14 and 2% of the genomes in Raji

Table 2. Correlation between number of EBV genomes per cell and amount of virus RNA in cells

Cell line	Amount of virus RNA		Virus genomes	
	n[a]	Ratio	Per cell[b]	Ratio
Raji	5.30×10^{-3}	1	50	1
D98/Raji	1.50×10^{-3}	0.28	17	0.34
D98/HR-1	7.45×10^{-4}	0.14	7	0.14
HR-1 clone No. 9	9.7×10^{-5}	0.018	1^{c}	0.02

[a] Equation $D/D_0 = \alpha(1-e^{kaR_0t})$ (Frenkel & Roizman, 1972) was used, where D_0 and D are the initial and hybridized amounts of EBV DNA, α is the transcribed fraction of virus DNA, k is a kinetic constant, a is the fraction of virus-specific RNA in the total cellular RNA (R_0) and t is the time for hybridization; $n = ka$

[b] The number of genome equivalents per cell was obtained by cRNA hybridization as described (Nonoyama & Pagano, 1971).

[c] Tanaka et al., 1976

cells.   The data clearly indicate that the amount of virus-specific RNA synthesized in EBV genome-carrying cells is proportional to the number of virus genomes in the cells.   Since this direct proportion is found in cells where the number of genomes ranges from one genome per cell to 50 genomes per cell, this demonstrates that all the copies of virus DNA in these cells participate in virus genome transcription. However, the fact that the characteristics of HR-1 clone No. 9 cell line are not significantly different from those of other lymphoblastoid cell lines (Tanaka et al., 1976) indicates that the existence and transcription of a single copy of virus DNA is sufficient for continuous cell growth.   It remains to be determined whether the single copy of virus DNA and its transcription is required for the maintenance of EBV-transformed cells.

SUMMARY

   Expression of latent Epstein-Barr virus genomes in lymphoblastoid
cells and somatic-cell hybrids of Burkitt's lymphoblastoid cells has
been studied.   IUDR treatment induced the formation of early antigen
(EA), virus capsid antigen (VCA) and virus DNA replication in D98/Raji
and D98/HR-1 cells whereas only EA was induced in Raji cells.   HR-1
clone No. 9 did not respond to IUDR treatment.   The pattern of transcription of virus genomes in these cell lines without IUDR treatment
was uniform with 20-25% of virus DNA transcribed.   IUDR treatment
enhanced the transcription of virus DNA to 50% in D98/Raji, D98/HR-1
and Raji cells but no enhancement of virus genome transcription was
observed in HR-1 clone No. 9.   The amount of virus RNA in the cells
calculated from DNA-RNA hybridization kinetics was found to be proportional to the number of virus genomes per cell indicating that
every copy of virus DNA in these cells is actively transcribed.

ACKNOWLEDGEMENTS

   We thank Dr Bernard Roizman for the use of his computer for
      the calculation of DNA-RNA hybridization kinetics.
         We thank Mr Toni Bibb, Ms Martha Whitman and
            Ms Justine Gorodecki for their technical
            assistance.   This work was supported by
              grants from the National Institutes of
               Health, CA 21665-01 and CA 15038, and
                  by Contracts NO 1 CP 53516 and
                   NO 1 CP 33205 within the Virus
                  Cancer Program of the National
                       Cancer Institute.

REFERENCES

Frenkel, N. & Roizman, B. (1972)   Ribonucleic acid synthesis in cells infected with herpes simples virus: Control of transcription and of RNA abundance. *Proc. nat. Acad. Sci. (Wash.), 69,* 2654-2658

Glaser, R. & Nonoyama, M. (1974)   Host cell regulation of induction of Epstein-Barr virus. *J. Virol., 14,* 174-176

Glaser, R. & O'Neill, F.J. (1972)   Hybridization of Burkitt lymphoblastoid cells. *Science, 176,* 1245-1247

Nonoyama, M. & Pagano, J.S. (1971)   Detection of Epstein-Barr viral genome in nonproductive cells. *Nature new Biol., 233,* 103-106

Tanaka, A., Nonoyama, M. & Hampar, B. (1976)   Partial elimination of latent EBV genomes from virus producing cells by cyclohexamide. *Virology, 70,* 164-170

STUDIES ON THE ASSOCIATION OF THE EPSTEIN-BARR VIRUS GENOME WITH CHROMOSOMES IN HUMAN (BURKITT)/MOUSE HYBRID CELLS

R. GLASER

Department of Microbiology and Specialized Cancer Research Center,
The Pennsylvania State University College of Medicine,
Hershey, Penn., USA

C. CROCE

Wistar Institute,
Philadelphia, Penn., USA

M. NONOYAMA

Life Sciences Research Laboratories,
St. Petersburg, Fla., USA

INTRODUCTION

We have used somatic-cell hybridization to study the association of the Epstein-Barr virus (EBV) genome with human chromosomes in mouse/Burkitt hybrid cells. Previous studies with mouse/Burkitt hybrid cells suggest that the EBV genome is not associated with all human chromosomes (Glaser et al., 1975; Klein et al., 1974). In this study we have examined additional mouse/Burkitt hybrid cells in order to further clarify the association between EBV DNA and human chromosomes.

RESULTS AND DISCUSSION

Mouse fibroblast cells deficient in thymidine kinase (CL1D) were fused to the Burkitt lymphoblastoid cell line P3JHR-1 (HR-1) according to previously published procedures (Glaser & O'Neill, 1972; Glaser et al., 1975). The resulting CL1D/HR-1 hybrid cells were selected for ability to grow in HAT selective medium[1] (Glaser & O'Neill, 1972; Littlefield, 1964). The cells were cloned in soft agar and examined for the presence of EBV early antigen (EA), virus capsid antigen (VCA) and EBV-associated nuclear antigen (EBNA) by immunofluorescence using pretested antisera and EBV DNA by DNA-DNA reassociation kinetics. Six of 10 clones of CL1D/HR-1 cells obtained were EBV-positive as determined by the EBNA assay. None of the EBNA-positive clones spontaneously expressed EA or VCA nor could the EBV genome be induced to express additional antigens after treatment of the cells with iododeoxyuridine.

One clone of the CL1D/HR-1 cells, designated M44, was subcloned and studied in detail for EBV-specific markers and human chromosomes. Approximately 90% of the M44 cells were EBNA-positive when assayed at passage 8 (Table 1). Cells assayed for EBV DNA by DNA-DNA reassociation kinetics (Nonoyama & Pagano, 1973) at the same passage level were found to contain 0.3-0.5 EBV genome equivalents per cell (Table 1). Clone M44 cells were examined for the presence of human chromosomes by karyological and isozyme analysis. Five intact human chromosomes (numbers 7, 11, 12, 15 and 17) were found in at least 10% of the M44 cells at passage 8 (Table 1); chromosome number 7 was found in 55% and chromosome number 17 was found in 100% of the cells studied.

The M44 cells were then counterselected by growing in complete Eagle's medium containing 100 µg/ml bromodeoxyuridine (BUDR) for approximately four months. The BUDR-counterselected M44 cells were then subcloned. A total of 30 subclones were isolated and examined for EBNA; all but subclone 5 cells were EBNA-positive. We selected three EBNA-positive subclones (2, 4 and 24) in addition to EBNA-negative subclone 5 cells for detailed study. Subclones 2 and 24 had > 90% EBNA-positive cells and contained 0.3-0.5 EBV genome equivalents per cell; subclone 4 had 2-3% EBNA-positive cells but less than detectable levels (< 0.1 genome equivalents per cell) of EBV DNA (Table 1). Karyological (Fig. 1) analysis suggests that no intact human chromosomes were present in any of the four subclones of clone M44 cells at the same passage levels examined for EBV DNA and EBNA.

---

[1] Medium containing hypoxanthine, aminopterin and thymidine

Table 1. Presence of EBNA, EBV DNA and human chromosomes in CL1D/HR-1 cells

Clone-subclone (passage level)	% EBNA-positive cells	Number of EBV genome equivalents per cell	Number of intact human chromosomes present[a]
M44 (8)	90	0.3-0.5	5[b] 2[c]
M44-2 (10)	> 90	0.3-0.5	0
M44-4 (10)	2-3	< 0.1	0
M44-5 (12)	0	< 0.1	0
M44-24 (11)	> 90	0.3-0.5	0

[a] At least a portion of human chromosome 14 is present since nucleoside phosphorylase activity was detected.

[b] Chromosomes numbers 7, 11, 12, 15 and 17 were found in at least 10% of the cells.

[c] Chromosome number 7 was found in 55% and chromosome 17 in 100% of the cells.

However, isozyme analysis for 23 of the 24 different human chromosomes indicates that all four subclones express human nucleoside phosphorylase activity. The gene for this enzyme has been assigned to human chromosome 14. It is of interest that every mouse chromosome was EBNA-positive when metaphase preparations of M44 cells were assayed using EBNA-positive serum; EBNA-negative, EA-negative and VCA-negative sera, and EBNA-negative, EA-positive and VCA-positive sera were used as controls (B. Hampar[1]).

---

[1] Personal communication

FIG. 1.   KARYOTYPES OF SUBCLONES OF CL1D/HR-1 M44 CELLS

(A) Karyotype of CL1D/HR-1 M44 subclone 2 cells.   More than 90% of
    cells of this subclone were EBNA-positive and contained EBV DNA.
    No intact human chromosome is present in this hybrid, but at
    least a portion of human chromosome 14 is present as determined
    by isozyme analysis;
(B) Karyotype of CL1D/HR-1 M44 subclone 5 cells which were negative
    for EBNA and EBV DNA.   No intact human chromosome is present in
    this hybrid, but at least a portion of human chromosome 14 is
    present as determined by isozyme analysis.

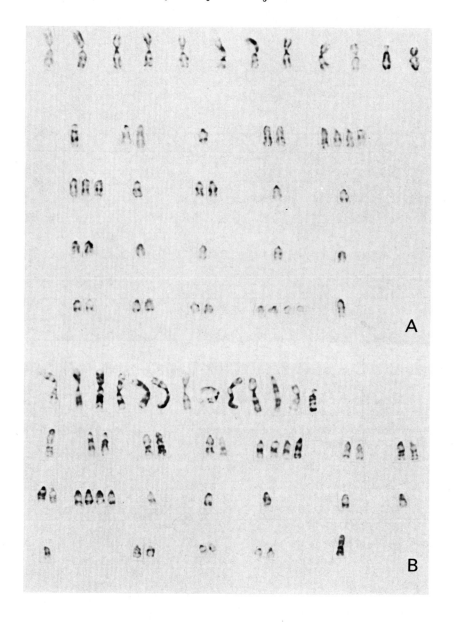

Several different interpretations of these data can be made. (1) EBV DNA may have become associated with mouse chromosomes since no intact human chromosomes can be identified by karyological analysis and human nucleoside phosphorylase activity was detected in both EBV genome-positive and genome-negative subclones. (2) EBV DNA may be associated with a human chromosome(s) which was lost leaving a portion of the virus genome behind. If true, then this suggests that the EBV genome can be maintained in the absence of intact human chromosomes, and can do so without a stable association with one or more specific human chromosomes. (3) It is possible that the EBV genome may not be associated with any specific human chromosome regardless of the type of association between EBV DNA and cellular DNA. (4) The maintenance of the EBV genome in the CL1D/HR-1 cells may be due to the association of EBV DNA with a small fragment of a human chromosome which was translocated on to a mouse chromosome and which cannot be detected using available techniques.

It is clear that these results have raised some interesting questions which need further study. Whether the association of the EBV genome and a human chromosome(s) exists in the classical sense in any cell type remains to be clarified.

SUMMARY

We have used somatic-cell hybrids of mouse fibroblast and Burkitt's lymphoblastoid tumour cells to continue our investigation of the association between Epstein-Barr virus (EBV) genome and human chromosomes. A mouse/Burkitt hybrid cell, designated CL1D/HR-1, was cloned in soft agar. Each of 10 clones was assayed for the spontaneous expression of EBV-associated nuclear antigen (EBNA), early antigen (EA) and virus capsid antigen (VCA). Six of 10 clones were EBNA-positive but negative for EA and VCA even after treatment with iododeoxyuridine. One clone, designated M44, contained approximately 90% EBNA-positive cells and 0.3-0.5 EBV genome equivalents per cell. Thirty subclones of clone M44 were obtained and analysed for EBV DNA, EBNA and human chromosomes. Four subclones (three EBNA-positive and one EBNA-negative) were studied in detail. Data obtained thus far indicate that none of the four subclones of clone M44 studied contained any intact human chromosomes. Isozyme analysis of these subclones indicated that all four subclones, regardless of the status of the EBV genome, synthesized nucleoside phosphorylase, an enzyme which has been linked to human chromosome number 14.

ACKNOWLEDGEMENTS

The authors thank Shendy Landis, Nanci Brown, Jean Letofsky,
Martha Whitman, Toni Bibb and Sandra Silver for their
excellent technical assistance. This investigation
was supported by Grant numbers CA 15038, CA 21665
and CA 18450 awarded by the National Cancer
Institute, and by contracts NO1 CP 53516
and NO1 CP 33205 within the Virus Cancer
Program of the National Cancer Institute.
R. Glaser is a recipient of a Leukemia
Society of America Scholar Award.

REFERENCES

Glaser, R. & O'Neill, F.J. (1972)   Hybridization of Burkitt lymphoblastoid cells. *Science, 176*, 1245-1247

Glaser, R., Nonoyama, M., Shows, T.B., Henle, G. & Henle, W. (1975)
   *Epstein-Barr virus: Studies on the association of virus genome
   with human chromosomes in hybrid cells.*   In: de-Thé, G.,
   Epstein, M.A. & zur Hausen, H., eds, *Oncogenesis and Herpesviruses,
   Part 1*, Lyon, International Agency for Research on Cancer (*IARC
   Scientific Publications* No. 11), pp. 457-466

Klein, G., Weiner, F., Zech, L., zur Hausen, H. & Reedman, B. (1974)
   Segregation of the EBV-determined nuclear antigen (EBNA) in somatic
   cell hybrids derived from the fusion of a mouse fibroblast and a
   human Burkitt lymphoma line. *Int. J. Cancer, 14*, 54-64

Littlefield, J.W. (1964)   Selection of hybrids from matings of fibroblasts *in vitro* and their presumed recombinants. *Science, 145*,
   709-710

Nonoyama, M. & Pagano, J.S. (1973)   Homology between Epstein-Barr
   virus DNA and viral DNA from Burkitt lymphoma and nasopharyngeal
   carcinoma determined by DNA-DNA reassociation kinetics. *Nature
   (Lond.), 242*, 44-47

ESTABLISHMENT OF SOMATIC HYBRID CELL CLONES FROM RAT EMBRYONIC FIBROBLAST CELLS WITH BURKITT'S LYMPHOBLASTOID CELLS USING POLYETHYLENE GLYCOL

G. DARAI, H.W. DOERR & B. MATZ

*Institut für medizinische Virologie der Universität Heidelberg,
Heidelberg, Federal Republic of Germany*

R.M. FLÜGEL, H. ZENTGRAF & K. MUNK

*Institut für Virusforschung,
Deutsches Krebsforschungszentrum,
Heidelberg, Federal Republic of Germany*

Several investigators have previously reported the establishment of somatic-cell hybrids between human Burkitt's lymphoma cells and either human, murine or monkey cells by using Sendai virus-mediated cell fusion (Glaser & Rapp, 1972; Klein et al., 1974; Tsang & Hann, 1977).

The aim of this study was to transfer the Epstein-Barr virus (EBV)-carrying chromosomes of human Burkitt's lymphoma cells to the cells of other mammals by using the polyethylene glycol (PEG) technique.

Burkitt's lymphoblastoid cell line (HR1K) (Pulvertaft, 1964), and rat embryo fibroblast cell cultures (REF-1-76) (Darai et al., 1977) were used. HR1K suspension cell cultures were grown in RPMI-1640 medium containing 20% fetal calf serum. Monolayers of REF-1-76 cell cultures were grown in Eagle's basal medium in Earle's balanced salt solution (BME) supplemented with 10% fetal calf serum (BME-FCS-10).

The technique used for cell fusion was essentially as described by Ahkong et al. (1975) and modified as follows:

HR1K cells (1×10^8 cells) and freshly trypsinized cells (5×10^7 cells)
were resuspended and thoroughly mixed in 1.0 ml 40% w/v PEG solution
(molecular weight 6000) in phosphate-buffered saline (PBS) (pH 7.4)
and incubated at 37°C for 30 minutes.   Thereafter, the cell mixtures
were centrifuged at 3000 rpm for 20 minutes.   The cell pellet was
resuspended finally in BME-FCS-10 and incubated at 37°C in a 5%
carbon dioxide atmosphere.

    Nuclear fusion of heterokaryons of rat plus HR1K cells was
immediately detectable by direct microscopic observation.   The
cultures were refed after 24 hours and thereafter every four days
with BME-FCS-10.   The cultures were subsequently grown as monolayers.
After 1-3 weeks, cytopathic (CPE)-like foci were formed in the
cultures, which typically showed rounded cells that started to detach
from the monolayer and to float in the culture medium (Fig. 1).

        FIG. 1.   PHOTOMICROGRAPHS OF MONOLAYERS OF BR-H2 CELL CLONE
The photomicrographs show the CPE-like foci which were formed and
produced floating cells.   ($\times$ 120)

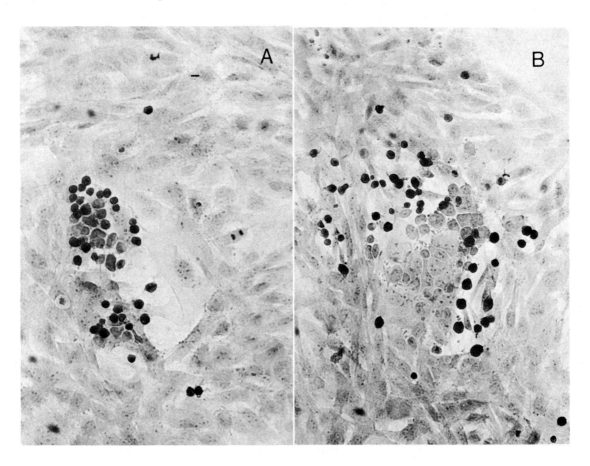

The floating cells were larger in size than the HRlK cells and could therefore be spun down at a lower centrifugation speed, namely 1000 rpm, for 10 minutes. These floating cells also grew in BME-FCS-10 and formed monolayers which again produced floating cells.

Some clones were isolated by picking cells from monolayer colonies which had originated from floating cells. Each clone was subsequently similarly cloned three times in succession and established in tissue culture. One Burkitt's lymphoma-rat hybrid cell clone (BR-H2) was studied in more detail. The BR-H2 hybrid cell clones retained their ability to grow both in monolayers and as floating cells.

In studies on the metaphase chromosomes, cells were incubated for 24 hours with 0.1 µg colchicine per ml of culture medium. Thereafter the cells were pelleted by low-speed centrifugation and resuspended in a hypotonic solvent (0.062 M potassium chloride) for 15 minutes at 37°C and fixed with methanol/acetic acid (3:1). The chromosome counts in the BR-H2 cell clone ranged from 38 to 92 with a modal number of 55.

The BR-H2 hybrid cell clone was studied for the presence of EBV intranuclear antigen (EBNA) by anticomplement fluorescence (Reedman & Klein, 1973) using an EBNA-positive reference serum, human complement from an EBV-negative donor (both from Dr F. Deinhardt) and a 1:40 diluted goat antihuman β_1C/β_1A conjugate (Hyland Laboratories). The fixation of cells was performed with methanol-acetone (1:1) at 4°C. Areas of monolayer cultures, which were in the process of producing floating cells, were consistently EBNA-positive (Fig. 2).

FIG. 2.   IMMUNOFLUORESCENCE PHOTOMICROGRAPH OF EBNA STAINING

Areas of monolayer cultures of BR-H2, which produced floating cells, showed positive EBNA staining. (× 360)

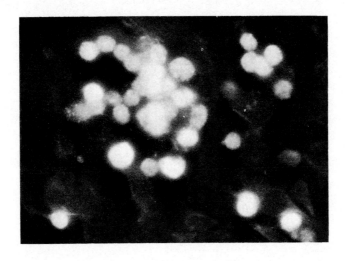

EBV-specific antigen (VCA) was also detectable in at least 1 out of
200 BR-H2 cells at 37°C by indirect immunofluorescence.

   Floating cells of BR-H2 were examined by electron microscopy for
spontaneous synthesis of EBV particles; nucleocapsid-like structures
comparable in size with EBV were observed in the cytoplasm and complete
EBV particles (110 nm in diameter) were also found in nuclei in at
least 1 out of 200 cells examined (Fig. 3).

      FIG. 3.   ELECTRON PHOTOMICROGRAPH OF BR-H2 CELL CLONE

EBV particles were spontaneously induced in cell hybrids after cell
fusion with PEG.

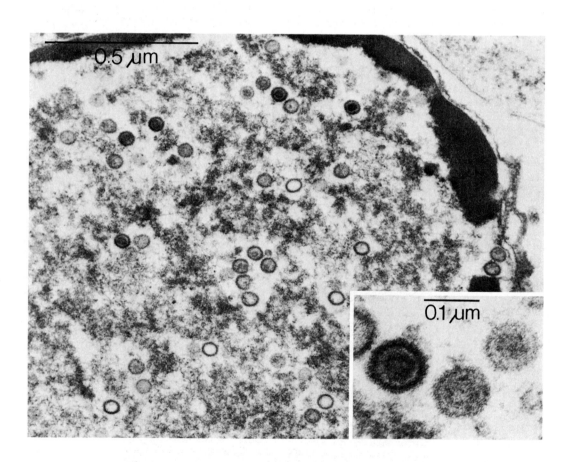

Supernatants of the BR-H2 cells were checked for reverse transcriptase activity and found to be positive, as compared to the
parental rat cell, indicating that type-C RNA viruses were also
activated in the BR-H2 cell clone.

We have also recently established hybrid cell clones from HR1K
cells and embryo fibroblasts of the primitive prosimian tupaia (tree
shrew) which had properties similar to those of the BR-H2 cell clone.

A study of the oncogenic capacity of hybrid cell clones in
syngeneic animals is in progress.

ACKNOWLEDGEMENTS

We should like to thank Dr F. Deinhardt for providing the HR1K
cell culture, EBNA-positive reference sera and human complement
from an EBV-negative donor.   This work was supported in part
by the Deutsche Forschungsgemeinschaft,
Sonderforschungsbereich 136.

REFERENCES

Ahkong, Q.F., Isobel Howell, J., Lucy, J.A., Safwat, F., Davey, M.R.
    & Cocking, E.C. (1975)   Fusion of hen erythrocytes with yeast
    protoplasts induced by polyethylene glycol. *Nature (Lond.)*,
    255, 66-67

Darai, G., Braun, R., Flügel, R.M. & Munk, K. (1977)   Malignant
    transformation of rat embryo fibroblasts by herpes simplex virus
    types 1 and 2 at suboptimal temperature. *Nature (Lond.)*, *265*,
    744-746

Glaser, R. & Rapp, F. (1972)   Rescue of Epstein-Barr virus from
    somatic cell hybrids of Burkitt lymphoblastoid cells.   *J. Virol.*,
    10, 288-296

Klein, G., Wiener, F., Zech, L., zur Hausen, H. & Reedman, B. (1974)
    Segregation of the EBV-determined nuclear antigen (EBNA) in
    somatic cell hybrids derived from the fusion of a mouse fibro-
    blast and a human Burkitt Lymphoma line. *Int. J. Cancer, 14*,
    54-64

Pulvertaft, R.J. (1964)   Cytology of Burkitt's tumour (African lymphoma). *Lancet, i,* 238-240

Reedman, B. & Klein, M. (1973)   Cellular localization of an Epstein-Barr virus (EBV) associated complement-fixing antigen in producer and non-producer lymphoblastoid cell lines. *Int. J. Cancer, 11,* 499-520

Tsang, K.Y. & Hann, W.D. (1977)   Activation of Epstein-Barr virus in hybrid cells. *J. nat. Cancer Inst., 58,* 1295-1299

DISCUSSION SUMMARY

P.A. SCHAFFER

*Sidney Farber Cancer Institute,
Harvard Medical School,
Boston, Mass., USA*

In an introductory review of transformation of non-lymphoid cells by herpesviruses, the unavailability for study of human cell lines transformed by herpesviruses, and the fact that transplantation rejection antigens have not yet been identified in herpesvirus systems, were stressed. The major problem associated with attempts to transform cells *in vitro* with herpesviruses remains the lack of a sensitive method for detecting and quantifying *oncogenic* transformation. The selection of thymidine kinase (TK) transformants by differential growth in HAT medium (hypoxanthine, aminopterin, thymidine) in the HSV system remains the most sensitive method for selecting biochemical transformants to date. The need to include the passage history and pedigree of transformed cell lines, when reporting results of studies aimed at characterization of these cell lines, was emphasized. Failure to do so has led to considerable confusion in the field.

The results of attempts to identify HSV DNA sequences in transformed cells by an improved nitrocellulose filter hybridization technique, were described. Results of studies with seven cloned HSV-2 transformed cell lines demonstrated that all lines contained less than one genome equivalent of HSV DNA. Advantages of the new technique include its apparently increased sensitivity and its suitability for rapid screening, while disadvantages include the present inability to quantitate the number of copies per cell of a given fraction of the viral genome. Although the data presented were preliminary and the lower limits of detectability of the technique

-577-

remained to be determined, the nitrocellulose filter
hybridization technique shows great promise.   Hopefully, this procedure will lead to the identification
of the viral DNA sequences present both in cells
transformed *in vitro* by herpesviruses and in human
cells putatively transformed by herpesviruses.

The subject of HSV-specific TK was considered and
the transformation of TK^- cells to the TK^+ phenotype,
following transfection with randomly sheared HSV-1 and
HSV-2 DNA fragments, was described.   Furthermore, an
increased transforming potential of cellular DNA
obtained from $HSV-TK^+$ transformed cells, as compared
with HSV-DNA alone was demonstrated.   The reasons for
this increased potential are presently unclear but
represent an interesting subject for further study.

Attempts to examine the biochemical basis for the
spontaneous loss of TK activity of $HSV-TK^+$ cells were
discussed.   Whether the loss of viral TK expression
is due to the repression or loss of the resident viral
gene, or whether it can occur for both reasons is not
known.   The molecular basis for this phenomenon is
clearly significant to studies of the mechanism of
maintenance of transformation.

The identification of a 3.4 kilobase *Bam*I-generated
HSV-1 DNA fragment which encodes the gene for HSV TK, was
reported.   In addition to the obvious implications of
this work for biochemical and genetic studies of HSV-
induced TK, these investigations have demonstrated the
feasibility of using restriction enzyme-generated fragments for studies of other viral genes.

The oncogenic transformation of non-permissive murine
cells by intact equine herpesvirus type 1 DNA represents
further evidence in support of the previous observation
that cells which are non-permissive for herpesvirus
replication remain susceptible to neoplastic transformation by the virus.

The studies of regulation of HSV TK gene expression
in transformed cells constitute an important new area in
the field of transformation by herpesviruses.   It has
been shown that the expression of a repressed viral TK
gene in HSV-transformed cells is subject to regulation by
the gene products of superinfecting HSV.   These investigations should ultimately lead to the identification of
the specific viral and/or cellular functions controlling
HSV gene expression in transformed cells.

The second major topic of the session concerned transformation of lymphoid cells by herpesviruses, and a comprehensive compendium of the characterics of lymphoblastoid cell lines transformed by Epstein-Barr virus (EBV) and other primate herpesviruses was presented. Two basic types of cell lines were described. Whether the differences between the two types of lines and the existence of intermediate types of cell lines is due to viral or cellular factors – such as differences in the levels of differentiation of transformed cell lines – remains to be determined. Suffice it to say that the problem of relating viral gene expression to the state of the viral genome in cells infected and transformed by these viruses is a considerable one. For those of us who are not EB-virologists, however, our understanding of this situation would be greatly enhanced if a published list of commonly used cell lines and their characteristics were readily available.

An attempt has been made to identify putative transforming sequences in EBV DNA. In one series of studies, polyadenylated cytoplasmic RNA corresponding to 5% of the genome has been identified in EBV-transformed cells and considerable progress has been made in mapping the templates for this DNA on the viral genome.

In a second study, the DNA sequences present in the genome of the non-transforming virus HR-1 were compared with those present in the transforming virus B95-8 by physical mapping procedures. This study has led to the identification of sequences unique to the transforming viral genome.

The transcription of EBV genomes in somatic cell hybrids of a HeLa cell variant line and Burkitt's lymphoma cells exhibiting a variety of characteristics has been examined. Iododeoxyuridine (IUDR) induction of hybrid cell lines and subsequent DNA-RNA hybridization showed that the control of gene expression differed at the transcriptional and post-transcriptional levels among the cell lines tested. The number of genomes and the amount of viral RNA transcribed were co-linear, indicating that all copies of latent EBV DNA are transcribed. It was concluded that plasmid DNA is transcribed, resulting in the production of EBV-determined nuclear antigen (EBNA), and that this sequence of events is sufficient for transformation.

Studies of the association of the EBV genome with chromosomes in human Burkitt's lymphoma/mouse cell hybrid lines have shown that expression of viral genetic information in some hybrid lines can be correlated with the presence of certain human chromosomes. In another hybrid line which had lost all human chromosomes, EBNA continued to be expressed suggesting either: (a) the transfer of the EBV genome to mouse cells; or (b) the transfer of a portion of the human chromosome bearing the EBV genome to a mouse chromosome.

New EBV-like viruses have been isolated from Old-World primates (the orangutan and the baboon). These viruses differ with regard to their ability to transform the lymphocytes of Old- and New-World primates. The baboon virus is able to transform human cord-blood cells.

Finally, the usefulness of the PEG method for inducing cell fusion between EBV-containing cells and cells of other species was described. A major advantage of the method is that it is not complicated by the introduction of RNA, as is the case when Sendai virus is used to induce fusion.

PUBLICATIONS OF THE INTERNATIONAL AGENCY FOR RESEARCH ON CANCER

SCIENTIFIC PUBLICATIONS SERIES

IARC MONOGRAPHS ON THE EVALUATION OF THE CARCINOGENIC RISK OF CHEMICALS TO HUMANS

WHO/IARC publications may be obtained, direct or through booksellers, from:

ALGERIA : Société Nationale d'Edition et de Diffusion, 3 bd Zirout Youcef, ALGIERS

ARGENTINA : Carlos Hirsch SRL, Florida 165, Galerías Güemes, Escritorio 453/465, BUENOS AIRES

AUSTRALIA : *Mail Order Sales :* Australian Government Publishing Service Bookshops, P.O. Box 84, CANBERRA A.C.T. 2600 ; *or over the counter from* Australian Government Publications and Inquiry Centres *at :* 113–115 London Circuit, CANBERRA CITY A.C.T. 2600 ; Shop 42, The Valley Centre, BRISBANE, Queensland 4000 ; 347 Swanston Street, MELBOURNE VIC 3000 ; 309 Pitt Street, SYDNEY N.S.W. 2000 ; Mt Newman House, 200 St. George's Terrace, PERTH WA 6000 ; Industry House, 12 Pirie Street, ADELAIDE SA 5000 ; 156–162 Macquarie Street, HOBART TAS 7000 — Hunter Publications, 58A Gipps Street, COLLINGWOOD VIC 3066

AUSTRIA : Gerold & Co., Graben 31, 1011 VIENNA I

BANGLADESH : The WHO Programme Coordinator, G.P.O. Box 250, DACCA 5 — The Association of Voluntary Agencies, P.O. Box 5045, DACCA 5

BELGIUM : Office international de Librairie, 30 avenue Marnix, 1050 BRUSSELS — *Subscriptions to World Health only :* Jean de Lannoy, 202 avenue du Roi, 1060 BRUSSELS

BRAZIL : Biblioteca Regional de Medicina OMS/OPS, Unidade de Venda de Publicações, Caixa Postal 20.381, Vila Clementino, 04023 São Paulo, S.P.

BURMA : *see* India, WHO Regional Office

CANADA : *Single and bulk copies of individual publications (not subscriptions) :* Canadian Public Health Association, 1335 Carling Avenue, Suite 210, OTTAWA, Ont. K1Z 8N8. *Subscriptions : Subscription orders, accompanied by cheque made out to the* Royal Bank of Canada, OTTAWA, Account World Health Organization, *should be sent to the* World Health Organization, P.O. Box 1800, Postal Station B, OTTAWA, Ont. K1P 5R5. *Correspondence concerning subscriptions should be addressed to the* World Health Organization, Distribution and Sales, 1211 GENEVA 27, Switzerland

CHINA : China National Publications Import Corporation, P.O. Box 88, PEKING

COLOMBIA : Distrilibros Ltd, Pio Alfonso García, Carrera 4a, Nos 36–119, CARTAGENA

CZECHOSLOVAKIA : Artia, Ve Smeckach 30, 111 27 PRAGUE 1

DENMARK : Ejnar Munksgaard, Ltd, Nørregade 6, 1164 COPENHAGEN K

ECUADOR : Librería Científica S.A., P.O. Box 362, Luque 223, GUAYAQUIL

EGYPT : Nabaa El Fikr Bookshop, 55 Saad Zaghloul Street, ALEXANDRIA

EL SALVADOR : Librería Estudiantil, Edificio Comercial B No 3, Avenida Libertad, SAN SALVADOR

FIJI : The WHO Programme Coordinator, P.O. Box 113, SUVA

FINLAND : Akateeminen Kirjakauppa, Keskuskatu 2, 00101 HELSINKI 10

FRANCE : Librairie Arnette, 2 rue Casimir-Delavigne, 75006 PARIS

GERMAN DEMOCRATIC REPUBLIC : Buchhaus Leipzig, Postfach 140, 701 LEIPZIG

GERMANY, FEDERAL REPUBLIC OF : Govi-Verlag GmbH, Ginnheimerstrasse 20, Postfach 5360, 6236 ESCHBORN — W. E. Saarbach, Postfach 101610, Follerstrasse 2, 5 COLOGNE 1 — Alex. Horn, Spiegelgasse 9, Postfach 3340, 6200 WIESBADEN

GREECE : G. C. Eleftheroudakis S.A., Librairie internationale, rue Nikis 4, ATHENS (T. 126)

HAITI : Max Bouchereau, Librairie "A la Caravelle", Boîte postale 111-B, PORT-AU-PRINCE

HONG KONG : Hong Kong Government Information Services, Beaconsfield House, 6th Floor, Queen's Road, Central, VICTORIA

HUNGARY : Kultura, P.O.B. 149, BUDAPEST 62 — Akadémiai Könyvesbolt, Váci utca 22, BUDAPEST V

ICELAND : Snaebjørn Jonsson & Co., P.O. Box 1131, Hafnarstraeti 9, REYKJAVIK

INDIA : WHO Regional Office for South-East Asia, World Health House, Indraprastha Estate, Ring Road, NEW DELHI 110002 — Oxford Book & Stationery Co., Scindia House, NEW DELHI 110000 ; 17 Park Street, CALCUTTA 700016 (*Sub-Agent*)

INDONESIA : M/s Kalman Book Service Ltd, Jln. Cikini Raya No. 63, P.O. Box 3105/Jkt., JAKARTA

IRAN : Iranian Amalgamated Distribution Agency, 151 Khiaban Soraya, TEHERAN

IRAQ : Ministry of Information, National House for Publishing, Distributing and Advertising, BAGHDAD

IRELAND : The Stationery Office, DUBLIN 4

ISRAEL : Heiliger & Co., 3 Nathan Strauss Street, JERUSALEM

ITALY : Edizioni Minerva Medica, Corso Bramante 83–85, 10126 TURIN ; Via Lamarmora 3, 20100 MILAN

JAPAN : Maruzen Co. Ltd, P.O. Box 5050, TOKYO International 100–31

KOREA, REPUBLIC OF : The WHO Programme Coordinator, Central P.O. Box 540, SEOUL

KUWAIT : The Kuwait Bookshops Co. Ltd, Thunayan Al-Ghanem Bldg, P.O. Box 2942, KUWAIT

LAO PEOPLE'S DEMOCRATIC REPUBLIC : The WHO Programme Coordinator, P.O. Box 343, VIENTIANE

LEBANON : The Levant Distributors Co. S.A.R.L., Box 1181, Makdassi Street, Hanna Bldg, BEIRUT

LUXEMBOURG : Librairie du Centre, 49 bd Royal, LUXEMBOURG

MALAYSIA : The WHO Programme Coordinator, Room 1004, Fitzpatrick Building, Jalan Raja Chulan, KUALA LUMPUR 05–02 — Jubilee (Book) Store Ltd, 97 Jalan Tuanku Abdul Rahman, P.O. Box 629, KUALA LUMPUR 01–08 — Parry's Book Center, K. L. Hilton Hotel, Jln. Treacher, P.O. Box 960, KUALA LUMPUR

MEXICO : La Prensa Médica Mexicana, Ediciones Científicas, Paseo de las Facultades 26, Apt. Postal 20–413, MEXICO CITY 20, D.F.

MONGOLIA : *see* India, WHO Regional Office

MOROCCO : Editions La Porte, 281 avenue Mohammed V, RABAT

MOZAMBIQUE : INLD, Caixa Postal 4030, MAPUTO

NEPAL : *see* India, WHO Regional Office

NETHERLANDS : N. V. Martinus Nijhoff's Boekhandel en Uitgevers Maatschappij, Lange Voorhout 9, THE HAGUE 2000

NEW ZEALAND : Government Printing Office, Mulgrave Street, Private Bag, WELLINGTON 1, *Government Bookshops at :* Rutland Street, P.O. Box 5344, AUCKLAND ; 130 Oxford Terrace, P.O. Box 1721, CHRISTCHURCH ; Alma Street, P.O. Box 857, HAMILTON ; Princes Street, P.O. Box 1104, DUNEDIN — R. Hill & Son, Ltd, Ideal House, Cnr Gillies Avenue & Eden St., Newmarket, AUCKLAND 1

NIGERIA : University Bookshop Nigeria Ltd, University of Ibadan, IBADAN — G. O. Odatuwa Publishers & Booksellers Co., 9 Hausa Road, SAPELE, BENDEL STATE

NORWAY : Johan Grundt Tanum Bokhandel, Karl Johansgt. 43, 1010 OSLO 1

PAKISTAN : Mirza Book Agency, 65 Shahrah–E–Quaid–E–Azam, P.O. BOX 729, LAHORE 3

PAPUA NEW GUINEA : WHO Programme Coordinator, P.O. Box 5896, BOROKO

PHILIPPINES : World Health Organization, Regional Office for the Western Pacific, P.O. Box 2932, MANILA — The Modern Book Company Inc., P.O. Box 632, 926 Rizal Avenue, MANILA

POLAND : Składnica Księgarska, ul Mazowiecka 9, 00052 WARSAW (*except periodicals*) — BKWZ Ruch, ul Wronia 23, 00840 WARSAW (*periodicals only*)

PORTUGAL : Livraria Rodrigues, 186 Rua do Ouro, LISBON 2

SIERRA LEONE : Njala University College Bookshop (University of Sierra Leone), Private Mail Bag, FREETOWN

SINGAPORE : The WHO Programme Coordinator, 144 Moulmein Road, G.P.O. Box 3457, SINGAPORE 1 — Select Books (Pte) Ltd, 215 Tanglin Shopping Centre, 2/F, 19 Tanglin Road, SINGAPORE 10

SOUTH AFRICA : Van Schaik's Bookstore (Pty) Ltd, P.O. Box 724, 268 Church Street, PRETORIA 0001

SPAIN : Comercial Atheneum S.A., Consejo de Ciento 130–136, BARCELONA 15 ; General Moscardó 29, MADRID 20 — Librería Diaz de Santos, Lagasca 95, MADRID 6 ; Balmes 417 y 419, BARCELONA 6

SRI LANKA : *see* India, WHO Regional Office

SWEDEN : Aktiebolaget C. E. Fritzes Kungl. Hovbokhandel, Regeringsgatan 12, 103 27 STOCKHOLM

SWITZERLAND : Medizinischer Verlag Hans Huber, Länggass Strasse 76, 3012 BERNE 9

SYRIAN ARAB REPUBLIC : M. Farras Kekhia, P.O. Box No. 5221, ALEPPO

THAILAND : *see* India, WHO Regional Office

TUNISIA : Société Tunisienne de Diffusion, 5 avenue de Carthage, TUNIS

TURKEY : Haset Kitapevi, 469 Istiklal Caddesi, Beyoglu, ISTANBUL

UNITED KINGDOM : H. M. Stationery Office : 49 High Holborn, LONDON WC1V 6HB ; 13a Castle Street, EDINBURGH EH2 3AR ; 41 The Hayes, CARDIFF CF1 1JW ; 80 Chichester Street, BELFAST BT1 4JY ; Brazennose Street, MANCHESTER M60 8AS ; 258 Broad Street, BIRMINGHAM B1 2HE ; Southey House, Wine Street, BRISTOL BS1 2BQ. *All mail orders should be sent to P.O. Box 569, LONDON SE1 9NH*

UNITED STATES OF AMERICA : *Single and bulk copies of individual publications (not subscriptions) :* WHO Publications Centre USA, 49 Sheridan Avenue, ALBANY, NY 12210. *Subscriptions : Subscription orders, accompanied by check made out to the* Chemical Bank, New York, Account World Health Organization, *should be sent to the* World Health Organization, P.O. Box 5284, Church Street Station, NEW YORK, NY 10249. *Correspondence concerning subscriptions should be addressed to the* World Health Organization, Distribution and Sales, 1211 GENEVA 27, Switzerland. *Publications are also available from the* United Nations Bookshop, NEW YORK, NY 10017 (*retail only*), *and single and bulk copies of individual* International Agency for Research on Cancer *publications (not subscriptions) may also be ordered from the* Franklin Institute Press, Benjamin Franklin Parkway, Philadelphia, PA 19103

USSR : *For readers in the USSR requiring Russian editions :* Komsomolskij prospekt 18, Medicinskaja Kniga, Moscow — *For readers outside the USSR requiring Russian editions :* Kuzneckij most 18, Meždunarodnaja Kniga, Moscow G-200

VENEZUELA : Editorial Interamericana de Venezuela C.A., Apartado 50785, CARACAS 105 — Libreria del Este, Apartado 60337, CARACAS 106

YUGOSLAVIA : Jugoslovenska Knjiga, Terazije 27/II, 11000 BELGRADE

ZAIRE : Librairie universitaire, avenue de la Paix Nº 167, B.P. 1682, KINSHASA I

Special terms for developing countries are obtainable on application to the WHO Programme Coordinators or WHO Regional Offices listed above or to the World Health Organization, Distribution and Sales Service, 1211 Geneva 27, Switzerland. Orders from countries where sales agents have not yet been appointed may also be sent to the Geneva address, but must be paid for in pounds sterling, US dollars, or Swiss francs.

Price: Sw. fr. 50.–   US $ 30.00   Prices are subject to change without notice.   IARC/2/78

D